AF573863

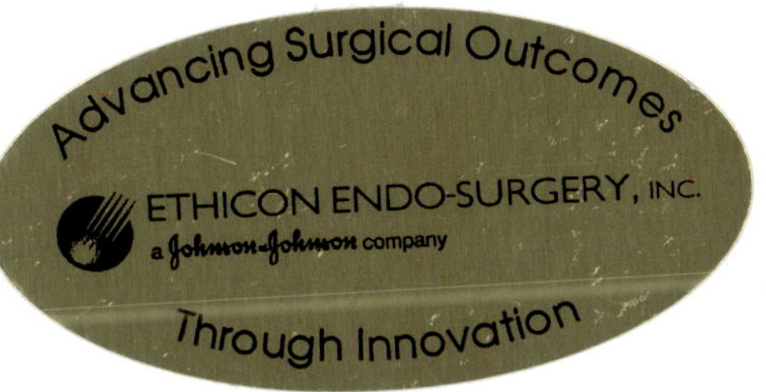
Advancing Surgical Outcomes
ETHICON ENDO-SURGERY, INC.
a Johnson&Johnson company
Through Innovation

Operative Gynecologic Laparoscopy

Principles and Techniques

CAMRAN R. NEZHAT, M.D.
Clinical Professor of Obstetrics and Gynecology
Mercer University School of Medicine
Macon, Georgia
Clinical Professor of Surgery
Clinical Professor of Obstetrics and Gynecology
Stanford University School of Medicine
Stanford, California
Director, Center for Special Pelvic Surgery
Atlanta, Georgia

FARR R. NEZHAT, M.D.
Clinical Professor of Obstetrics and Gynecology
Mercer University School of Medicine
Macon, Georgia
Clinical Professor of Obstetrics and Gynecology
Stanford University School of Medicine
Stanford, California
Director, Center for Special Pelvic Surgery
Atlanta, Georgia

ANTHONY A. LUCIANO, M.D.
Professor of Obstetrics and Gynecology
University of Connecticut School of Medicine
Director, New Britain General Hospital
Director, Center for Fertility and Reproductive Endocrinology
New Britain, Connecticut

ALVIN M. SIEGLER, M.D., D.SC.
Professor
Department of Obstetrics and Gynecology
Health Science Center at Brooklyn
Brooklyn, New York

DEBORAH A. METZGER, PH.D., M.D.
Associate Clinical Professor of Obstetrics and Gynecology
University of Connecticut Health Center
Director, Reproductive Medicine Institute of Connecticut
Hartford, Connecticut

CEANA H. NEZHAT, M.D.
Assistant Clinical Professor of Obstetrics and Gynecology
Mercer University School of Medicine
Macon, Georgia
Assistant Clinical Professor of Obstetrics and Gynecology
Stanford University School of Medicine
Stanford, California
Director, Center for Special Pelvic Surgery
Atlanta, Georgia

OPERATIVE GYNECOLOGIC LAPAROSCOPY

PRINCIPLES AND TECHNIQUES

CAMRAN R. NEZHAT, M.D.
FARR R. NEZHAT, M.D.
ANTHONY A. LUCIANO, M.D.
ALVIN M. SIEGLER, M.D., D.SC.
DEBORAH A. METZGER, PH.D., M.D.
CEANA H. NEZHAT, M.D.

ILLUSTRATED BY CHARLES H. BOYTER, C.M.I.

McGRAW-HILL, INC.
Health Professions Division

New York St. Louis San Francisco Auckland Bogotá
Caracas Lisbon London Madrid Mexico City Milan Montreal
New Delhi San Juan Singapore Sydney Tokyo Toronto

Operative Gynecologic Laparoscopy
Principles and Techniques

234567890 KGPKGP 98765

ISBN 0-07-105422-7

This book was set in Caslon 224 by Digitype, Inc.

The editors were William Lamsback, Martin J. Wonsiewicz, and Susan Finn.

The production supervisor was Clare Stanley.

The cover designer was Barolini Computer Graphics.

Quebecor Printing/Kingsport Press was printer and binder.

This book is printed on acid-free paper.

Library of Congress Cataloging-in-Publication Data

Operative gynecologic laparoscopy : principles and techniques / Camran R. Nezhat . . . [et al.].
p. cm.
Includes bibliographical references and index.
ISBN 0-07-105422-7
1. Generative organs, Female — Endoscopic surgery.
2. Laparoscopic surgery. I. Nezhat, Camran.
[DNLM: 1. Genital Diseases, Female — surgery. 2. Surgery, Laparoscopic. WP 660 0613 1995]
RG104.7.064 1995
618.1′45 — dc20
DNLM/DLC
for Library of Congress 94-42847

To our patients who have entrusted their care to our judgment and surgical skills.

NOTICE

Medicine is an ever-changing science. As new research and clinical experience broaden our knowledge, changes in treatment and drug therapy are required. The authors and the publisher of this work have checked with sources believed to be reliable in their efforts to provide information that is complete and generally in accord with the standards accepted at the time of publication. However, in view of the possibility of human error or changes in medical sciences, neither the authors nor the publisher nor any other party who has been involved in the preparation or publication of this work warrants that the information contained herein is in every respect accurate or complete, and they are not responsible for any errors or omissions or for the results obtained from use of such information. Readers are encouraged to confirm the information contained herein with other sources. For example and in particular, readers are advised to check the product information sheet included in the package of each drug they plan to administer to be certain that the information contained in this book is accurate and that changes have not been made in the recommended dose or in the contraindications for administration. This recommendation is of particular importance in connection with new or infrequently used drugs.

CONTENTS

	FOREWORDS	ix
	PREFACE	xi
	ACKNOWLEDGMENTS	xii
	SECTION I	
CHAPTER 1	Introduction	1
CHAPTER 2	Patient Education and Informed Consent	7
	SECTION II	
CHAPTER 3	Equipment	15
CHAPTER 4	Lasers in Endoscopic Surgery	47
CHAPTER 5	Electrosurgery	57
CHAPTER 6	Comparative Studies with Electrosurgery and Lasers	65
	SECTION III	
CHAPTER 7	Anesthesia	71
CHAPTER 8	Laparoscopy	79
	SECTION IV	
CHAPTER 9	Laparoscopic Adhesiolysis	97
CHAPTER 10	Ectopic Pregnancy	107
CHAPTER 11	Laparoscopic Treatment of Endometriosis	121
CHAPTER 12	Ovarian Cysts	149
CHAPTER 13	Ovarian Surgery	167
CHAPTER 14	Tubal Surgery	185
CHAPTER 15	Uterine Surgery	205
CHAPTER 16	Appendectomy	239
CHAPTER 17	Presacral Neurectomy and Uterosacral Transection and Ablation	245
CHAPTER 18	Reconstructive Pelvic Surgery	255
CHAPTER 19	The Role of Laparoscopy in the Management of Gynecologic Malignancy	273
CHAPTER 20	Complications	287
	SECTION V	
CHAPTER 21	Questions and Answers	311
	COLOR APPENDIX	
	INDEX	325

FOREWORDS

Dr. Nezhat's textbook on endoscopic surgery is a timely contribution and has all the trappings of being extremely successful. The competition is keen at this point in time with regards to textbooks and atlases on endoscopic surgery but none will rival Dr. Nezhat's.

In the past decade, gynecologic surgery, because of endoscopic surgery, has undergone a tremendous revolution. There are few cases now remaining in the gynecologist's surgical armamentarium that cannot be carried out through an endoscopic approach. Many of these changes are due to the courage, innovativeness, and technical skill of Dr. Camran Nezhat. Just as in Star Trek, he dared to go where no man went before and, by doing this, he opened up unimagined vistas to endoscopic surgeons all over the world. For his courage, Camran has over the years suffered, but he has persevered.

This book brings to a culmination many of Dr. Nezhat's techniques, innovations, and most importantly, thought processes. All of the characteristics necessary for an excellent textbook of surgery are included. The text is well-written, provocative, clear, and demonstrates editorial consistency. The illustrations are superb and would provide the novice in endoscopic surgery with enough information to carry out many of the procedures proposed.

I've chosen as an illustrative chapter, the chapter on endometriosis. It demonstrates many of the things that have been conjured up by Dr. Nezhat and have become part of what we do as endoscopic surgeons. These include hydrodissection, ureteric resection, reanastomosis, bowel resection, repair, and reanastomosis with a stapler. If one could learn all of the techniques suggested in the chapter on endometriosis, one could become, as Dr. Nezhat has, a master endoscopic surgeon.

The book is encyclopedic in that it covers not only all surgical techniques, but also various kinds of equipment, laser and electrosurgical physics, adhesion formation, and most importantly, complications.

Dr. Nezhat has synthesized his years of experience in this text. It will become a classic in the field and is a testimony to his skill, intelligence, and perseverance.

Alan DeCherney, M.D.
Louis E. Phaneuf Professor and Chairman
Department of Obstetrics and Gynecology
Tufts University
Boston, Massachusetts

Excellence in any human activity always commands admiration and respect. In the case of surgical techniques, excellence commands not only the admiration and respect of professional colleagues, but the gratitude of patients as well. Those who have had the opportunity to see the "Nezhat Orchestra" operate and simultaneously conduct the endoscopic operating team, recognize that they have seen a performance of excellence. It is a unique combination of manual dexterity, innovation, creativity, and team work.

The rapid proliferation of laparoscopic procedures in the last two decades originated in gynecology, but crossed the borders of this discipline to several other applications below and above the diaphragm. Many new devices have been introduced into the armamentarium of the endoscopic operating room. However, if there was a single factor that contributed to the increased interest, quality of patient care, and education of new generations of surgeons, it was the incorporation of video equipment as an integral part of the standard endoscopic set. This was promulgated and pioneered by Dr. Camran Nezhat. In so doing, the secrets behind the curtain of the "single eye–single hand" procedures were revealed and broadened the horizons of operative laparoscopy.

In this book, "The Nezhats" review the instrumentation and general principles of laparoscopy and elucidate the management of various procedures in gynecology and gastrointestinal and genitourinary surgery. The uniformity of text and illustration format of this book contribute to the clear message that comes from the "Nezhat School of Laparoscopic Surgery," and is complementary to the high quality educational video-library that originated in the same school.

I regard it as an honor to have this opportunity to be associated with this special project that will find an important place in the literature of our specialty.

Yona Tadir, M.D.
Department of Surgery
Beckman Laser Institute & Medical Clinic
Irvine, California

PREFACE

Enormous technical advances have taken place since reflected light was first used to look into body cavities for diagnostic purposes. The rapid improvement in endoscopic technology has led to important changes in the quality and reliability of the available equipment so that an increasing number of gynecologic operative procedures can be performed endoscopically. Indeed, laparoscopy has become one of the most frequently performed operative procedures in gynecologic practice. The interest in minimally invasive surgery has been ignited by video monitoring, the use of safe automatic high flow insufflators, and effective methods of hemostasis that involve intra-abdominal suturing, electrosurgery, lasers, and stapling devices. These advances have extended the safety and efficiency of operative laparoscopy.

Laparoscopy is valuable to the patient and her physician when performed accurately for proper indications. The purpose of this book is to familiarize the reader with the instruments that are currently available and to describe their appropriate use for the management of uterine, tubal, and ovarian abnormalities. The authors have described these procedures so that gynecologists may become familiar with the possibilities of correcting many pelvic diseases without the need for conventional laparotomy. The benefits of this approach are fewer postoperative adhesions and a decrease in morbidity, disability, and health costs. Data are accumulating to substantiate these impressions.

The first three sections of this book describe the importance of informed consent, the proper use of mechanical and power instruments including lasers and electrosurgery, and the special requirements for anesthesia associated with laparoscopy. The chapter on laparoscopy includes a thorough description of pelvic anatomy and the important landmarks viewed through the laparoscope. The photographs and artistic drawings will help the reader form the appropriate visual image of the normal anatomy as well as anatomic distortions caused by the disease.

In Section IV, the principles and techniques of specific operative procedures are described, including the prevention and treatment of pelvic adhesions, the selection of patients for the management of tubal pregnancy, and the myriad approaches to pain and infertility associated with endometriosis. The criteria for the proper endoscopic treatment of ovarian cysts has been described, always keeping in mind the pitfalls in the differential diagnosis of benign and malignant ovarian neoplasms. The selection of patients for the surgical approaches for pelvic pain that is unresponsive to medical management is included in another chapter. Less commonly performed procedures such as sacral colpopexy, retropubic urethral suspension, and the repair of vesicovaginal fistula are described and illustrated. One chapter is directed to the contemporary use of videolaparoscopy for the treatment of several types of gynecologic malignancies including para-aortic node biopsy, radical hysterectomy, and the value of laparoscopy as a second look procedure in patients treated for ovarian malignancy. In the final section, we have included a list of questions that have been asked by students, colleagues, and patients concerning advanced operative laparoscopy. The authors have answered them based on their experience.

Laparoscopic surgery requires the acquisition of new skills because there is the loss of depth perception and the inability to digitally feel the lesions. Even after training with laboratory animals, with preceptors and in postgraduate courses, minimally invasive surgery requires continued practice to maintain the skill and to minimize complications. The incorporation of operative laparoscopy into the training program of gynecologic residents should proceed expeditiously so that the young gynecologist of the twenty-first century will be able to perform most gynecologic operative procedures laparoscopically.

In this book, we share our experiences in learning and adopting operative laparoscopy in our clinical practice, and we offer our philosophy in its safe and effective application and describe our methodology in minimizing and resolving complications. Although this book is directed mostly to the gynecologist, it is likely to be helpful to other surgeons who wish to make the transition from laparotomy to the less invasive and more cost effective laparoscopy.

ACKNOWLEDGMENTS

We appreciate the support and cooperation of our operating room staff who have been essential to the development and maintenance of our endoscopic units. We are grateful to our colleagues who have stimulated us to write this book. We thank Clayton S. White, M.D., for his advice and support of our work. We would like to express our special appreciation to Dr. Ceana Nezhat for his excellent review of several chapters. No book on operative gynecology could be written without the help of illustrators. We are grateful to Charles Boyter and Christopher Wikoff for their superior artistic work, attention to detail, and documentation of procedures. We are grateful to American Hydrosurgical Instruments, Circon, Coherent, Karl Storz, Richard Wolf Instruments, and Valleylab for generously providing us with photographs of endoscopic instruments. We would like to acknowledge Melanie Barstad, Director of Marketing, Surgical Specialties, Johnson and Johnson Medical Inc. We are grateful to Ethicon Endosurgery, specifically, Nick Valeriani, Vice President of Marketing, and Bill Weldon, President, for their photographs and generous grant supporting the artistic work in the book. We would like to thank William Lamsback of McGraw-Hill for his confidence, support, and encouragement during the development of this textbook. Finally, we wish to thank our assistants Marian C. Garrison, Juliane Whitehead, Marian Bekker, and Audrey M. Bergenty.

1

Introduction

During the early decades of the 20th century, physicians developed an interest in exploring body cavities with various forms of speculums and optics. Almost a century before in 1807, Bozzini[1] described a light conductor in which a candle served as the illumination for a special "vase-like" instrument whose purpose was to enable the physicians to explore the cavities of various organs. At the time, the medical profession was opposed to this type of "curiosity." Not until 1880 when Nitze[2] developed the cystoscope were such investigations begun again. This new instrument could be passed into the bladder so that the physician could locate bladder stones and remove them without the need for an abdominal incision. In 1901, Kelling[3] reported his findings of a celioscopic examination of a living dog after pneumoperitoneum had been created with filtered air. Jacobaeus[4] coined the term *laparoscopy* after having explored the peritoneal cavity in human beings by "direct" insertion of a Nitze cystoscope without pneumoperitoneum. He described the use of the laparoscope in 17 patients who had ascites. Kelling and Jacobaeus should be regarded as the pioneers of early laparoscopy.

The technique of the abdominal entry was varied and controversial. The early laparoscopes were primitive, the lens systems were of inferior quality, and adequate light and image transmission could be achieved only with wide lenses requiring large-bore telescopes. Distally placed incandescent light bulbs generated heat within the abdominal cavity and they had the disconcerting habit of failing just at the critical point of a procedure. In 1938, Veress[5] described a new needle for inducing pneumothorax for the treatment of tuberculosis, and this instrument currently is used most frequently for the creation of pneumoperitoneum. Ruddock[6] described a good optic system including a built-in biopsy forceps with the capability of electrocoagulation. He was able to report on its use in over 2000 patients. Apparently, the first gynecologic report was published by Hope[7] on the use of the laparoscope for the diagnosis of tubal pregnancy. In the same year, Anderson[8] suggested tubal fulguration as a method for tubal sterilization but did not report the description of any cases. Decker[9] was able to achieve good observation of the pelvic organs with the patients in the knee-chest position using a culdoscope. Indeed, this endoscopic method was practiced almost exclusively in the United States for the next 25 years. In 1941, Power and Barnes[10] reported the performance of tubal sterilization by coagulation of the isthmic portions of the fallopian tubes under laparoscopic control. In France, Palmer[11] adopted the deep Trendelenburg position and designed a forceps for ovarian biopsy. In 1947, he published the results of his first 250 laparoscopic operations. Laparoscopy and other endoscopic procedures in general attained a wider acceptance after the introduction in 1952 of the "cold light" concept by Fourestier and colleagues.[12] In the same year, Hopkins and Kapany[13] in England introduced fiberoptics to the field of endoscopy. Frangenheim[14] and Albano and Cittidini[15] incorporated the new techniques of laparoscopy and published their findings in textbooks on the subject. The first book on this topic published in the English language was written by Steptoe[16] describing the instruments available at the time. Details of many endoscopic procedures including tubal sterilization, ovarian biopsy, uterine suspension, appendectomy, and lysis of adhesions were included. Books by Cohen,[17] Semm,[18] and Gomel[19] also included discussions on laparoscopy, culdoscopy, hysteroscopy, and gynecography.

In response to the worldwide interest in sterilization and population control with the use of the laparoscope and concern about potential complications, the American Association of Gynecologic Laparoscopists was formed in 1972. The initial enthusiasm for laparoscopy was based largely on the fact that for the first time female sterilization was available at a reasonable cost and the procedure could be accomplished in large numbers of women on an outpatient basis. Advanced operative endoscopic surgery represents a continuation of these early developments.

The evolution of modern diagnostic and operative laparoscopy has been reviewed by Semm,[20] Cushieri and Buess,[21] Murphy,[22] Gomel,[23] and Nezhat and colleagues.[24] These authors discussed essential instruments, the utility of multiple puncture sites, insufflation equipment, light sources, endoscopic photography, and the use of video monitors for endoscopic procedures. Initially, videolaparoscopy was difficult because available cameras were cumbersome and offered poor resolution, and light sources were inadequate. The use of video was not widespread and was opposed by some gynecologists. However, technologic improvements and surgical advances accelerated the development of videolaparoscopy as a safe, effective, and reasonable alternative to laparotomy. These advances enable surgeons and assistants to stand comfortably while observing a monitor that provides a magnified view of the operative field.

The surgeon must learn hand, eye, and foot coordination to optimize the options available with trocar sleeves that contain the videolaparoscope, graspers, suction-irrigator, and bipolar forceps. The surgeon uses one hand to control the videolaparoscope and the other to manipulate selected instruments. With the foot control, either the laser placed through the operative channel of the laparoscope or the bipolar forceps inserted through an ancillary trocar sleeves can be activated. Alternatively, with an assistant holding the videolaparoscope, the surgeon may use instruments in both hands for procedures, such as suturing or cutting. Surgeons must learn monocular depth perception, as does an individual with sight in only one eye who can operate a motor vehicle safely. The loss of depth perception initially may hamper inexperienced trainees as well as experienced videolaparoscopists when they evaluate experimental video equipment purporting to provide binocular depth perception.[21] Proficient videolaparoscopists work successfully in three dimensions using cues displayed on a two-dimensional screen.

An essential part of the learning process is mastering the coordinate use of the videolaparoscopists' feet, with the common setup using the left foot pedal to fire the laser and the right foot pedal to energize the bipolar coagulator. It is essential that switching be timely because lasers and electrocoagulators are potentially hazardous. To avoid associated complications, both energy sources should not be in the peritoneal cavity simultaneously.

Operative laparoscopy offers shorter hospitalization, less postoperative pain and morbidity, and shorter recuperation time compared to laparotomy. Nevertheless, findings during diagnostic endoscopy of intraoperative complications such as severe hemorrhage may require immediate laparotomy. Patients must be appropriately informed and the proper consent obtained preoperatively.[25] Laparoscopists must be competent in laparotomy or have qualified personnel available.

Learning videolaseroscopy and videolaparoscopy and maintaining skill requires continual experience with different procedures of various levels of difficulty. The frequency with which they are repeated and the manual dexterity, patience, motivation, dedication, and clinical acumen of the surgeon all influence the learning process. Data to assess positive and negative learning (conditioning and deconditioning) in such multifactorial situations often are elusive. Accumulation of this data is hampered further by sparse information about neurophysiologic alterations causally accompanying variations in both long- and short-term memory. Thompson and coworkers[26] noted that learning is accompanied by structural and chemical changes in the nervous system, some being more time dependent and durable than others with varied relations between practice sessions and improved performance. Some skills learned early are influenced slightly by subsequent training, whereas other skills require additional repetition over long periods.

Similar time-related findings for visual learning were reported by Karni and Sagi[27] who found that processes serving learning occur after practice sessions over periods of several hours to the end that performance is enhanced. Such data clearly offer collaborative opportunities for neurophysiologists, psychiatrists, and other biomedical personnel to improve the efficiency of teaching complicated procedures to physicians who choose to become proficient in laparotomy and videolaparoscopic surgery. It is relevant that some of the known basics of memory and learning processes have been applied in the design of training aids and equipment intended to simulate specific videolaseroscopic and videolaparoscopic techniques and procedures. Examples are Semm's "Pelvi-Trainer" and the Tübingen trainer (a closed anatomic phantom); their roles in training along with teaching specific endoscopic procedures (appendectomy, cholecystectomy, etc.) are described in a text edited by Cushieri, Buess, and Perissat.[21] Summarco and Youngblood[28] emphasize hands-on simulation exercises requiring eye-hand coordination. They are particularly beneficial when used early in teaching operative endoscopy to residents.

As proficiency is achieved, the complication rate for each procedure should fall. The findings of Götz and associates[29] in their initial use of videolaparoscopy for appendectomy are of interest. They converted 12 of their first 50 cases to laparotomy because lack of experience with the method made it difficult to deal with bleeding in 3 cases, adhesions in 3, and an abnormal position of the appendix in 4. Additional contributing factors included adiposity in 3, perforation in 1, and abscesses in 3; 2 patients had multiple reasons for laparotomy. No deaths or severe complications occurred. Operative time was 15 to 20 minutes. Generally, patients were discharged one day after operation. The authors concluded that laparoscopic appendectomy with the described modification was a safe, practical method of removing the appendix and can be learned quickly. Within 18 months, four of the seven surgeons at their hospital learned this operative technique.

Nezhat and Nezhat[30] reported the results of 100 incidental appendectomies. These surgeons were proficient in videolaparoscopy when the study was initiated. Except for a transient, 24-hour fever in one patient and mild periumbilical ecchymosis, there were no intraoperative or postoperative complications. Appendectomy time ranged from 4 to 21 minutes, and all patients were discharged within 24 hours of surgery.

Although the above data have general and specific applications to learning curves, they only indirectly address the issue of whether laparotomy or videolaparoscopy with or without the CO_2 laser is the preferred option for appendectomy. Tate and colleagues[31] reported data on 140 patients equally divided between appendectomy by laparotomy and laparoscopy. They reported no difference in the postoperative course between the two groups; the higher-than-expected conversion rate to laparotomy was probably related to experience because other studies showed contrary findings. Thus, the benefits of appendectomy by laparotomy or laparoscopy remain controversial. Tate and coworkers[31] stated that ". . . the ability to perform a diagnostic laparoscopy should be advantageous in the longer term and there should be a reduction in wound infection rates; we believe these are major benefits that justify a laparoscopic approach."

For many more complex surgical problems, particularly wherein laparotomy requires larger incisions for uncomplicated appendectomy, future randomized trials are unlikely for ethical reasons. Examples are procedures to treat gallbladder disease and intractable midline pelvic pain. In the former instance, the benefits of laparoscopic cholecystectomy are clear both for patients and physicians.[32] A prospective randomized trial to evaluate presacral neurectomy was terminated by the monitoring committee because they deemed it unethical "to continue to deprive patients with midline dysmenorrhea of the benefit of pain relief that could be afforded with presacral neurectomy."[33]

Credentialing

Over the period during which most of the data cited thus far were evolving, surgical endoscopy followed by videoendoscopy and subsequently videolaseroscopy emerged much as a consequence of patient demands for minimally invasive procedures. The results of videolaseroscopy in 600 cases of endometriosis were reported in 1986.[34] Correcting the severely distorted anatomy in many women with extensive endometriosis poses a great challenge to every experienced surgeon performing laparotomy. Successful laparoscopic treatment of these patients implies that most abdominal and pelvic surgery can be performed laparoscopically. The success of the improved camera-CO_2 laser laparoscope has been demonstrated in more than 6000 patients, including many with extensive endometriosis.[24,35,36]

The Committee on Gynecologic Practice of the American College of Obstetricians and Gynecologists (ACOG) released credentialing guidelines for operative laparoscopy[37] that stimulated the interest of the American Board of Obstetricians and Gynecology. They suggested that residents should document their training in gynecologic endoscopic procedures.[38] The realization that such data were not available and that the need for changes in training was important was highlighted in a survey undertaken by the Council on Resident Education in Obstetrics and Gynecology (CREOG) of Junior Fellows who had finished their residencies between 1987 and 1992.[38] Most residents regarded their training in advanced surgical techniques, including endoscopic procedures, as inadequate. The council noted no consensus concerning the best method to simultaneously train gynecologists in laparotomy and endoscopic techniques. In many instances, the properly trained postgraduate faculty was not available. Two other conclusions were that it would be necessary to "teach the teachers" and that an experimental training program should be conceived and initiated. Subsequent implementation of such a program at the Truman Medical Center in Kansas City was described by Sammarco and Youngblood.[28] Other centers similarly have upgraded resident training programs.

A memo concerning laparoscopic hysterectomy was issued by the Advisory Council of ACOG.[39] The council considered guidelines for diagnostic laparoscopy (level I), minor operative laparoscopy (level II), moderately advanced operative laparoscopy (level III), and advanced operative laparoscopy (level IV). Specific training and performance criteria including the number of human operations done under supervision and a list of complications over 2 years were described, but final decisions will evolve through consensus that will be influenced by participating gynecologic surgeons.

Opinions regarding the time to acquire competence vary. For a relatively simple laparoscopic appendectomy, Götz and colleagues[29] noted that 18 months was responsible. To become proficient in advanced laparoscopy (level IV), 4 to 5 years[24,40] is needed with the opportunity to practice regularly. In the future, specific criteria recognizing the relationship between the number and difficulty of operations, frequency of performance, complications encountered, and periodic quality assessment will evolve to refine credentialing guidelines. Because preceptors judge proficiency, it is essential to ensure availability of such personnel. A relationship between supply and demand needs to be recognized by hospital administrations, medical boards, and department chairpersons.

Cass and coworkers[41] described their findings with esophagogastrodoudendoscopy and colonoscopy, showing that success was a function of the number of procedures performed. Cecal intubation was successful in 84% of patients after 100 procedures. Comparable figures for upper gastrointestinal endoscopy were 90% after 100 procedures. The authors also noted that the relationship between experience and competence in mastering and using cognitive and technical skills has not been researched adequately.

The proportion of operations by laparotomy and videolaparoscopy is changing. As surgeons gain experience in laparoscopy, laparotomy will be used less often. Video technology offering magnification, excellent visibility, and taping procedures for teaching purposes will enhance surgical resident training. As models and simulators improve, they will mimic more accurately the contemplated "live" procedure.

Tadir and Fisch[42] have been active in advancing the use of technology in gynecologic laparoscopy since 1980. They noted that even after new techniques emerge as feasible and safe, caution is advised in assessing their appropriate use because feasibility may or may not indicate that it should be done. Surgical skill and prudent patient selection remain major elements in pacing the changing balance between laparotomy and videolaparoscopic techniques.

Operative endoscopy is one of the most innovative surgical advances of this century. It can be modified for application to almost any existing cavity in the body, and as instruments and techniques continue to improve, endoscopy will become more practical. Virtual reality, tele-endoscopy, distant live surgery, and teaching are not outside the realm of possibility. In this book, the authors share their experiences with endoscopy in pelvic surgery and describe appropriate techniques. Information is included pertaining to the laparoscopic treatment of a variety of pelvic abnormalities by basic and complex procedures. Future residents will have more opportunities to learn operative endoscopy than their predecessors, but all practicing physicians must begin with simple procedures and advance to more complicated ones.

REFERENCES

1. Bozzini P. Der Lichtleiter oder Beschreibung einer einfachen Vorrichtung und ihrer Anwendung zur Erleuchtung innerer Höhlen und Zwischenräume des lebenden animalischen Körpers. Weimar: Landes Industrie, Comptoir; 1807.
2. Nitze M. Über eine neue Beleuchtungsmethode der Höhlen des menschlichen Körpers. *Wien Med Presse.* 1879; 20:251.

3. Kelling G. Über Osophagoskopie, Gastroskopie und Zoelioscopic. *Munch Med Wochenschr.* 1902;49:21.
4. Jacobeaus H. Über die Möglichkeit, die Zystoskopie bei Untersuchunger seröser Höhlungen anzuwenden. *Münch Med Wochenschr.* 1910; 57:2090.
5. Veress J: Neues instrument zur Aüsfuhrung von Brust-oder Bauchpumktionen und Pneumothorax behandlung. *Dtsch Med Wochenschr* 1938;64:1480.
6. Ruddock JC. Peritoneoscopy. *West J Surg.* 1934;42:392.
7. Hope R. The differential diagnosis of ectopic gestation by peritoneoscopy. *Surg Gynecol Obset.* 1937;64:229.
8. Anderson ET. Peritoneoscopy. *Am J Surg.* 1937; 35:36.
9. Decker A, Cherry T. A new method in the diagnosis of pelvic disease. *Am J Surg.* 1944;64:40.
10. Power FH, Barnes AC. Sterilization by means of peritoneoscopic tubal furguration: a preliminary report. *Am J Obstet Gynecol.* 1941;41:1038.
11. Palmer R. La coeloscopie gynecologique, ses possibilités et ses indications actuelles. *Sem Hop Paris.* 1954;30:441.
12. Fourestier M, Gladau A, Voulmiere J. Perfectionments de l'endoscope medicale. *Presse Med.* 1952;60:1292.
13. Hopkins HH, Kapany NS. Flexible fiberoscope using static scanning. *Nature.* 1954;173:39.
14. Frangenheim H. *Die Laparoskopie und die Culdoscopie in der Gynäkologie.* Stuttgart: G Thieme; 1959.
15. Albano V, Cittidini E. *La celioscopia in Ginologia.* Palermo: Denaro; 1962.
16. Steptoe PC. *Laparoscopy in Gynaecology.* Edinburgh: Livingstone; 1967.
17. Cohen M. *Laparoscopy, Culdoscopy, and Gynecography.* Philadelphia: WB Saunders; 1970.
18. Semm K. *Atlas of Gynecologic Laparoscopy and Hysteroscopy.* Philadelphia: WB Saunders; 1975.
19. Gomel V. *Laparoscopy and Hysteroscopy in Gynecologic Practice.* Chicago: Yearbook Medical Publishers, 1986.
20. Semm K. *Operative Manual: Endoscopic Abdominal Surgery.* Chicago: Yearbook Medical Publishers, 1987.
21. Cuschieri A, Buess G. Introduction and historical aspects. In: Cuschieri A, Buess G, Perissat J, eds. *Operative Manual of Endoscopic Surgery.* Berlin: Springer-Verlag; 1992.
22. Murphy AA. Diagnostic and operative laparoscopy. In: Thompson JD, Rock JA, eds. *Te-Linde's Operative Gynecology*, 7th ed. Philadelphia: JB Lippincott; 1992.
23. Gomel V. Operative laparoscopy: Time for acceptance. *Fertil Steril.* 1989;52:1–11.
24. Nezhat C, Nezhat F, Nezhat C. Operative laparoscopy (minimally invasive surgery): state of the art. *J Gynecol Surg.* 1992;8:111–141.
25. Donovan JF, Van Voorhis BI. Legal issues in operative laparoscopy. *Contemp Obstet Gynecol.* 1993;August 31–39.
26. Thompson RF, Berger TW, Madden J. Cellular processes of learning and memory in the mammalian CNS. *Am Rev Neuro Sci.* 1983; 6:447–491.
27. Karni A, Sagi D. The time course of learning a visual skill. *Nature.* 1993;365:250–252.
28. Sammarco MJ, Youngblood JP. A resident teaching program in operative endoscopy. *Obstet Gynecol.* 1993;81:463–466.
29. Götz F, Pier A, Bacher C. Modified laparoscopic appendectomy in surgery. *Surg Endosc.* 1990;4:6–9.
30. Nezhat C, Nezhat F. Incidental appendectomy during videolaseroscopy. *Am J Obstet Gynecol.* 1991;165:559–564.
31. Tate JTT, Dawson JW, Chung SCS, et al. Laparoscopic versus open appendectomy: prospective randomized trial. *Lancet* 1993;342: 633–637.
32. Neugebauer E, Troidl H, Dierich A, et al. Conventional versus laparoscopic cholecystectomy and the randomized trial. *Br J Surg* 1991;78:150–154.
33. Tjaden B, Schlaf WD, Kimball A, et al. The efficacy of presacral neurectomy for the relief of midline dysmenorrhea. *Obstet Gynecol.* 1990;76:89–91.
34. Nezhat C. Videolaseroscopy: a new modality for the treatment of endometriosis and other diseases of reproductive organs. *Colposc Gynecol Laser Surg.* 1986;2:221–224.
35. Nezhat C, Crowgey SR, Garrison DP. Surgical treatment of endometriosis via laser laparoscopy. *Fertil Steril.* 1986;45:778.
36. Nezhat C, Crowgey S, Nezhat F. Videolaseroscopy for the treatment of endometriosis associated with infertility. *Fertil Steril.* 1989;51:237–240.
37. Committee on Gynecologic Practice. "Cre-

dentialing Guidelines for Operative Laparoscopy." ACOG Committee Opinion No. 106, April, 1992.

38. Youngblood JP. Advanced surgical techniques in obstetrics and gynecology. Correspondence released by the Council on Resident Education in Obstetrics and Gynecology. 409 12th St SW, Washington, DC, November 18, 1992.
39. Nusbaum ML. Memorandum to the Advisory Council of the American College of Obstetricians and Gynecologists regarding laparoscopic hysterectomy. District II NYS, 152 Washington Ave, Albany NY 12210, July 28, 1993.
40. Nezhat C. Stanford University Hospital Medical Staff Update. 1993;17:3.
41. Cass OW, Freeman ML, Craig JP, et al. Objective evaluation of endoscopy skills during training. *Ann Intern Med.* 1993;118:40–44.
42. Tadir Y, Fisch B. Operative laparoscopy: a challenge for general gynecology? *Am J Obstet Gynecol.* 1993;169:7–12.

2

Patient Education and Informed Consent

Before any operation, a surgeon is required by law, and bound by moral and ethical standards, to explain the procedure, its risks, and expected outcome to the patient. The purpose of this chapter is to provide a guide for discussing the proposed laparoscopic operation with the patient, the legal implications, and the concept of informed consent and disclosure as it relates to laparoscopy.

Although laparoscopy has gained widespread acceptance among gynecologists and general surgeons, a gap may exist between patient expectations and actual results from advanced operative laparoscopic procedures. For example, some patients believe that lasers are essential for a thorough operation, although most surgeons acknowledge that lasers are used similarly to scissors and electrosurgical instruments. Patients tend to consider laparoscopic procedures minor operations, a perception reinforced by such terms as "same-day surgery," "band-aid surgery," or "laser surgery." Patients and physicians tend to underestimate the risks of complex operative endoscopy, which are potentially as serious as those associated with laparotomy.

Concept of Informed Consent

Since 1914, physicians have been required to obtain a patient's written consent before a surgical procedure. This process should allow the patient to participate in decisions with an understanding of the factors relevant to the proposed operation. Obtaining proper consent requires that the patient be informed of the diagnosis, the proposed treatment, the probability of success, alternative forms of therapy, and risks involved with the planned operation. The information should be precise and presented in an understandable manner. Audiovisual material may be used to supplement the physician's explanation. This dialogue forms an intrinsic part of the doctor–patient relationship. Through these discussions, the physician can make intraoperative decisions consistent with the patient's desires and goals. The circumstances under which the consent is obtained are also important. The patient should not be under the influence of a medication that might interfere with her rational judgment.

Essentials of an Informed Consent

Although the principle of obtaining an informed consent is the same regardless of the surgical procedure, the following discussion concerns issues relevant to laparoscopic surgery.

Operative laparoscopy often is performed immediately following a diagnostic laparoscopy because, in some instances, a precise diagnosis cannot be made preoperatively, particularly in infertile women or those complaining of pelvic pain. The preoperative discussion should include possible diagnoses because some infertile patients have no clinical evidence of adhesions, endometriosis, or any other pelvic abnormalities, but significant disease is found laparoscopically, requiring an extensive operation.

The anticipated procedures should be explained so that the patient has realistic expectations about the type and duration of the anesthesia, the planned operation, and the length of hospitalization. Postoperative complaints following laparoscopic operations vary with the type of procedure[1] and are influenced by the geographic setting.[2] Most women are informed that they can return to normal activity within a week after advanced operative procedures and a few days following a diagnostic laparoscopy. Many return to work before they have experienced full relief from postoperative complaints.[1]

The surgeon provides information about the chance of success and the possible need for follow-up therapy. Even if the patient does not decline the proposed laparoscopic surgery, alternatives are offered and explained. Patients undergoing operations for the relief of pain require extensive preoperative evaluation and counseling because these women may be disappointed if they experience postoperative pain.

If the findings provide a range of options, the patient can elect to have only diagnostic laparoscopy. A woman suspected of having an ectopic pregnancy needs to understand the relative risks and benefits of salpingectomy, salpingostomy, and expectant management. Her obstetric history, clinical findings, desire for fertility, and acceptance of assisted reproductive technology influence the type of operation. The need for laparotomy because of hypovolemic shock is mentioned. Salpingostomy for tubal pregnancy is associated with a 5% to 10% incidence of persistent trophoblastic tissue. The need for postoperative serum serial β-human chorionic gonadotropin titers is emphasized.

Myomectomies by laparoscopy can be associated with bleeding or injury to adjacent organs and a laparotomy may be required. When initial laparoscopy reveals severe pelvic disease, a laparotomy may be safer than laparoscopy. Severe endometriosis, particularly in women with cul-de-sac obliteration, is associated with a risk of bowel injury.

Ideally, most questions are answered in the physician's office during the preoperative consultation, but the patient should be given ample time preoperatively to discuss additional concerns such as fertility, in case intraoperative decisions affect future childbearing. Although some patients will request a laparotomy under the same anesthesia, others will want to schedule a laparotomy at a later date if the abnormalities cannot be corrected laparoscopically.

Adequacy of Informed Consent

Three legal standards define the adequacy of an informed consent.[3] In states that use the majority rule, disclosure is decided by a professional medical standard based on the customary disclosure practices of physicians of the same specialty. Other states have adopted the minority rule, in which physicians must divulge those risks that a reasonably prudent patient needs to understand to make a decision. The minority rule has been modified to either a subjective test or the informational requirements of a specific patient (ie, the plaintiff).

Sensitivity to the patient and a commonsense approach to the informed consent are practical. Good communication is essential and must be encouraged. The patient expects her physician to assess the problem, propose treatment, and address her concerns with compassion. Patients are anxious preoperatively; the physician can ease that apprehension by carefully explaining the anticipated consequences of the procedure. When describing the frequency of complications, use terms such as rare, uncommon, or unusual. Do not attempt to provide precise complication rates. Explain precautions that will be taken to minimize the risks. Additional consent is required for photographic documentation.

Exceptions to Informed Consent

Clinical conditions can create exceptions to a full disclosure such as a life-threatening emergency in the unconscious patient and if the risks of failure to treat are greater than the risks of treatment. If possible, the patient's family should be informed.

Obtaining an informed consent implies that the patient is competent to give it. No clear standard exists for competency, but patients with severe mental retardation, psychiatric disorders, or those intoxicated by drugs or alcohol are unable to give an informed consent. Criteria for ascertaining incompetency include the inability to make decisions; making decisions for irrational reasons; making irrational decisions; or the inability to know, appreciate, or understand the information provided. If the physician believes a patient to be partially or totally incompetent, it is important to involve the family, a guardian, or even the courts to get proper informed consent. Sometimes, a patient may waive her right for full disclosure of the risks, but the reasons must be documented and discussed with the family. However, the physician should not decide that disclosing some or all of the risks would upset the patient and prevent her from making a rational decision because such a claim may be difficult to prove. The court may view the physician's self-interest as an overriding factor.[4]

Malpractice (Civil Liability)

Although operative laparoscopy is relatively new, the number of malpractice suits related to complications from this procedure is increasing. Regardless of the type or route of the surgical procedure, the basis for malpractice is the same. Most cases are launched after the patient experiences an unanticipated, unfavorable result.[5]

Gynecologic surgeons are trained to perform routine vaginal and abdominal operations in residency programs. To minimize sequelae, gynecologists must improve their skills in operative laparoscopy with postgraduate courses and by gradually undertaking increasingly difficult procedures. Knowing when to stop a complicated procedure represents commonsense and good judgment. Despite proper training and judgment, sequelae can occur. The cause of the complication should be explained to the patient. When the surgeon does not communicate adequately, the patient may seek another physician to explain the untoward result. Physicians should be restrained in criticizing colleagues unless all of the facts are known. In a recent review of adverse outcomes, less than 2% resulted in a malpractice claim.[6]

Four elements must be present to legally prove malpractice: duty, dereliction of duty (negligence), damage, and direct causality. The physician's duty, in a legal sense, is decided by the community standard of practice that exists for a particular procedure. Negligence is defined as a deviation from the accepted standard of care, custom, or common practice. Negligence may result from a number of acts or failures to act, including the following: failure to conduct adequate examinations and tests, careless execution of medical and surgical procedures, inappropriate prescription or administration of drugs, inadequate monitoring of the patient, failure to refer patients to other specialists as needed, and unethical conduct that harms a patient. If an injury results, the patient needs to prove that the negligence was the proximate cause of the damage to claim malpractice.

Operative laparoscopy is becoming more complex and the levels of experience and expertise vary widely. In many instances, the standard of care is not defined clearly. Laparoscopic surgeons must comprehend their own level of skill. A difficult laparoscopic operation may be performed more safely by laparotomy, a colleague with more endoscopic experience may be requested to help, or the patient may be referred to a more accomplished endoscopist. Most patients respect concern for consultation.

Malpractice cases usually are instituted because of delayed diagnosis or inadequate treatment. Many injuries can be identified intraoperatively and repaired. Once the injury is identified, the physician must be able to either repair it or seek proper consultation.[7] Hemorrhage, ureteral damage, and postoperative infection have been significant causes of liability. Patients who complain postoperatively of increasing abdominal pain should be examined promptly and their clinical condition evaluated. Postoperative infection is rare and a careful examination is needed to ascertain the cause of fever. Hypotension caused by intraoperative hemorrhage is managed by promptly diagnosing and locating the vascular injury, obtaining hemostasis, and replacing blood as needed.

Although performing an appendectomy incidental to other authorized abdominal and pelvic operations is acceptable, the physician can be liable for assault and battery if proper consent is not obtained. If a complication arises, the lack of consent can become the source of a malpractice claim.[7]

Avoiding Malpractice

Although it is impossible to guarantee that a surgeon can avoid malpractice claims, Roberts and colleagues[8] suggest several steps to reduce the risk.

1. Engage in good-quality, careful medical practice.

2. Be sure that you are adequately trained before attempting a diagnostic procedure or treatment.
3. Refer a patient to other physicians for care of consultation if the care required is not within your area of expertise.
4. Make sure that your knowledge is current, especially in the rapidly advancing areas of diagnostic and operative laparoscopy.
5. Perform the procedure only if the facility in which care is given is equipped to provide good emergency care should a complication occur during treatment.
6. Exercise caution when using nonstandard treatments, that is, those not generally condoned and used by the medical community at large.
7. Obtain adequate informed consent as described above. Sample consent forms are seen (Figures 2-1, 2-2, and 2-3).

CONSENT TO LAPAROSCOPIC SURGERY

Patient's Name____________________ Date________________

I authorize and direct ____________________M.D., and/or associates or assistants of his choice to treat the condition/s believed to exist in my case.

The laparoscope, a surgical instrument similar to a telescope is inserted through a small incision in the belly button. The abdomen is distended with a gas called carbon dioxide. The scope allows the doctor to visualize the pelvic organs and allows other instruments to be used under direct vision. Small second, third and fourth incisions are occasionally made at the pubic hairline for scissors, coagulator, or laser to perform major closed surgery at laparoscopy.

Hysteroscopy (the use of a small optical tube that is inserted through the vagina into the uterus without incision to visualize the uterine cavity) is usually performed with laparoscopy in order to determine: (1) the size and depth of the uterine cavity: (2) the presence of congenital abnormalities within the uterus, such as a septum that divides the inside of the uterus, or a double uterus; (3) the presence of polyps or fibroid tumors in the uterine cavity; (4) whether specific abnormalities of the endometrium (lining of the uterus) are present, e.g. hyperplasia (build up lining of the uterus), tuberculosis, or cell changes that indicate early cancer. D&C (dilatation and curettage) may also be performed if indicated.

Video and/or pictures may be taken during surgery and used to show you what was seen and done. They are also used for teaching other patients and other surgeons these techniques.

Your doctor performs advanced laparoscopic surgery that includes procedures considered investigational and may include modified instrumentation. These are relatively new techniques not commonly undertaken elsewhere and can include laparoscopic oophorectomy, hysterectomy, and tubal reversal. Laparoscopic treatment of ovarian neoplasms, benign or malignant is considered investigational.

Antibiotics, anticoagulants, and other medications may be used with surgery to aid in healing. These medications are not labeled (neither approve nor disapproved) by the FDA for adhesion prevention.

Although laparoscopy is generally an outpatient procedure, you may be asleep from 1-4 hours, occasionally longer.

1. Plan to avoid any activities that will require concentration for at least 2 days.
2. You can usually return to work and moderate activities by the third day.
3. You may need 1-3 weeks to return to heavy activities and for full recover.

Shoulder pain from the carbon dioxide gas and abdominal distention are common. Your throat may be sore from the endotracheal tube. About 1 in 40 patients are admitted for overnight stay due to nausea, drowsiness, or pain.

Figure 2-1.

Complications from laparoscopy surgery are very uncommon, but they do sometimes occur. It is also possible that because of complications, or because of the discovery of life-threatening abnormalities, immediate major abdominal surgery might be necessary. The chance of severe complications such as hysterectomy, colostomy, paralysis, or death is rare. With respect to your life, this operation is six times safer than driving a car and two to three times safer than being pregnant.
Some of the possible complications are the same as those of regular surgery. Complications include bleeding; infection, particularly of the navel; generalized disease; inflammation of the lining of the abdomen; injury to the stomach or intestines; gas embolism to the lining from the carbon dioxide; abnormal gas collections underneath the skin and in the chest; ruptures or hernias in the surgical wound and through the breathing muscles (diaphragm); burns on the skin of the abdomen and inside the abdomen; damage to the kidney and urinary system; blood clots in the pelvis and lungs; damage to the kidney and urinary systems; blood clots in the pelvic and lungs; and allergic and other bad reactions to one or more substances used in the procedure.

Some of the complications of this procedure may require major surgery; some of the complications can cause poor healing wounds, scarring and permanent disability, and very rarely, some of the complications can even cause death.

The alternative procedure to the laparoscopic surgery is major surgery. However, this alternative method also carries the same risks, and requires a much longer period to recover and more pain and discomfort. Therefore, in those patients in whom laparoscopic surgery is possible, the procedures provide the patient with diagnosis and treatment at low risk and less discomfort. Your doctor cannot and does not guarantee the success of this procedure, but believes that the procedure is in your best interest.

I further understand that during the course of the operations or treatment, unforeseen conditions may be revealed requiring an extension of the original procedure/s or different procedures than those specifically discussed. I hereby authorize the above named surgeon, his associates, and assistants to perform such other laparoscopic surgical procedures and if necessary laparotomy (abdominal surgery) and to remove any tissue or organs that may be necessary or medically desirable as determined by the surgeons professional judgement. This authority shall extend to treatment of conditions not previously known by my physicians.

My signature below constitutes my acknowledgment: 1. that I have read or had read to me the contents of this form, 2. that I understand and I agree to the foregoing, 3. that the proposed operation/s or procedures/s have been satisfactorily explained to me including possible risks and alternatives, 4. that I have all the information that I desire and have had ample opportunity to ask questions on specific points, 5. and that I hereby give my authorization and consent.

DO NOT SIGN THIS FORM UNLESS YOU HAVE READ IT, UNDERSTAND IT, AND AGREE WITH WHAT IT SAYS.

Date: Signature:

Time: Witness:

Since Drs. are considered pioneers in advanced laparoscopic surgery, visiting surgeons may observe and/ or participate in my operative care, always under the direct supervision of my doctor. I am aware that visiting surgeons may observe and/or participate during my operation.

Signature:

Witness:

Figure 2-1 (continued).

PHOTOGRAPH CONSENT AND RELEASE FORM

I, ____________________, hereby irrevocably authorize
, their successors, assigns, and those acting with their permission upon their authority to copyright, use and publish for art, advertising, medical, trade, commercial and other lawful purpose, any depiction or likeness for me or which I may be included in whole or part, including, but not limited to, motion pictures, video tapes and still photographs, and further including any composite photograph or photograph distorted in character or in form, and any motion picture or video tape edited by addition thereto or deletion of any part thereof, whether in conjunction with my name, a fictitious name or no name, or any reproduction or variation thereof by whatever medium made, taken at Hospital during the period of ______________________.

I hereby waive any right which I may have to inspect or approve any such photograph, motion picture, video tape or other likeness or the use to which it is put, and acknowledge that except for the consideration recited I shall receive no payment or remuneration for the use of any such photograph, motion picture, or video tape or likeness.

I hereby release their successors and assigns, and those acting with their permission and upon their authority, of and from every liability, responsibility and claim which may arise by reason of any exercise of the authority granted above or any blurring, distortion, alteration, optical illusion, or use in composite form, whether intentional or otherwise, which may occur or result in the taking or publication of such photograph, motion picture, video tape or other likeness unless it can be shown that publication
thereof was for the purpose of subjecting me to conspicuous, ridicule, scandal or indignity.

I understand that my tape(s) may be used for medical studies and instructional purposes for the advancement and increase expertise of videolaseroscopy.

The condition of the pelvis will be videotaped before, in some parts during, and after the procedure. This tape could be misplaced or erased. If I personally receive a tape, it will be an edited version, approximately 5-10 minutes in length, and the and staff cannot be held responsible for any mechanical failure that might occur during the original filming or reproduction of the video.

______________________	______________________
SIGNATURE	DATE
______________________	______________________
WITNESS	DATE

Figure 2-2.

CONSENT AND APPLICATION FOR OBSERVATION OF MEDICAL PROCEDURE RELEASE AND INDEMNITY

PATIENTS CONSENT TO OBSERVER

I hereby authorize ________________ Hospital to permit the presence of such observers as they may deem fit while I am undergoing surgery, childbirth, examination, or other treatment or diagnostic procedure at the Hospital. I hereby consent to being observed by any such persons.

This consent and authorization is expressly limited to the following conditions:

____

____

____

________________		________________	
Patient's Signature	Date/Time	Witness	Date/Time
________________			
Patient's Representative	Date/Time	Patient unable to consent because ________________ ________________	

I. OBSERVER'S REQUEST AND RELEASE

I ________________, hereby request ________________ Hospital to permit me to observe certain medical and/or surgical procedures to be performed at the Hospital. I understand that I will be under the physician's direct supervision and agree to follow the physician's instructions to abide by all Hospital rules and regulations governing such observations. I recognize that I will be under the supervision of the physician, and not the hospital.

In consideration for the physician and hospital allowing me to observe, I hereby expressly release the physician, the hospital, their agents and employees of and from any and all claims, damages, responsibilities and liabilities which may arise, directly or indirectly, from or in connection with my activities at the Hospital. I further agree to indemnify and hold harmless the physician, the hospital, their agents and employees from and against any and all claims, liabilities and damages arising directly or indirectly out of or in connection with my observation of medical and/or surgical procedures at the Hospital.

If I am under eighteen year of age, my parent or legal guardian has consented to my observation of the medical and/or surgical procedures and agrees to release, indemnify and hold harmless the physicians, the hospital, their agents and employees from and against any and all claims, liabilities and damages arising directly or indirectly out of or in connection with my observation of medical and/or surgical procedures at the Hospital.

________________		________________	
Observer	Date	Witness	Date
________________		________________	
Parent or Guardian	Date	Witness	Date

II. PHYSICIAN'S INDEMNITY FOR OBSERVER

I have agree to let ________________ (the "observer") accompany me during certain medical and/or surgical procedures at the Hospital and to observe such procedures. I agree that I will be completely responsible for the Observer and that he or she will be within my control at all times and will abide by all Hospital rules and regulations relating to his or her observing such procedures at the hospital.

In consideration of the Hospital's permitting the observer to accompany me, I agree to indemnify and hold harmless the hospital, its agents and employees from and against any and all claims, liabilities and damages arising, directly or indirectly, out of or in connection with the observation by such observer of medical and/or surgical procedures at the Hospital.

________________ ________________

Figure 2-3.

References

1. Azziz R, Steinkampf MP, Murphy A. Postoperative recuperation: relation to the extent of endoscopic surgery. *Fertil Steril.* 1989; 51:1061.
2. Semm K. *Operative Manual for Endoscopic Abdominal Surgery.* Chicago: Yearbook Medical Publishers; 1987;22.
3. Stenchever MA. Too much informed consent? *Obstet Gynecol.* 1991;77:631.
4. Meisel A. The "exceptions" to the informed consent doctrine: striking a balance between competing values in medical decision making. *Conn Med.* 1981;45:(pt 1):107; 45:(pt 2):27.
5. Barr JR. Following a few simple rules may help prevent malpractice claims. *Can Med Assoc J.* 1991;114:355.
6. Localio AR, Lawhters AG, Brennan TA, et al. Relation between malpractice claims and adverse events due to negligence: results of the Harvard Medical Practice Study III. *N Engl J Med.* 1991;325:245.
7. Mills, HM. Medical lessons from malpractice cases. *JAMA.* 1963;183:1073.
8. Roberts DK, Shane JA, Roberts ML. *Confronting the Malpractice Crisis: Guidelines for the Obstetrician-Gynecologist.* Kansas City: Eagle Press; 1985.

Bibliography

Borten M. Informed consent and counseling. In: *Laparoscopic Complications.* Philadelphia: BC Decker; 1986:415–428.

Cassileth BR, Zupkis RV, Sutton-Smith K, March V. Informed consent—why are its goals imperfectly realized? *N Engl J Med.* 1980;302:896.

Roberts DK. Informed consent and medicolegal problems. In: Sciarra JJ, ed. *Gynecology and Obstetrics.* Philadelphia: JB Lippincott; 1990; 99:1–10.

Shindell S. Medicolegal aspects of pelvic surgery. In: Mattingly RF, ed. *Operative Gynecology*, 5th ed. Philadelphia: JB Lippincott; 1977:13.

3

Equipment

Many instruments have enabled surgeons to increase the diversity of laparoscopic procedures and, although some have multiple functions, others are specialized. They are designed to fit through trocar sleeves 3 to 30 mm in diameter. Many ancillary instruments have a unipolar electrosurgical capability.

Successful operative laparoscopy requires proper basic instruments, whereas specialized instruments make difficult procedures technically possible and safer. Most procedures can be performed with two or three forceps, a suction-irrigator probe, a bipolar electrocoagulator, a pair of scissors, and the CO_2 laser. With the rapid growth of operative laparoscopy, disposable, semireusable, and reusable instruments have become available. In selecting the appropriate instruments, cost and effectiveness of each one should be considered because too many instruments clutter the field and increase operative time.

With the technique of videolaseroscopy, the operation is observed by the surgeon and operating room staff on multiple video monitors. The CO_2 laser is used through the operative channel of the laparoscope for cutting and hemostasis of small blood vessels.[1] Electrocoagulation with a bipolar forceps is used to control bleeding from larger blood vessels. The CO_2 laser can be replaced by another cutting instrument, and the bipolar forceps can be replaced by another instrument to control bleeding.

Disposable or Reusable Instruments

When choosing instruments, several factors must be considered, including initial cost, cost per use, ease of use, and reliability. Reusable instruments involve initial and maintenance expenses, such as handling, sterilizing, sorting, and storing. For some reusable instruments, such as scissors, performance declines with use and they must be replaced periodically. However, most instruments perform reliably, and their construction and materials allow a certain level of indelicate handling.

In contrast, disposable instruments cost the patient as much as $100 to $200 per instrument. The use of the stapler may add $1000 to $3000 to the operation, thus offsetting the cost savings achieved by laparoscopy. There remains the expense of handling and storing disposable instruments. The main advantage is high performance, including sharpness and a theoretically reduced risk of transmission of disease. However, once discarded, environmental concerns are raised about disposal and biodegradability. The materials used are not durable and they are not reliable with repeated use. The combination of disposable and reusable instruments helps maintain high performance standards.

Essential Instruments

Laparoscope

The endoscope must be in optimal condition for the procedure. Although the diameters of laparoscopes vary from 1 to 12 mm and the angle of view from 0 to 90 degrees, the most commonly used laparoscopes are the straight, diagnostic, and right angle operative laparoscopes (Figure 3-1). A direct 10-mm, 0-degree diagnostic laparoscope, and an 11-mm, 0-degree operative laparoscope for operative laparoscopy with the CO_2 laser are preferable (Figure 3-2). The image transmitted by the

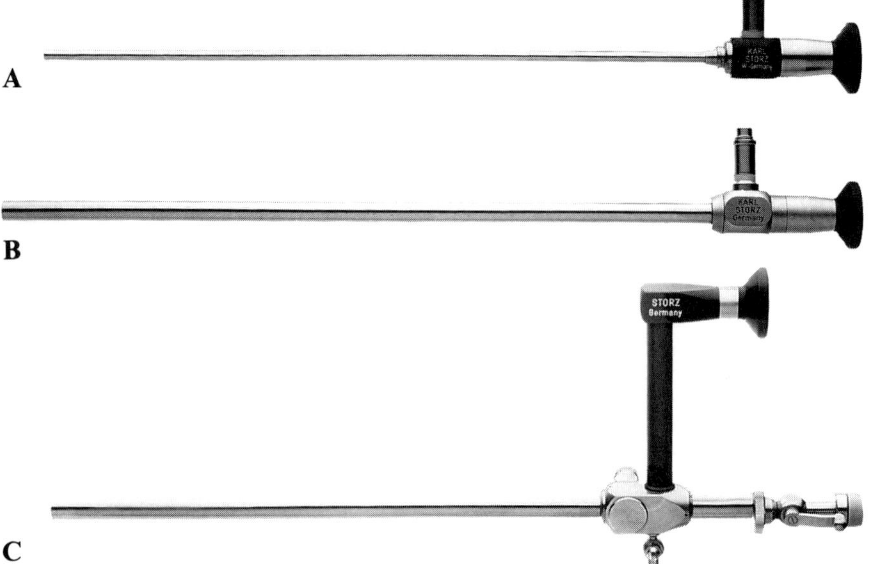

Figure 3-1 A, A 4-mm straight diagnostic laparoscope. B, An 11-mm straight diagnostic laparoscope. C, A 10-mm right angle operative laparoscope.

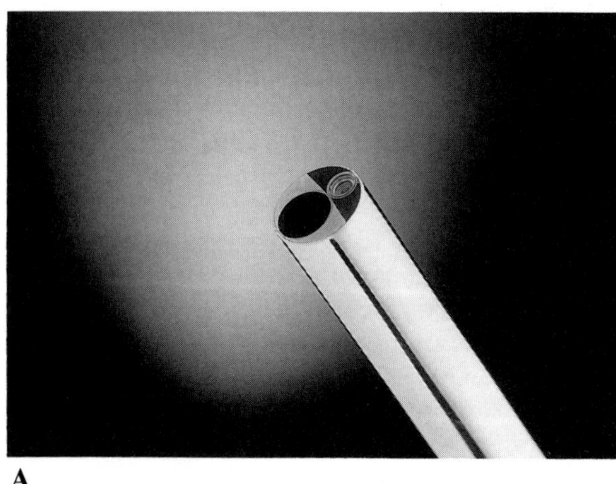

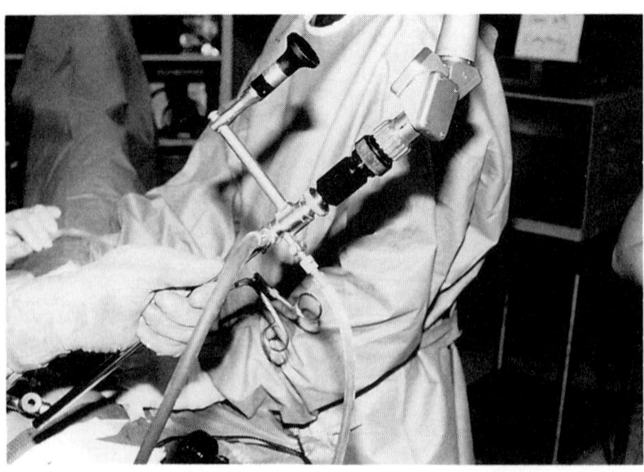

Figure 3-2 A, The laser laparoscope has two channels: one for the CO_2 laser and one for the light source. B, Connection of the CO_2 laser to the operative channel of the laparoscope.

diagnostic scope is superior because of the absence of an operative channel where its presence requires a reduction in the size of the lens system and number of fiberoptic bundles. The endoscope is the access to the abdominal and pelvic cavity and the most important piece of equipment.

With a Hopkins rod lens system, the shaft of the laparoscope contains quartz rods with concave ends, a configuration that is known to provide excellent clarity. Further, this type of lens rarely is dislodged during handling.

Primary Trocar

Reusable and disposable trocars are constructed of a combination of metal and plastic (Figure 3-3). A feature common to all cannulas is a flapper or trumpet valve to prevent gas leakage as the laparoscope or other instruments are removed from the abdomen. Unfortunately, in reusable trocars, this valve mechanism creates friction on the laparoscope. After a long procedure, the trocar tends to move with the laparoscope, often resulting in inadvertent removal of the trocar from the abdominal cavity and a loss of pneumoperitoneum. By removing the spring from the valve, there is less friction and the problem can be avoided. A new feature of disposable cannulas is a retention screw (Ethicon) (Figure 3-4A) or an inflatable balloon (Marlow Surgical Technologies, Willoughby, OH) (Figure 3-4B). The latter can tamponade abdominal wall bleeding that may obscure the operating field.

Various disposable trocar tips are available, including spring-loaded safety shields that retract into the cannula as the trocar is inserted into the

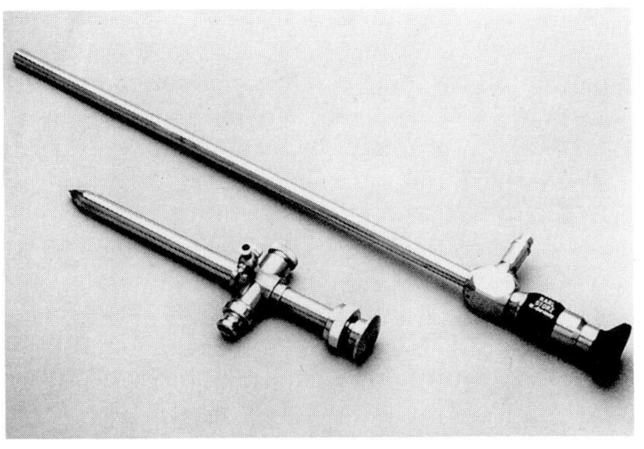

A

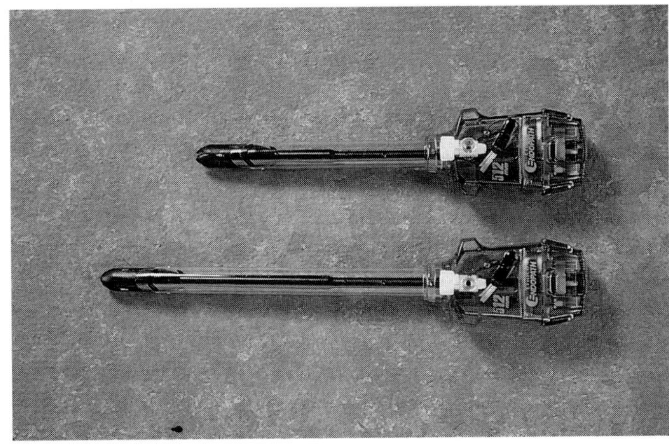

B

Figure 3-3 A, A reusable 10-mm trocar. B, Tristar 10-mm and 12-mm disposable trocars (Ethicon).

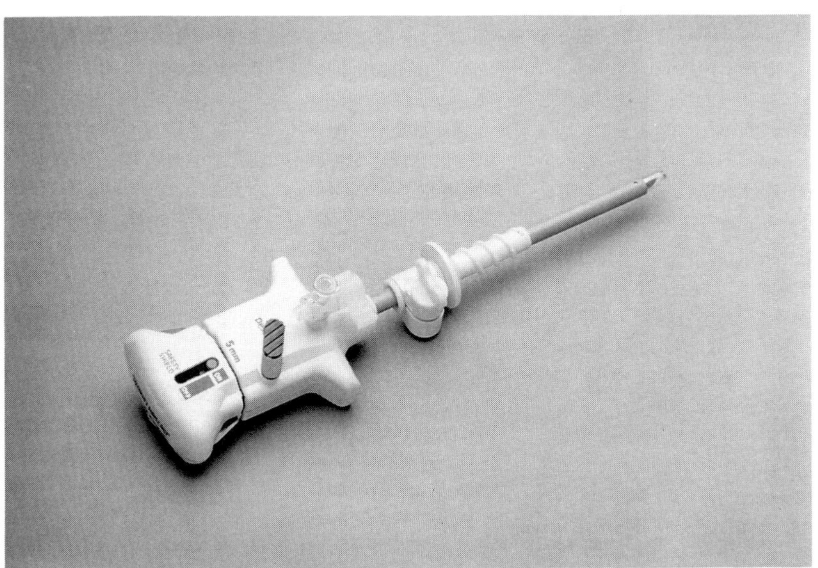

A

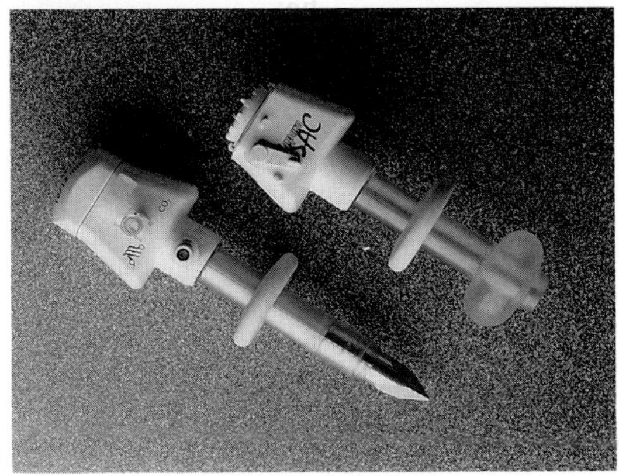

B

Figure 3-4 A, A 5-mm trocar with a retention screw (Ethicon). B, Trocar with an inflatable balloon (Marlow Surgical Technologies).

abdomen (Ethicon). This exposes the sharp trocar for entry, but the plastic shield is released automatically inside the peritoneal cavity to cover the sharp tip and protect intra-abdominal organs. Another trocar uses the same principle as the Veress needle. After the peritoneal cavity is penetrated, the blunt stylet moves beyond the tip to prevent injury. The bullet tip disposable trocar (Ethicon) minimizes the possibility of tissue being caught between the trocar and sleeve and muscle injury. In the presence of adhesions to the anterior abdominal wall, under the umbilicus, the reusable devices offer no advantage.

Secondary Trocars

Like primary trocars, reusable and disposable accessory trocars and sleeves are available. They come in a variety of lengths and range in diameter from 3 to 30 mm; the most common size is 5 mm (see Figure 3-4A). Some are threaded so that they can be screwed into the abdominal wall, making them relatively immobile during manipulation.

Veress Needle

Disposable and reusable Veress needles are available (Figure 3-5). The needle consists of a blunt-tipped, spring-loaded inner stylet and a sharp outer needle. As the needle passes through the abdominal layers, the stylet retracts to allow penetration. Once the peritoneal cavity is entered, the absence of tissue resistance allows the blunt stylet to protrude. A lateral hole on this stylet enables CO_2 gas to be delivered intra-abdominally. The new disposable Veress needle has several added safety points.

Insufflator

To adequately observe the contents of the abdominal and pelvic cavity, the abdomen must be insufflated. Only CO_2 is used for operative laparoscopy. Advanced procedures require an automatic, electric insufflator (Figure 3-6) that can deliver up to 15 L of gas per minute, or two insufflators, each delivering 9 to 10 L of gas per minute. The insufflator will compensate for any change when the intra-abdominal pressure is preset. Intra-abdominal pressure should not exceed 16 mm Hg to avoid complications such as subcutaneous emphysema.

Although a mechanical abdominal wall lifter can replace establishing a pneumoperitoneum, exposure is poor and complications including femoral nerve injury have been reported with the new device.

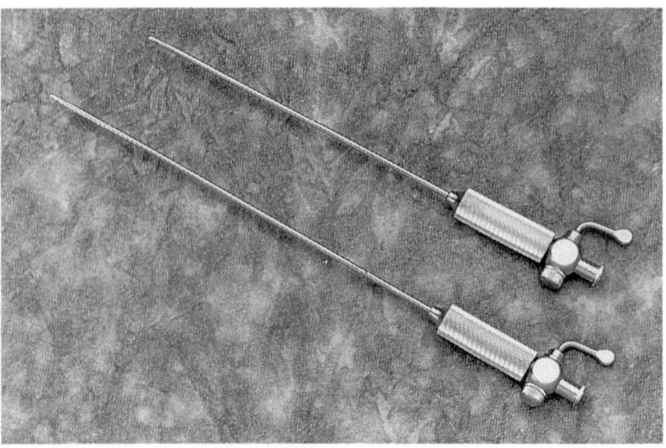

Figure 3-5 Reusable Veress needles.

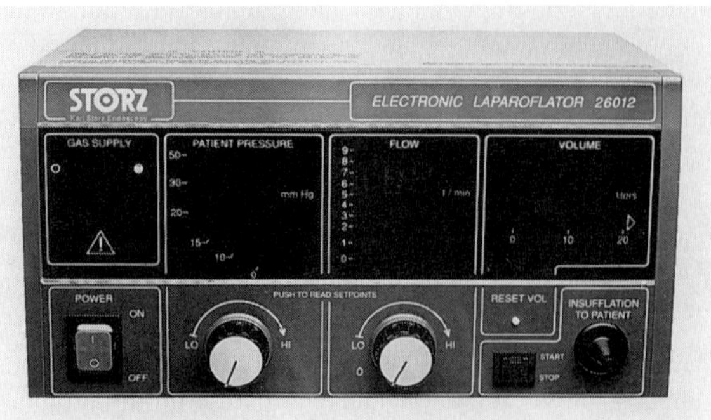

A

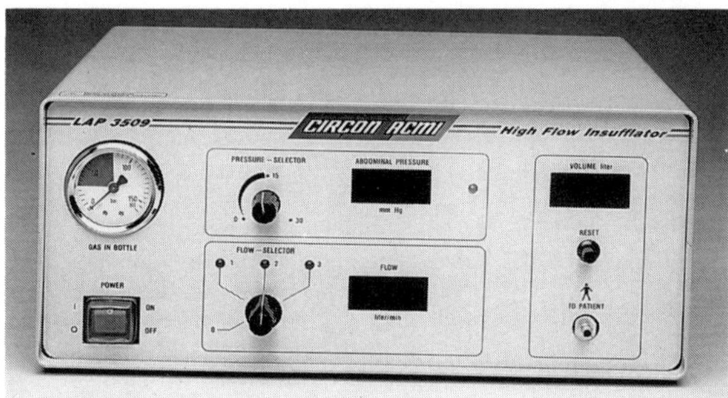

B

Figure 3-6 A and B, Automatic insufflators that deliver up to 10 L/min (Karl Storz) and 9 L/min (Circon).

Camera Equipment

In early endoscopic surgery, no medical video cameras were available and endoscopists adopted cameras from the television trade. Camera tubes and single- and three-chip cameras followed the introduction of similar advancements in commercial cameras. However, that trend began to change with the introduction of equipment specific for endoscopy, including the breakthrough of digital processing and chip-on-a-stick, three-dimensional, and virtual reality technologies.

Historical development. The first medical camera, introduced by Circon Corporation in 1972, had three tubes and weighed 18 lb. It used a fiberoptic image guide to transfer a microscopic image to the camera, which in turn transferred the image to a video monitor. In 1973, a single-tube camera weighing 3.8 lb was introduced (Figure 3-7). Although the weight was reduced, the camera remained heavy and counterweights were needed. To its credit, this camera advanced surgical video technology because it was the first camera that could be attached directly to the microscope or endoscope without using a fiberoptic image guide. In addition, the single one-inch tube had a specially striped filter to produce, for the first time, a full color picture. From this point on, surgical video camera manufacturers continued to make improvements in size, weight, and image quality (Figure 3-8).

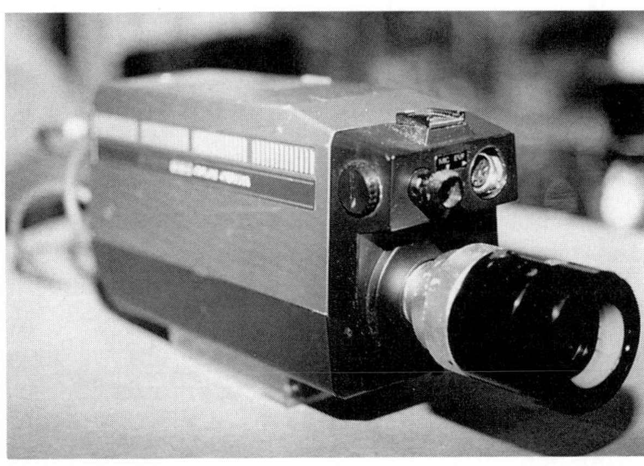

A

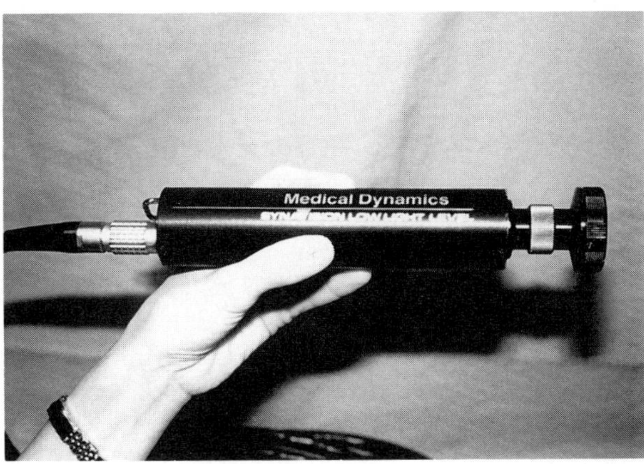

B

Figure 3-7 A and B, Two early cameras used in videolaparoscopy.

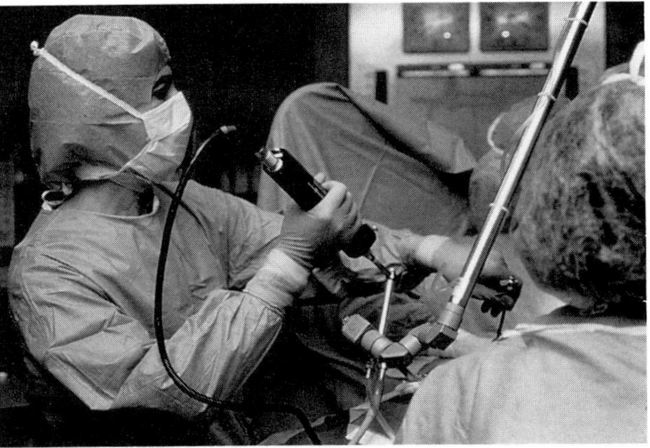

Figure 3-8 Camran Nezhat performing videolaparoscopy in early 1980.

In 1975, a camera weighing 1.25 lb was introduced and, in the following year, a low light feature enabled it to be 10 times more light sensitive. In 1980, a new 6-oz camera was small enough to be held in the palm of the surgeon's hand and yet produced excellent color separation and image resolution. Another milestone was achieved 2 years later with the first solid-state charged coupled device (CCD) camera. This camera weighed 3 oz and, with the change from tubes to solid-state CCD sensors, two major achievements were accomplished. First, the camera could be disinfected in solutions, so the need to bag the camera was gone. Second, the colors produced by solid-state construction were more consistent than the colors produced by the tube cameras.

Since 1982, all surgical camera manufacturers have switched to solid-state construction. New developments include low lux levels (enhancing the quality of the image in low light situations), buttons on the cameras to start and stop VCRs, field replaceable camera cables, and increased lines of resolution (S-Video and red-green-blue, or RGB signal output as opposed to just National Television Systems Committee, or NTSC). Cameras also became more durable. The technology of the 1990s has added digitally processed signals, three-chip cameras, chip-on-a-stick, and more to surgical video (Figure 3-9).

Basic video knowledge. Within the camera is a CCD that "sees" an optical image through the camera lens. The CCD then converts that optical image into an electrical image that is sent through camera cables to the CCU (camera control unit), or camera box, and on to the monitor input. The monitor converts the electrical image back to the original optical image, an image that the human

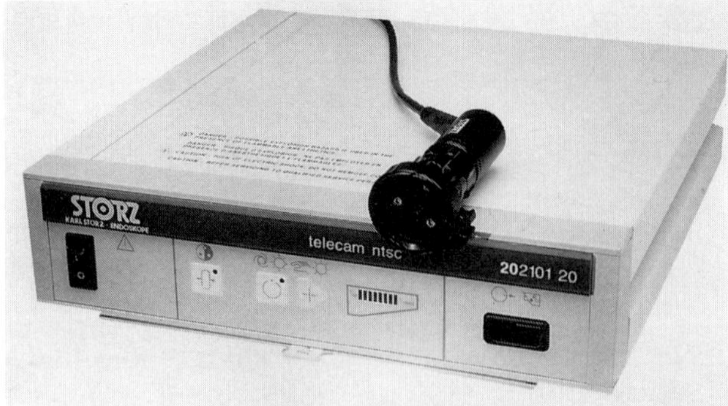

A

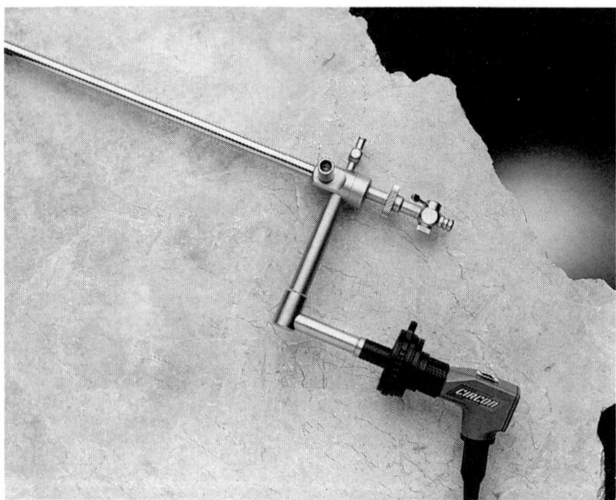

B

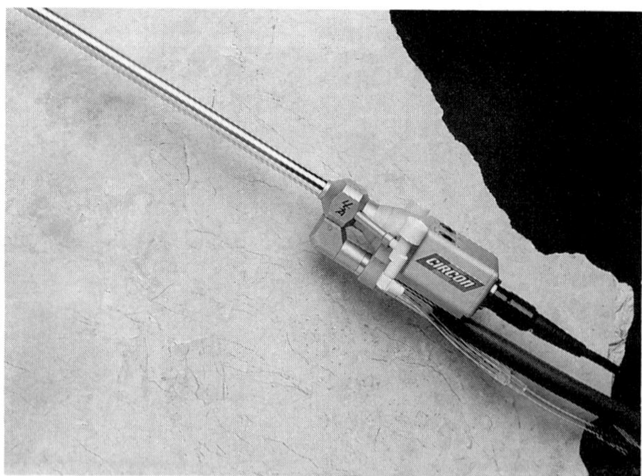

C

Figure 3-9 A, NTSC camera by Karl Storz. B, The camera is attached to the laparoscope. C, The camera is built into the laparoscope. The eyepiece is omitted.

eye can see. The electrical image may be directed to components other than the monitor after leaving the CCU. It could be relayed by a cable to a VCR and from the VCR to a printer and then on to a monitor.

How is the optical image converted to an electrical image and how is it sent from one video component to another? The answer lies in the CCD, where the optic to electronic conversion occurs. The CCD is composed of rows of tiny picture elements called pixels. The more pixels per row in a CCD, the better the resulting picture. Each pixel is capable of sensing either red, green, or blue light (the three primary colors of video) to produce color information. At this point, the CCD has both color and light intelligence.

This video information, color and light (or luminance), is scanned to generate a signal frequency. The scanning is performed at a rate of 525 lines per frame, and there are 30 frames per second of video information. The scanning rate is that of television broadcast, standardized by the NTSC. NTSC scanning rate is used in the United States, Canada, Japan, and most of South America and Asia. Russia and France use a different scanning rate called "Secam." PAL, a third type of scanning rate, is used in other European nations. These scanning rates are not compatible with NTSC standards. Videotapes made in the United States must be converted before they can be viewed in countries with non-NTSC scanning rates, and the process of converting one scanning rate to another is expensive.

When the NTSC scanning rate was created, technicians were using a limited band width to send the video signal and both color and luminance information were sent simultaneously. Therefore, the format of the NTSC signal is referred to as a "composite signal." There are inherent problems with this method of transference because a camera first processes color and luminance information separately, then combines the two to create a signal. One problem with this method is referred to as "cross-talk," a signal noise that generates grainy images with soft edges and causes colors to have less consistency from one use to the next. (In the business, NTSC is also known as "Never Twice Same Color.") Thus, of the three signal-carrying formats, the first format, NTSC, is the least desirable. The second and third formats carry much clearer signals with less noise.

The second format is called a "component signal," meaning that the color and luminance are carried separately. Y/C (Y stands for luminance or light brightness and C refers to color) is a common name for the format. SVHS and Super VHS are tape formats that accept this type of signal. Because there is less cross-talk, pictures generated by component signals appear cleaner, with sharper edges and truer colors than pictures generated by composite signals. The Y/C format, like the NTSC format, carries the video signal in a single cable, even though color and luminance are separate.

The third format style, RGB, is also a component signal. It is distinct from the Y/C format in that the video information (color and luminance) is separated into four signals, a red signal, a green signal, a blue signal, and a timing signal. Each signal carries its own luminance information. The separation occurs in the camera head and is performed electrically. Because the colors and luminance are separate from the start, the RGB format requires less electronic processing than do the NTSC and Y/C formats. Therefore, the ultimate quality of the image is enhanced. In the back of a three-chip camera CCU (camera box), there are cables for RGB and a fourth cable for "sync." There are four separate cables from the camera box, so a monitor that accepts RGB input is needed. These monitors are more expensive than most other types of monitors, but they have higher resolution capabilities than NTSC and often accommodate both RGB and Y/C input.

Terms referred to thus far include resolution, pixels, and signal noise. What exactly do these terms mean? Picture resolution determines the clarity and detail of the video image. Resolution specification refers to a set number of horizontal lines of resolution. Horizontal resolution measurements are ascertained by the number of distinct vertical lines that can be seen in a picture. Vertical resolution is the number of horizontal lines that can be seen in a picture. The higher the resolution numbers, the sharper and cleaner the image will be. However, resolution is a subjective measurement within certain limits as set forth by the camera's pixel count and by the formula used to achieve the resolution number. No resolution number can be higher than that of the pixel count. In addition, the ability of the video system to carry and process signals, the attributes of the components that transmit signals, and the resolution numbers of the monitor together determine the ultimate picture quality.

Relying only on resolution specifications when purchasing video equipment is problematic because the resolution number is established by the equipment manufacturer, not an independent tester. The industry standard is to measure horizontal resolution using 75% of the chip. However, some manufacturers have been known to use 100% of the chip. This results in a higher resolution number that is not true resolution, so never make a purchasing decision based on specifications alone.

Each line of resolution is composed of pixels, and the more pixels per line, the better the image. It is akin to a computer printer in which the more dots of ink per letter, the crisper each letter looks, contributing to the overall appearance of the document. Another way to understand the pixel effect is to compare a large screen television with a small (13-inch) monitor. The smaller monitor will have a sharper, crisper image, especially at the edges of an image because pixels are placed more closely together on the small screen.

Signal-to-noise ratio is a measurement that differentiates between video noise (cross-talk) and useful video information. The higher the signal-to-noise ratio, the better the detail at the edge and the better the overall image. Signal noise value is measured in decibels. A quick way to evaluate noise is not to allow any light to reach the camera chip. With the absence of picture information, the image contains only noise. Another way to see picture noise is to adjust the camera to place color bars on the monitor screen. Select first an NTSC signal, then a Y/C signal, and finally an RGB signal. Look at the edge of each bar color and notice that movement from NTSC to Y/C to RGB makes the edges progressively sharper because NTSC has the most noise and RGB has the least. Specifications (lines of resolution, pixels, signal-to-noise ratios) set the parameters of the video components, but always test the monitor.

Endoscopes. Biomedical Business International, a medical marketing research firm, estimates the number of laparoscopic general surgical procedures will reach 1.7 million by the year 1997. An estimate that includes all specialties using a rigid or flexible scope is expected to exceed 4 million by 1997.

There are essentially two types of scopes, rigid and flexible. The rigid scopes are based on the Hopkins rod lens system, which provides good resolution and depth of field. The flexible scopes rely on a set number of fiberoptic bundles. The rigid scopes range in diameter from 10-mm laparoscopes down to 1.9-mm arthroscopes with a range of angles cut into the distal lens (eg, 70 degree, 45 degree, 30 degree).

Most rigid scopes are focused with the camera coupler. With a videoscope (camera and scope together), there will be either a focus control on the scope or the focus will occur automatically inside the camera. The image is magnified so that it appears larger on the monitor. With flexible scopes, when the bundle image is magnified, so are the bundles. This makes the end of the bundles visible along with the image. The scopes are relatively fragile, and small cracks may allow water to seep through the lens and distort the image.

The light cord is as important as a high-resolution camera and a precision scope because if light does not move properly from the light source to the scope through the cord, the value of the camera is limited and poor images appear. Some light cords focus the light in the center, whereas others focus it on the edges of the image. Light dispersed evenly across its diameter is preferred. Light cords are either fiberoptic or liquid filled. Fiberoptic light guide cables are available in varying lengths (6, 8, and 10 ft) with little diminished light loss. Light cords are fragile; avoid dropping them and do not wind them into small bundles. Liquid-filled light guide cables produce more light and are more durable than fiberoptic cables. However, liquid-filled cables are more expensive and produce more heat at the endoscope. Liquid-filled cables also are limited by their standard 6-foot length.

Light sources. All light sources use similar types of bulbs, either xenon, halogen, or mercury. Each type of bulb generates light of a slightly different color and intensity. The most common bulbs are halogen and xenon, with xenon available in 150, 175, or 300 watts (Figure 3-10). Xenon bulbs generate a higher intensity of light, last longer, and are more expensive to replace but provide consistent levels of light intensity. It is capable of generating even higher levels of light, and when more light is needed, it is instantly available.

The camera. The camera includes two components: the camera head with its cable and the CCU or camera controller. The cable is plugged into the camera controller. The lens on the medical camera is referred to as a "coupler." The coupler screws onto the camera head and is available in several sizes that magnify the image. A 35-mm coupler will produce a larger image on the monitor than a 28-mm coupler. Two styles of couplers are available, the direct coupler and the beam-splitter coupler. With a direct coupler, the image travels directly to the camera. With a beam splitter, part of the image travels to the camera and part of the image travels to a porthole or eye cup. The porthole enables the surgeon to view the image directly.

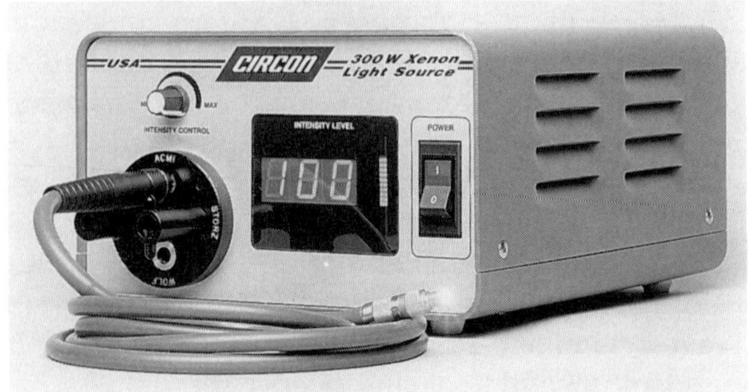

Figure 3-10 Xenon light source by Circon.

Couplers can be mounted and fixed on the camera head and are unremovable. Removable couplers allow the purchase of a camera with interchangeable direct couplers and beam splitters. Although the removable coupler provides flexibility and economy, its quality of being removable is a potential problem because the coupler must be screwed to the camera head. If it is not completely attached or if its O ring is worn, liquids may seep between the coupler and the camera head, causing internal fog. A coupler with internal fog is not usable and must be repaired. A fixed coupler eliminates this problem.

Most cameras are either a single chip or a three chip, and both images are equal in quality. One unique video camera (Circon) has proprietary RGB 24-bit digital enhancement circuits, so that the signals coming from the CCD sensor are sampled at equal time intervals and the amplitude of each sample is classified into a discrete level system and converted to a binary code. Thus, all of the video information is encoded into a stream of noise-free digital numbers. These numbers are used as variables in mathematical equations (algorithms) to manipulate and shift in time and value through digital signal processing. Digital electronics is the leading edge in video technology and it will be the new standard of performance just as digital compact discs have replaced records and audio cassettes. Digital signals take up less band width than do analog signals currently in use. Moreover, digital-processed signals can be applied to three-chip and high-definition television (HDTV).

Another breakthrough in medical cameras is chip-on-a-stick, a technology that combines the camera and scope on one piece of equipment. The camera chip is taken out of the camera head and placed at the distal end of the scope. This technology does away with all of the optical lenses that an image passes through when the chip is in the camera head. Chip-on-a-stick cameras require less light than do standard cameras because light is not lost in the light cord and rod lens.

One of the more common features of the camera heads is the ability to manipulate peripheral equipment using buttons that accomplish a variety of tasks, including activation of the video printer and VCR. Some cameras have a single button that activates both the video printer and VCR. This feature is possible with a main control switch that can be manipulated to command several desired functions. Another variation includes separate buttons on the camera head that increase or decrease the camera gain level. With this arrangement, the first button can operate the video printer, VCR, and additional components. An infrared remote control is required for all components to make the buttons operable. One company offers a camera with two buttons on the camera head that can control any two components. This is a hard-wire system, meaning that actual cables run from the CCU (camera box) to two selected components, the video printer and VCR, or the video printer and the still video recorder. With this particular system, infrared remote control is not required. Another camera feature is field replaceable camera cables. Because most camera problems occur in the camera cable, replacing cables at the hospital rather than sending the camera out for repair saves time and expense.

The camera box (CCU). The CCU component offers many different configurations (Figure 3-11). The most common features include a color bar button and a white balance button. Some CCUs have manual and automatic white balance features. The most important feature of the CCU is an automatic shutter that automatically adjusts each pixel's exposure time up to 1/15,000 of a second. The circuit can react to varying light conditions as fast as the human eye. Compared to electronic shutter control, the automatic light source is slow and deceived by arbitrary highs and lows caused by the flaring of instruments. Although an electronic shutter can be deceived, it is quick to recover and no harm is done. The electronic shutter is essential when purchasing a surgical video camera.

The monitor and accessories. The size of the screen varies from 8 to 20 inches. The closer the surgeon is to the monitor, the smaller the monitor should be because it provides the better picture. Monitors last a long time so purchase a high-end product with at least 600 lines resolution, and ensure that the monitor accepts all three video formats (NTSC, Y/C, and RGB).

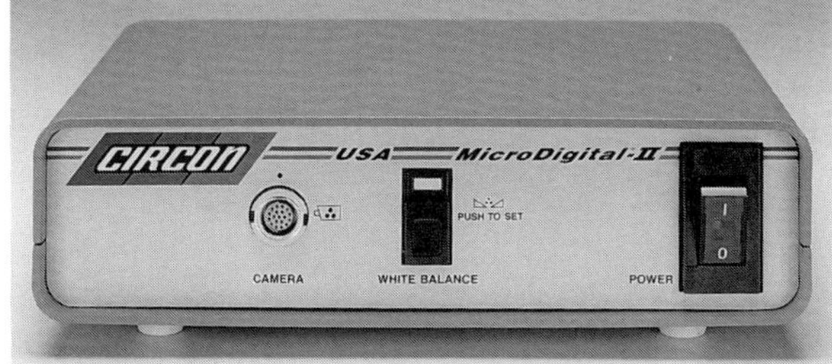

Figure 3-11 An example of a modern camera box.

When purchasing a VCR, do not rely on a consumer model even though they do cost less because durability is a major concern. Moreover, consumer models generally have unnecessary features, but Y/C inputs and outputs are important and Y/C-type VCRs are called SVHS VCRs.

Additional equipment includes the video printer, which costs a few thousand dollars, but it is an excellent method for recording and documenting the findings. Video prints easily can fit into a patient's chart.

Another component in surgical video is the 35-mm slide-making system that can produce 35-mm slides from any standard video signal and is designed to work in unison with video printers. The systems make 35-mm slides more quickly and efficiently than does the traditional method of fastening a 35-mm camera to the end of an endoscope in the middle of an operation. With 500 lines of resolution, it also produces high-quality images.

Equipment problems and troubleshooting techniques. After the video system is moved to the operating room, plug it in and test the components. Plug in the camera, note the image, put color bars on the monitor screen, and evaluate the accuracy of the colors. Look at the monitor, check the buttons, turn on the light source, and check the light cord for damaged light bundles. Look through the scope with the naked eye before it is hooked up and illuminated because light hides defects. Hold the scope with the distal end pointed at a normal ceiling light, then look through the eye piece. Is the scope clear? Next, check both the distal end and the eye piece for cracks or other visible damage. By following this routine, unexpected events can be minimized.

If a problem occurs during a surgical procedure, start with the scope end of the video chain because most defects are located in either the scope, light cord, or camera. If the picture is poor, check the color and light level to ascertain the best solution. If there is no picture, be certain that the equipment is turned on or adjust the button. If this does not solve the problem, turn on the room's overhead lights, detach the camera from the scope, and focus it on an object in the room. If the picture is good, the camera is functioning properly and the scope or the light cord is at fault. If the picture is poor, the camera could be defective, and either a button change on the CCU or a new camera may be required. A methodical piece-by-piece examination of the components makes it easier to locate the faulty equipment so that it can be fixed or replaced and the operation can proceed.

Changing times in health care. New endoscopic procedures are performed with increasing frequency so that hospitals will need more video equipment to keep up with demand, and purchases must justify the cost. As medical services move from a large hospital-based facility to smaller community-based surgical centers, patients residing 2 hours from the main hospital could have a knee arthroscopy or laparoscopy performed much closer to home.

The future. The leading edge of technology includes three dimensional, virtual reality, and HDTV. HDTV expands the scanning rate from 525 lines of resolution to 1100 or 1200 lines per frame, and the quality of current pictures would more than double. Broadcast television has been considering this technology. It is already in use in some Japanese facilities, and HDTV will soon be available for practical use in the United States. The challenge is to reduce the cost to make it affordable for hospitals.

With virtual reality, a three-dimensional computer image is presented to the user through liquid crystal glasses. This technique is used in the United States by public institutions like the Central Intelligence Agency and by architects—so that clients can "see" a building inside and out before construction. In a way, this is similar to a surgeon's use of virtual reality, but cost continues to be a major obstacle.

The future of three dimensional imaging is upon us, and many medical equipment companies have prototypes in the field. This technology attempts to provide depth to the image that is not available with monocular endoscopic systems. The increased perception of depth of field enables the surgeon to locate instruments in relation to tissues and organs. These systems rely either on active or inactive eyewear.

Suction-Irrigator Probe and Hydrodissection Pump

A suction-irrigation probe can be a versatile instrument (Figure 3-12). Controlled suction and irrigation enhance observation and improve operative technique. This device serves as an extension of the surgeon's fingers and a backstop for the CO_2 laser, and facilitates hydrodissection, division of tissue planes and spaces, lavage, blunt dissection, and smoke and fluid evacuation. A properly designed suction-irrigation system has the following characteristics (see Figure 3-12).

1. The trumpet valve should be ergonomically designed and versatile so that electrosurgical accessories, lasers, and hand instruments can be inserted through the probe (Figure 3-13).

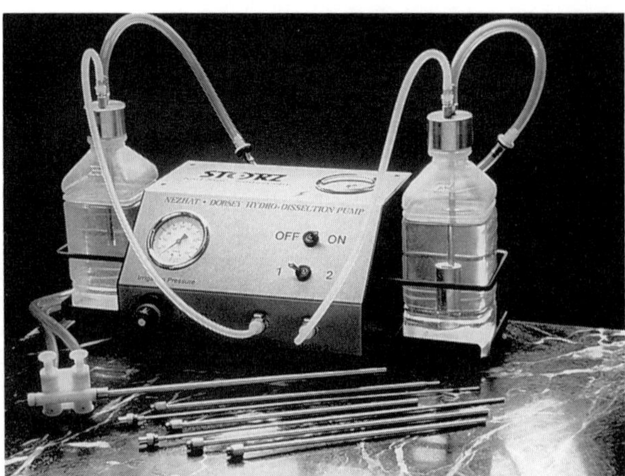

Figure 3-12 Nezhat-Dorsey hydrodissection pump and probes.

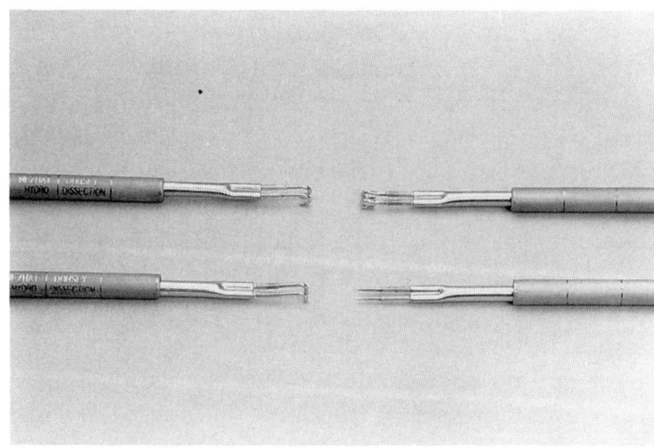

A

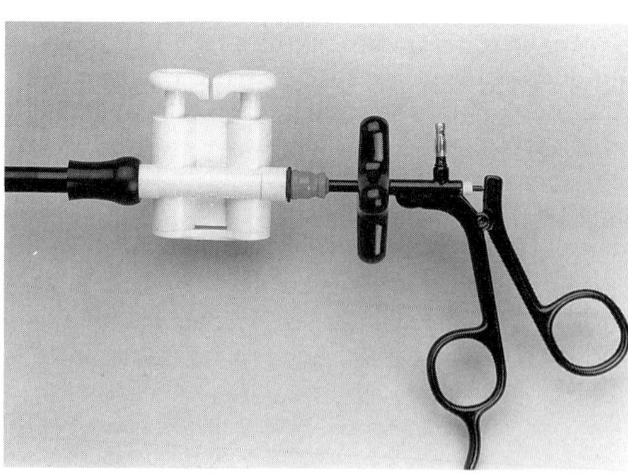

B

Figure 3-13 A, Nezhat-Dorsey hydrodissection probe with different electrosurgical accessories. B, Hydrodissection probe that can accommodate hand instruments.

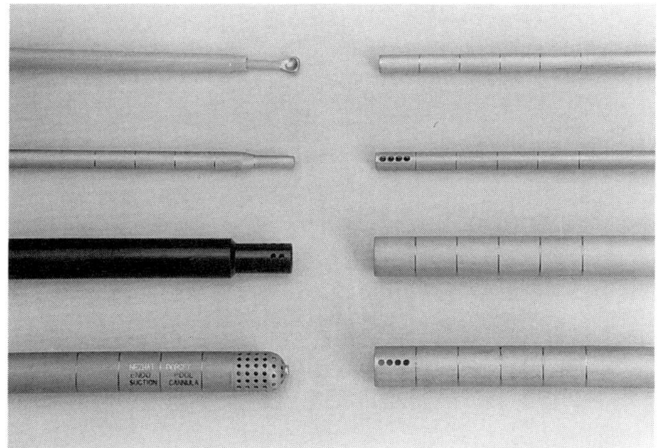

Figure 3-14 Different size probe tips, which are smooth and nonreflective, can be used for blunt dissection and laser backstops.

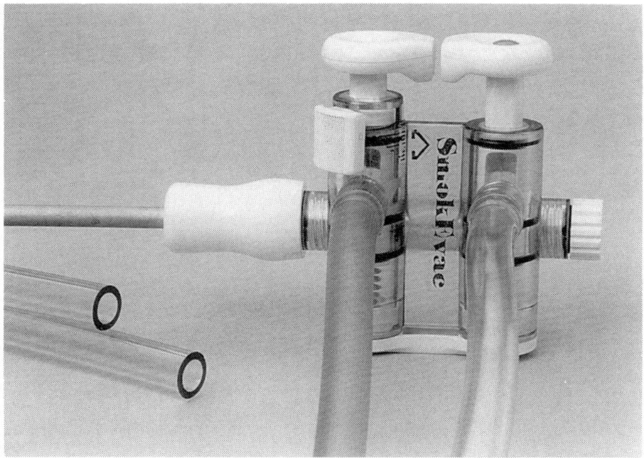

Figure 3-15 Trumpet valve with a control-metered adjustment pad that allows smoke evacuation.

2. The trumpet valve must be easy to use and provide constant control of fluid or suction including valve regulation rather than an on/off mechanism.
3. The internal valve diameters must be large enough to allow blood and tissue to pass easily through the canister and must provide sufficient irrigation flows.
4. Probe tips must be smooth, strong, and nonreflective so that they can be used for blunt dissection and laser backstops (Figure 3-14).
5. The irrigation pump must provide precise and variable irrigation pressure.

One system has a trumpet valve that incorporates a metered adjustment feature allowing smoke evacuation without manual intermittent depression of the suction piston. To activate smoke evacuation, a control pad is rotated counterclockwise by the surgeon allowing variable evacuation of 0 to 10 L/min (Figure 3-15). Additional suction capability remains by depressing the suction piston button. Laser or electrosurgical accessories inserted through the rear access port may be combined simultaneously with continuous smoke evacuation, maintaining a clear field of vision. Several probe tips are available in various lengths and configurations (Figure 3-16). A quick-disconnect mechanism probe tip speeds the changing of tips. An aspiration/injection needle accessory with 5 mm/28 cm probe tip without fenestrations allows a precise closed-chambered aspiration of ovarian cysts or injection of fluid (Figure 3-17). This system has reusable probe tips.

Although the pump should be able to deliver fluid with a pressure up to 775 mm Hg, 300 mm Hg is used for routine irrigation (Figure 3-18). Higher pump pressures are used to dissect areas near the bowel, ureter, bladder, and major blood vessels. A gravity flow or an IV bag wrapped with a blood pressure cuff may not provide enough pressure to

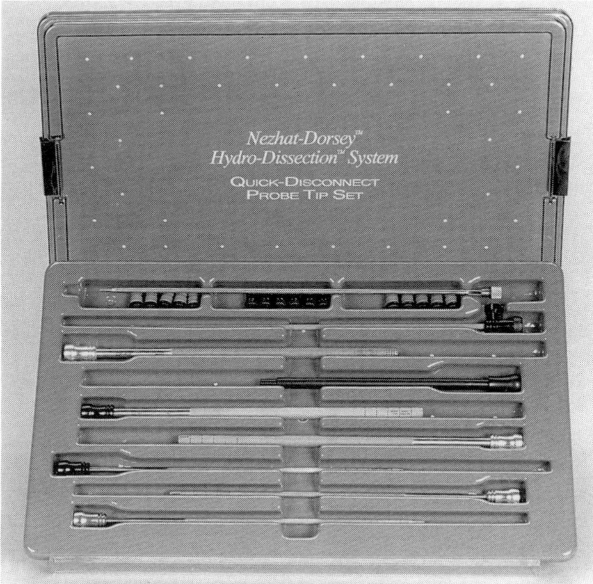

Figure 3-16 Designed specifically for use with the Nezhat-Dorsey Hydrodissection System, the "Quick-Disconnect" probe tip set contains one 5-mm probe tip without irrigation holes, one Micro-Probe tip, one 10-mm probe tip with irrigation holes, one Endopool suction cannula, one Instrument Insert Probe, 12 instrument insert adapters, and 6 "Quick-Disconnect" adapters. All probe tip sets are available in lengths of 23 cm, 28 cm, and 33 cm.

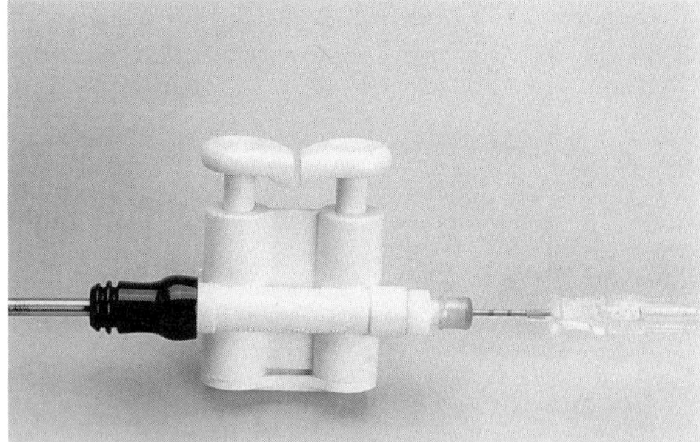

Figure 3-17 The aspiration/injection needle is inserted through the back of the trumpet valve. At distal end of the needle, there is a Luer-Lock that allows connection to a syringe so that suction and irrigation are not interrupted.

perform hydrodissection or wash away debris. The irrigation fluid consists of warmed 1-L bottles of lactated Ringer's and wall suction is used as the aspirated material initially enters a Vac-Rite canister. A laser plume filter removes particles that might clog the wall suction. A higher pneumatically powered pressure pump with adjustable pulsations has been developed (American Hydro-Surgical Instruments System II Pump). It incorporates the cost effectiveness and convenience of bag irrigation with the precision and effective delivery of pressurized pump irrigation (Figure 3-19). It does not use electric current, electric circuitry, electronics, or any type of computer software, but offers irrigation control. It has a "pump cartridge chamber" into which a disposable cartridge is inserted (Figure 3-20). Because compressed gas does not come in contact with the irrigation fluid at any time, this design eliminates the potential for procedural contamination during setup and the possibility of gas inadvertently entering the abdominal cavity. Irrigation bags replace bottled solution. As the bag is depleted, it collapses on itself, stopping the pump and alerting the staff to switch to the second fluid supply. The fluid is delivered in a continuous flow or pulsed irrigation mode. The rate of pulsation and irrigation pressure are adjustable. The latter setting ranges from 0 to 2500 mm Hg. Pulsatile irrigation cleanses the surgical site more effectively than normal continuous flow irrigation, enabling a more thorough removal of blood clots and char.

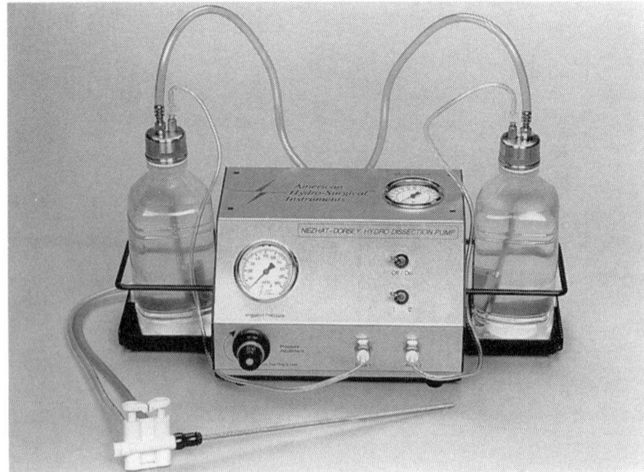

Figure 3-18 The hydrodissection pump holds two bottles of irrigation fluid and delivers up to 775 mm Hg. For routine irrigation, 300 mm Hg is used and is provided by pressurized CO_2 that is connected to the bottles.

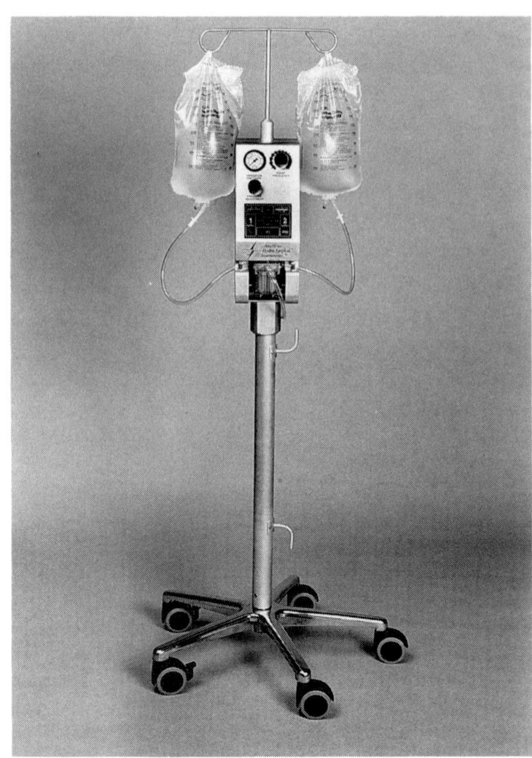

Figure 3-19 The System II Pump (American Hydro-Surgical Instruments) uses bag irrigation as effectively as pressurized pump irrigation.

Forceps

Atraumatic and grasping forceps with jaws are available in sizes from 3 to 10 mm (Figure 3-21). Atraumatic stabilization of structures is important for many procedures and several types of forceps are available for this purpose. The preferred type is medium sized with a rounded tip and serrated jaws. It can grasp tissue for exposure, act as a

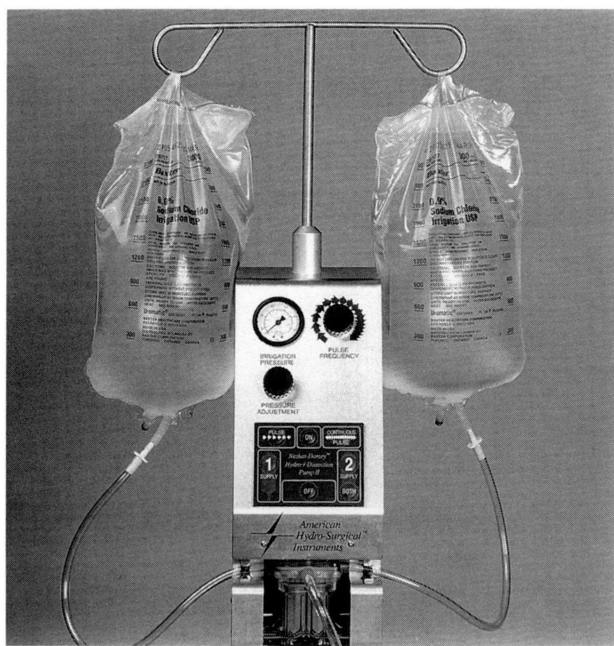

Figure 3-20 The System II Pump (American Hydro-Surgical Instruments) has a "pump cartridge chamber" into which a disposable cartridge is inserted.

blunt probe with jaws closed, affect traction with jaws open for more tissue surface area, serve as a needle holder, and tie suture (Figure 3-22). Forceps can grasp and remove tissue from the peritoneal cavity. Those made of titanium with a polished finish can serve as a backstop for the CO_2 laser, whereas others have monopolar electroco-

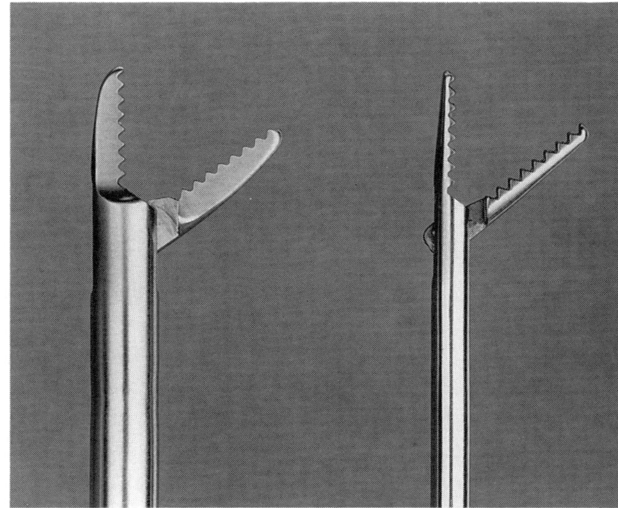

Figure 3-22 Serrated jaws of 3-mm (*left*) and 5-mm (*right*) needle-holders.

agulating capabilities. Creating a neosalpingostomy in a hydrosalpinx requires two grasping forceps for traction and countertraction. Fine forceps are used in delicate work such as ovariolysis, fimbrioplasty, and tubal exploration during salpingostomy for ectopic pregnancy (Figure 3-23).

Scissors

This instrument can be curved, straight, or hooked (Figure 3-24). Some have an electrical adaptor so they can be combined with unipolar or bipolar electrocoagulation (Figure 3-25). Scissors must be

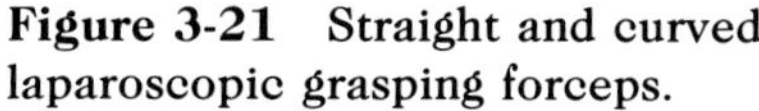

Figure 3-21 Straight and curved laparoscopic grasping forceps.

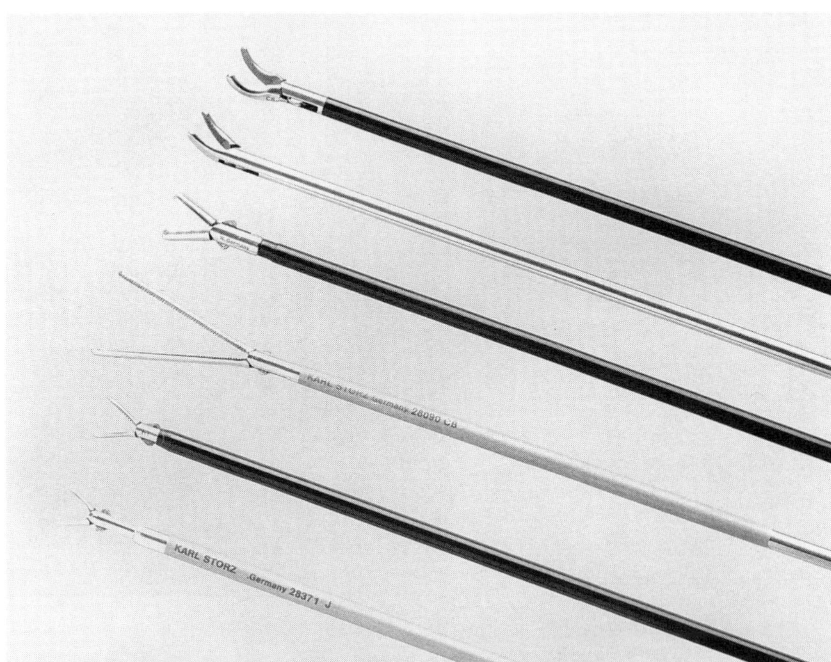

Figure 3-23 Fine forceps can be used for delicate procedures such as ovariolysis, fimbrioplasty, and tubal exploration for ectopic pregnancy.

used cautiously, particularly when being inserted into the secondary trocar. This maneuver should be done under direct observation to avoid injury to pelvic structures. Hooked scissors have overlapping tips and even closed can cause damage.

Scissors can lyse adhesions, divide coagulated tissue, cut sutures, and open a fallopian tube for salpingostomy. They become dull and cannot be sharpened, so they should be discarded after eight to ten operations. Disposable scissors are useful particularly for patients who have extensive adhesions.

Biopsy Forceps

These instruments can sample suspected endometrial implants, ovarian lesions, or peritoneum (Figure 3-26). The jaws should be sharp and overlap slightly when closed to avoid tearing tissue and causing unnecessary bleeding. Some have a small tooth on the upper or lower jaw and are ideal for taking a tissue sample from hard or slippery surfaces (Figure 3-27). Bleeding from the biopsy site can be controlled by a defocused laser or bipolar electrocoagulation.

Aspiration/Injection Needle

A 16- or 22-gauge calibrated aspiration/injection needle can be used to precisely aspirate and inject fluids (Figure 3-28). When used in conjunction with a 28-cm probe tip without fenestrations, closed-chambered ovarian cyst aspiration can be performed. When the suction is activated and the

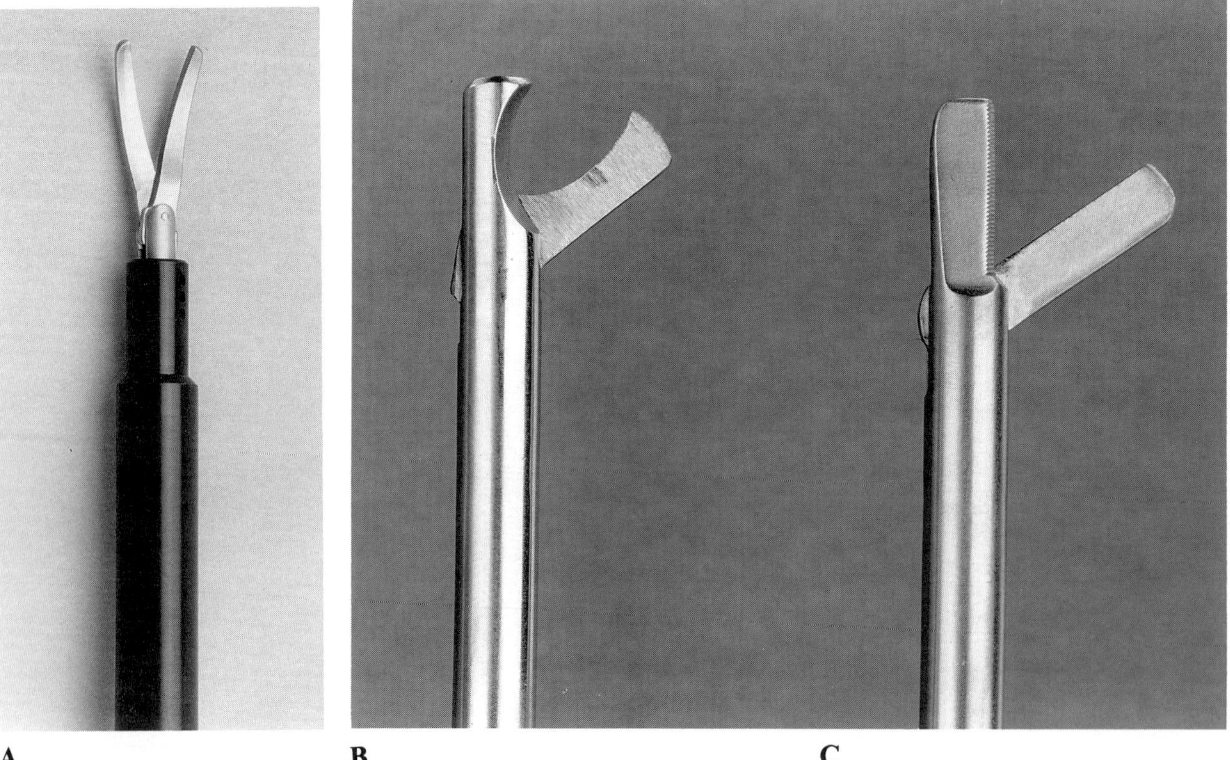

A B C

Figure 3-24 Laparoscopic scissors. A, Curved. B, Hooked. C, Straight.

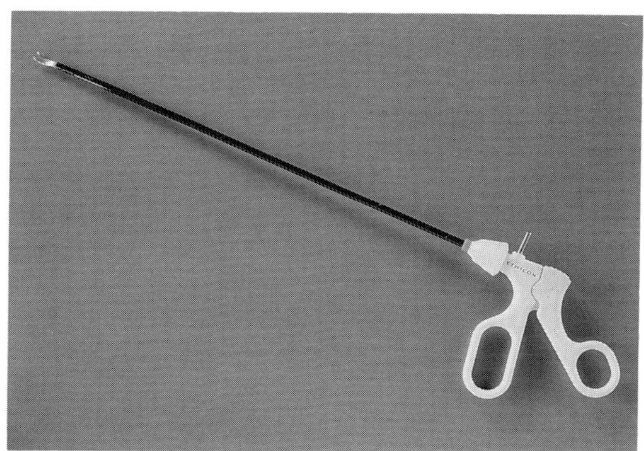

Figure 3-25 Laparoscopic scissors with unipolar electrocoagulation capability.

probe tip is placed on tissue, suction-retraction of that tissue results. The needle is inserted into the cyst and leakage of contents is avoided. The 2-cm exposed portion of the needle is etched with 0.5-cm markings to accurately gauge tissue penetration. By attaching a 60-mL syringe to the needle, the fluid from the aspirated cyst can be sent for cytologic examination.

This needle also may be used to inject dilute vasopressin into the base of fibroids prior to myomectomy or into the mesosalpinx or tube prior to salpingostomy for ectopic pregnancy. A syringe is attached to the needle by a connecting tube before injection to verify that intravascular injection does not occur.

Figure 3-26 A 5-mm biopsy forceps for endometrial implant on ovarian lesions.

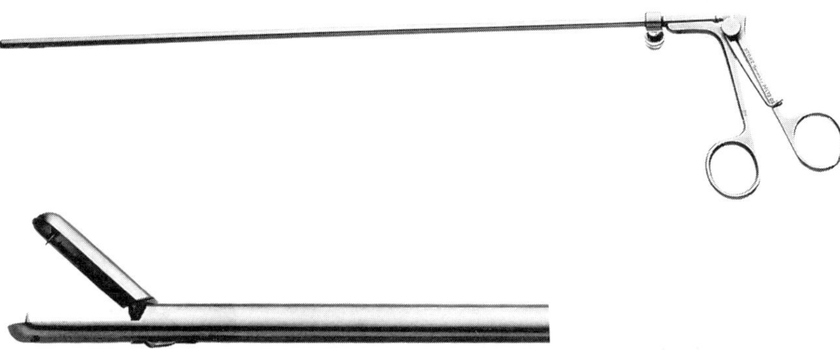

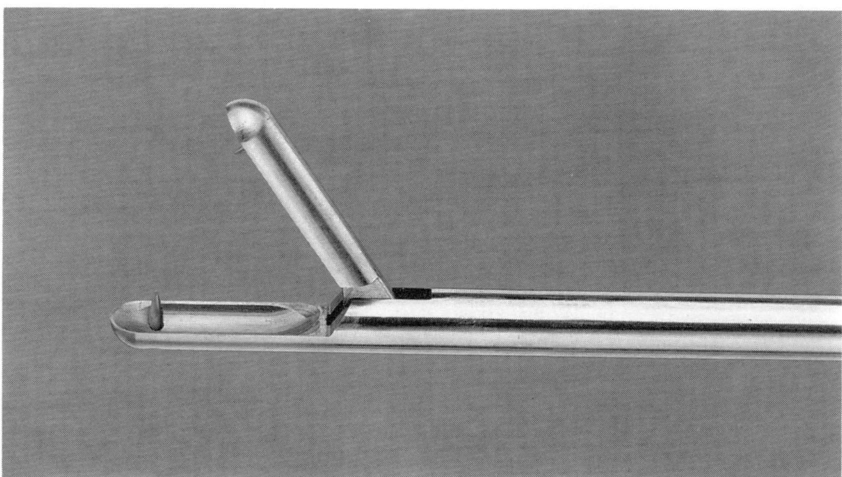

Figure 3-27 Biopsy forceps with small teeth on the upper and lower jaws for biopsy of hard and slippery surfaces.

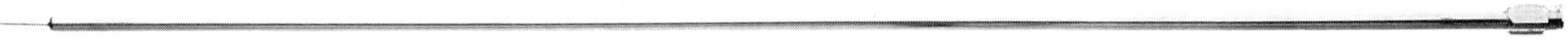

Figure 3-28 Laparoscopic aspiration/injection needle. It can be used for aspiration of ovarian cysts (16 or 18 gauge), injection of diluted vasopressin in the base of a myoma, or hydrodissection (22 gauge).

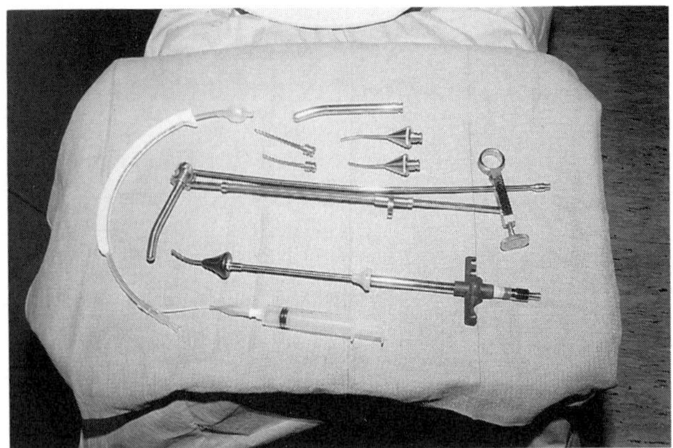

Figure 3-29 Three different uterine manipulators: HUMI; Cohen cannula; and Valtchev cannula.

Uterine Manipulator

Safe, effective endoscopy requires adequate mobilization and stabilization of the uterus and associated organs. Various combinations of uterine sounds, cannulas, and dilators are available. The most useful manipulators are the HUMI (Unimar, Wilton, CT) and the Cohen cannula in combination with a single-toothed tenaculum applied to the anterior cervical lip (Figure 3-29). The HUMI has a balloon at its tip to minimize the chance of uterine perforation, but when uterine manipulation is vigorous, the HUMI can twist within the uterine cavity, making it difficult to stabilize the uterus. The Cohen cannula is inserted as far as the internal os and is rigid, allowing excellent control of the uterine position. Although a large acorn tip limits its uterine entry, the cervix may dilate, resulting in uterine perforation by the acorn tip. Therefore, it is crucial to continually monitor the position of uterine manipulators.

Valtchev and Papsin[2] (Conkin Surgical Instruments, Ltd., Toronto) devised an instrument consisting of an acorn-shaped head with a cannula connected to a rod by an articulation point. This arrangement allows the angle between the rod and the cannula to be changed, providing various degrees of uterine anteversion, which can be adjusted with a screw. The Hulka tenaculum and sound combination is a good uterine manipulator but lacks a channel for chromopertubation.

Electrogenerator and Bipolar Forceps

Our primary instrument used for hemostasis during operative laparoscopy is the bipolar electrocoagulator (Figure 3-30). Do not begin a procedure without preparing and testing this instrument because it is essential for hemostasis during oophorectomy, hysterectomy, or even during bowel resection to desiccate the mesenteric artery without complication.

Several types of jaws are available (Figures 3-30 and 3-31). Fine tips are used for coagulating small blood vessels during delicate surgery involving the tubes, bowel, or ureter. More flat jaws are appropriate for use on large blood vessels or pedicles, including the uterine artery of infundibulopelvic ligaments.

Specialized Instruments

Claw-toothed and Spoon Graspers

These 10-mm graspers require a 10- to 11-mm sleeve and are used during myomectomy to remove relatively large pieces of tissue such as a section of tube and ovary or ectopic pregnancy (Figure 3-32).

Clips

The laparoscopic clip applicators are used through 10- to 11-mm sleeves for reapproximation of peritoneal surfaces or hemostasis of medium-sized vessels. Disposable loaded applicators and reusable single-chip applicators are available (Figures 3-33 and 3-34.)

Linear Stapler

The stapler designed for gynecologic use is similar to the one for bowel surgery and fits through a 12-mm trocar sleeve[3] (Figure 3-35). Ethicon and U.S. Surgical produce endoscopic surgical staplers with slightly different designs, but their function is essentially the same. The available staplers are disposable and can be reloaded with cartridges for use in gynecologic, general, and thoracic surgery (Figure 3-36). The stapler is introduced through a 12-mm port. Each cartridge contains 54 (Ethicon) or 48 (U.S. Surgical) titanium staples. They are arranged in two sets of triple-staggered rows. The instrument also contains a push bar knife assembly, which cuts between the two sets of triple rows, ligating both ends of the incised tissue. The cut line usually is shorter than the staple line. For example, the laparoscopic linear cutter 35 (Ethicon) cut line is approximately 33 mm with a staple line of 37 mm.

The tissue to be clipped is placed on stretch with grasping forceps and the Endoclip applicator's jaws are placed at the desired incision site.

Figure 3-30 A, Electrogenerator with two different types of bipolar forceps. B, Electrogenerator by Valley Laboratories.

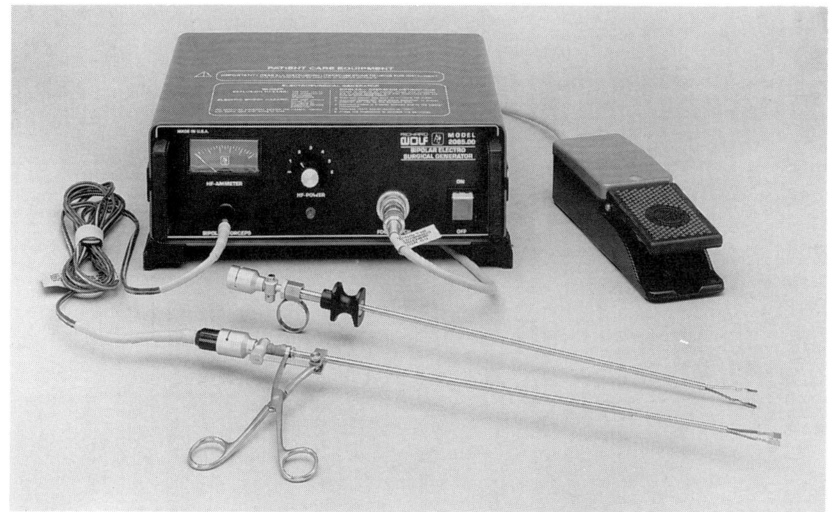

A

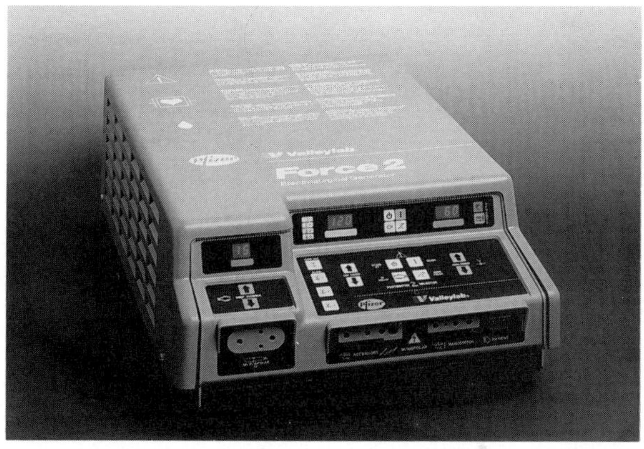

B

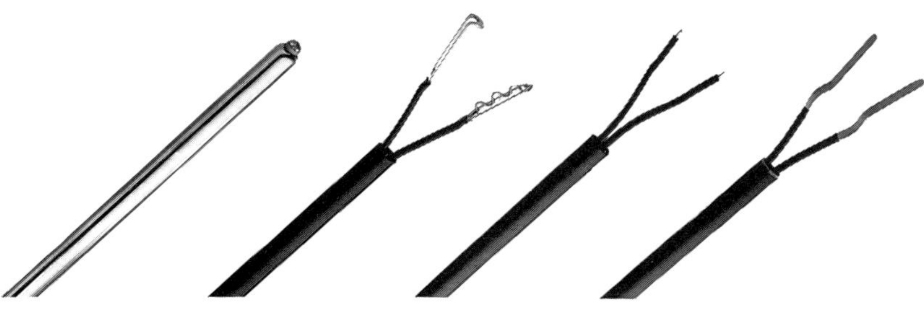

Figure 3-31 Bipolar forceps with different tips.

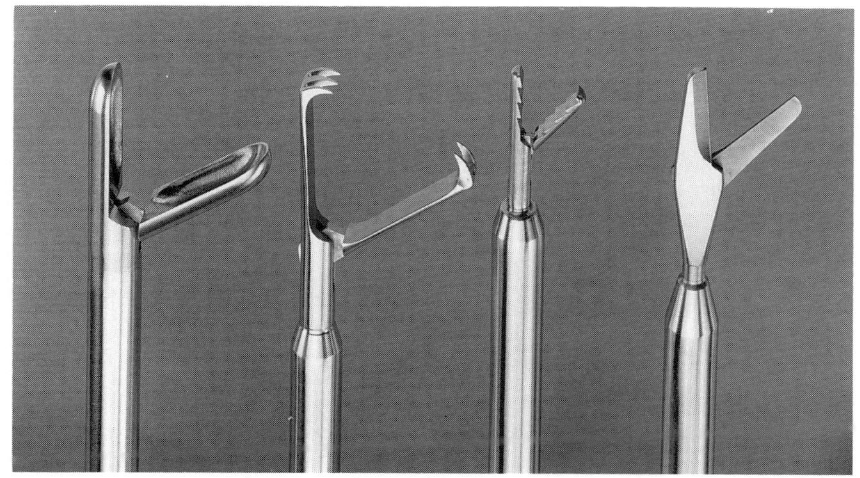

Figure 3-32 Different 10-mm instruments used during operative laparoscopy. From left to right: spoon forceps, claw graspers, serrated grasper, and scissors.

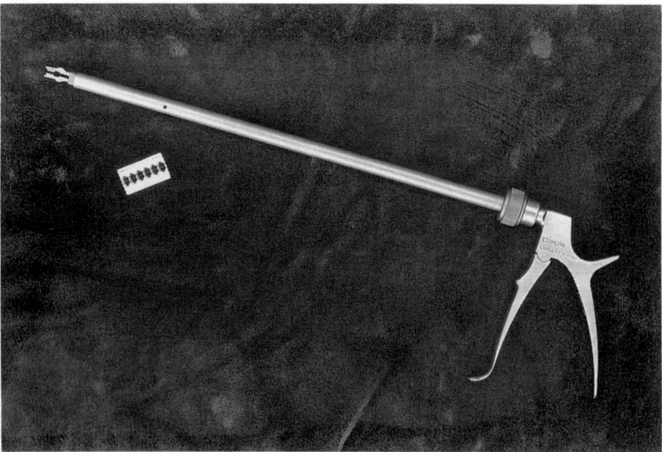

Figure 3-33 Reusable 10-mm laparoscopic clip applicators.

When fired, it simultaneously places six rows of small titanium clips and cuts along the center, leaving three rows of clips on the edge of each pedicle (Figure 3-37). This instrument can be used to seal blood vessels and cut pedicles, but should be used with extreme caution. A number of complications have resulted during the use of this device by untrained surgeons.[4]

Suture

The ability to suture laparoscopically increases the laparoscopic surgeon's versatility. Suturing can be used for both hemostasis and to oppose tissues during reconstructive procedures. Different types of suture are available for endoscopic use. The Endoloop (Ethicon) suture, a preformed slipknot attached to a rigid, disposable 5-mm applicator, is available in 0-chromic, polyglactin, polydioxanone, and polypropylene (Figure 3-38A). The loop is positioned around the pedicle by grasping the structure to be removed, and pulling it through the loop. The loop is tightened against the applicator and the suture cut with either scissors or the laser beam against a backstop.

Suture material is available with a straight or slightly curved swaged needle, specifically designed for laparoscopic use. It is available in 0-chromic catgut, 4-0 polydioxanone with a swaged ST-4 needle (PDS; Ethicon), and polyglactin. The suture is grasped with forceps several centimeters from the needle. The grasper with suture is inserted intra-abdominally through the 5-mm accessory trocar sleeve with a 3-mm suture introducer (Figure 3-38B).

Surgeons also can use any suture with a swaged needle of any size. To place the needle intra-abdominally, the grasper or needle driver is removed along with the trocar sleeve, which remains around the grasper's shaft. The suture is grasped about 5 cm from the needle and the grasper is reintroduced with the trocar sleeve, into the suprapubic incision site. The needle follows the

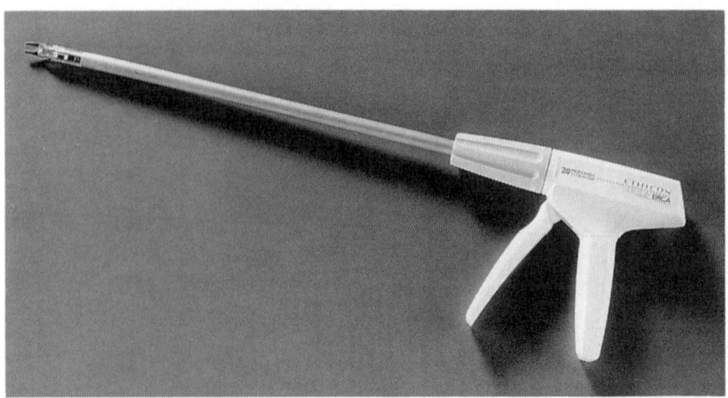

Figure 3-34 Disposable loaded 10-mm laparoscopic clip applicator.

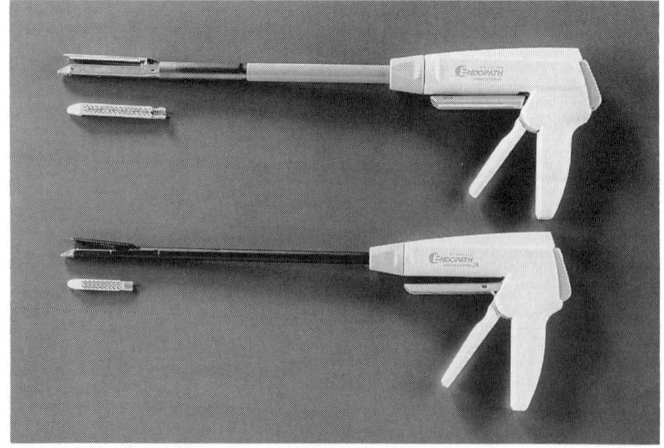

Figure 3-35 Endo-path linear cutters (Ethicon) used in laparoscopic bowel surgery and gynecologic surgery.

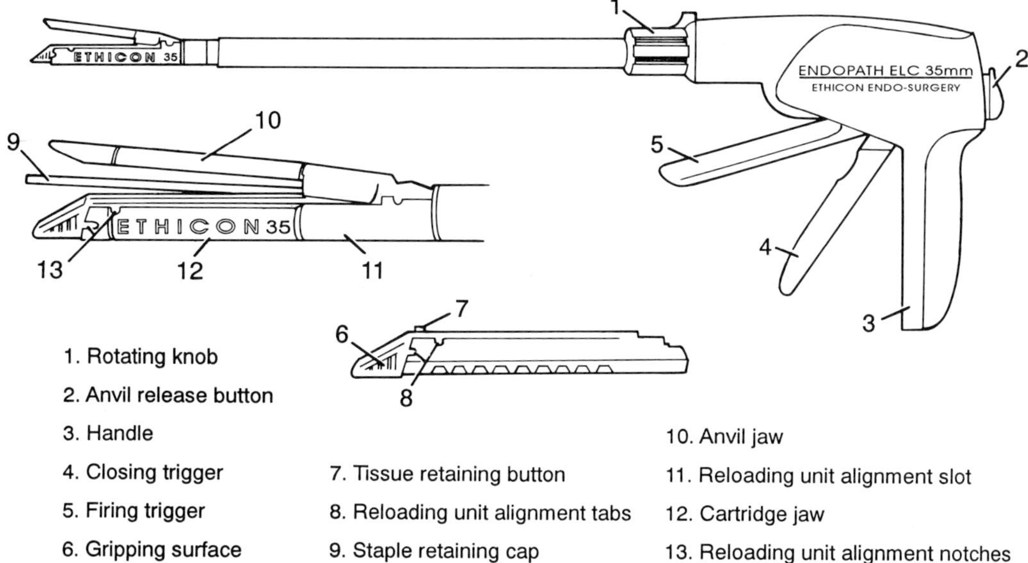

Figure 3-36 Endo-path linear cutter 35 (ELC 35, Ethicon) formation.

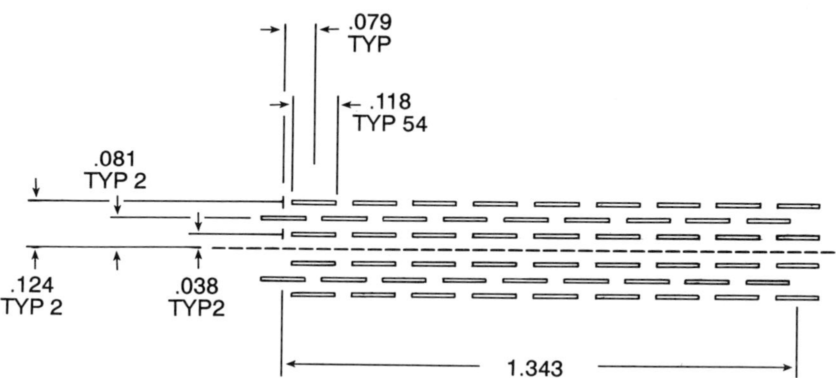

Figure 3-37 The stapler places six rows, a total of 54, small titanium staples.

Figure 3-38 A, Endoloop suture, a pretied slipknot attached to a rigid disposable applicator. B, A 3-mm suture introducer.

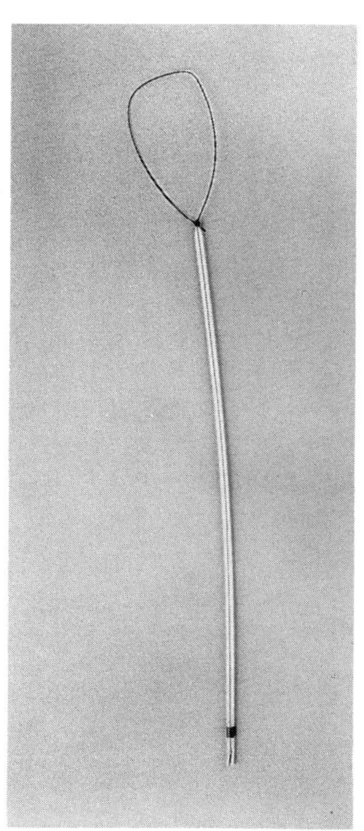

A

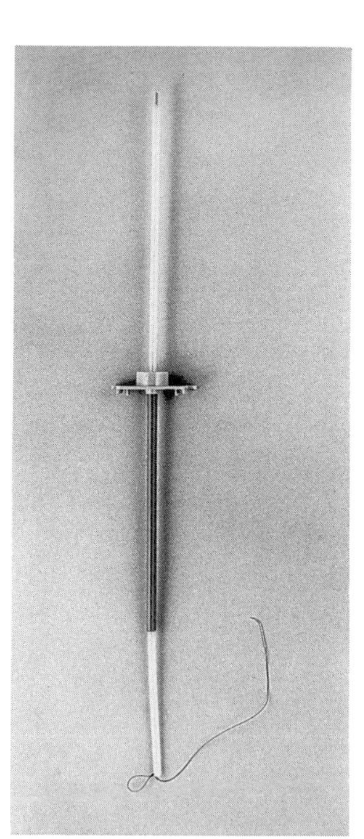

B

grasper into the abdominal cavity. A needle larger than a CT-1 is awkward to use intra-abdominally. Once the suture is placed, several techniques can secure the knot. An Endoloop (Ethicon) with a premade knot can be tightened around the pedicle with the plastic knot pusher.

Other types of extracorporeal knots are the Duncan[5] and clinch knot, but their closure depends on a single knot, which may slip. The knot may not slide because of suture friction. Tissue trauma can result from the suture being pulled in opposite directions through transfixed tissue when the needle is withdrawn from the abdomen and when a sliding knot is applied.

An instrument tying method within the abdomen uses two forceps and any suture material. Intracorporeal knotting is difficult and requires practice. The suture can get caught in the articulation point of the forceps and break. However, variations of the Fisherman's clinch knot may prevent some difficulties. Use of the knot pusher was originally described in 1972.[6] The principles of this instrument do not differ from those of tying suture deep in the pelvis, where the surgeon uses a finger to push and secure the knot.

Extracorporeal knot tying. Extracorporeal knot tying simplifies laparoscopic suturing. Instruments to facilitate this process include a needle-holder, needle-driver, suture introducer, and scissors. Suture is loaded into the needle-holder, holding the suture below the swage point so the needle will collapse into the introducer. The needle-holder is inserted into the introducer (Figure 3-39). The introducer is placed into a 5-mm sleeve and the needle-driver into a contralateral sleeve.

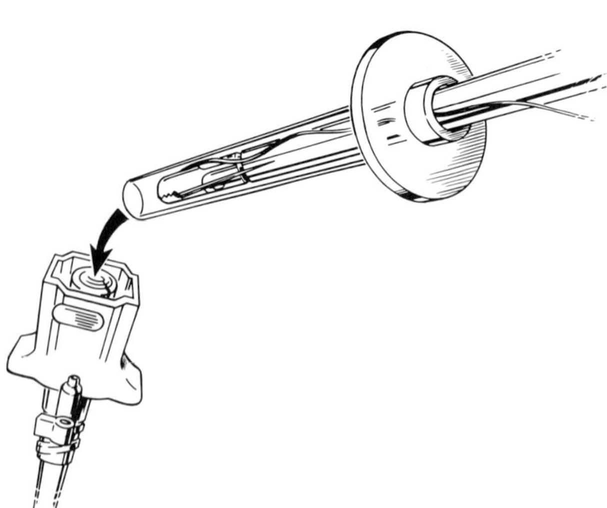

Figure 3-39 The needle-holder is inserted into the introducer.

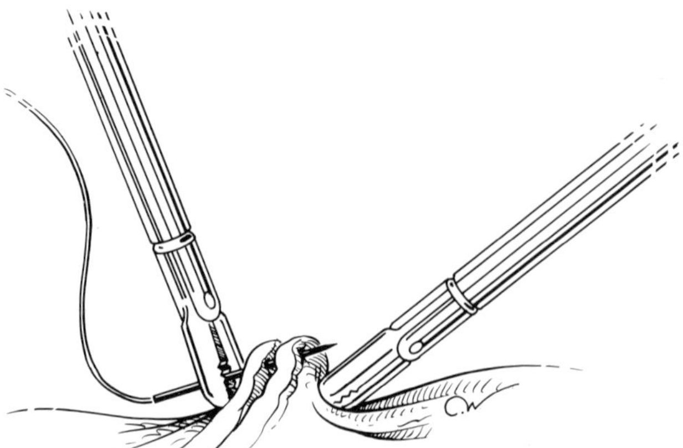

Figure 3-40 The suture is passed through the tissue.

The needle is advanced into the abdominal cavity and passed from the holder to the driver. While steadying the needle with the driver, the holder is repositioned to the desired location. The needle is tapped with the driver to lock it into a right angle position. The needle is rearmed with the driver. The driver is used to pass the needle through the tissue, then grasp the tip and pass the needle to the holder (Figure 3-40). To reduce the risk of pulling the suture out of the tissue, tension on the suture line is kept to a minimum. The needle holder and excess suture line are withdrawn from the abdominal cavity through the introducer. An assistant covers the introducer channel to maintain pneumoperitoneum. The surgeon cuts the suture below the swage point and makes a single-throw knot with the two suture ends (Figure 3-41).

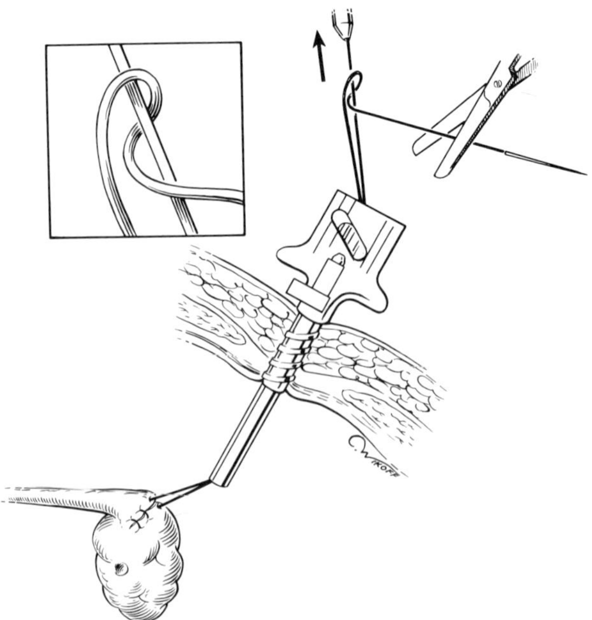

Figure 3-41 The surgeon makes a single-throw knot.

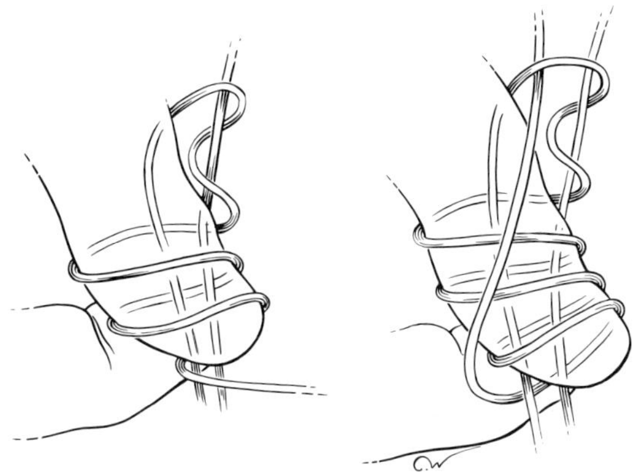

Figure 3-42 Three revolutions are made around both suture strands with the free end of the suture. The tail of the suture is inserted through the first loop.

The knot is held securely with the thumb and third finger while three revolutions are made around both suture strands with the free end of the suture (Figure 3-42). The tail of the suture is inserted through the first loop directly above the surgeon's thumb (Figure 3-42). After the tail is passed through the loop, the operator pulls up on the tail to form the knot and cuts the tail approximately 0.6 cm above the knot (Figure 3-43). The end of the Endoknot shaft is snapped off at the colored band, allowing the shaft to slide the knot downward (Figure 3-43, inset). Placing the shaft perpendicular to the knot minimizes suture breakage and ensures knot security. The Endoknot cannula is placed in the introducer. By pulling back on the small end piece of the Endoknot shaft while sliding the plastic shaft forward, the knot is allowed to move forward as the loop decreases in size. The Endoknot cannula acts as an integral knot pusher for placement of the formed knot (Figure 3-44). Scissors inserted through the contralateral trocar are used to cut the excess suture (Figure 3-45).

Extracorporeal pretied suture knot. An endoscopic pretied suture knot device can be used for extracorporeal knot tying. The pretied Endoknot (Ethicon) consists of a synthetic absorbable suture material with a hollow plastic tube that is narrowed at one end and scored at the other. The center of the plastic tube has a 4-0 stainless steel suture that is looped at the narrow end and swaged at the surgical needle. The scored end of the device serves as the handle. As with all extracorporeal knot tying techniques, the endoscopic pretied suture knot can be used to ligate vessels, reconstruct organs, approximate opposing tissue surfaces, and suture anastomoses. The primary advantage of these devices is that the knot is already

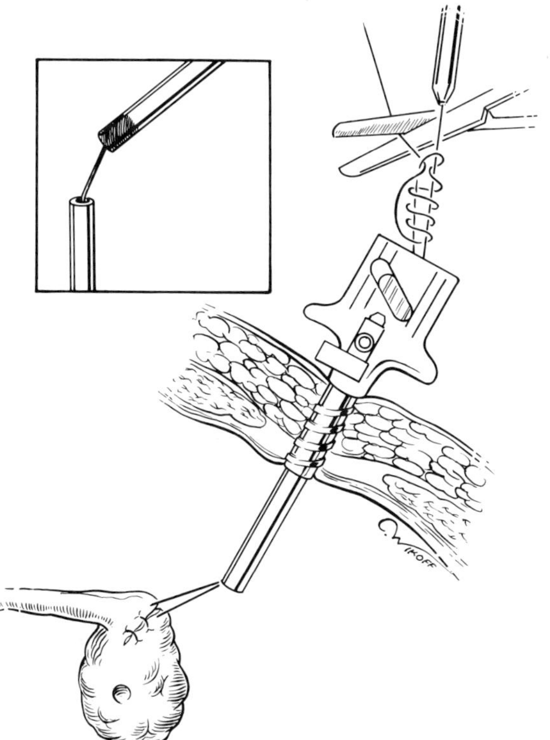

Figure 3-43 The suture tail is cut approximately 0.6 cm above the knot. The end of the Endoknot shaft is snapped off at the colored band, allowing the shaft to slide the knot downward.

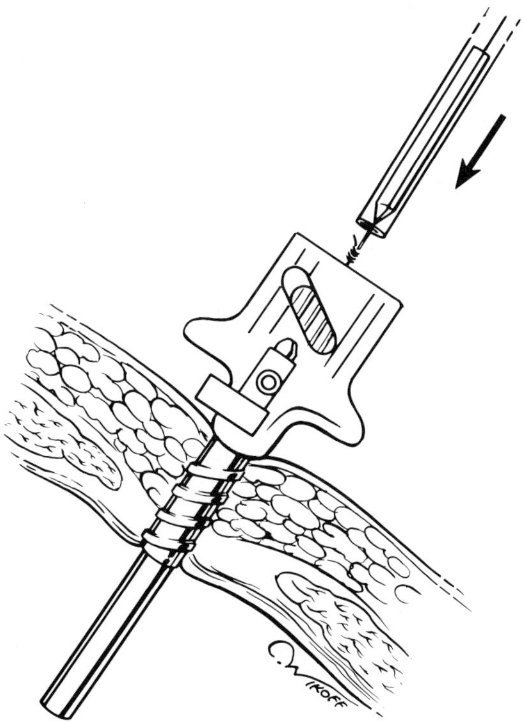

Figure 3-44 The Endoknot cannula acts as a knot pusher to place the formed knot.

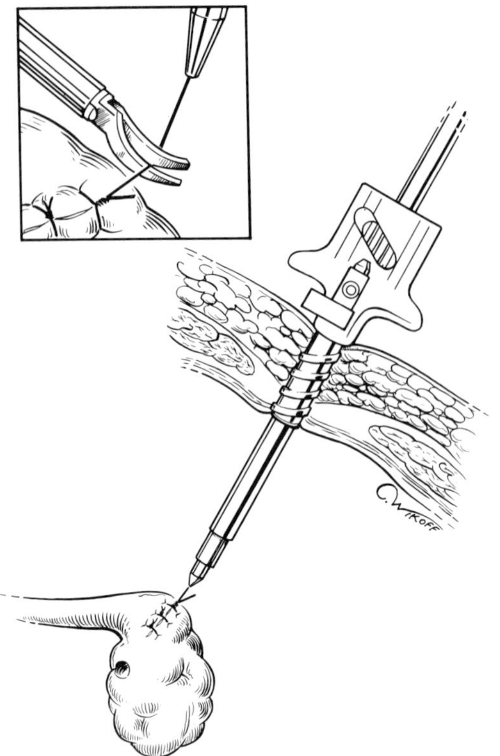

Figure 3-45 The knot is placed over the tissue and the suture above the knot is cut.

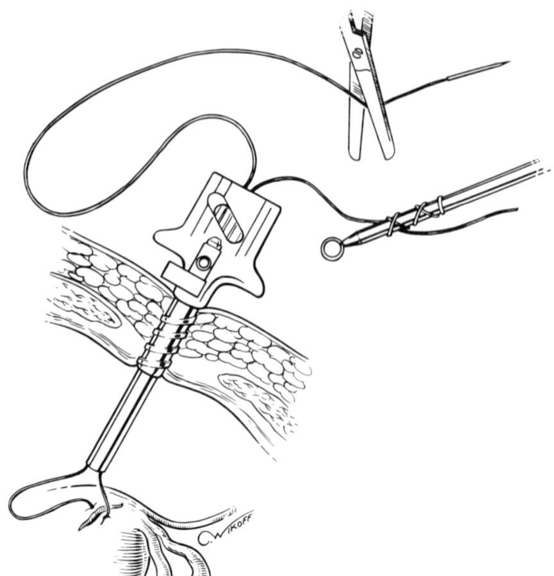

Figure 3-46 The needle and suture are placed in the 3-mm suture introducer as previously described. After the needle is passed through the tissue, the needle and suture are brought out of the cannula and the needle is cut off.

made and does not have to be manually tied by the surgeon (Figures 3-46 to 3-49).

Intracorporeal knot tying. Intracorporeal knot tying, which is used during microsurgery and fine suturing, is more difficult and time consuming than extracorporeal knot tying. The instructions for introducing the needle and suture to the abdomen are the same as for extracorporeal knot tying. The needle and entire suture are placed in the abdominal cavity. After the needle is positioned, it is grasped with the needle-holder (Figure 3-50). While the grasping forceps apply pressure or hold the tissue being sutured, the suture is inserted through the tissue (Figure 3-51). The graspers hold the needle, and the needle holder applies counterpressure to the tissue (Figure 3-52). The needle is removed from the tissue (Figure 3-53). Enough suture to form a knot is pulled through, leaving a sufficient tail (Figure 3-53). The needle is grasped with a grasping forceps and two or three loops are made around the needle-holder (Figure 3-54). The free end of the suture is grasped with the needle-holder and brought inside the formed loops (Figure 3-54, inset), and using both grasping forceps and the needle holder, the suture is tied over the tissue (Figure 3-55).

Additional knots are applied over the suture, reversing the direction of the sutures with each successive knot (Figures 3-56, 3-57).

Myoma Screw

When performing a laparoscopic myomectomy, it is difficult to stabilize a smooth, hard fibroid. Five and 10-mm myoma screws allow the surgeon to maneuver the myoma and apply traction with improved visibility and access.

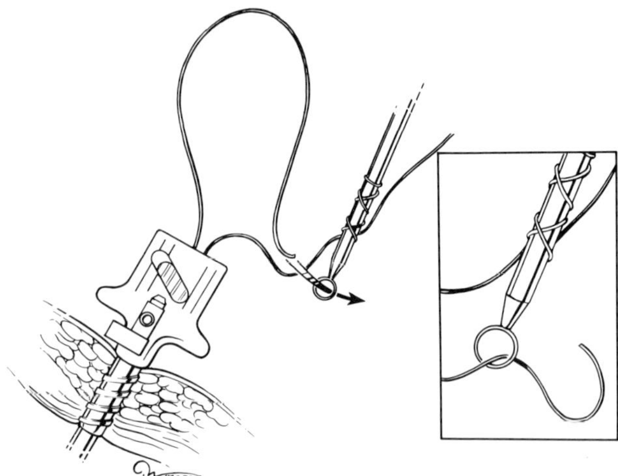

Figure 3-47 Push about 2 inches of the longest end of the suture through the wire loop near the tapered end of the cannula.

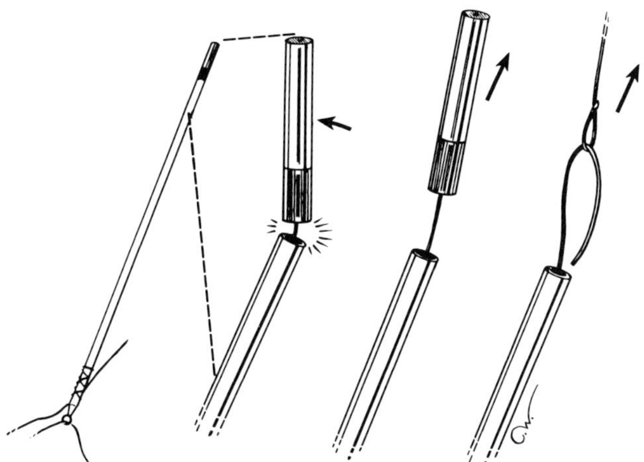

Figure 3-48 Grasp the scored end of the cannula and snap it off. Pull the wire and suture completely through the cannula. Discard the scored end of the cannula and the wire.

Tissue Morcellator

The morcellator grasps and cores the tissue to be removed and cuts it into small bits, which are forced into the hollow part of the instrument. It is designed for removal of a myoma or an ovary, in pieces, through 5- or 10-mm trocar sleeves or through a colpotomy incision. If removal of a large myoma is attempted, the effort to morcellate it mechanically may outweigh the amount of time saved, particularly if the myoma is calcified. Although different manual and electronic morcellators have been introduced for operative laparoscopy, none are ideal at the present time.

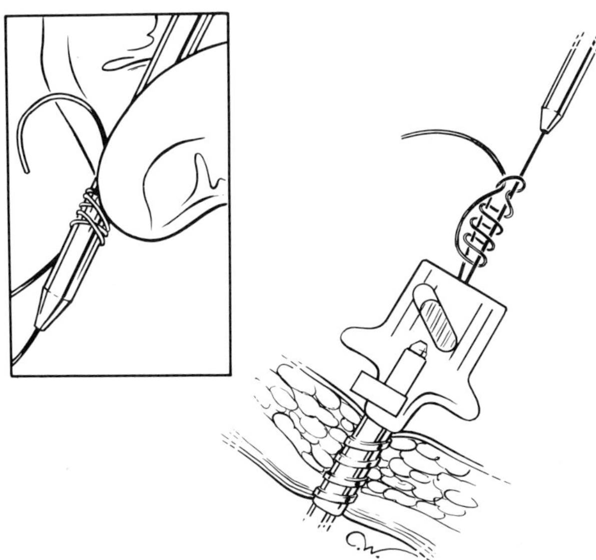

Figure 3-49 Push the pretied slip knot off the conical end of the cannula. Tighten the knot by pulling both ends of the slip knot. Trim off excess suture at the end of the slip knot. Push the slip knot into the trocar port and onto the area to be closed.

Laparotomy-type Instruments

Babcocks, atraumatic bowel grasping forceps, Allis clamps, and Metzenbaum scissors have been adapted for laparoscopic use. The acquisition of these instruments should depend on whether they would improve a procedure's efficiency.

Needle-Holders

Standard grasping forceps hold needles for most procedures, but stronger needle-holders are necessary when precise placement is required or when suturing thick tissue (ie, myometrium or periosteum). Some needle-holders have handles similar to those used in laparotomy (Figure 3-58). Straight and curved narrow tip needle-holders are available for fine intra-abdominal suturing (Figure 3-59).

Specialized Graspers

Three-pronged forceps specifically designed to atraumatically immobilize adnexal structures[7] can hold the ovary; the four-pronged forceps are designed to hold more delicate structures, such as fallopian tubes. The force applied by the prongs can be adjusted and maintained by tightening a screw in the handle. Three-prong graspers with teeth also are available. Large spoon forceps can be used to extract tissue excised during the course of the procedure.

Laparoscopic Specimen Retrieval Bag

To facilitate the retrieval of specimens from the abdominal cavity and avoid contamination of abdominal and pelvic cavity with cyst contents, a disposable retrieval bag (Endo-pouch, Ethicon) has been introduced (Figure 3-60). It is composed of a flexible plastic bag with a cannula, introduction sleeve, and introduction cap (Figures 3-61 to 3-68). The bag is pushed by hand into the introducer before being loaded into a 10/11-mm trocar (Figures 3-61 and 3-62A). During loading, the cannula should not be pulled to retract the Endo-pouch bag. The introducer cap and introducer sleeve are inserted into the abdomen through the trocar (Figure 3-62B). The introducer cap should remain flush against the top of the trocar. The cannula is pushed until the bag is fully exposed. A closed grasper is used to expand the bag opening (Figure 3-63). The specimen is placed in the bag

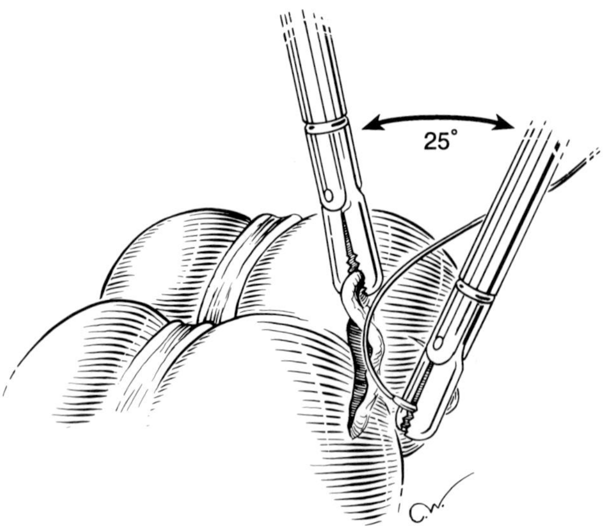

Figure 3-50. In Figures 3-50 through 3-57 intracorporeal knot tying is demonstrated (see text for details).

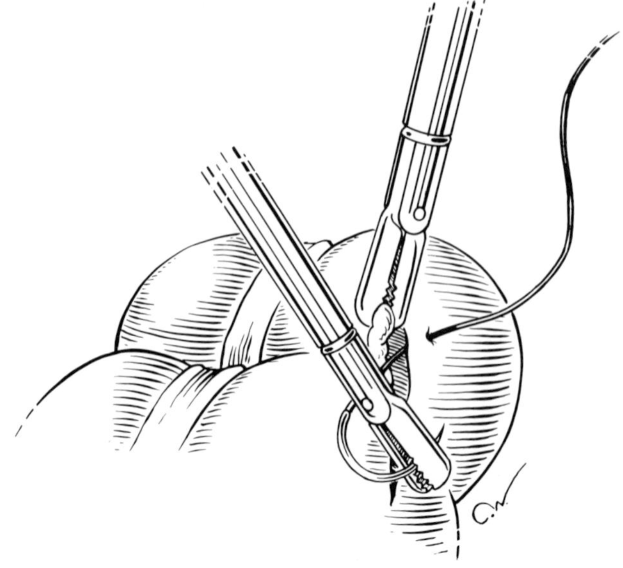

Figures 3-52.

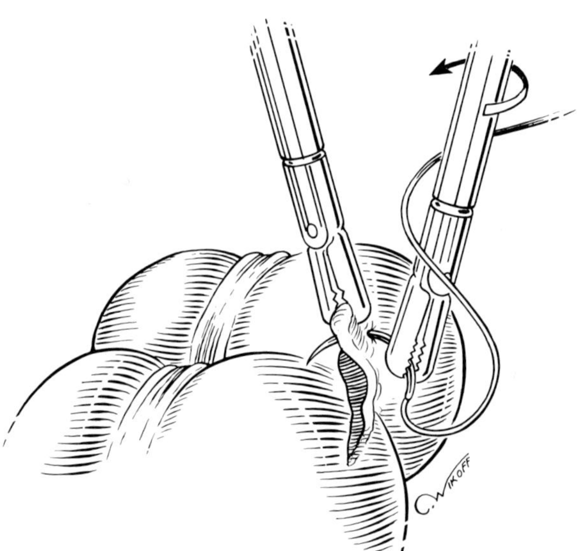

Figures 3-51.

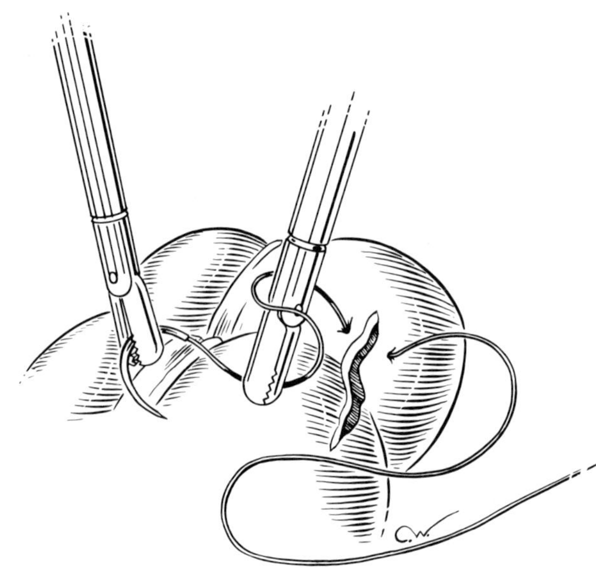

Figures 3-53.

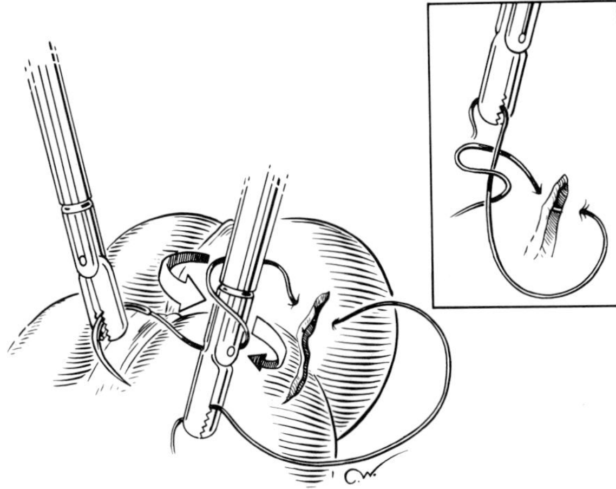

Figures 3-54.

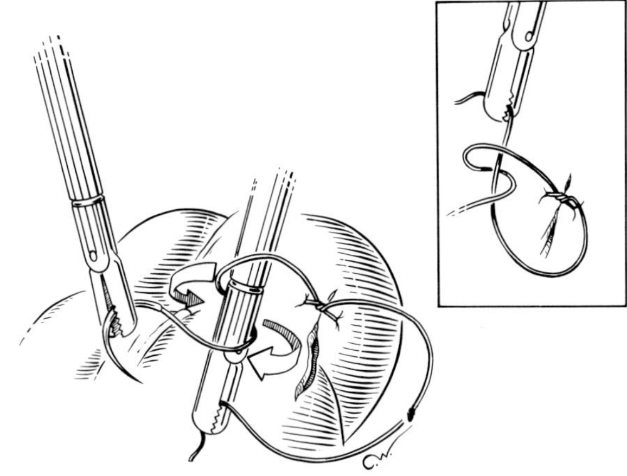

Figures 3-56.

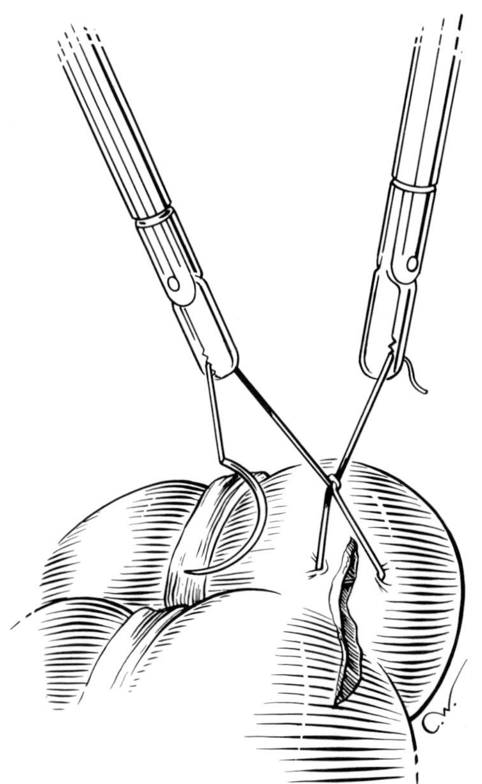

Figures 3-55.

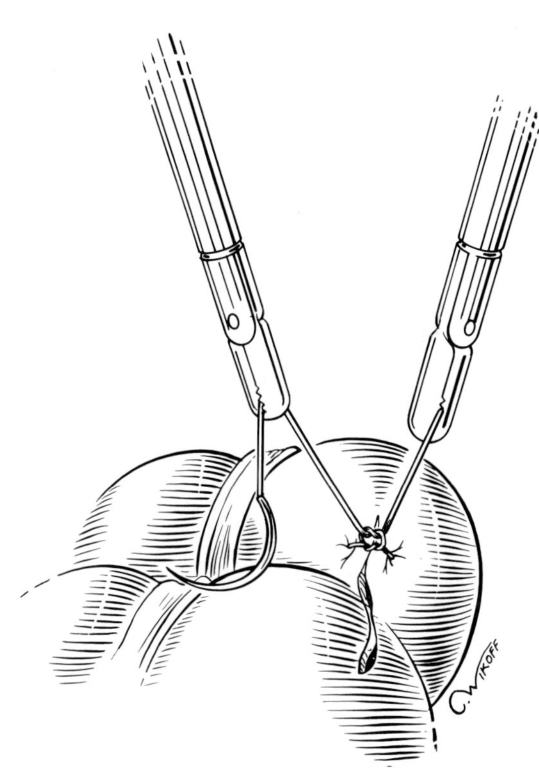

Figures 3-57.

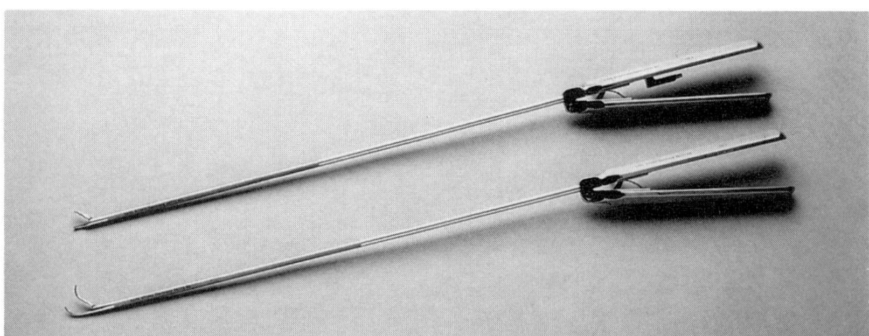

Figure 3-58 This needle-holder is similar to that used at laparotomy with locking capability.

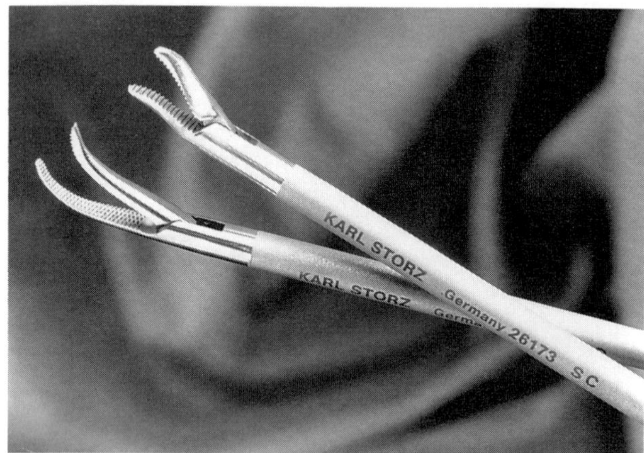

Figure 3-59 Curved and straight fine serrated tips will provide a better grip of straight or curved needle.

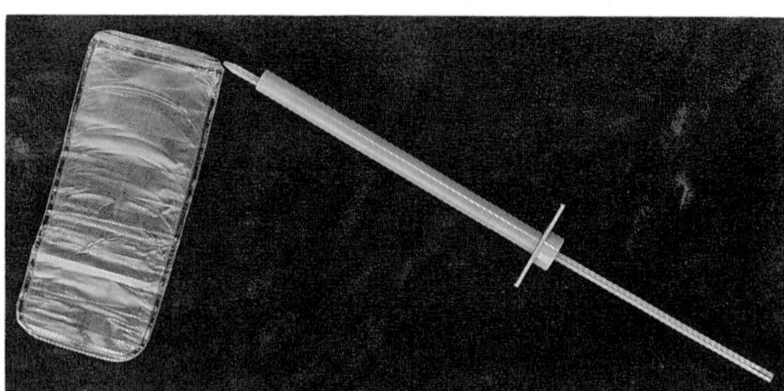

Figure 3-60 Specimen retrieval bag (Endo-pouch, Ethicon).

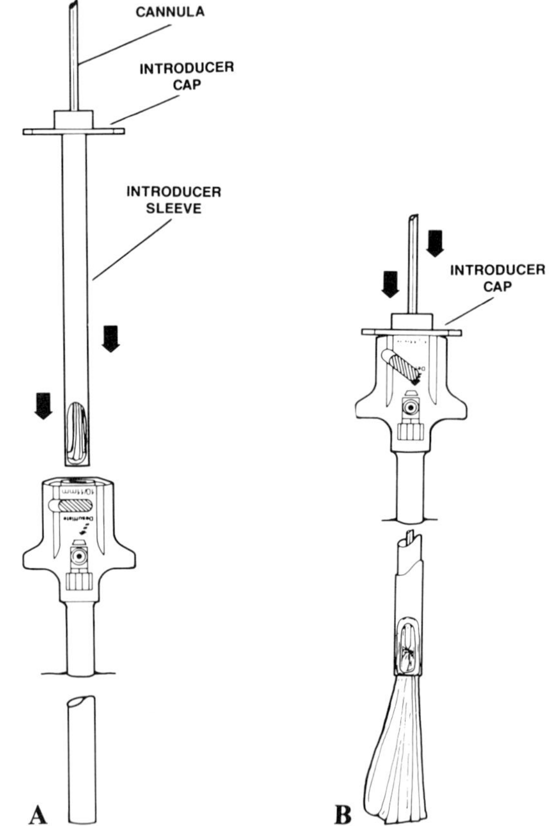

Figure 3-62 A, The introducer is placed into the trocar. B, the bag is pushed into the abdominal cavity.

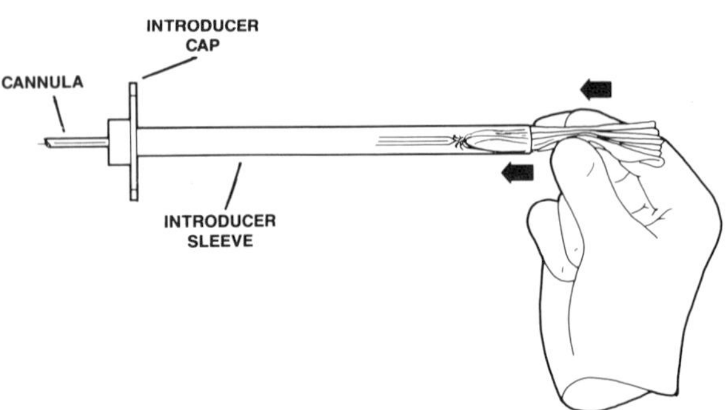

Figure 3-61 The bag is put into the introducer.

(Figure 3-64A), and the cannula broken at the scored point (Figure 3-64B), allowing the suture to be pulled through the cannula and close the top of the bag (Figure 3-65). The bag is retracted to the base of the trocar sleeve by carefully pulling the suture strand. Small masses may be retracted into the introducer and extracted through the trocar sleeve. If the bag and contents cannot be extracted, the bag is pulled into the trocar until resistance is felt (Figures 3-66 and 3-67). The trocar is removed and the bag brought to the incision.

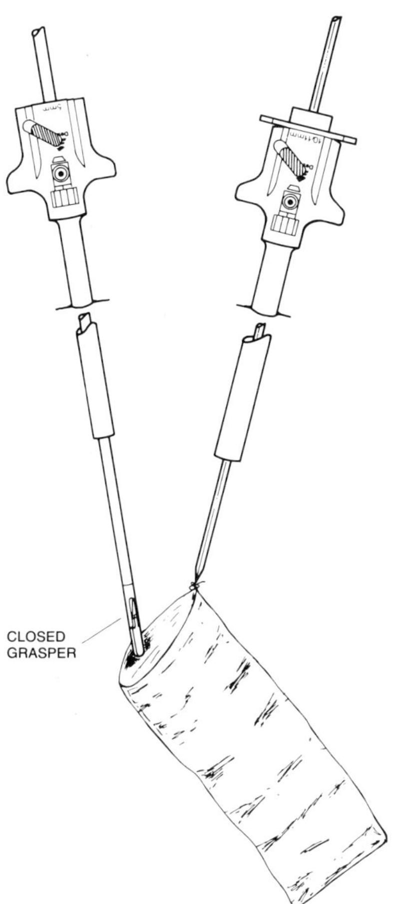

Figure 3-63 A closed grasper is used to open the bag.

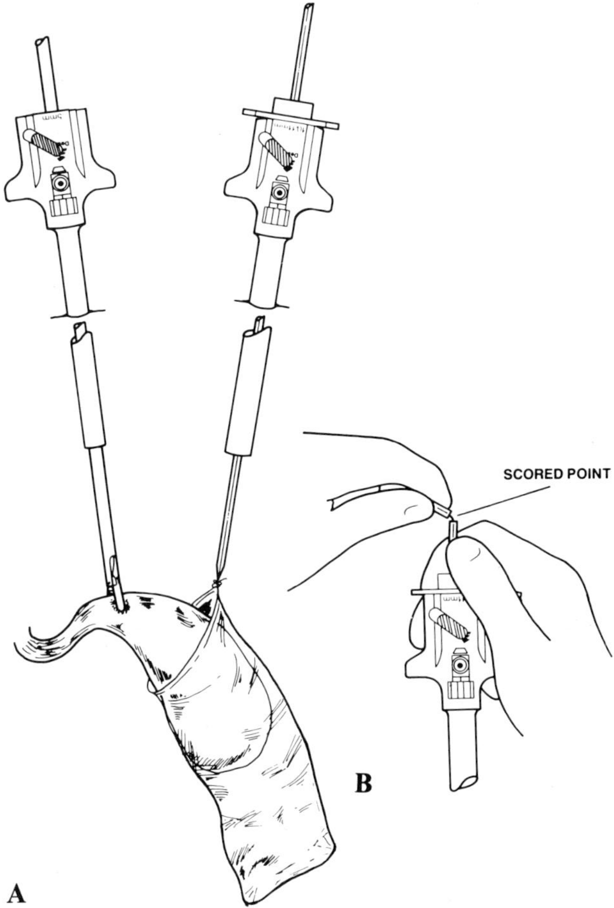

Figure 3-64 A, The specimen, in this case a cyst, is placed in the bag. B, The cannula is broken at the scored point.

The contents may be aspirated or removed with forceps (Figure 3-68). If necessary, a larger incision may be required to remove the bag with contents from the body.

Instruments for Dilation

On occasion, a 10- or 12-mm instrument must be inserted through incisions made for 5-mm instruments. Dilator rods for this purpose allow placement of a 10- or 12-mm trocar. The operator withdraws the smaller trocar and replaces it with a larger one.

Operating Room Set-up

An organized and well-equipped operating room is essential for successful laparoscopy. The surgical team and the operating room staff should be familiar with the instruments and their function. Each instrument must be inspected periodically; check scissors, graspers, trocars, trocar sleeves, etc. for

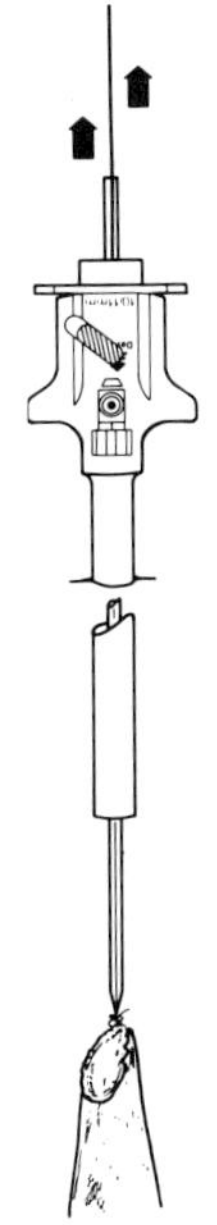

Figure 3-65 The bag is closed around the cyst.

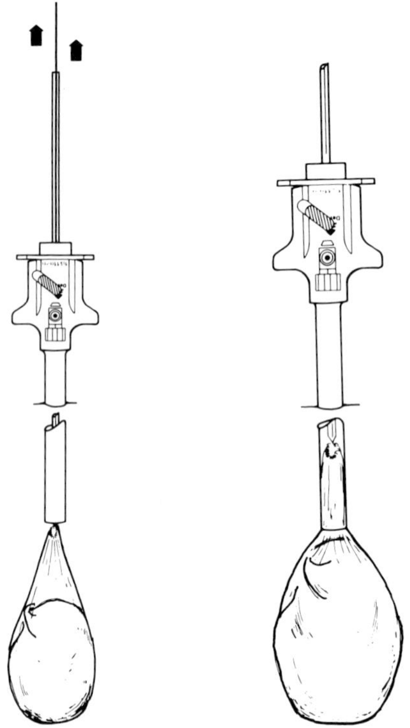

Figures 3-66 and 3-67. The bag is pulled to the base of the trocar sleeve until resistance is felt.

loose or broken tips even if the same instruments were used during a previous procedure. It is necessary to confirm that all instruments have been cleaned. The surgeon ultimately is responsible for the proper functioning of all instruments and equipment.

Before using a new instrument, it should be tested by the surgeon. Although the total cost of operative laparoscopy is decreased by the shortened hospital stay and recovery, the cost of the operating room is higher for operative laparoscopy because of increased cost of instruments and the longer operating time. Every effort should be made to have sufficient instruments and an efficient operating room with reasonable costs.

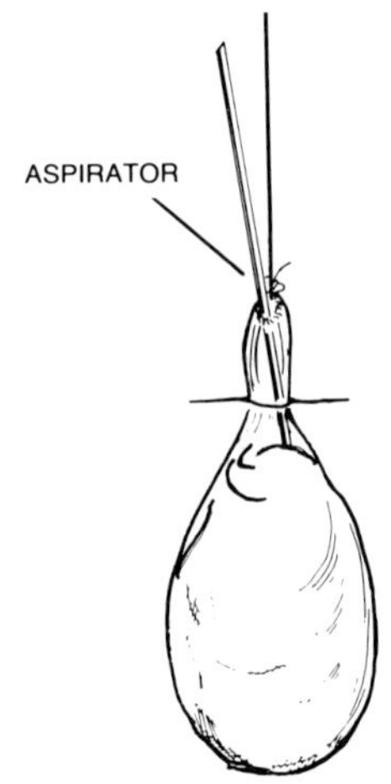

Figure 3-68 The cyst is pulled to the abdominal wall and aspirated.

Positioning of Equipment

The equipment positioning (Figure 3-69) varies according to the surgeon's preference. The following arrangements are suggested.

A. Operating Tables

Before the patient is brought to the operating room, the operating tables are set.

1. Mayo stand #1 contains a D & C set-up with instruments for video-augmented hysteroscopy (videohysteroscopy). Included are a long-bladed weighted speculum, double- or single-toothed tenaculum, dilators, a uterine sound, a small Kervorkian curet, a uterine manipulator, Raytec (Baxter Healthcare, Deerfield, IL), Telfa and a Foley catheter. The videohysteroscopy equipment includes a Circon (Circon-ACMI, Santa Barbara, CA) or a Storz (Karl Storz, Culver City, CA) diagnostic and operative hysteroscope along with its appropriate scissor and grasper. The adaptive sleeve is available for passing a scissor, grasper, or the fiber laser when it is used in the uterus. For more complicated procedures like resection of intrauterine leiomyomas and endometrial ablation, electrosurgical wire loops and roller balls (Circon, Karl Storz) are added.
2. The back table is positioned behind the surgeon and next to the first assistant (see Figure 3-69). The table contains a Veress needle, a scalpel, an Allis clamp, an 11-mm trocar and sleeve, a 10-mm laparoscope, a fiberoptic light cord, 5.5-mm secondary trocars and sleeves, a suction-irrigator probe (American Hydro-Surgical Instruments) with irrigation and suction tubing, tubing for the CO_2 insufflator with a CO_2 connector, atraumatic grasping forceps with teeth, bipolar forceps with cord, aspirating needles each with a 60-mL syringe, and Telfa and Raytec (Baxter Healthcare). A small amount of diluted Pitressin is made available (1 ampule in 100 mL of bacteriostatic sterile water). Pitressin (1 to 2 mL) is injected through the laparoscopic needle before removing a large fibroid or endometrioma to reduce bleeding. Vicryl suture (3-0) on a cutting needle for closing the pri-

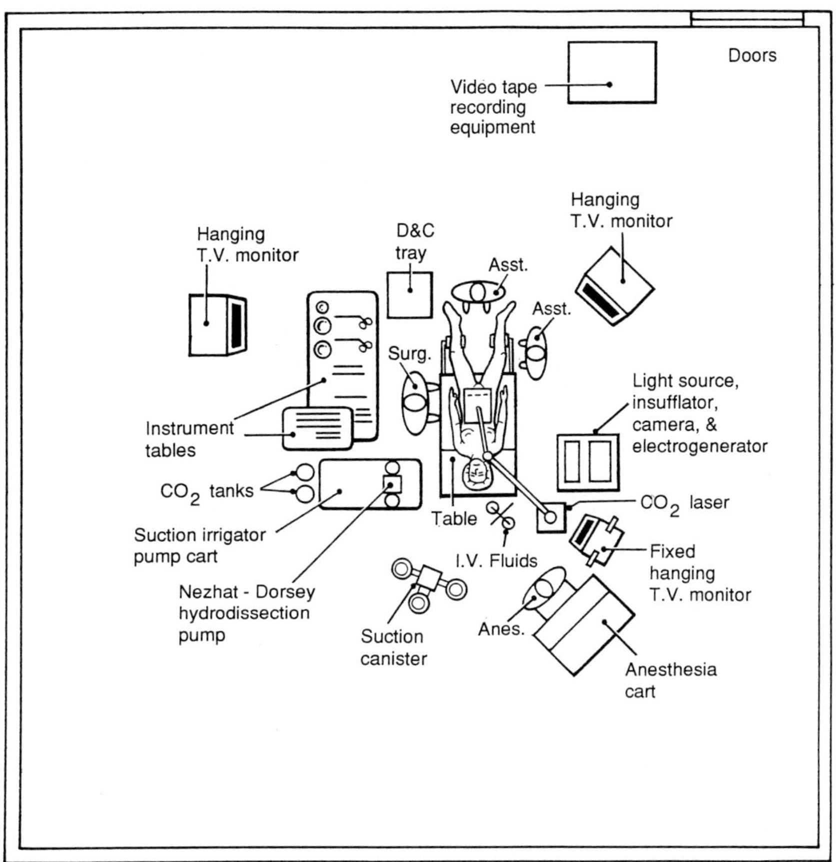

Figure 3-69 Position of patient, assistants, surgeon, and equipment.

mary trocar site and 1.5-inch Steristrips to be used with Mastisol (Ferndale Laboratories, Inc., Ferndale, MI), eye pads, and 3M tape for dressing care are placed on the back table.

3. Mayo stand #2 is positioned so that the surgeon and first assistant can reach the endoscopic scissors and grasping forceps, with and without teeth (see Figure 3-69).

B. Hydrodissection Pump

The Nezhat-Dorsey hydrodissection pump (American Hydrosurgical Instruments, Del Ray, FL) provides pressure during hydrodissection and is located behind the surgeon on a cart or specially designed stand. The plastic tubing is connected to the pump, brought to the operative field, and attached to the suction-irrigator probe.

C. Light Sources, Insufflator, Electrogenerator

Other items kept on the side of the room opposite the surgeon include a storage table that holds the insufflator, electrosurgical equipment, camera boxes, and light sources. This equipment can be stored in a specially designed stand opposite the surgeon, close to the patient, toward her head. This cart should be placed so that it does not interfere with the assistants' position and does not obstruct the surgeon's view of the insufflator and light source. The camera is covered with a sterile cover, connected to the camera box, brought to the operative field, and attached to the laparoscope. Video cabinets are manufactured with removable backs, making adjustments of the machines easy.

D. Video Monitors

Video monitors should be positioned within view of the surgeon and the two assistants, one of whom stands between the patient's legs and the other one is opposite the surgeon. Three video monitors provide adequate views for the surgeon, assistants, and other observers (Figure 3-70). The monitor is the surgeon's view of the operative site and should be set for maximal clarity and true color transmission.

The video monitors can be fixed to the ceiling, placed on a portable stand, or attached to a mobile stand via an articulating arm. The latter can be positioned for optimal viewing from any area in the operating room and can be pushed from the operative area at the end of the day.

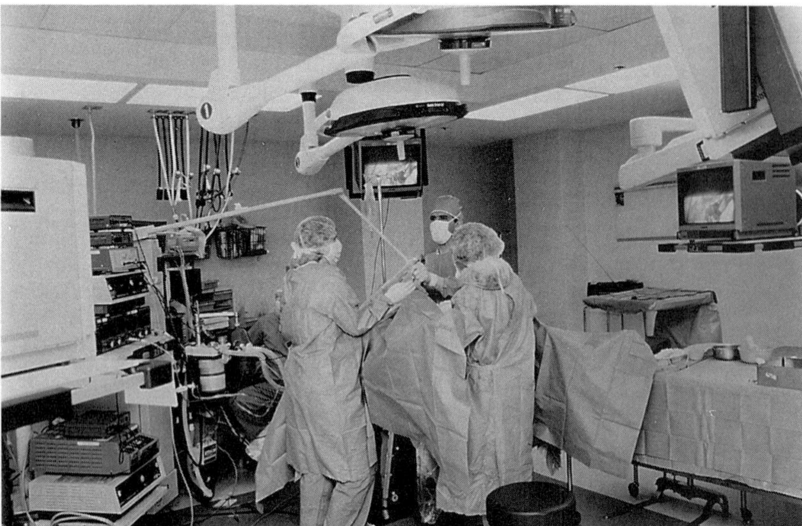

Figure 3-70 View of monitor, instrument placement.

E. Video Recording
Depending on the surgeon's preference, one or two VCRs are located in the room. Two are recommended if a videotape of the procedure will be provided for the patient or referring physician. The recorders are stored in a cabinet near a wall and are wired to the camera box. When surgery is not in progress, the cabinet can be locked to prevent damage and tampering. For those who videotape procedures for educational purposes, a Beta recorder is recommended and kept in the same cabinet.

F. Lasers and Laser Equipment
Three different lasers are available in the operating room: a CO_2 laser (with a coupler), argon or potassium-titanyl-phosphate (KTP) laser, and a neodymium yttrium-aluminum-garnet (YAG) laser. These are used through the operative channel of the laparoscope or a suprapubic trocar. The CO_2 laser is on the patient's lateral side, opposite the surgeon. The articulating arm is extended appropriately so as not to weigh too heavily on the surgeon's hand. The YAG and argon lasers are used less frequently than the CO_2 laser and are located behind the first assistant standing between the patient's legs. This allows laser fibers to be passed from the back table through the second puncture site. Appropriate electrical outlets and special water connections are necessary when using the fiber lasers. Typically, an outlet supplying a 220-volt, 30-amp circuit is required. The YAG laser can be either three phase or single phase and air or water cooled, depending on the peak wattage required for a particular procedure. The CO_2 laser can be operated from a 100-volt circuit supplied by any standard electrical outlet.

Individually wrapped sterile fibers are kept with the fiber lasers, each with its own cleaver for sharpening fiber tips. Because the fibers break quite easily, they must be handled carefully and repeatedly checked.

Safety precautions must be strictly followed when using lasers. One risk of fiber-equipped lasers that does not exist when using a CO_2 laser is the possibility of fiber breakage in or outside of the patient's abdomen. In the CO_2 laser, the beam is transmitted through and reflected by mirrors contained in the articulating arm. When using fiber lasers, the appropriate tinted eye protection must be worn by both the patient and staff. Regular glasses can be worn when using the CO_2 laser but are not necessary during videolaseroscopy. The patient's eyes are covered with moistened eye pads when using the CO_2 and with the appropriate tinted goggles when using other lasers.

Preparation and Termination of the Procedure

All the setup tables are brought close to the operating table and both hysteroscope and laparoscope are connected to the light sources and cameras.

After they have been checked to be sure they are functioning, they are placed over the patient. After the videohysteroscopy is completed, and as the laparoscopic portion begins, the first Mayo stand is moved out of the way and the surgeon moves to the side of the patient for the laparoscopy.

The anesthesiologist covers the patient's eyes with moistened 4 × 4 pads when the laser is to be used and places a foam pad over her neck to protect her if lightweight camera equipment is placed on the sterile field during the procedure.

On completing the procedure, instruments are handled carefully so that laparoscopes and other delicate equipment are not damaged. The disposable equipment is discarded and the reusable instruments given to the circulating nurses for cleaning. Care must be taken to ensure that reusable instruments are not mixed with disposables and inadvertently thrown out.

The patient's abdomen is washed thoroughly and her legs are lowered. Even though patients may not be fully alert, they often can hear conversation as they are being extubated and are in the process of awakening. A professional demeanor should be maintained and conversation limited.

References

1. Nezhat F, Nezhat C, Silfen SL. Videolaseroscopy for oophorectomy. *Am J Obstet Gynecol.* 1991;165:1323-1330.
2. Valtchev KL, Papsin FR. A new uterine mobilizer for laparoscopy: its use in 518 patients. *Am J Obstet Gynecol.* 1977;127:738.
3. Nezhat C, Nezhat F, Silfen SL. Laparoscopic hysterectomy and bilateral salpingo-oophorectomy using multifire GIA surgical stapler. *J Gynecol Surg.* 1990;6:287–288.
4. Nezhat C, Nezhat F, Bess O, et al. Injuries associated with the use of a linear stapler during operative laparoscopy: review of diagnosis, management, and prevention. *J Gynecol Surg.* 1993;9:145–150.
5. Weston PV. A new clinch knot. *Obstet Gynecol.* 1991;78:144.
6. Clarke HC. Laparoscopy—new instruments for suturing and ligation. *Fertil Steril.* 1972; 23:274.
7. Hasson HM. Ovarian surgery. In: Sanfilippo JS, Levine RL, eds. *Operative Gynecologic Endoscopy.* New York: Springer Verlag; 1989:19–37.

4

Lasers in Endoscopic Surgery

Often referred to as "the light that heals," the surgical laser was first introduced in 1969 by Fox.[1] In 1979, Bruhat and colleagues and Tadir and coworkers introduced the use of the CO_2 laser via laparoscopy,[2,3] which increased its role in gynecologic surgery.[4–6] Use of video and laser as introduced by Nezhat further expanded the use of the laser via laparoscope.[7,8] Like all innovations, the laser has had both strong advocates who have made glowing and sometimes unrealistic claims regarding its usefulness and also its share of skeptics who quickly dismissed it as just another gimmick. As is often the case, the truth lies somewhere in the middle and, although they have not replaced either the scalpel or electrosurgery, lasers play an important role in gynecologic surgery. In this chapter, we review the relevant physics of the various lasers in their clinical applications so that they may be used safely and effectively in endoscopic surgery.

Physical Properties of Lasers

Laser is an acronym for "light amplification by stimulated emission of radiation." The device produces and amplifies light energy to create intense, coherent electromagnetic radiation. However, unlike the ionizing radiation of x-rays and gamma rays, which result from nuclear destruction, the energy emitted by laser results from the release of photons that occurs when stimulated electrons circling their nuclei return from their "excited" (E2) to their "resting" (E1) states (E2 − E1 = photon; Figure 4-1). These intermediate energy photons induce molecular vibration and create heat when they interact with tissue. Therefore, although laser light is powerful and penetrating, it is neither mutagenic nor carcinogenic.

Because each lasing substance has a unique atomic and molecular structure with its characteristic electron orbits, the wavelength and frequency of emitted photons will be unique and uniform for each particular substance (CO_2, potassium titanyl phosphate (KTP), argon; Figure 4-2, see also Plate 44). Laser light is monochromatic, consisting of a single wavelength that cannot be separated into any other components, unlike regular light that can be separated into the colors of the spectrum when passed through a prism. When all the light waves are exactly in phase with each other, the light is said to be coherent and when all waves are parallel, the light is collimated. Because the light waves of lasers have exactly the same length (monochromatic), are in phase with each other (coherent), and always run parallel (collimated), the laser can be focused precisely by lenses into a very small spot, which can develop an extremely high power density (Figures 4-3A and 4-3B).

Power Density

The amount of power delivered by lasers is measured in watts, which may be adjusted at various settings by turning the power dial on the machine. However, the penetrating power of the laser, which is determined by the power density, depends mostly on the diameter of the laser beam hitting the tissue. The power density is related directly to the wattage but inversely related to the

1. Absorption

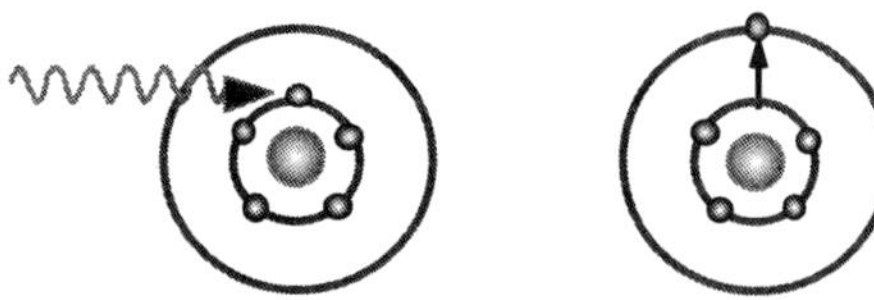

2. Spontaneous Emission

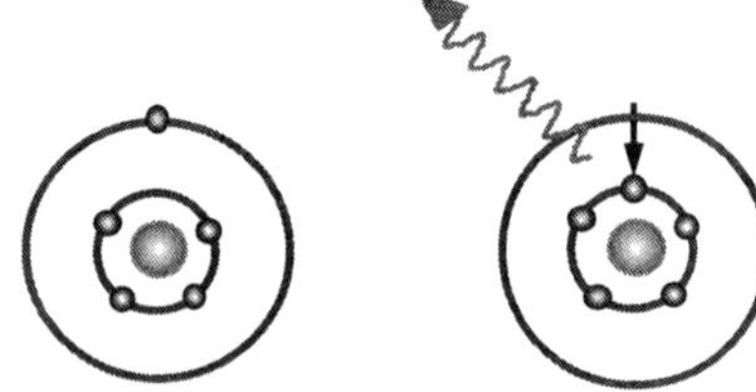

3. Stimulated Emission

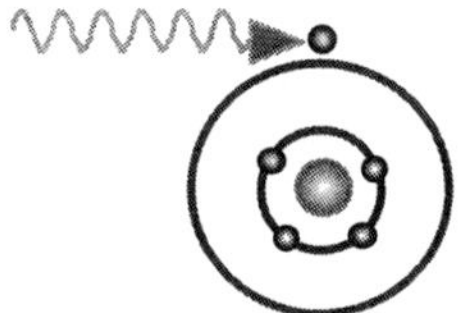
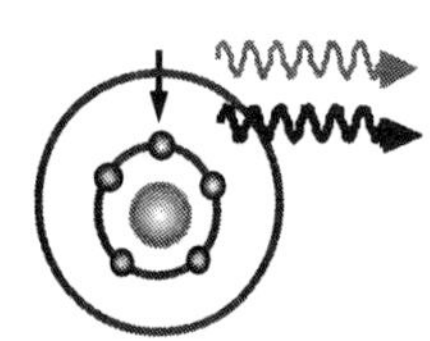

Figure 4-1 Laser energy results from the release of photons when electrons return from their "excited" phase to their "resting" phase during stimulated emission.

square of the spot size, as illustrated by the following formula:

$$\text{Power Density (W/cm}^2\text{)} = \frac{\text{Watts} \times 100}{\text{Spot Diameter}^2 \text{ (mm)}}$$

As the laser beam strikes the tissue, the cells at the site of impact are heated rapidly and vapor-

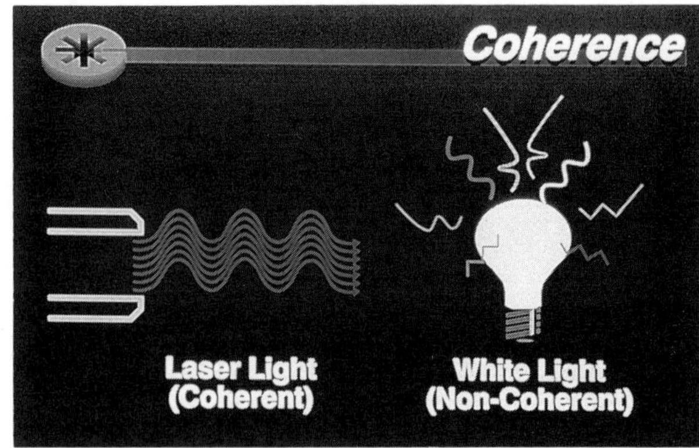

Figure 4-3A Laser light waves are exactly the same length (coherent) unlike white light (noncoherent).

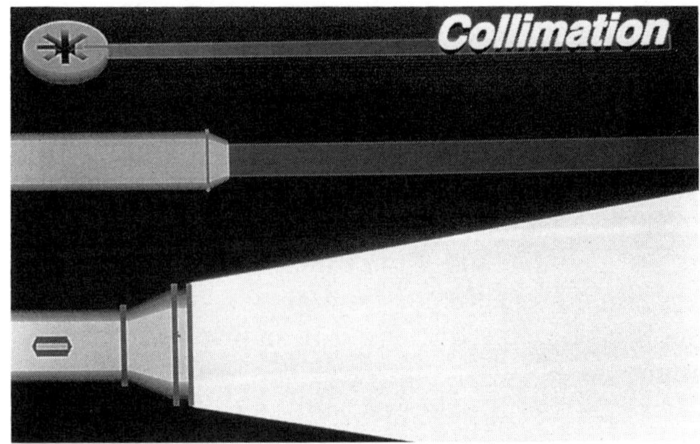

Figure 4-3B Because laser light waves are collimated, they can be focused by lenses into a very precise spot.

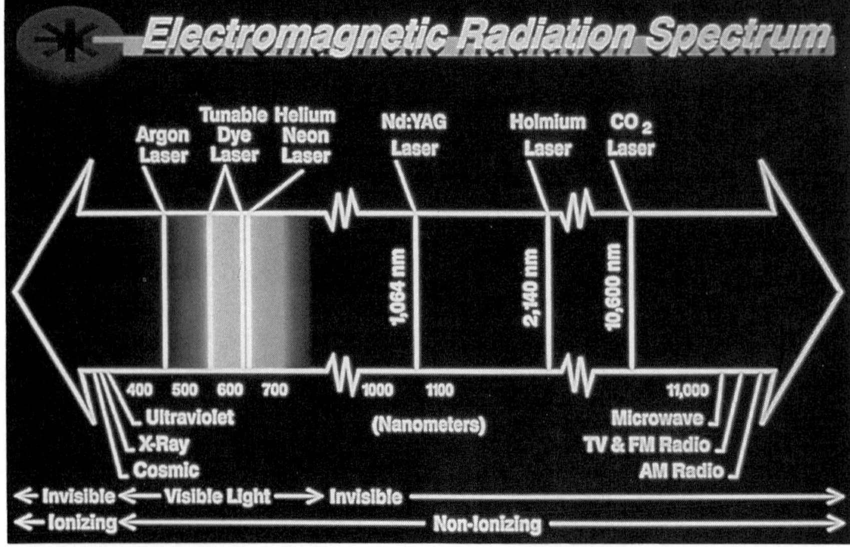

Figure 4-2 Laser light is unique and uniform unlike regular light, which is divided into the colors of the electromagnetic spectrum (see Plate 44).

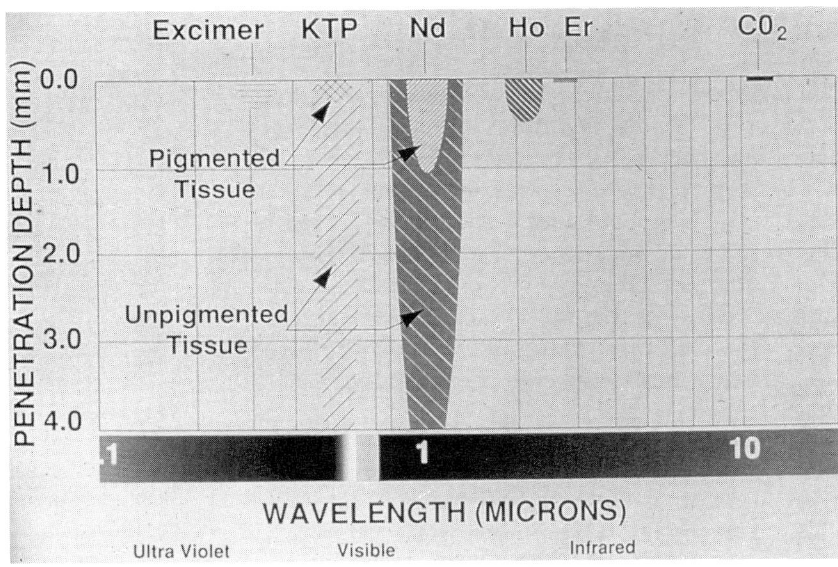

Figure 4-4 Argon, KTP, and Nd:YAG lasers are absorbed by pigmented tissues containing hemoglobin but pass through water and clear tissues (see Plate 45).

ized, ablated, or coagulated, depending on the power density used. Power densities of less than 200 W/cm^2 result in surface heating and serosal contraction. Such lower power densities are useful to coagulate superficial endometriosis on bowel serosa or to evert the ampullary stoma at salpingostomy. Power densities between 1200 and 4000 W/cm^2 result in wide vaporization and less hemostasis. Power densities greater than 4000 W/cm^2 result in rapid, narrow vaporization with minimal coagulation or thermal damage.

Although these general guidelines for power densities and tissue effects were developed for the CO_2 laser,[9] they can be applied equally to electrosurgery, radiosurgery, and, to a lesser degree, to other types of lasers.

Tissue Effects

In addition to the power density, the other major determinants of tissue effects include the degree to which each laser is absorbed, refracted, or reflected by the targeted tissue. For example, the CO_2 laser, which is not color dependent, is absorbed by water. Because tissue is mostly water, all tissues regardless of color will absorb the laser energy, boil, and vaporize immediately. Argon, KTP, and neodymium: yttrium-aluminum-garnet (Nd-YAG) lasers are absorbed by pigmented tissues containing hemoglobin, but are not absorbed by and penetrate deeply through water and clear tissues (Figure 4-4, see also Plate 45). Consequently, they vaporize tissue less efficiently[5] but are much better at coagulating bleeding esophageal varices[10] and ablating pigmented tissue such as endometrium[11] and vascular tumors.[12] The property of fiber lasers to be refracted and transmitted but not absorbed by clear tissues has been used successfully to coagulate bleeding vessels on the retina of the eye without affecting the clear structures in front of it. The commonly used lasers in gynecologic surgery, their physical properties, and tissue effects are listed (Table 4-1).

TABLE 4-1 Physical Properties and Characteristics of Surgical Lasers

Type of Laser	CO_2	Argon	KTP	Nd-YAG
Wavelength (μm)	10.6	0.458–0.515	0.532	1.064
Color	Infrared	Blue-green	Green	Infrared
Delivery	Air or endoguide	Fiber	Fiber	Fiber
Absorption	All tissues and fluids	Color dependent	Color dependent	Color dependent
Pass through fluids	No	Yes	Yes	Yes
Cutting	Excellent	Good	Good	Good
Coagulation	Fair	Good	Good	Excellent

Laser Components

The basic components of lasers consist of a pumping system, lasing medium, optical cavity, and operating system.[9] The pumping system is the power source that energizes the atoms or molecules of the lasing medium to higher energy states. The ultimate power source of all lasers is the electrical outlet, which either stimulates the lasing medium directly or induces electrochemical reactions which, in turn, pump energy into the lasing medium to stimulate its electrons to higher energy levels.

The lasing medium consists of a selected assembly of atoms, molecules, or ions, which may be distributed in a solid crystal matrix (ruby, Nd-YAG), a gas (CO_2, helium-neon [He-Ne]), or a liquid (gallium arsenide diode). Each lasing substance has a unique atomic or molecular structure, with its characteristic electron orbits and energy levels. Thus, the wavelength and frequency of photons emitted will be uniform and unique for each lasing substance, CO_2, KTP, YAG, and so forth.

The optical cavity, also referred to as a resonator cavity, consists of a tube with parallel mirrors on either side, which allow continuous reflection of photons back and forth in all directions as they strike other excited atoms to effect "stimulated emission of radiation" (Figure 4-5). At one end of the optical cavity, the mirror is partially reflective, thus allowing escape of those photons that are exactly in phase (coherent) and are traveling in the same parallel direction (collimated). As the photons are reflected repeatedly back and forth between the parallel mirrors of the optical cavity, the intensity of the laser beam inside the cavity builds. This amplification is similar to the amplification in the resonator chamber of a musical instrument. The small portion of the beam that is transmitted through the partially reflective mirror provides the laser energy for surgery.

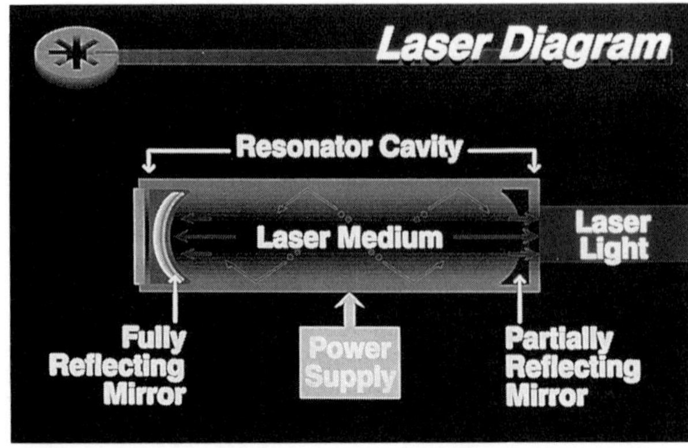

Figure 4-5 The resonator cavity of a laser consists of one reflective mirror and one partially reflective mirror to both reflect the photons, thus producing stimulated emission, and allow coherent and collimated photons to escape, creating the laser energy.

The operating system controls the delivery of laser energy to the tissue. It determines the power in watts and the mode at which the laser is delivered from the unit. The power is adjusted by the power control knob. The mode of delivery of the laser energy is continuous, pulsed, superpulsed, or ultrapulsed. In the *continuous mode*, the laser energy is delivered to the tissue without interruption as long as the control pedal remains depressed. The pulsed mode is in single or repeated pulses (Figure 4-6, see also Plate 46). With single

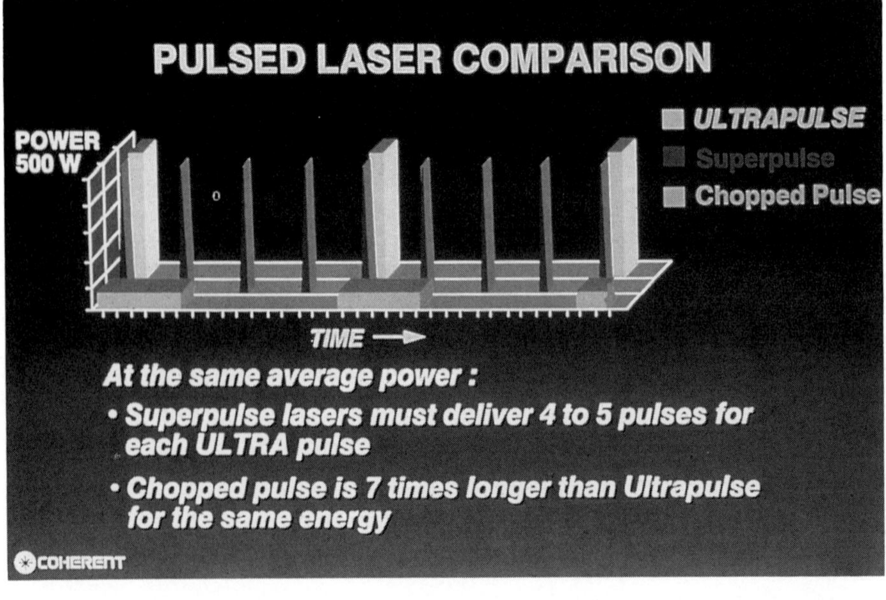

Figure 4-6 Comparison of ultrapulse, superpulse, and chopped pulse modes (see Plate 46).

pulses, the operating system releases one burst of energy for a specified interval (range, 0.05 to 0.5 seconds) with every depression of the pedal. To discharge a second laser pulse, the pedal must be released and depressed again. The single-pulse mode gives a controlled, precise penetration of the laser beam. It is used by surgeons with less experience in laser surgery to ablate endometriosis over the bowel to avoid perforating the bowel wall and, on the pelvic sidewall, to avoid perforating the blood vessels and ureter. The repeat pulse mode delivers intermittent bursts of laser of predetermined width and intervals (number of pulses per second), for as long as the pedal remains depressed.

The *superpulse mode* of the CO_2 laser releases rapid pulses at short intervals alternating with refractory, short periods when the laser energy is not delivered. During the pulse, the peak power is extremely high (up to 10 times the continuous output). By releasing "bursts" of peak power, the power density is increased fourfold or more over the average obtainable with a continuous mode. The refractory periods between laser output allow heat dissipation and prevent heat buildup in adjacent tissues, minimizing thermal injury. The use of the superpulse mode results in precise and rapid vaporization with decreased tissue desiccation, carbonization, thermal injury, and smoke plume. Although the same tissue effects are obtained using the continuous mode, this usually proves impractical. The continuous mode must be delivered in a small spot with high power density and the resulting rapid tissue vaporization is difficult to control. The benefit of the superpulse mode is that it allows the surgeon to use the high power density necessary for clean tissue vaporization and minimal thermal damage at a controlled rate of delivery.

Baggish and Elbakry[13] ascertained from animal studies that pulse durations between 0.6 and 0.2 milliseconds, at rates below 700 pulses per second, permit effective ablation with minimal thermal injury. Thus, for the superpulse mode, it is recommended that the pulse duration be less than 0.6 milliseconds and the frequency should be approximately 300 pulses per second. Superpulse lasers can be very effective when used with spot sizes less than 0.75 mm. At larger spot sizes, the tissue effect with the superpulse mode becomes more thermal with increasing tissue desiccation, carbonization, and thermal injury. The superpulse mode cannot sustain the high power density long enough in a single pulse to vaporize all of the tissue exposed to the larger spot. In endoscopy, the full advantages of the superpulse mode cannot

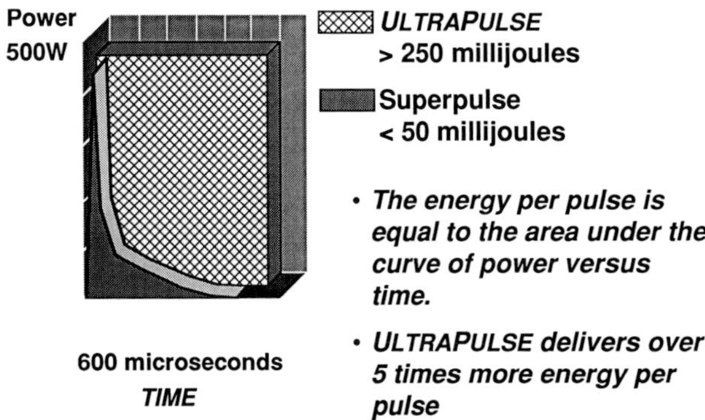

Figure 4-7 Pulse energy comparison of ultrapulse and superpulse modes.

be obtained because the spot sizes are too large (typically 1.0 to 1.5 mm).

More recently, the *ultrapulse mode* for the CO_2 laser has been introduced by Coherent Inc.,[14] and delivers pulses with the highest power density available for laparoscopy. These high power densities are desirable whenever thermal tissue injury should be minimized and coagulation effects of the laser are not important. The ultrapulse mode displays both the average power output of the laser and the energy delivered in each pulse (Figure 4-7). The pulse energy is related to the peak power in the pulse and the pulse duration and determines the amount of tissue each pulse can vaporize. High pulse energy means that the laser can sustain the high peak power long enough to vaporize all of the tissue exposed by a larger spot. The ultrapulse mode delivers up to five times more energy per pulse than conventional superpulse mode. This feature allows clean tissue vaporization with decreased tissue desiccation, carbonization, and thermal injury. For example, 200 mJ/pulse can ablate spot sizes up to 2.5 mm. The ultrapulse mode provides separate controls for adjusting pulse energy and average power, allowing the surgeon to control the laser–tissue response at different operating speeds (Figure 4-8). By lowering the pulse energy, the surgeon can increase hemostasis by increasing the amount of thermal injury. Because the pulse energy reaching the tissue remains constant at different average power settings, the ultrapulse mode can produce char-free tissue ablation in laparoscopy at the slow working speeds that accompany low average power and the rapid working speeds that accompany high average power. This gives the surgeon a new level of control.

Another significant problem associated with delivery of the CO_2 laser through the operating chan-

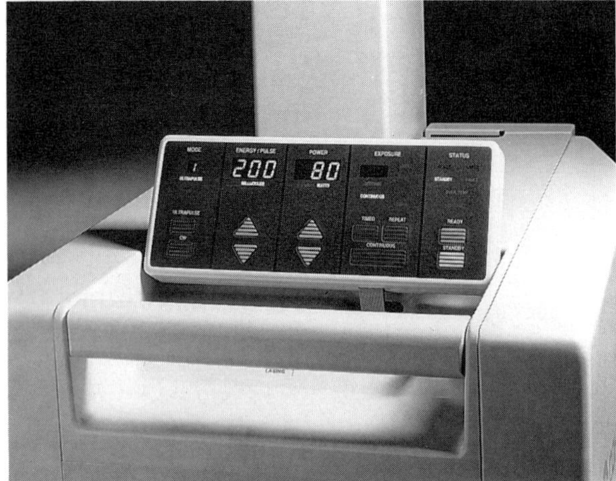

Figure 4-8 Control panel for ultrapulse mode.

nel of the laparoscope is thermal blooming. When used through the operative channel of the laparoscope, the CO_2 laser energy is absorbed by the CO_2 insufflation gas in the channel (Figure 4-9A), causing the CO_2 laser spot size to increase and reducing the transmitted energy by up to 30% to 60% at high power settings (Figure 4-9B). This "blooming effect" at high power settings (20 to 100 W) can provide effective coagulation. However, for most applications it is a disadvantage, because the larger spot size decreases precision and results in more carbonization and thermal damage. The new ultrapulse laser eliminates the "thermal blooming" problem. This laser uses the carbon 13 isotope in the laser gas mix instead of the carbon 12 isotope, which is used in both conventional CO_2 lasers and CO_2 insufflation gas. No noticeable effect on tissue attributable to distortion or power loss from absorption in the insufflation gas was noted. The surgeon can work with minimal charred tissue (Figure 4-10, see also Plate 47).

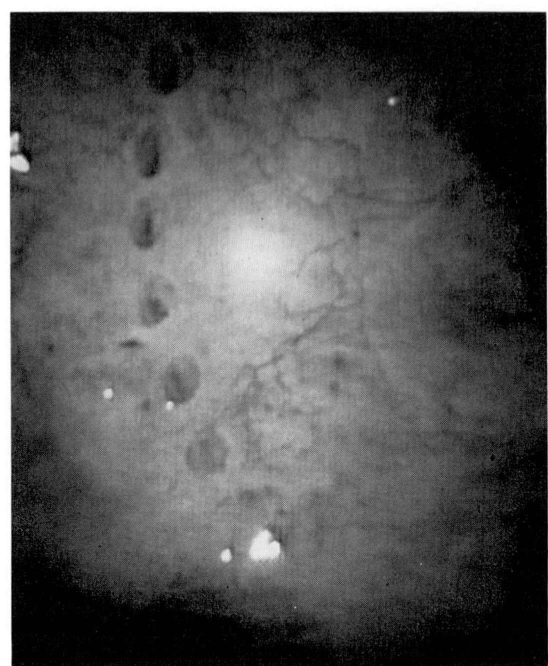

Figure 4-10 The new ultrapulse laser eliminates the "thermal blooming" effect and side effects such as the formation of charred tissue (see Plate 47).

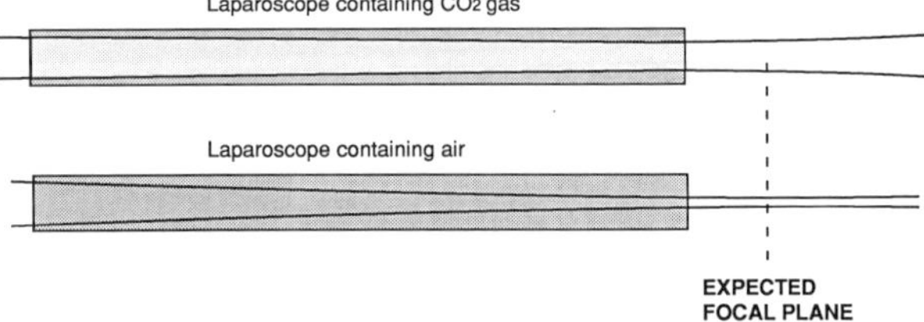

Figure 4-9A When used in the laparoscope, the CO_2 insufflation gas in the chamber absorbs the CO_2 laser energy and is heated, causing the "thermal blooming" effect. Warmer gas in center of lumen is less dense than gas near lumen walls. The density gradient forms a thermal lens increasing the laser spot size at the focal plane.

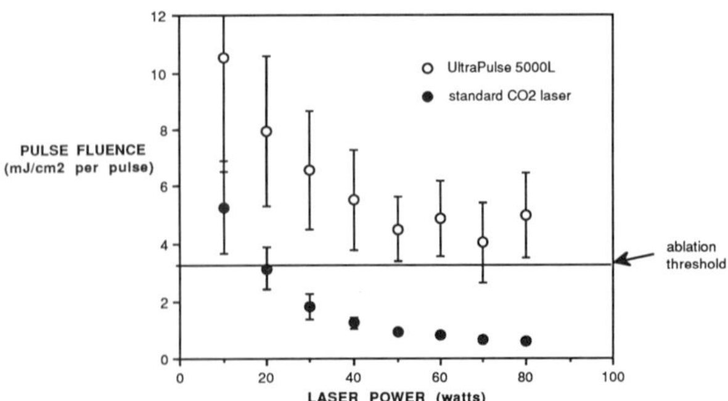

Figure 4-9B The increase in spot size reduces transmitted energy up to 30% to 60% at high power settings.

Delivery Systems

The CO_2 laser beam leaves the optical resonator and is delivered to the end of an articulated arm by several specially coated mirrors that are aligned precisely to preserve the configuration and power of the beam as it leaves the generator (Figure 4-11). Since the CO_2 laser beam is invisible, a visible, low-power He-Ne laser beam is provided as an aiming beam. At the output of the arm, the CO_2 laser beam and the He-Ne beam are composed of

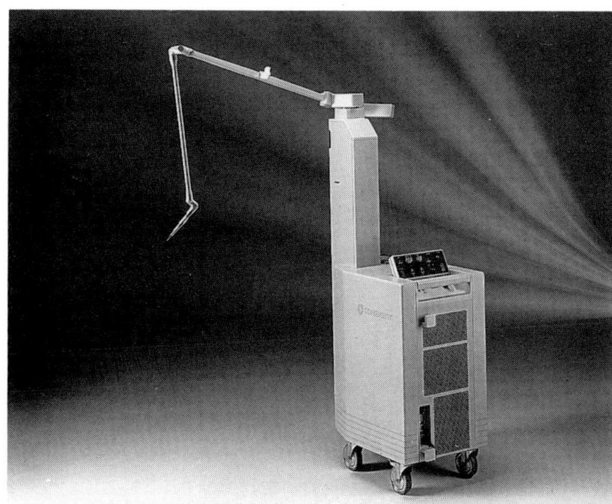

Figure 4-11 The CO_2 laser generator and articulated arm are shown.

parallel waves that need to be focused to increase power density. Coupling lenses of various focal length are used to focus the beams at the end of either the handheld probe or laparoscope. One type of coupling lens is a fixed lens, which is assembled easily between the arm of the laser and the laparoscope (Figure 4-12). Its focal length may be set at 28 cm if the laser is delivered through the operating channel of the laparoscope or at 18 cm if the laser is delivered through a second puncture site to focus at the end of the shorter accessory trocar. In laparoscopic procedures, the focal point is usually 2.0 cm from the tip of the laparoscope.

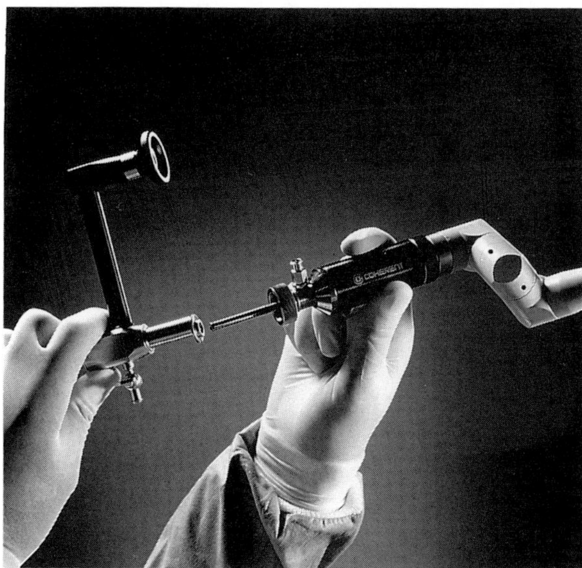

Figure 4-12 Coupling lens is assembled between the arm of the laser and the laparoscope.

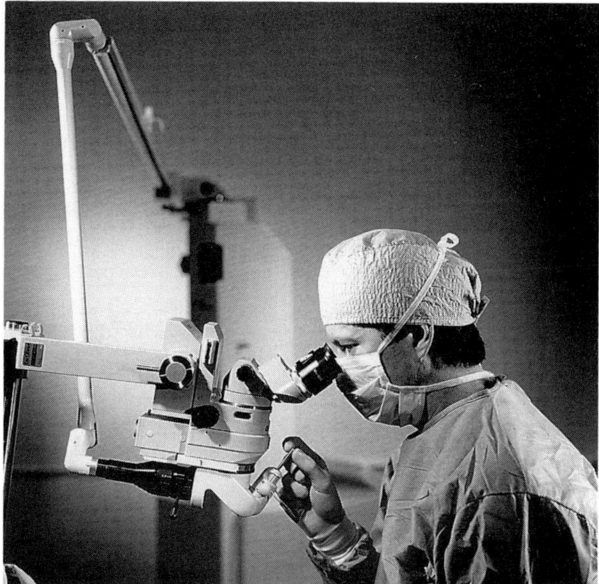

Figure 4-13 Laser coupler with multiple lens system enables the surgeon to focus and defocus the laser beam by simply turning a knob on the coupler.

Instead of a fixed lens, the laser couplers can have a multiple lens system with variable focal lengths enabling the surgeon to focus and defocus the laser beam and change the spot size by turning a knob on the coupler (Figure 4-13). This system allows for the spot size to be varied between 0.5 to 2.0 mm in diameter.

It is obvious from the foregoing that the quality of the CO_2 laser output depends largely on the proper alignment of the directing mirrors in the articulated arm of the laser, on the quality and performance of the coupling lens, and on the integrity of the operative channel of the laparoscope. A disturbance of any part of these three systems will result in poor beam alignment and loss of laser power. A number of approaches have been taken to minimize these problems. Manufacturers continually improve the design and stability of the laser, articulated arm, and laparoscope coupling system. New laparoscope couplers, such as the Coherent-Nezhat laparoscope coupler, eliminate a major source of alignment error by aligning the laser beam directly to the operating channel of the laparoscope. Finally, rigid wave guides have been developed to guide the focused laser beam from the articulated arm through the operative channel of the laparoscope or through a second puncture site. The beam exits the wave guide in perfect focus and close to the tissue. Rigid wave guides are usually composed of ceramics with a low index of refraction so that high power densities are transmitted with less than a 10% power loss. A purge of continuous CO_2 of up to 1000 mL/min flows down the wave guide channel to keep it cool and clear of smoke. This CO_2 is an additional source of insufflation to replace the gas evacuated with suctioning of the smoke.

The availability of fiber delivery systems is a major advantage of the argon, KTP, and Nd-YAG lasers. These quartz fibers are flexible, light, and thin. They can be delivered at a greater distance from the laser generator than the CO_2 laser, which needs to be close to the operative field because of its relatively short articulated arm. The laser beam is at maximal focus at the tip of the fiber, which may deliver the laser with or without contact with the tissue. By varying the diameter of the fiber, or the distance between the fiber and the targeted tissue, the power density of the argon or KTP lasers may be adjusted to vaporize, ablate, or coagulate. The Nd-YAG laser may be modified with sapphire tips to effect coagulation or vaporization.

In addition to providing a delivery system for the laser beam, fiberoptics also may be used in the future to monitor laser surgery. Sensor data can be returned to console computers for an analysis of tissue effects through the same fiberoptic bundles used to deliver the beam. This type of back and forth transmission of light is common in the communications industry today and may make laser application in surgery much safer and more useful in the future.

Surgical Lasers Used in Gynecology

The major types of lasers currently used in surgery are the CO_2, argon, KTP-532, and Nd-YAG. Developmental work involves the use of the krypton, excimer, free electron, and tunable lasers, which may have surgical applications in the future.

The CO_2 laser was the first laser to be used in our specialty. The CO_2 laser emits photons with a wavelength of 10.6 μm, which is within the infrared portion of the electromagnetic spectrum and therefore cannot be seen. Thus, the CO_2 laser is delivered together with the visible He-Ne laser, which serves as the aiming beam. The CO_2 laser offers high power density and high efficiency and is ideally suited for cutting and vaporizing. It is absorbed by nonreflective solids and liquids, is not dependent on the color of tissue for absorption, and is not scattered from the target point. Thus, the impact of the laser is limited to the target tissue, sparing adjacent tissue layers. CO_2 laser cannot be delivered through fluids, is a poor coagulator, and cannot be delivered by true fibers. However, the wave guide delivery system offers a fair alternative to reflective mirrors. By varying the output wattage or the diameter of the laser spot, a large range of power densities is available with the CO_2 laser. Low power densities, being more hemostatic, are used for the cervix and myomata where hemostasis is important and thermal damage is not a major concern. Higher power densities are preferred for reconstructive adnexal surgery where thermal damage must be minimized.

The argon and KTP-532 lasers are similar in their characteristics and clinical applications because they have similar wavelengths of 0.532 and 0.458 to 0.515 μm, respectively. Both release a visible green light that travels through clear fluids and is absorbed by dark-pigmented tissue. Both can be delivered through flexible fibers, making them suited for endoscopic use. Since they are not absorbed by clear fluids or unpigmented tissue, these lasers are ideal for coagulation of retinal bleeding or for ablation of peritoneal endometriosis where tissue coagulation can be effected without disrupting the clear overlying tissue. The argon laser is available in two models, the 5 W and 16 W for abdominal and pelvic surgery. The more powerful model is more useful for reproductive surgery and ablation of endometriosis. This model requires high electrical current energy, three phase, in excess of 200 V at 60 A. The laser fibers range in size from 300 to 600 μm in diameter and are introduced through the small channels of the operating laparoscope or ancillary trocars, and steered toward the target with special bridges. The laser beam is focused at the tip of the fiber. As the distance from the tissue is increased, the spot size increases (the beam diffuses) and the power density diminishes. In addition to protective goggles for the specific laser wavelength through the laparoscope, the operator may choose to cover the eyepiece of the laparoscope with the "monoshutter," an electronically triggered eyepiece that attaches to the laparoscope and interposes a protective filter between the operator's eye and the laparoscope when the laser is fired. The monoshutter is used with the videocameras for videosurgery and documentation.

The Nd-YAG laser is a crystal laser with an infrared wavelength of 1.064 μm, in the near infrared spectrum. The YAG laser is invisible and highly color dependent and passes through fibers and clear fluids. The YAG laser penetrates deeply into tissue, an advantage in coagulating tumors or hemorrhaging ulcers or in endometrial ablation. Although it is an excellent coagulator, the YAG laser cuts poorly unless used with sapphire tips. The sapphire tips completely absorb the laser energy, reaching very high temperatures resulting in a "hot tip" for cutting. The YAG laser is not a good choice for reconstructive adnexal disease because of the large amount of scatter and excessive thermal damage to tissue.

Clinical Applications

Lasers have several unique characteristics that differentiate them from other medical instruments. The primary difference is that, with some exceptions, the tissue is not touched by surgical instruments but only by the laser beam. Thus, the depth of the incision is not controlled by the pressure exerted on the tissue but by the power density and the time that the laser is focused on any one spot. This "action at a distance" allows for greater accessibility to the target tissue and perhaps less tissue trauma. When used at laparotomy, the CO_2 laser is delivered with a handheld probe or attached to the operating microscope. The former has the advantage of a shorter focal distance and therefore a smaller spot size resulting in greater power density. The greater power density yields much higher penetrating power and significantly less thermal damage to the contiguous normal tissue. The handheld probe is subject to hand tremor and less accurate beam delivery. Attaching the laser to the microscope increases precision because of the magnification and the absence of hand tremor; however, because of the longer focal length, the spot size is larger. With more precise lasers, very high power density is achievable through the laparoscope.

Although each laser has unique properties and tissue effects determined by wavelength and tissue absorption, by varying the power density or mode of delivery (sapphire tips, fiber diameter), desired tissue effects such as ablation, coagulation, or vaporization can be achieved with most lasers.

The most effective use of the CO_2 laser beam is through the operative channel of the laparoscope as a "long knife"; the beam does not obstruct the view and works well for delicate dissection. The CO_2 laser is stopped easily by a water backstop. This characteristic of the CO_2 laser gives high precision for dissection in sensitive areas like bowel, bladder, ureter, and blood vessels. The low morbidity and absence of mortality in more than 7000 advanced operative procedures is attributable in part to videolaseroscopy.

References

1. Fox G. The use of laser radiation as a surgical "light knife." *J Surg Res.* 1969;9:199.
2. Bruhat H, Mage C, Manhes M. Use of the CO_2 laser via laparoscopy. In: Kaplan I, ed. *Laser Surgery III.* Proceedings of the Third International Society for Laser Surgery. Tel Aviv: 1979:275.
3. Tadir Y, Ovadia J, Zuckerman Z, et al. Laparoscopic application of the CO_2 laser. In: Proceedings of the 4th Congress of International Society for Laser Surgery. Tokyo: Japanese Society for Laser Medicine; 1981:25.
4. Nezhat C, Crowgey S, Garrison C. Surgical treatment of endometriosis via laser laparoscopy. *Fertil Steril.* 1986;6:778–783.
5. Luciano AA, Frishman GN, Kratka SA, Maier DB. A comparative analysis of adhesion reduction, tissue effects and incising characteristics of electrosurgery, CO_2 laser and Nd-YAG laser at operative laparoscopy: an animal study. *J Laparoendoscopic Surg.* 1992;2:287.
6. Nezhat C, Winer WK, Nezhat F. A comparison of the CO_2 argon, and KTP/532 laser in the videolaseroscopic treatment of endometriosis. *Colposcopy Gynecol Laser Surg.* 1988;4:41.
7. Nezhat C. Videolaseroscopy: a new modality for the treatment of endometriosis and other diseases of reproductive organs. *Colposcopy Gynecol Laser Surg.* 1986;2:221–224.
8. Nezhat C, Crowgey S, Nezhat F. Videolaseroscopy for the treatment of endometriosis associated with infertility. *Fertil Steril.* 1989;512:23.
9. Martin DC. Tissue effects of lasers. *Semin Reprod Endocrinol.* 1991;9:118.
10. Fuller TA. Fundamental of lasers in surgery and medicine. In: Dixon J, ed. *Surgical Applications of Lasers.* Chicago: Year Book Medical Publishers; 1983:11–28.
11. Keye WR, Hansen LW, Astin M, et al. Argon laser therapy of endometriosis: a review of

92 consecutive patients. *Fertil Steril.* 1987; 47:208.

12. Joffe SN, Brackett KA, Sankar MY, Daikuzono N. Resection of the liver with Nd-YAG laser. *Surg Gynecol Obstet.* 1986;163:437.
13. Baggish MS, Elbakry MM. Comparison of electronic superpulsed and continuous wave CO_2 laser on the rabbit uterine horn. *Fertil Steril.* 1986;45:20.
14. Nezhat C, Nezhat F. Laparoscopic surgery with a new tuned high-energy pulsed CO_2 laser. *J Gynecol Surg.* 1992;8:251–255.

5

Electrosurgery

The rapid expansion of operative endoscopy has created an increasing demand for new instruments and applications. Electrosurgery was initially used during laparoscopy for tubal sterilization. The basic principles of microsurgery and electrosurgery are applied in reconstructing oviducts, resecting ovarian cysts, or ablating endometriosis endoscopically. If used incorrectly, electrosurgery can cause serious complications from unintended electrical injury to vital organs.[1] In this chapter, the basic principles and clinical applications of electrosurgery are reviewed so that it can be used safely and effectively.

Electrical energy comes from the flow of electrons or current. *Ampere* (A) is the rate that electrons flow; *volt* (V) is the unit of force (pressure) driving the electrons; *ohm* (Ω) is the tissue resistance to the electrons; *watt* (W) is the amount of work produced. A current of 1A is produced by 1 V applied across a resistance of 1Ω (Table 5-1). A high impedance (resistance) of tissue to electron flow generates heat that boils (vaporizes) or denatures (coagulates) tissue. Wattage, the amount of work produced by the electron flow (current), is equal to volts multiplied by amperes.

Voltage is measured by the electrosurgical generator and tissue resistance is measured in ohms. It ranges from 100 to 1000 Ω and changes during the use of electrical energy. With tissue coagulation, water evaporates from cells and results in tissue desiccation, leading to progressively increased resistance until current no longer flows. At this point, if higher voltage is applied, the electrical energy will seek other outlets and sparking can occur. Under normal circumstances, a pressure greater than 15,000 V is required to cause sparking, that is, to push electrons 1 cm in room air.[2,3] This is above the maximal voltage (peak-to-peak voltage) of 1200 V produced by the high-frequency electrogenerators currently recommended for laparoscopy by the Food and Drug Administration. With these generators, when the tissue resistance exceeds the driving force of 1200 V maximum, flow stops, provided the desiccated tissue is not in contact with bowel, blood vessels, or ureter.

With DC, electron flow is unidirectional while the flow of electrons with AC constantly is changing direction, increasing to maximum in one direction, dropping to zero, and then increasing to maximum in the other direction, resulting in a waveform (Figure 5-1). The frequency with which the current changes direction (oscillation) is measured in hertz (Hz). Normal household current is 60 Hz and nerves and muscles are stimulated by frequencies below 10,000 Hz. With electrosurgery, AC is converted into a higher frequency to avoid unwanted neuromuscular stimulation. A "step-up" transformer increases the voltage and frequency (oscillation) of the electric circuit to between 500,000 and 4,000,000 Hz (Figure 5-2). Because these frequencies are within the AM radio frequency range, the term radiofrequency surgery has been used.

Types of Waveforms

Different electrical waveforms produce different tissue effects (Figure 5-3). A *cutting current* is a continuous high-frequency flow of electrons delivered from one peak polarity to the opposite peak without pausing at the zero polarity in the middle. Electrons are delivered constantly to the tissue

TABLE 5-1 Definitions of Electrical Terms

Terms	Units	Description
Current	Ampere (Å)	Volume of electron flow/s
Voltage	Volt (V)	Force (pressure) driving the current
Resistance	Ohm (Ω)	Resistance (impedance) to flow
Power	Watt (W)	Amount of work produced by the flow

without interruption. Pure cutting, undamped current cuts through tissue by exploding the cells at their boiling point of 100°C (vaporization), without elevating the tissue temperature to high levels, thereby avoiding unintended thermal damage. It is similar to the superpulse delivery mode of the CO_2 laser.

A *coagulating* or *damped current* results when peak polarity alternates with zero polarity. Bursts of rapidly increasing current interrupted by intervals without current result in denaturation and dehydration with hemostasis and charring but no cutting. Many generators provide a blended current, combining undamped and damped waveforms where there is a continuous but altering waveform that cuts and coagulates simultaneously.

Unipolar and Bipolar Systems

In a unipolar system, current flows from the small electrode to the tissue being cut or coagulated, through the patient, and to a return electrode attached to the buttock or leg. As the electrical energy spreads, the current density is diffused and the tissue is not heated under the return electrode. A situation that inadvertently concentrates electron flow can result in tissue damage caused by an incompletely applied return plate. Electrical injuries at the ground pad can be avoided by using generators with return electrode monitors. These circuits monitor the electrical contact between the pad and the skin and if inadequate, the electrosurgical unit is deactivated.

Capacitive coupling occurs when electrical energy is transferred from an insulated active electrode to nearby conductive material. Figure 5-4 diagrams a suction irrigator that is an effective capacitor. The electrical energy from the "insulated" electrode will transfer to the surrounding suction–irrigator cannula. If the cannula is inserted through a metal trocar, the transferred energy will disperse through the skin to the return pad without causing injury. However, if the cannula is inserted through a plastic, nonconductive trocar, the transferred energy is not dispersed and thermal injury becomes possible. The capacitive effect is avoided by using metal (conductive) trocar sleeves or the electroshield monitor system, which measures and shunts all capacitively coupled current back to the generator's return plate,

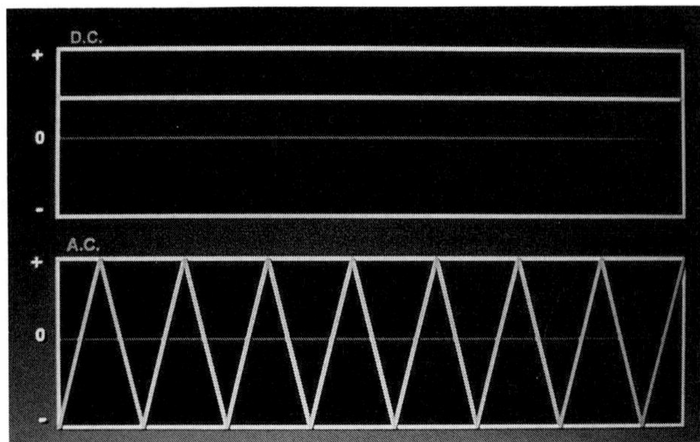

Figure 5-1 Current is either unidirectional (direct) or alternating.

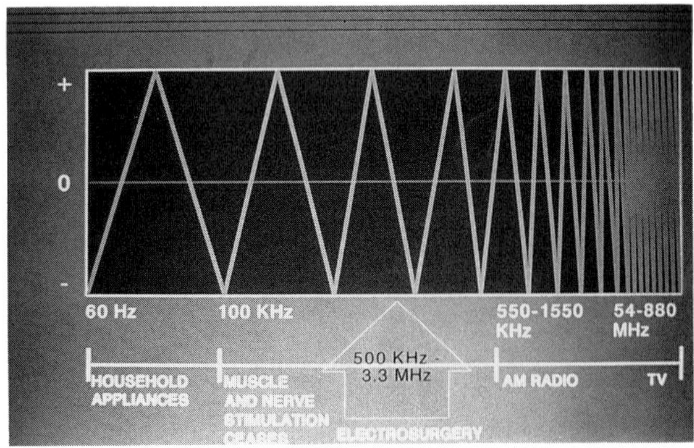

Figure 5-2 The frequency spectrum illustrates the variations in AC from household appliances to a television, with electrosurgery at the midpoint.

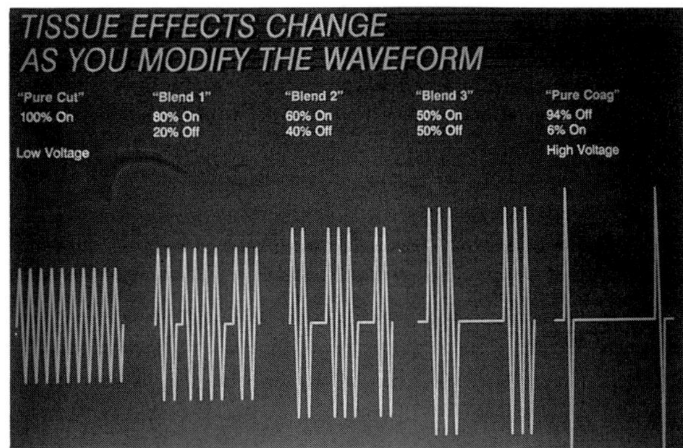

Figure 5-3 As shown on this diagram of various modes of delivering electrical energy to tissue, note that at a fixed power setting, the voltage increases as the current flow interval decreases. Therefore, the cutting current delivers the lowest voltage, is the least penetrating, and inflicts the least thermal damage.

avoiding transmission through the cannula to biologic tissue. If the electroshield cannot handle the capacitively coupled current, it will automatically shut off the generator.

Besides capacitive coupling, unintended electrical injuries also result from direct coupling or insulation failure. Direct coupling occurs if the active electrode touches other metal instruments within the abdomen; the energy is transferred to the second instrument, injuring tissue with which it comes in contact. For example, if the active electrode touches the laparoscope, the latter can burn bowel or other juxtaposed organs. To avoid thermal damage from direct coupling, never activate the electrode until it is in full view and in contact with the intended target.

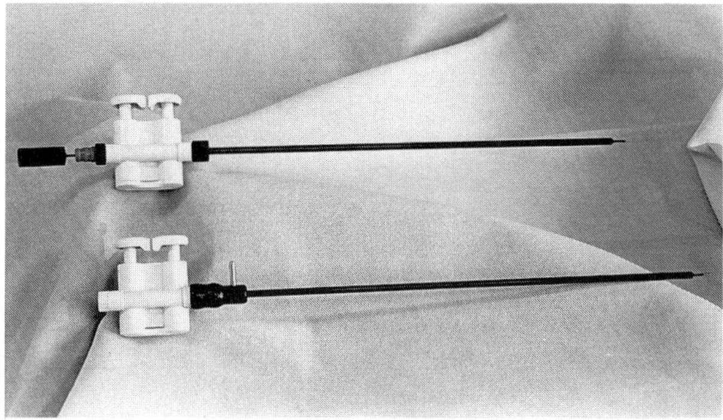

Figure 5-4 An electrode within a suction–irrigator cannula is an effective capacitor. When activated, the electrode induces an electromagnetic field along the entire length of the surrounding cannula. If the cannula is inserted through a nonconductive trocar sleeve, the coupled energy may be discharged to adjacent tissue, causing electrical burns.

Insulation failure occurs if the insulation shield of the electrode is compromised from wear, poor handling, or mechanical accidents. Defective insulation, too small to be recognized, can deliver the full current of the generator to unintended tissue at the end of the electrode. The defect could be on the shaft of the electrode contained within the trocar sleeve. Even new disposable unipolar instruments can have small defects.

A bipolar system does not require a return plate because only the small amount of tissue between the two electrodes is included in the circuit. With these forceps, one prong of the forceps is the active electrode and the other is the return electrode. However, some heat is transmitted to surrounding tissue. Bipolar coagulation requires that the tissue being coagulated be surrounded by the forceps, making the instrument more difficult to use with retracted vessels. Grasping tissue can coapt the walls of vessels before the current is passed, helping to seal the vessels. Bipolar current desiccates but does not cut tissue. As with unipolar systems, the tissue to be coagulated must not be in contact with other organs so as to avoid unintended thermal injury. During laparoscopy, the focus is on the target tissue and the tendency is to ignore vital structures that may be in physical (electrical) contact with the electrode.

Clinical Application

Electrosurgery is used to cut (vaporize) or coagulate deeply (desiccate) or superficially (fulgurate) tissue. The cutting waveform is characterized by high-frequency and low-voltage sine waves (see Figure 5-3). A needle electrode yields very high current density and generates intense intracellular heat, causing the intracellular water to boil, thereby vaporizing the cell. The vaporization has a cooling effect that prevents thermal damage to adjacent tissue and prevents heat transfer to deeper tissue. Activation of the electrode prior to touching the tissue produces a plume of vapor between the electrode and the tissue, resulting in cutting with the least thermal damage (Figure 5-5). For adhesiolysis or for vaporization of ovarian endometriosis or bladder reflection, cutting current is used with a small needle electrode just before making contact with the target tissue.

Desiccation is effective for coagulating tissue and is achieved with electrodes used with a high

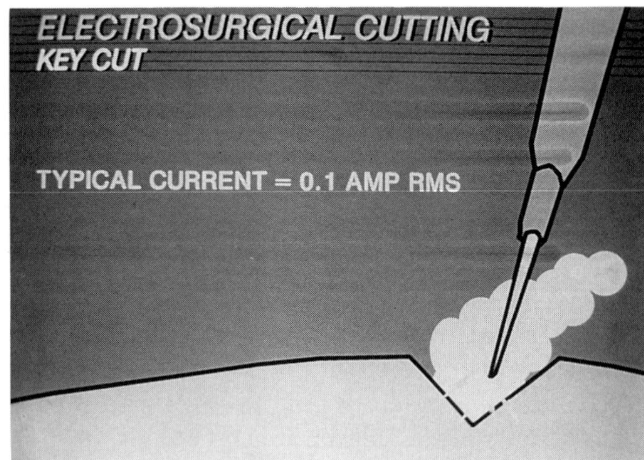

Figure 5-5 Activation of the electrode prior to touching the tissue produces a plume of vapor between the electrode and tissue, resulting in cutting with the least thermal damage.

frequency and low voltage with nonmodulated current. The extent of lateral damage observed with desiccation is reproduced in depth (Figure 5-6). Coaptive coagulation involves clamping a bleeding vessel with a conductive clamp and applying cutting current to coagulate and promote a collagen weld.

The ammeter of the electrogenerator is used to ascertain the end point of desiccation and assurance for hemostasis. The flowmeter measures the flow of electrons as they pass through the tissue contained between the electrodes and its intensity depends on the resistance of the tissue between the field of the forceps. Excessive heating or inadequate hemostasis can be noted using this device. Observing the tissue before it becomes charred and decreasing the pneumoperitoneum after transection of vessels to ensure hemostasis also are adequate.

Fulguration is superficial coagulation of small capillaries, usually over a large surface area, such as the ovarian capsule following cystectomy or a uterine defect following a myomectomy. An electrode is activated with modulated current and placed over the bleeding area without touching it (Figure 5-7). This type of current requires a high peak-to-peak voltage and produces intermittent sparks of electricity that strike the bleeding tissue, causing superficial coagulation. The sparks lose some of their energy as they travel through the air, but deeper desiccation is produced if the tissue is touched by the electrode. With fulguration, the risk of stray current from capacitive coupling or insulation failure is increased.

Electrosurgery provides the surgeon with a wide range of options: types of waveform, wattage, unipolar or bipolar systems, and various electrodes. With the proper equipment and an understanding of the electrosurgical principles, electrosurgery is useful therapeutically.[1]

Bipolar forceps are safer than monopolar instruments. At present, bipolar is used mainly for coagulation and desiccation, but with future technology, bipolar will be capable of cutting and vaporizing tissue. The current bipolar scissors do not have significant advantages over available alternatives.

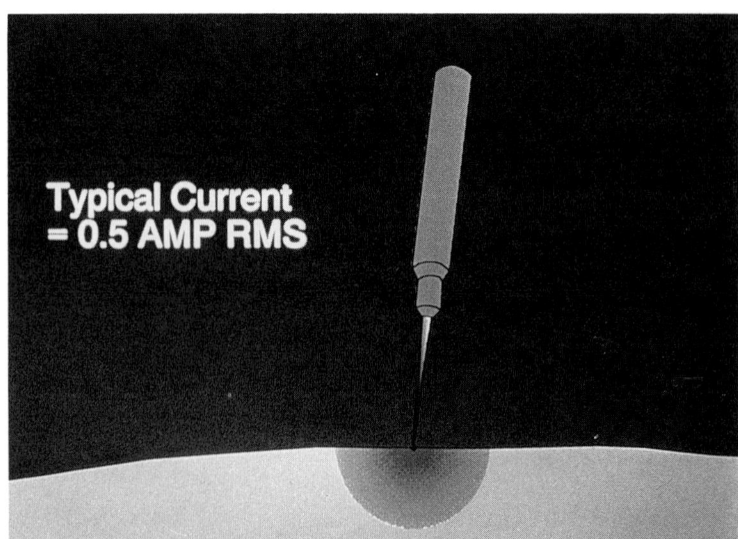

Figure 5-6 The extent of lateral damage observed with desiccation is exactly reproduced in depth.

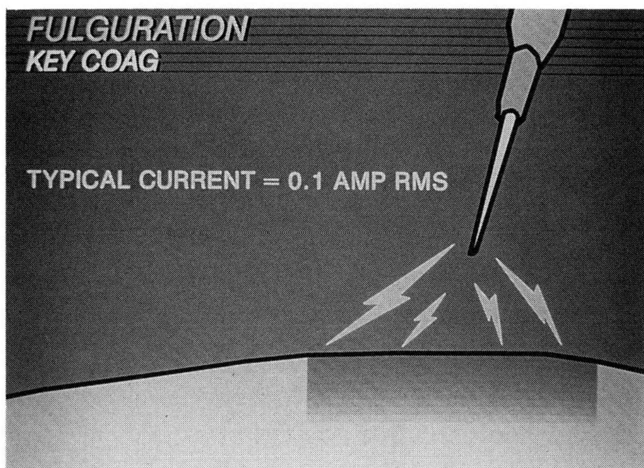

Figure 5-7 An electrode, activated with coagulating current, is placed over the bleeding area, without touching it.

Laparoscopic Ultrasonic Surgery

Ultrasonic surgery is the rapid mechanical vibration of a metal surgical tip. As the vibrating tip contacts tissue, cellular collapse occurs through the process of cavitation. Ultimately, the pressure differentials become so great that cellular implosions occur. Ultrasonic devices were used initially by dentists as the Cavitron dental scalar to clean tartar and plaque. In this situation, the rapidly vibrating tip strips away tartar and plaque, leaving teeth and gums unaffected.

Another application of ultrasonic technology was the phacoemulsifier used by ophthalmologists to remove lenses from patients undergoing cataract extraction. The rapidly vibrating tip fragments and aspirates unwanted lens material. It was not until the mid 1970s that a full-powered ultrasonic surgical aspirator, known as the CUSA (Cavitational Ultrasonic Surgical Aspirator), was used by neurosurgeons in the removal of intracranial tumors. More recently the CUSA has been applied by surgical and gynecologic oncologists during operative laparoscopy.

The CUSA consists of a console that regulates the amplitude or intensity, an operative handpiece connected to the console, and a foot pedal to activate the system. The functional end of the handpiece consists of a hollow titanium tip that moves in and out (longitudinally) of the tissue at 23,000 Hz. This action fragments and removes tissue within a 1- to 2-cm radius of the vibrating tip. The amplitude setting on the console corresponds to the excursion of the tip into the tissue and therefore to the depth of tissue disruption. A setting of 1 produces cellular fragmentation to a depth of 30 μm, at 5 to a depth of 150 μm, and at 10 to a depth of 300 μm. The operative field is irrigated continuously with normal saline through the functioning tip, thus reducing the heat produced by the vibrating tip and suspending tissue fragments to allow their aspiration through the hollow tip. The specimen is collected in a filter trap and sent for cytopathologic and histopathologic examination. The CUSA simultaneously fragments, irrigates, and aspirates through the functional tip. All three activities are controlled from the front of the console.

The vibrating tip selectively fragments and removes tissue with high water content and spares tissue with high collagen content such as blood vessels, nerves, and ductal structures.[4,5] This selectivity is ascertained by the rate at which different tissues are fragmented. The selectivity of the ultrasonic aspirator provides visual and tactile feedback so that the surgeon sees and feels structures as they present themselves in the surgical field. By gently applying differing amounts of pressure, the tip dissects unwanted tissue from vital structures without risk of perforation or damage.

Ultrasonic surgical aspiration is not hemostatic but electrosurgical capabilities, such as cutting and coagulation currents, are administered from the vibrating tip. The combination of rapid, selective ultrasonic tissue dissection with electrosurgical cutting and coagulation offers a unique synergistic effect with the added advantage of hemostatic control. With the introduction of a laparoscopic handpiece in 1992, ultrasonic dissection became feasible. The 31.2-cm extended laparoscopic tip is attached to a standard autoclavable CUSA handpiece. The laparoscopic tip is used with the electrosurgical accessory. The laparoscopic tip will fit through most 10-mm trocar cannulas. The CUSA provides selective tissue dissection without the use of heat, and it can provide precise tissue dissection with minimal trauma to surrounding tissues. However, if hemostasis is needed, the built-in electrosurgical energy source is activated. Additionally, laparoscopic ultrasonic dissection affords improved views since there is no plume or monitor interference, and reduced intraoperative blood loss.

Laparoscopic ultrasonic surgery provides safety and precision. Laparoscopic ultrasonic dissection has been used for laparoscopic cholecystectomy, bowel resection, liver and kidney biopsies, pelvic lymph node dissections, myoma resection, vagotomy, adhesion dissection, hernia repair, ovarian cyst resection, and endometriosis.

Safe Use of Electrosurgery

Electrosurgical energy has been used during laparotomy for more than 50 years. Potential problems are associated with the laparoscopic use of electrosurgical energy because it is passed through cannulas and long insulated active electrodes which can change its physics.

Problems can result from insulation failure, direct coupling of current, and capacitive coupling.

Insulation Failure

Insulation failure is caused by damage to the insulation during reprocessing or the use of high-voltage coagulation current. The breaks in the insulation provide an alternative pathway for the current to leave the electrode as it completes the circuit to the return electrode. If the generator is being activated while the portion of the electrode with defective insulation encounters adjacent tissue, the current can complete the circuit by jumping from the electrode, through the insulation break to adjacent tissue. If the point of exit is small, current density can be high enough to produce significant tissue damage outside the surgeon's field of vision and can go undetected.

Intact insulation can be broken during the operation and is most likely to occur with coagulation current. Coagulation current was designed primarily to fulgurate. Fulguration is "spray" coagulation through the high impedance of air. Such a current has a very high level of voltage, sometimes more than 10,000 V. This high voltage can push the current through the otherwise intact insulation. High-voltage coagulation current can blow holes in otherwise intact insulation. If the breakage touches a small amount of tissue, significant current densities may result in full-thickness burns of bowel or other vital structures.

To avoid open circuit activation, do not activate the generator until the active electrode is near to or touching the target tissue. The high impedance created by the open circuit is interpreted by the generator as a need to increase the voltage because the generator tries to provide enough voltage to push the current to the intended target tissue to complete the circuit. Maximal voltage is built up throughout the length of the active electrode and may be high enough to blow a hole through the insulation. By doing so, the current has found a way to complete the circuit to the return electrode. The laparoscopist has no way of controlling the current density of this exit point.

To eliminate these potential hazards, inspect the insulation or instrument for small cracks and defects and use the cut waveform whenever possible. The cut waveform is lower in voltage and it can be used to coagulate when the electrode contacts with tissue. Make sure the generator is able to complete the circuit through the target tissue. This will make "blowing holes" in insulation next to impossible and even when holes are present, it will be unlikely that the current will find these defects to be the path of least resistance.

Direct Coupling of Current

Direct coupling of current is defined as the unintended contact of the energized active electrode with another metal instrument or object within the abdomen. Never activate the electrode while it is touching or close to another metal object. Three potential problems arise from direct coupling. Sparking to metal clips could cause necrosis of underlying tissue and clips can fall off the vessel as the tissue begins to slough. Metal-to-metal sparking can cause frequency demodulation. This demodulation is noticed as neuromuscular stimulation of surrounding muscles. Third, metal-to-metal sparking can cause current to flow to unintended sites. If the electrode is activated while touching the laparoscope, the metal laparoscope may become energized. To complete the circuit to the return electrode, the current dissipates through the relatively large surface area between the laparoscope and the abdominal wall, and likelihood for damage is small. However, if the laparoscope is insulated from the abdominal wall by a plastic collar, the current finds another point of exit from the laparoscope to complete the circuit. The degree of tissue damage is related directly to the amount of current density. A large point of contact has a low current density and no tissue damage should occur. However, if the energized laparoscope touches a small area of tissue, a high current density results and thermal injury is more likely.

To avoid direct coupling, the electrosurgical generator is not activated while the electrode touches or is near another piece of metal. Capacitively coupled current is the inducement of currents through the intact insulation of electrodes to surrounding cannulas or instruments and are increased with high-voltage coagulation current, more than low-voltage cutting current. Activating the generator in open circuit increases the probability that capacitance will occur. In addition, by isolating the electrosurgical instrument from the abdominal wall by nonconductor, the possibility for thermal injury is increased. The smaller the cannula and the longer the electrode, the greater the potential for capacitance.

Monopolar current is used during laparoscopy because it is effective, versatile, and relatively safe. The guidelines listed below can reduce the incidence of thermal injury.

1. Inspect insulation in electrosurgical instruments for defects.
2. Avoid metal-to-metal sparking (direct coupling).
3. Use the cut waveform whenever possible. The cutting current uses less voltage, thereby reducing the likelihood of causing defects in insulation.
4. Activate the generator only as the electrode touches the tissue because capacitance is minimal during a closed circuit. Even with defective insulation the current will use the tissue as the pathway of choice.
5. Use either *all* metal or *all* plastic for the operative channel. All-metal systems allow safe dispersement of capacitively coupled current through the abdominal wall and all-plastic systems eliminate capacitors.
6. Use the lowest power setting to achieve the desired results to reduce the likelihood of insulation failure, capacitance, and thermal injury.

References

1. Levy BS, Soderstrom RM, Dail DH. Bowel injury during laparoscopy: gross anatomy and histology. *J Reprod Med.* 1985;30:168.
2. Soderstrom RM. Preventing adhesions—electrosurgery: advantages and disadvantages. In: DiZerega GS, Malinak LR, Diamond MP, Linsky CB, eds. *Progress in Clinical and Biological Research.* vol. 358. New York: Wiley-Liss Publishers; 1990:59.
3. Soderstrom RM. Electrosurgery's advantages and disadvantages. *Contemp Ob/Gyn.* 1990; 35:35.
4. Addonizio JC, Choudhury MS. Cavitrons in urologic surgery. *Urol Clin North Am.* 1986;13:445.
5. Hurst BS, Awoniyi CA, Stephens JK, et al. Application of the cavitron ultrasonic surgical aspirator (CUSA) for gynecological laparoscopic surgery using the rabbit as an animal model. *Fertil Steril.* 1992;58:444.

6

Comparative Studies with Electrosurgery and Lasers

Since their introduction to gynecologic surgery, lasers have been purported to be superior to electrosurgery and scissors because lasers are allegedly less traumatic, more precise, and associated with reduced postoperative adhesions.[1–5] The results published from experiments in animals[6–11] and clinical trials in patients[12–18] do not always support these claims. In addition, lasers are usually expensive and not without hazards.[19]

Early Studies

The initial studies comparing tissue effects of electrosurgery and lasers used electrosurgical generators and electrodes intended for coagulation or tissue destruction.[2,3,8] Some results indicated that the laser was superior although other reports claimed that the two energy forms had similar tissue effects and healing patterns.[6,9–11] The important determinants of tissue effects for CO_2 laser and electrosurgery are similar (Table 6-1).

In one experiment, twenty sexually mature female rabbits underwent bilateral ovarian wedge resection and uterine segmental resection using standard microsurgical techniques with the CO_2 laser or electrosurgery, and microsurgical anastomosis with 8-0 polyglactin sutures (Figure 6-1).[9] To ensure the optimal use of each surgical instrument, similar power densities were used for electrosurgery and the CO_2 laser, so that the desired tissue vaporization was obtained with both energy sources. The removed ovarian wedges and the uterine segments were evaluated histologically to assess the extent of acute thermal damage beyond the line of incision. To evaluate and compare the healing pattern and adhesion formation that followed each technique in the presence or absence of suture material, each uterine horn was subjected to a single transverse and two longitudinal incisions, one loosely approximated with 8-0 polyglactin sutures and the other not sutured. Four weeks later, the animals were euthanized, the abdomen was opened, and the adhesions were graded by the same observer. Fibrosis at the injury sites with and without sutures after laser and electrosurgery was assessed histologically.

The results obtained from these studies are summarized in Tables 6-2 through 6-4. There was no difference in the depth of thermal damage, extent of collagen deposition, or postoperative adhesion formation between CO_2 laser and electrosurgery at any site. These data support the concept that the power density is the major determinant of tissue penetration and thermal damage and that comparable power densities for the CO_2 laser and electrosurgery probably will produce similar results. Interestingly, thermal damage was significantly greater to the uterus than the ovary, suggesting that the ovaries are less susceptible to thermal injury than the uterus, regardless of the energy source used.

Racette and colleagues reported that ovarian incision with the CO_2 laser inflicted more damage to oocytes than either electrosurgery or scalpel.[20] Luciano and coworkers evaluated the relative damage to ovarian follicles and the consequences on ovarian function when a surgical incision was

TABLE 6-1 Determinants of Tissue Effects of Electrosurgery and CO_2 Laser

Electrosurgery	Laser
1. Size and shape of electrode	1. Spot size
2. Power (watts)	2. Power (watts)
3. Peak-to-peak voltage	3. Pulse mode
4. Output impedance	4. Tissue absorption

made on the ovary with scalpel, CO_2 laser, or microelectrode.[10] Thirty sexually mature female rabbits were randomly assigned to one of three surgical groups. The injury consisted of a linear incision along the entire long axis of both ovaries, from the cortex to the hilum. One ovary was removed and fixed immediately for histologic evaluation of the acute tissue damage to the follicular apparatus, oocytes, and stromal cells. The other ovary was left in situ to evaluate subsequent healing, steroidogenesis, folliculogenesis, ovulation, and ovum pickup. Blood samples were assessed weekly for estradiol and progesterone concentrations. Two weeks postoperatively, the remaining ovary was removed from five animals of each group, cut in 10-μm sections and histologically evaluated for stromal and follicular morphology. Five other animals were injected with human chorionic gonadotropin (hCG) and 18 hours later subjected to salpingo-oophorectomy to assess ovarian histology and to count the number of corpora lutea and ovulated eggs.

Histologic evaluation revealed minimal (0.041 mm) but equal tissue damage along the incision made by the laser and microelectrodes. The laser and electrical incisions had straight, sharp edges as opposed to the uneven incision line made by the scalpel. No architectural disruption of the ovary was evident in the acute or healed specimens. The follicular apparatus and the oocytes, unless transected by the surgical instrument, showed no difference among the three surgical groups. Postoperatively, the mean adhesion scores were the same for the three groups. Steroidogenesis was normal and similar among the three groups. The progesterone levels 8 hours after hCG administration, the number of antral follicles, number of corpora lutea on the remaining ovary, and the number of oocytes collected in the oviduct from each of the three study groups are summarized in Table 6-5. Except that more oocytes were found in the oviduct of the electrosurgical group, no differences were noted among any of the parameters studied. The ova that did not appear in the oviduct were found at histologic evaluation entrapped in unruptured luteinized follicles, usually covered by thin, microscopic adhesions, which formed just above the ruptured, luteinized follicle with the entrapped oocytes. These findings confirm previous studies that showed acute injury, subsequent healing, steroidogenesis, folliculogenesis, and ovum pickup by the oviduct do not differ following ovarian incision by microscalpel, CO_2 laser, or microelectrode. Moreover, finding the entrapped oocytes within partially ruptured corpora lutea covered by microscopic adhesions emphasizes the role that periovarian adhesions may play in oocyte release and perhaps infertility.

Further studies were conducted to ascertain the advantages of lasers over electrosurgery at operative laparoscopy. Thirty rabbits underwent surgical procedures to create extensive intraperitoneal adhesions.[11] Then the animals were assigned randomly to undergo laparoscopic adhesiolysis using electrosurgery, CO_2 laser, or neodymium-yttrium

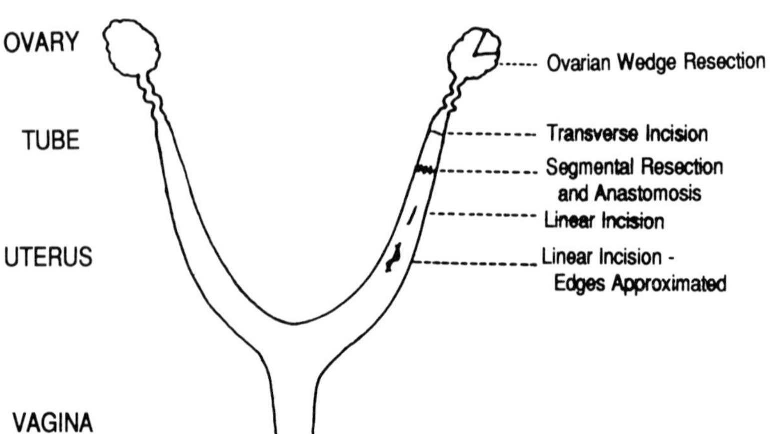

Figure 6-1 Operative procedure. The procedure was performed bilaterally, using only the CO_2 laser or electrosurgery for each side, randomly, and at comparable power densities.

TABLE 6-2 Mean (±SD) Depth of Thermal Injury on the Ovarian and Uterine Tissues Immediately Following Resection*

	Ovary	Uterus
	mm	mm
CO_2	0.041 ± 0.02	0.16 ± 0.04 $P = .007$
Electrosurgery	0.041 ± 0.02	0.095 ± 0.01 $P < .05$

*Depth of thermal injury was significantly greater on the uterus than the ovary with either CO_2 laser or electrosurgery. No difference was observed in the extent of thermal damage between the CO_2 laser and electrosurgery on either the ovarian or uterine tissue.

aluminum garnet (Nd-YAG) laser exclusively for the assigned group. Each instrument was used at its optimal power density. Changes in adhesion scores, the depth of thermal injury to ovarian and uterine tissues, and the speed at which each instrument transected various segments of the uterine horn were compared among the groups. All three modalities significantly and equally reduced intraperitoneal adhesions by approximately 50% (Table 6-6). The depth of thermal injury was three times higher with the Nd-YAG laser compared to electrosurgery and the CO_2 laser on ovarian and uterine tissue. The transection speed across the uterine horn was slower with the Nd-YAG than either CO_2 laser or electrosurgery. The results at operative laparoscopy are similar to those at laparotomy, confirming the concept that the CO_2 laser and electrosurgery, when optimally used at comparable power densities, exert similar tissue effects.

TABLE 6-3 Width of Fibrosis at the Site of Injury 4 Weeks Postoperatively

	CO_2 Laser*	Electrosurgery*
	mm	mm
Transverse incision	0.96 ± 0.25	0.97 ± 0.4
Site of anastomosis	1.73 ± 0.3	0.96 ± 0.3
Longitudinal incision† with suture	0.76 ± 0.4	0.80 ± 0.2
Longitudinal incision† without suture	1.6 ± 0.4	1.6 ± 0.2

*Differences insignificant (P > .05) for laser versus electrosurgery for all sites.

†Statistically significant (P < .05). Wider areas of fibrosis when edges not approximated in either CO_2 laser or electrosurgery group.

Although the Nd-YAG laser was found to be equally effective at laparoscopic adhesiolysis, it caused more tissue damage and was less efficient at incising tissue than either CO_2 laser or electrosurgery, despite the application of the small sapphire tip, which yielded a higher power density than either the CO_2 laser or electrosurgery. Power density alone does not explain the different tissue effects of the Nd-YAG laser. Increased thermal damage was found when the tissue was incised at slower speed.[11,21] It is possible that thermal damage reflects the duration of tissue exposed to laser energy. This finding is consistent with the decreased thermal effects of the superpulse CO_2 laser and cutting electrical current. The total duration of tissue exposure to the laser or electrical energy is less than the continuous or blended delivery modes.

The less efficient cutting ability of the Nd-YAG laser is caused by its selective absorption by pigmented tissues and lack of absorption (reflection) by clear tissues. The unpigmented tissue fibers transmit rather than absorb the laser energy and are not vaporized or severed until heated by adjacent pigmented tissue. Contact between the laser energy and tissue is prolonged, resulting in greater thermal damage.

TABLE 6-4 Mean (±SD) Scores of Postoperative Adhesions at the Site of Surgery with CO_2 Laser or Electrosurgery

	CO_2 Laser	Electrosurgery
Ovary	1.7 ± 1.3	1.6 ± 1.9
Transverse incision	1.8 ± 1.3	1.6 ± 1.9
Site of anastomosis	1.2 ± 1.1	1.75 ± 1.2
Longitudinal incision with suture	1.1 ± 1.0	1.2 ± 1.0
Longitudinal incision without suture	1.7 ± 1	1.2 ± 1.0

TABLE 6-5 Serum Progesterone Level, Number of Antral Follicles, Number of Corpora Lutea, and Number of Ova in the Oviduct of Animals From Three Surgical Groups

	Scalpel	CO_2 Laser 58,964 (W/cm²)	Electrosurgery 88,888 (W/cm²)
Progesterone after hCG ng%	2.5 ± 5	1.9 ± 3	2.8 ± 6
Number of antral follicles in each ovary	33 ± 3.3	28 ± 3.3	32 ± 4.5
Number of corpora lutea in each ovary	4.4 ± 0.8	6.5 ± 0.8	6.8 ± 0.6
Number of ova in the tube	2 ± 0.8*	4 ± 0.8*	7 ± 1.2

*$P < .01$ indicates significant difference between number of corpora lutea and ova found in the ipsilateral oviduct.

The results from these studies show no difference in the outcome of the treatment of periadnexal adhesions with CO_2 laser and electrosurgery.[5,22] The intra-abdominal laser study group, which includes several gynecologic laser surgeons in North America, reported in 1984 that "nonlaser infertility surgery appeared to have equal or greater efficacy in the prevention of adhesion formation at most sites. Thus the CO_2 laser does not appear to be a panacea for the treatment of tuboperitoneal causes of infertility."[5,23] In 1986, this same group reported ". . . that use of CO_2 laser for neosalpingostomy at laparotomy with early second look laparoscopy provides a term pregnancy rate similar to that previously achieved by nonlaser microsurgical techniques. . . ."[22] The earlier studies by Bellina[2] and Chong and Baggish[13] suggesting that the CO_2 laser may be more effective than electrosurgery in tubal reconstructive surgery and in endometriosis, respectively, were neither randomized nor controlled and should be considered anecdotal. In prospective controlled studies by Tulandi and Vilos, randomized infertile patients scheduled to undergo adhesiolysis and tubo-ovarian reconstruction showed no difference in either postoperative adhesion formation or pregnancy rates between the CO_2 laser and the electromicrosurgery groups.[17,18]

When optimally used, lasers, microelectrodes, and mechanical instruments are equally effective in gynecologic surgery and perhaps in any surgery, whether performed by laparoscopy or laparotomy. The choice and preference should be based on the instrument with which the surgeon has the most experience or skill for a particular procedure. These instruments are used to ablate, coagulate, cut, or dissect.

The most effective use of the CO_2 laser beam is through the operative channel of the laparoscope as a "long knife." The beam does not obstruct the view and allows delicate dissection. Further, the area to be treated may be effectively contained by water, reducing the risk of thermal damage.[24] The CO_2 laser may be used to safely and thoroughly operate with high precision near sensitive areas like bowel, bladder, ureter, and blood vessels.

References

1. Baggish MS, ElBakry MM. Comparison of electronic super pulsed continuous wave CO_2 laser in the rat uterine horn. *Fertil Steril.* 1986; 45:120.

TABLE 6-6 Reduction of Peritoneal Adhesions, Depth of Thermal Injury, and Speed of Transection of Each Surgical Modality Used at Operative Laparoscopy

	Electrosurgery 66,666 (W/cm²)	CO_2 Laser 6000 (W/cm²)	Nd-YAG laser 75,000 (W/cm²)
Reduction of adhesions	−61%	−57%	−44%
Depth (μm) of thermal injury on uterus	102 ± 11.3	109.9 ± 6.5	358.4 ± 42*
Depth (μm) of thermal injury on ovary	43.7 ± 2.6	41.7 ± 4.1	175.6 ± 45*
Time (s) to transect uterine horn	1.5 ± 0.2	1.4 ± 0.2	2.60 ± 0.4*

*$P < .001$ signifies differences compared to electrosurgery and CO_2 laser.

2. Bellina JF. Microsurgery of the fallopian tube with the carbon dioxide laser: analysis of 230 cases with a 2 year follow-up. *Laser Surg Med.* 1983;3:255.
3. Bellina JH, Hemmings R, Voros IJ, et al. Carbon dioxide laser and electrosurgical wound study with an animal model. A comparison of tissue damage and healing patterns in peritoneal tissue. *Am J Obstet Gynecol.* 1984; 148:327.
4. Daniel JF, Brown DH. Carbon dioxide laser laparoscopy: initial experience in animals and humans. *Obstet Gynecol.* 1982;159:761.
5. Diamond MP, Daniel JF, Martin DC, et al. Tubal patency and pelvic adhesions at early second look laparoscopy following intraabdominal use of the carbon dioxide laser: initial report of the intraabdominal study laser group. *Fertil Steril.* 1984;42:717.
6. Filmar S, Gomel V, McComb P. The effectiveness of CO_2 laser and electromicrosurgery in adhesiolysis: a comparative study. *Fertil Steril.* 1986;45:407.
7. Filmar S, Jetha N, McComb P, et al. A comparative histologic study on the healing process after tissue transaction I. Carbon dioxide laser and electromicrosurgery. *Am J Obstet Gynecol.* 1989;160:1062.
8. Pittaway DE, Maxson WAS, Daniell JF. A comparison of the CO_2 laser and electrocautery on postoperative intraperitoneal adhesion formation in rabbits. *Fertil Steril.* 1983;40:366.
9. Luciano AA, Whitman G, Maier DB, et al. A comparison of thermal injury healing patterns and postoperative adhesion formation in rabbits. *Fertil Steril.* 1983;40:366.
10. Luciano AA, Marana R, Kratka S, et al. Ovarian function after incision of the ovary by scalpel, CO_2 laser and microelectrode. *Fertil Steril.* 1991;56:349.
11. Luciano AA, Frishman GN, Maier DB, et al. A comparative analysis of adhesion reduction, tissue effects and incising characteristics of electrosurgery, CO_2 laser and Nd-YAG laser at operative laparoscopy. *J Laparoendoscopic Surg.* 1993;2:305.
12. Bruhat H, Mage C, Manhes M. Use of the CO_2 laser via laparoscopy. In: Kaplan I, ed. *Laser Surgery III.* Proceedings of the Third International Society for Laser Surgery. Tel Aviv: 1979:275.
13. Chong AP, Baggish MS. Management of pelvis endometriosis by means of intraabdominal carbon dioxide laser. *Fertil Steril.* 1984;41:14.
14. Keye WR, Hansen LW, Astin M, et al. Argon laser therapy of endometriosis: a review of 92 consecutive patients. *Fertil Steril.* 1987;47:208.
15. Mage G, Bruhat MA. Pregnancy following salpingostomy: comparison between CO_2 laser and electrosurgery procedures. *Fertil Steril.* 1983;40:472.
16. Nezhat C, Winer WK, Nezhat F. A comparison of the CO_2 argon, and KTP/532 laser in the videolaseroscopic treatment of endometriosis. *Colposcopy Gynecol Laser Surg.* 1988;4:41.
17. Tulandi T, Vilos GA. A comparison between laser surgery and electrosurgery for bilateral hydrosalpinx: a 2 year follow-up. *Fertil Steril.* 1985;44:846.
18. Tulandi T. Salpingo-ovariolysis: a comparison between laser surgery and electrosurgery. *Fertil Steril.* 1986;45:48.
19. Nezhat C, Winder WK, Nezhat F, et al. Smoke from laser surgery; is there a health hazard? *Laser Surg Med.* 1987;7:376.
20. Racette N, Filmar S, Jetha N, et al. The viability of oocytes after incision of the ovary by CO_2 laser, microelectrode and scalpel. Presented at the 44th Annual Meeting of The American Fertility Society, Atlanta, Georgia, October 10–13, 1988. Published by the American Fertility Society in the Program Supplement 1988:S50. Abstract PO-18.
21. Joffe SN, Brackett KA, Sankar MY, et al. Resection of the liver with Nd-YAG laser. *Surg Gynecol Obstet.* 1986;163:437.
22. Diamond MP, Daniell SF, Feste J, et al. Adhesion reformation and de novo formation after reproductive pelvic surgery. *Fertil Steril.* 1987;47:864.
23. Nezhat C, Crowgey S, Garrison C. Surgical treatment of endometriosis via laser laparoscopy. *Fertil Steril.* 1986;45:778.
24. Nezhat C, Nezhat F, Nezhat CH. Operative laparoscopy (minimally invasive surgery): state of the art. *J Gynecol Surg.* 1992;8:111.

7

Anesthesia

Most women having laparoscopic surgery are young and in good health; however, as endoscopic procedures increase and applications expand, these characteristics will not always prevail. The factors involved in advanced operative laparoscopy that can compromise the patient intraoperatively are important. This chapter describes the general guidelines regarding anesthesia specific to operative laparoscopy.

Preoperative Evaluation and Preparation

Some patients undergoing laparoscopy will have had a previous experience with anesthesia. Women who had postoperative nausea, vomiting, or other complications may be quite anxious. Meeting the anesthesiologist preoperatively will allay some of the patient's anxiety.[1–4] If necessary, anxiolytics or sedatives are prescribed for the night before surgery.[5,6]

A complete blood count, electrolyte analysis, and urinalysis are obtained routinely. Unless specifically indicated by prior disease or age over 40 years, routine chest radiography and electrocardiogram (ECG) are not required. If significant blood loss is anticipated, the patient is encouraged to arrange autologous blood donation. An intraoperative cell saver can be planned preoperatively if the patient is anemic and is not a suitable candidate for autologous transfusion. The patient is instructed not to eat or drink after midnight before surgery.

A frequent disorder in women of reproductive age is mitral valve prolapse.[7,8] Ampicillin (2 g) and gentamicin (80 mg), or vancomycin if she has a penicillin allergy, are prescribed preoperatively. A preoperative ECG is not required unless the patient is symptomatic. If she is taking a prescribed β blocker (eg, Inderal), it is continued preoperatively, including the morning of the operation.[9]

Preinduction Medications

Once intravenous fluids are started, midazolam (Versed) is given in 1-mg increments until the patient is calm.[10] If needed, a narcotic is added to the sedation regimen,[11,12] but postoperative nausea and vomiting and respiratory depression can result.[13] Sufentanil (Sufenta) in 5-μg increments or morphine in 1- to 2-mg increments can be added to midazolam. Demerol can be equally effective. The goal is a calm and unafraid patient.

Anesthetic Considerations Specific to Laparoscopy

The management of general anesthesia for laparoscopic procedure is associated with three factors usually absent from laparotomy: steep Trendelenburg position, high-pressure insufflation of the abdomen with CO_2, and intraoperative irrigation with lactated Ringer's solution. The head down positioning shifts intestinal weight against the diaphragm, compromising full diaphragmatic excursion and optimal ventilation (Figure 7-1). Moreover, it has significant effects on cardiovascular function (Figure 7-2). Accumulation of irrigating solution in the abdominal cavity against the dia-

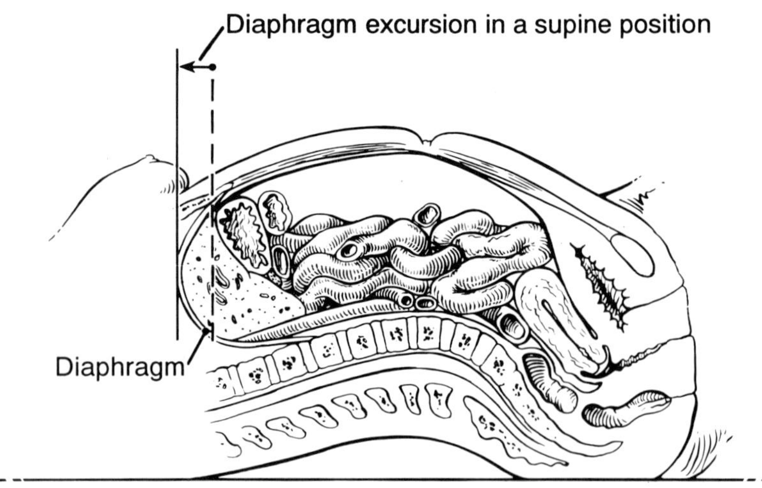

Figure 7-1 Note effect on diaphragm after repositioning of abdominal contents with Trendelenburg position.

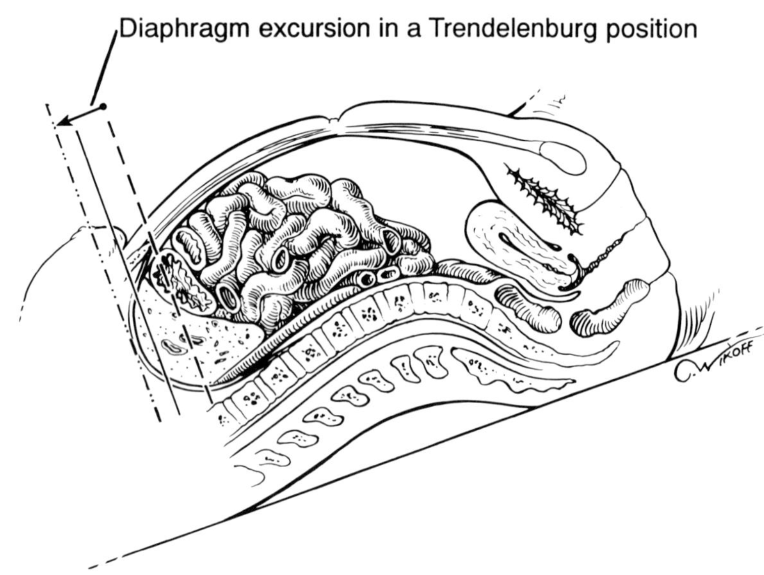

Figure 7-2 Effect of position and CO_2 insufflation on pH and P_{CO_2} is noted.

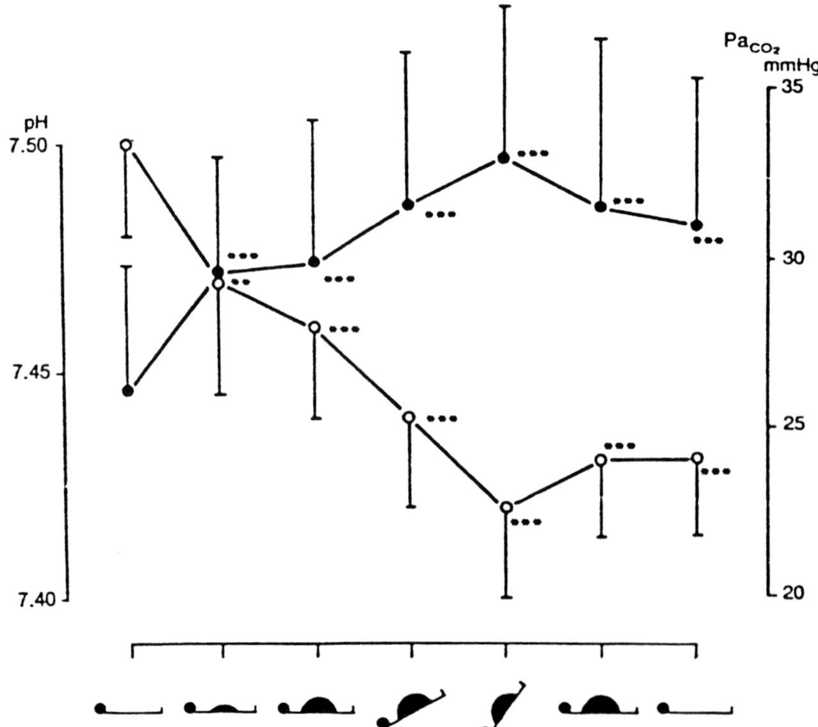

Figure 7-3 Effect of position and establishment of pneumoperitoneum on cardiovascular measurements is seen.

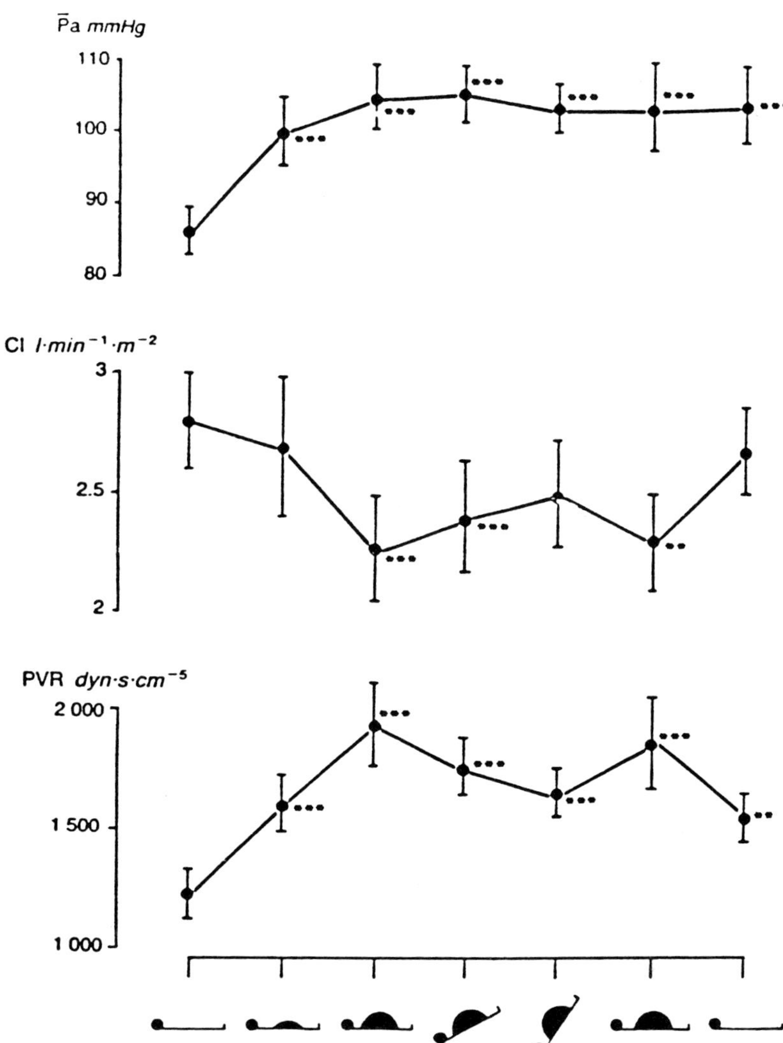

phragm further reduces ventilation. CO_2 not only generates a visceral sensation of abdominal and thoracic pressure, but also elevates the patient's P_{CO_2} (Figure 7-3). Based on these factors and the need for muscle relaxation, general anesthesia with controlled ventilation through an endotracheal tube is required.

Despite the constraints that laparoscopic operations place on anesthetic management, Bridenbaugh[14] reported good results with epidural anesthesia. A combination of rectus sheath block with general anesthesia has been advocated.[15] Although regional anesthesia may allay the fears of patients who want to avoid general anesthesia, these women often require so much sedation and attention during the procedure that the adequacy and safety of the surgical procedure may be diminished.

All patients have a single-lead ECG (usually lead II), a Dinamapp to monitor blood pressure, a pulse oximeter to follow hemoglobin/O_2 saturation, a combined esophageal stethoscope with a thermometer (placed after induction), a nerve stimulator, and an in-line oxygen analyzer with a disconnect alarm as part of the anesthesia machine. In addition, a mass spectrometer with capnograph capabilities is used on all patients.

Induction and Maintenance

Once all monitors are applied in the operating room, induction is begun. Although thiopental sodium (Pentothal) is still the most common induction agent, some anesthesiologists prefer propofol. This drug has proven effective for outpatient procedures because of its rapid onset of action, distribution, and elimination.[16,17] The drug possesses a short half-life and some antiemetic qualities.[18] Unconsciousness follows within 30 to 45 seconds in a manner similar to the natural onset of sleep. This agent lends itself to a continuous infusion technique for short procedures as the primary anesthetic.[19] Patients frequently are awake at the conclusion of surgery, often with a euphoric sensation. Morphine or sufentanil (Sufenta) are the narcotics primarily used, although Demerol is a reasonable substitute.

Muscle relaxation can be achieved in several ways. Some anesthesiologists prefer the depolarizing agent succinylcholine (Anectine). Its rapid action allows tracheal manipulation soon after induction. However, the reports of postoperative myalgias associated with the use of succinylcholine raised questions regarding its appropriateness in an ambulatory setting.[20] Atracurium (Tracrium), 0.5 mg/kg, and vecuronium (Norcuron), 0.1 mg/kg, are nondepolarizing agents of intermediate duration that provide relaxation that extends into the surgical procedure. Continued anesthesia can be maintained by additional increments of these drugs.

Intraoperative muscle paralysis is only possible with controlled ventilation. Adjustments in the ventilatory rate can control the hypercarbia that results from absorption of the insufflated CO_2 (see Figure 7-2). Depending on the amount of CO_2 absorbed, hyperventilation may be indicated. The end-tidal CO_2 of all patients is followed and ventilation adjusted to maintain a normal value.

Anesthetic maintenance is accomplished with 70% N_2O, 30% O_2, and 1% to 1.5% isoflurane (Forane). The combination of isoflurane with a propofol induction proves satisfactory.[21] Narcotic adjuvants may be used. Enflurane rather than isoflurane, or a propofol infusion, may be used. Narcotic infusions have been used with satisfactory results.

Spontaneous intestinal activity during the surgical procedure can make proper exposure of the operative field difficult. In addition, the use of N_2O for anesthetic maintenance may compound the problem because of the potential expansion of bowel gas by N_2O.[22] To overcome this effect, air is often substituted for N_2O. Further, some studies have implicated the use of N_2O with increased postoperative nausea and vomiting.

Before extubation, the patient's stomach is emptied with an orogastric tube. Muscle relaxation is reversed with neostigmine (3 mg) and glycopyrrolate (0.6 mg) or equivalent agents. Because of concerns about postoperative nausea and vomiting, the routine use of preoperative and intraoperative narcotics has been questioned (Figure 7-4). Ketorolac (Toradol) 60 mg intramuscularly, a parenteral nonsteroidal anti-inflammatory drug (NSAID), may be administered perioperatively for prophylactic pain management.

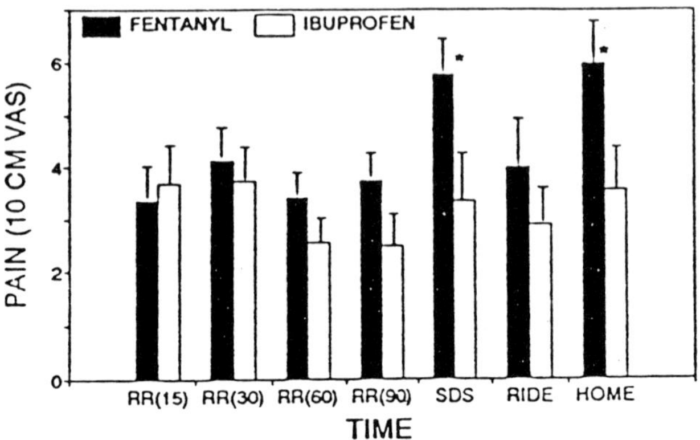

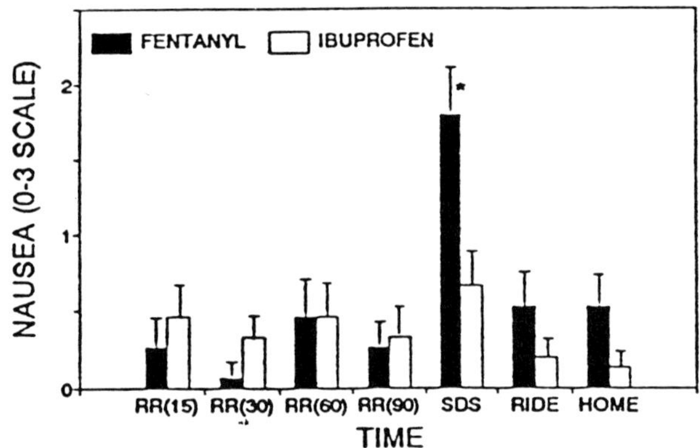

Figure 7-4A Comparison of fentanyl and ibuprofen on postoperative pain and nausea is seen.

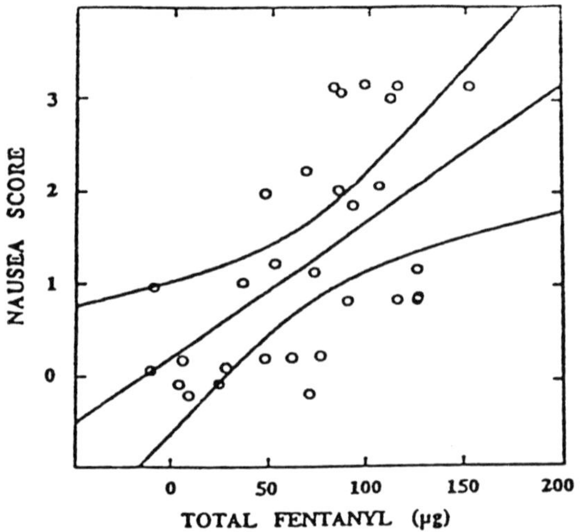

Figure 7-4B Relationship between total perioperative dose of fentanyl and nausea is noted.

Intraoperative Complications

Various arrhythmias have been associated with laparoscopy, including junctional rhythms, bigeminy, and asystole.[23,24] Bradycardia has been detected during initial abdominal insufflation and develops more frequently in older patients. The insufflating gas generates pressure on the peritoneum, increasing vagal tone, and hypercarbia secondary to absorption of the insufflation gas may be implicated. Bradycardia rarely needs treatment. However, if blood pressure drops, atropine has proven effective in restoring vagal tone. CO_2 gas is immediately released and when the patient is reinsufflated, cardiac rate returns to normal.

The development of a CO_2 gas embolus is a rarely encountered emergency. It develops as a result of the CO_2 used for insufflation. Some apparent signs include a sudden drop in end-tidal CO_2, a drop in blood pressure, development of an arrhythmia, and a classic "mill-wheel murmur." Should such an event be suspected, the patient should be hyperventilated with 100% O_2 and given necessary cardiovascular support. If a central venous line is present, aspiration of the embolus should be attempted.

Pulmonary edema can result from aggressive fluid replacement or irrigating fluid absorption. Fluid management can be further complicated in gynecologic procedures in which large volumes of Hyskon or other vascular fluids are used during hysteroscopy. Pulmonary edema is prevented by monitoring fluid intake and output. Intraoperative diuretics are advisable if there is a large discrepancy between fluid input and output or with a continued rise in thoracic fluids. If a patient develops respiratory distress in the recovery room, pulmonary edema is considered. Rales coupled with classic chest radiographic findings will confirm the diagnosis. Often respiratory support, supplemental oxygen, and furosemide are required until fluid balance is restored.

Abdominal distention coupled with steep Trendelenburg position result in increased pressure on the stomach but no significant increased incidence of regurgitation has been demonstrated.[25]

Postanesthesia Recovery

Patients spend a minimum of an hour in the recovery room, where vital signs and O_2 saturation are monitored and supplemental O_2 is administered by mask or nasal prongs, as indicated. Adequately alert and oriented patients leave the recovery room for the short-stay facility where they are monitored for several hours before their intravenous fluids are discontinued.

Nausea is a frequent side effect of general anesthesia, although the incidence seems lower with the use of propofol and the avoidance of narcotics (see Figure 7-4B). If nausea persists in the recovery room, intravenous droperidol (Inapsine) is recommended. Intravenous metoclopramide 10 mg (Reglan) can be added if nausea persists.[26–30]

Regardless of efforts to expel the intra-abdominal CO_2 following a laparoscopic procedure, referred shoulder pain from gas collected under the diaphragm is a common postoperative problem.[31–33] Some patients describe chest wall pressure or restriction but generally the gas is absorbed in 24 to 48 hours. The patient may obtain fairly prompt relief by lying in a supine position with a pillow under the abdomen so that CO_2 collects in the pelvis and shoulder pain is minimized.

Intraoperative use of narcotics reduces the need for analgesia in the recovery room. Fentanyl is administered intravenously as needed during the recovery period. In the short-stay center, oral medications may be prescribed. NSAIDs are appropriate for postoperative pain management and may have significant advantages over narcotics (see Figure 7-4). Pain control is important and will reduce the incidence of nausea. However, all narcotics can cause nausea.

Parenterally, the NSAID ketorolac tromethamine (Toradol), is helpful.[34] For postoperative analgesia, it is best used as an intraoperative loading dose, followed by supplements as needed postoperatively. Initial loading dose recommendations are 30 to 60 mg intramuscularly or intravenously, followed by one half the loading dose as needed every 6 hours. (The parenteral form of this medication has not been approved for intravenous administration.) Because it is not a narcotic, the risk of respiratory depression is decreased. It is recommended primarily for short-term therapy because long-term use evokes the same concerns about gastrointestinal bleeding as other NSAIDs. Like other NSAIDs, it also decreases platelet aggregation.[34]

References

1. Lichtor JL, Johanson CE, Mhoon D, et al. Preoperative anxiety: does anxiety level the afternoon before surgery predict anxiety

level just before surgery? *Anesthesiology.* 1987;67:594.
2. Egbert LD, Battit GE, Turndorf H, et al. The value of the preoperative visit by the anesthetist. *JAMA.* 1963;185:553.
3. Leigh JM, Walker J, Janaganathan P. Effect of the anesthetist's preoperative outpatient visit on anxiety. *Br Med J.* 1977;2:987.
4. Roizen MF. Routine preoperative evaluation. In: Miller RD, ed. *Anesthesia.* New York: Churchill Livingstone; 1990:743.
5. Short TAG, Galletly DC. Double-blind comparisons of midazolam and temazepam as oral premedicants for outpatient anesthesia. *Anaesth Intensive Care.* 1989;17:151.
6. Hargreaves J. Benzodiazepine premedication in minor day case surgery: comparison of oral midazolam and temazepam with placebo. *Br J Anaesth.* 1988;61:611.
7. Lang S, Morris A. Infective endocarditis—current recommendations for prophylaxis. *Drugs.* 1987;34:279.
8. Clemens JD, Horwitz RI, Jaffe CC, et al. A controlled evaluation of the risk of bacterial endocarditis in persons with mitral valve prolapse. *N Engl J Med.* 1982;307:776.
9. Swartz MH, Teicholz LE, Donnoso F. Mitral valve prolapse: a review of associated arrhythmias. *Am J Med.* 1982;62:377.
10. White PF. The role of midazolam in outpatient anesthesia. *Anesth Rev.* 1985;125:55.
11. Shafer A, White PF, Urquhart ML, et al. Outpatient premedication: use of midazolam and opioid analgesics. *Anesthesiology.* 1989; 71:495.
12. White PF, Chang T: Effect of narcotic premedication on the intravenous anesthetic requirement. *Anesthesiology.* 1984;61:A389.
13. Rosenblum M, Weller RS, Conrad PL, et al. Ibuprofen provides longer lasting analgesia than fentanyl after laparoscopic surgery. *Anesth Analg.* 1991;73:255.
14. Bridenbaugh LD. Regional anesthesia for outpatient surgery: a summary of 12 years' experience. *Can Anaesth Soc J.* 1983; 30:548.
15. Smith BE, Such M, Sigh D, et al. Rectus sheath block for diagnostic laparoscopy. *Anaesthesia.* 1988;43:947.
16. Sung YF, Fremiere S, Tillette T. Comparison of propofol and thiopental anesthesia in outpatient surgery: speed of recovery. *Anesthesiology.* 1988;69:A562.
17. Johnston R, Noseworthy T, Anderson B, et al. Propofol vs thiopental for outpatient anesthesia. *Anesthesiology.* 1987;67:431.
18. Korttila K, Faure E, Apfelbaum J, et al. Less nausea and vomiting after propofol than after enflurane or isoflurane anesthesia. *Anesthesiology.* 1988;69:A578.
19. Shafer A, Doze VA, Shafer S, et al. Pharmacokinetics and pharmacodynamics of propofol infusions during general anesthesia. *Anesthesiology.* 1988;69:348.
20. Berry F. The pros and cons of succinylcholine for routine intubation and ambulatory surgery. *Anesth Rev.* 1990;17:13.
21. de Grood GM, Harbes JB, von Eymond J. Anaesthesia for laparoscopy. *Anaesthesia.* 1987;42:815.
22. Eger EI, Saidman LJ. Hazards of nitrous oxide anesthesia in bowel obstruction and pneumothorax. *Anesthesiology.* 1965;26:61.
23. Harris MN, Plantevin OM, Crowther A. Cardiac arrhythmias during anesthesia for laparoscopy. *Br J Anaesth.* 1984;56:1211.
24. Doyle DJ, Mark PW. Laparoscopy and vagal arrest. *Anaesthesia.* 1989;44:448.
25. Jones MJ, Mitchell RW, Hindocha N. Effect of increased intra-abdominal pressure during laparoscopy on the esophageal sphincter. *Anesth Analg.* 1989;68:63.
26. Madej TH, Simpson KH. Comparison of the use of domperidone, droperidol, and metoclopramide in the prevention of nausea and vomiting following gynaecologic surgery in day cases. *Br J Anaesth.* 1986;58:884.
27. Doze VA, Shafer A, White PF. Nausea and vomiting after outpatient anesthesia—effectiveness of droperidol alone and in combination with metoclopramide. *Anesth Analg.* 1987;66:541.
28. Cohen SE, Woods WA, Wyner JA. Antiemetic efficacy of droperidol and metoclopramide. *Anesthesiology.* 1984;60:67.
29. Hardley AJ. Metoclopramide in the prevention of postoperative nausea and vomiting. *Br J Clin Pract.* 1967;21:460.
30. Manchikanti L, Grow JB, Colliver JA, et al. Bicitra (sodium citrate) and metoclopramide in outpatient anesthesia for prophylaxis against aspiration pneumonitis. *Anesthesiology.* 1985;63:378.
31. Alexander JI, Hull MG. Abdominal pain after laparoscopy: the value of a gas drain. *Br J Obstet Gynaecol.* 1987;94:267.
32. Collins KM, Docherty PW, Plantevin OM, et al. Postoperative morbidity following gynae-

cologic outpatient laparoscopy. A reappraisal of the service. *Anaesthesia.* 1984;39:819.

33. Hodgson C, McClelland RM, Newton JR. Some effects of the peritoneal insufflation of carbon dioxide at laparoscopy. *Anaesthesia.* 1970;25:382.

34. O'Hara DA, Fragen RJ, Kinzer M, et al. Ketorolac tromethamine as compared with morphine sulfate for treatment of postoperative pain. *Clin Pharmacol Ther.* 1987;41:556.

8

Laparoscopy

Since the first recorded optical inspection of the abdominal cavity with a culdotomy in 1901,[1] the number of techniques has increased for observing the pelvic cavity to endoscopically diagnose and correct pelvic abnormalities. The modern era of laparoscopy began in 1954 when Palmer[2] reported no sequelae in endoscopic procedures on 250 patients. His technique included producing a pneumoperitoneum with CO_2 at a rate of 300 to 500 mL/min. He warned that the intra-abdominal pressure should not exceed 25 mm Hg. Palmer concluded that the advantages of laparoscopy over culdoscopy were a decreased chance of infection, a better view of the pelvis, improved access to the pelvic organs and cul-de-sac, and easier application.

Although the basic principles of laparoscopy are the same, the instruments and the complexity of operative procedures have changed significantly since 1954. This chapter presents information that is important for the resident who is learning laparoscopic surgery and for clinicians who are updating their information on operative laparoscopy.

Preoperative Evaluation

Advanced operative laparoscopy should be considered a major intra-abdominal procedure. Careful preoperative evaluation will maximize the operative outcome and decrease the chance of injuries and complications. Appropriate preoperative consultation with surgeons of other disciplines (colorectal, urology, oncology) may be necessary. Patients often have misconceptions about operative laparoscopy with the procedures referred to as "Band-aid," painless, or laser surgery; none is accurate. The patient must be informed about the different aspects of her upcoming operation, the possible outcome and results, possible complications, and the surgeon's experience in performing the particular procedure.

The following preoperative work-up is suggested:

History and physical

Complete blood count with differential

Serum electrolytes

Urinalysis

Pap smear

Thrombin time, partial thrombin time, bleeding time (if appropriate)

Transvaginal sonography

The following studies are performed in selected patients:

Endometrial biopsy

Cervical culture

Hysterosalpingogram

Barium enema and intravenous pyelogram

Type screen or type and crossmatch

Bowel preparation

Two different regimens for bowel preparations are suggested (Tables 8-1 and 8-2).[3]

TABLE 8-1. One-Day Bowel Preparation

1. Clear liquid the day before surgery
2. One gallon of Go-LYTELY consumed over 3 h the evening before surgery or 45 mL of Fleet Phospho-Soda PO at bedtime
3. One Fleet enema at bedtime and AM
4. 1 g metronidazole (Flagyl) PO at 11:00 PM
5. 1 g cefoxitin (IV) 30 min before the procedure

The one-day bowel preparation is used for women who have had a previous laparotomy or who have an adnexal mass, pelvic endometriosis, or adhesions. The 3-day bowel preparation is used for a patient who may need extensive procedures such as bowel resection and in patients with several previous laparotomies and severe adhesions.

Patient Preparation and Position

The anesthesiology team and circulating nurses coordinate the patient's transfer to the operating table. The operative site is cleansed and shaved preoperatively by an operating room nurse. The table must be designed to provide a 25-degree Trendelenburg position. After the induction of endotracheal anesthesia, the patient's legs are placed in padded Allen stirrups to provide good support and to allow proper position. Padding near the perineal nerve is essential. To avoid nerve compression, no leg joint is extended over 60 degrees. The buttocks must protrude a few centimeters from the edge of the table to enable uterine manipulation. The patient's arms are placed at her side, padded with foam troughs, and secured by a sheet, allowing the surgeon and assistants to stand unencumbered next to the patient. The anesthesiologist should have easy access to the patient's arm (Figure 8-1).

TABLE 8-2. Three-Day Bowel Preparation

Day 1
100 mL Fleet Phospho-Soda PO at bedtime
Day 2
Clear liquid diet
Day 3
Clear liquid diet
10 mg prochlorperazine PO at noon
Begin drinking 1 gal Go-LYTELY at 2:00 PM
1 g neomycin PO at 6:00 PM and 11:00 PM
1 g erythromycin base PO at 6:00 PM and 11:00 PM
One Fleet enema at bedtime
Day of surgery
Two tap water enemas before reporting to the hospital

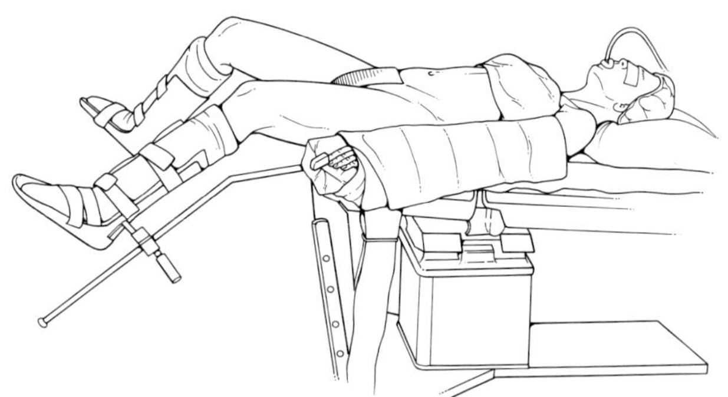

Figure 8-1 Position of patient for operative laparoscopy. The patient is in a dorsolithotomy position but her thighs are not flexed so that the suprapubic trocars may be maneuvered properly.

Once the patient is positioned, her abdomen, perineum, and vagina are prepared with a suitable bactericidal solution and a Foley catheter is inserted. She is draped to expose her abdomen and perineum and a pelvic examination is performed. Diagnostic hysteroscopy is suggested for patients undergoing diagnostic and operative laparoscopy unless there is a contraindication. After withdrawal of the hysteroscope, a uterine manipulator is inserted into the cervical os to manipulate the uterus and allow chromopertubation.

Rectal and vaginal probes are used to manipulate and separate tissue planes of the cul-de-sac or an assistant may perform simultaneous rectal and vaginal examination.[4] A sponge on a ring forceps is placed in the posterior fornix to outline the posterior cul-de-sac or anteriorly to identify the vesicouterine space. A sigmoidoscope or rectal probe can be used to outline the rectum and sigmoid colon. The sigmoidoscope can insufflate the rectum with air to facilitate identification of a bowel perforation by observing the air-inflated rectum to look for air bubbles as they pass into the posterior cul-de-sac filled with irrigation fluid.[4]

Placement of the Veress Needle

Insertion of the Veress needle, the primary trocar, and the secondary trocar is the most critical and important aspect of diagnostic and operative laparoscopy because the most serious complications and injuries can occur during this portion of the procedure. The following factors increase the risk of injury and should not be overlooked: previous abdominal and pelvic operations, body weight (whether patient is obese or very thin), a large uterus, and the presence of a large pelvis mass. Although the primary and secondary trocars usually are inserted at the subumbilical and suprapubic areas, respectively, these sites sometimes must be modified. Examples include an enlarged uterus caused by uterine leiomyoma or pregnancy, or for para-aortic node dissection, in which the primary trocar is introduced approximately 4 to 6 cm above the umbilicus. The optimal location for the Veress needle and primary trocar is the umbilicus because the skin is attached to the fascial layer and anterior parietal peritoneum with minimal intervening subcutaneous fat or muscle (Figure 8-2). The infraumbilical approach is the shortest distance between the skin and the peritoneal cavity, even in obese patients.

Before needle insertion, a transverse or vertical cutaneous incision is made, large enough to accommodate the primary trocar. A deep vertical umbilical incision may provide better cosmetic results.[5] When incising the umbilicus, an Allis clamp is used to grasp and evert the base of the umbilicus, raising it from the abdominal structures.

There is some debate surrounding the angle of insertion for the Veress needle and umbilical trocar, and patient positioning during these instruments' insertion. Premature Trendelenburg can alter the usual landmarks (Figure 8-3). Palpating the abdominal aorta and sacral promontory aids in determining the distance between the abdominal wall, spine, and aorta (Figure 8-4). Some authors have suggested that the Veress needle and trocar be inserted at an angle between 45 and 90 degrees, based on the patient's body weight (Figure 8-5).[6,7] Recently, we have conducted extensive observation and research on the relationship between the aortic bifurcation and abdominal wall, as well as abdominal wall elevation by different methods (using towel clips or hands of the surgeon and assistant). Based on our findings, we strongly believe that the 90-degree insertion angle can be safe in all patients if the surgeon maintains the adequate control of the insertion force and the abdominal wall is adequately elevated (keeping its thickness in mind) (see also Insertion Technique). While the patient is in supine position, two towel clips are placed 4- to 5-cm lateral to the umbilicus and while the surgeon and assistant lift the skin and fat, the Veress needle, held at the shaft, is inserted directly into the abdominal cavity at a 90-degree angle (Figure 8-6).

Verification of Intraperitoneal Placement

Failure to achieve and maintain a suitable pneumoperitoneum is a common error, and misplacing the Veress needle predisposes the patient to complications. Correct needle placement can be verified by the "hanging drop" technique. A drop of saline is placed on the hub of the Veress needle after inser-

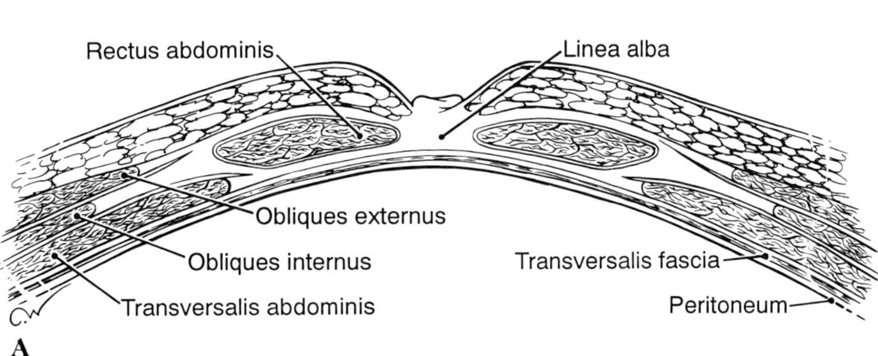

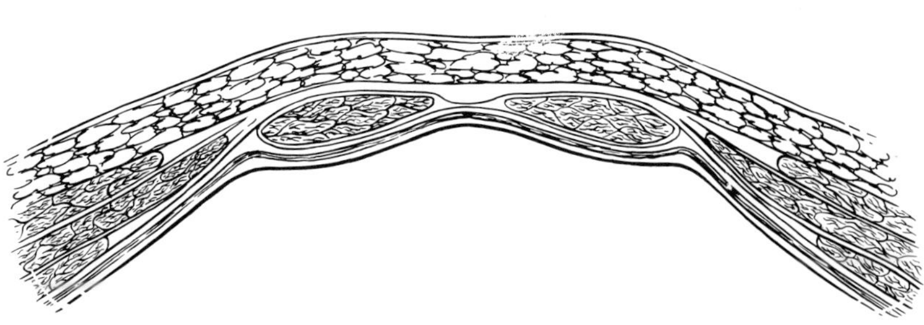

Figure 8-2 Transverse sections through the anterior abdominal wall. A, Immediately above the umbilicus. B, Below the arcuate line.

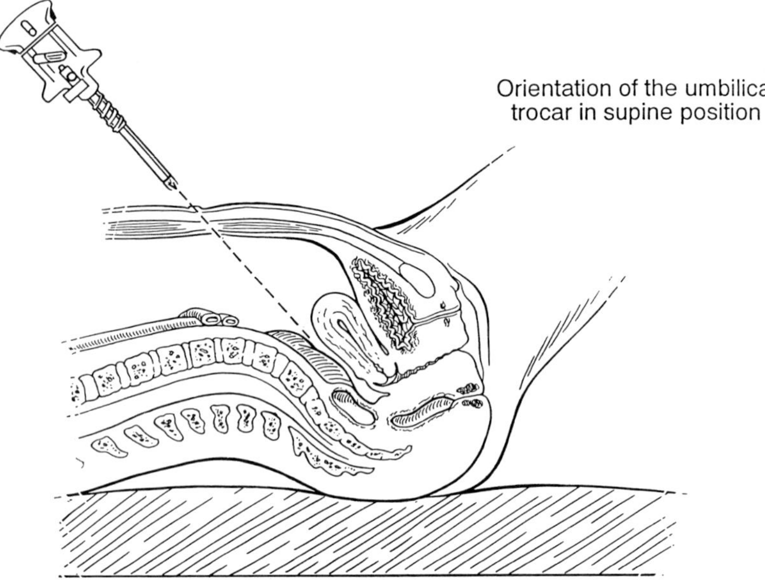

A

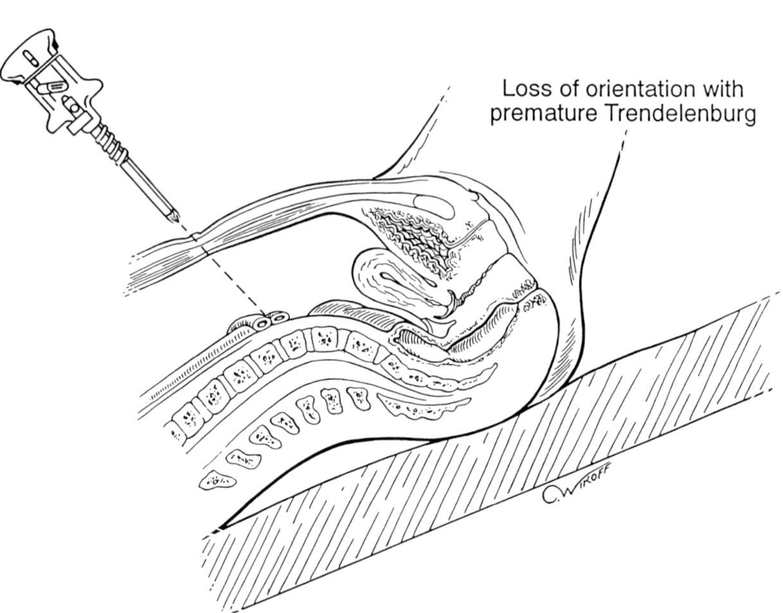

B

Figure 8-3 Angle of trocar insertion with operating table in flat (A) and in Trendelenburg position (B).

tion through the abdominal wall; lifting the abdominal wall establishes negative pressure within the abdomen, drawing the drop of fluid into the needle. Absence of this sign indicates improper placement of the Veress needle. Alternatively, a 10-mL syringe with normal saline is attached to the Veress needle and aspiration verifies the absence of bowel contents or blood (Figure 8-7). The saline is injected into the peritoneal cavity, and if the needle placement is correct, the fluid cannot be withdrawn because it is dispersed intraperitoneally. If the needle is placed within adhesions or the preperitoneal space, the fluid usually can be recovered by aspiration. If the needle has been placed intravascularly, or in the intestine or bladder, characteristic contents are obtained. Methods of ascertaining proper placement of the Veress needle are summarized in Table 8-3.

Alternative Sites

Different sites have been used for insertion of the Veress needle (Figure 8-8). The site most often used other than the umbilicus is the left subcostal margin, in the midclavicular line. This site is palpated and percussed to rule out splenomegaly or an insufflated stomach from a misplaced endotracheal tube. This site is useful especially in patients who have had multiple previous laparotomies.

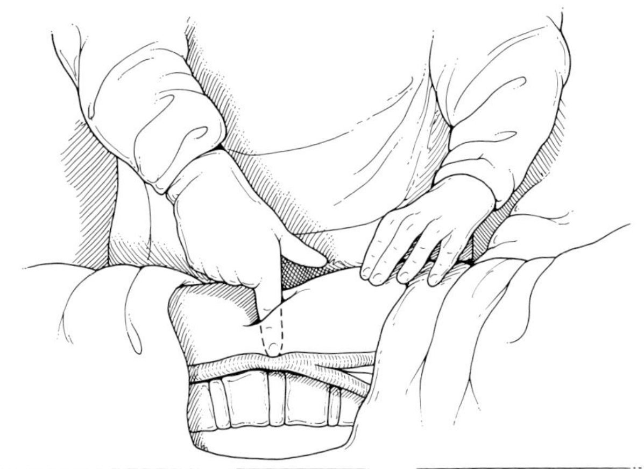

Figure 8-4 Palpating the aorta and sacral promontory.

The transvaginal approach is used by inserting the needle through the posterior cul-de-sac, providing there is no evidence of pelvic thickening or masses in the cul-de-sac and the uterus is mobile.[8] This technique is effective in patients who have developed preperitoneal emphysema from unsuccessful attempts to insert the needle through the umbilicus or other abdominal sites.

Another technique is the transcervical or transabdominal route through the uterine fundus.[9,10] In the latter procedure, the fundus is pushed up against the abdominal wall using the uterine manipulator. The needle is passed through all layers of the abdomen and into the uterine fundus. The uterus is pulled away from the tip of the needle, which theoretically achieves its intra-abdominal placement. Alternatively, the Veress needle is inserted transcervically through the fundus into the abdominal cavity. These alternative methods have questionable margins of safety. Puncture of the uterus with this technique can result in persistent low-grade bleeding throughout the laparoscopy. Inadvertent perforation of the bladder can occur and broad ligament perforation and hemorrhage are possible. An intrauterine or intramyometrial position during insufflation risks gas embolism. The technique is contraindicated if fundal adhe-

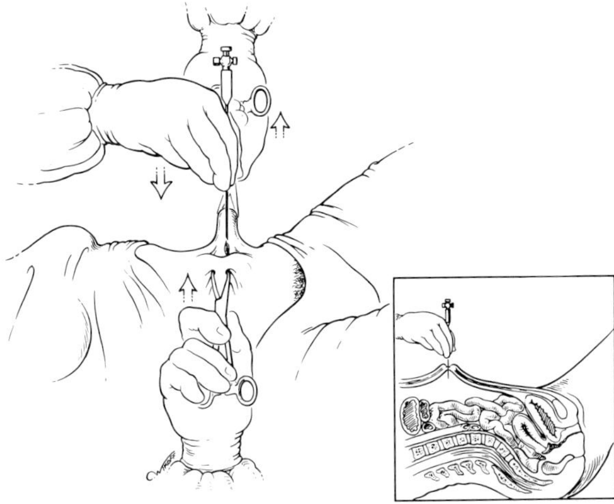

Figure 8-6 As the surgeon and assistant lift the abdominal wall with two towel clips placed 4- to 5-cm lateral to the umbilicus, the Veress needle is inserted at a 90-degree angle.

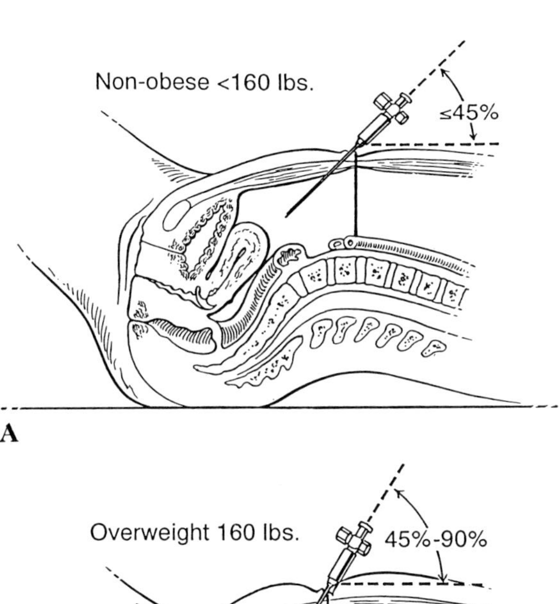

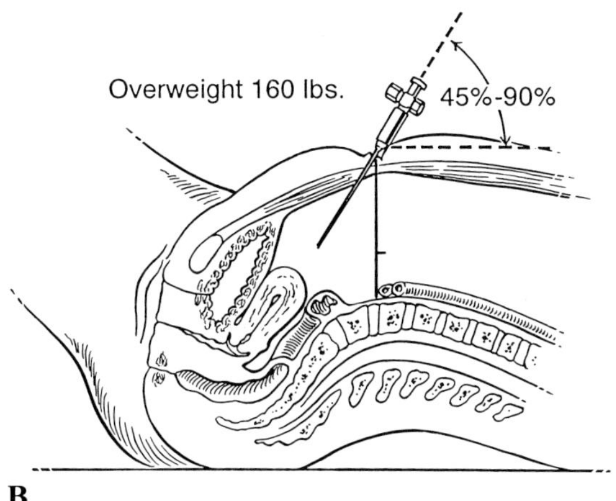

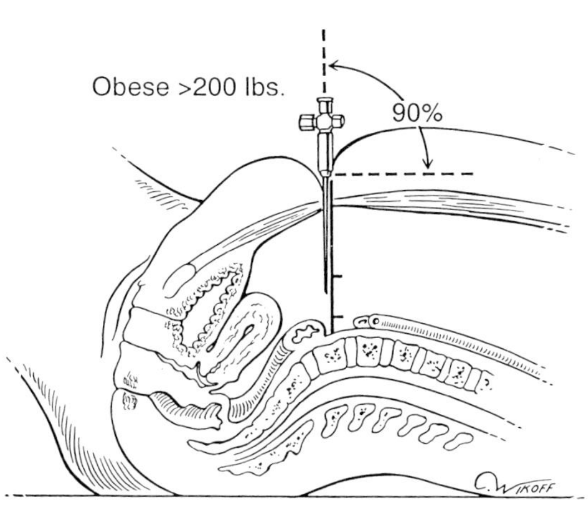

Figure 8-5 Anatomic location of umbilicus and abdominal aorta in nonobese (A), overweight (B), and obese (C) patients.

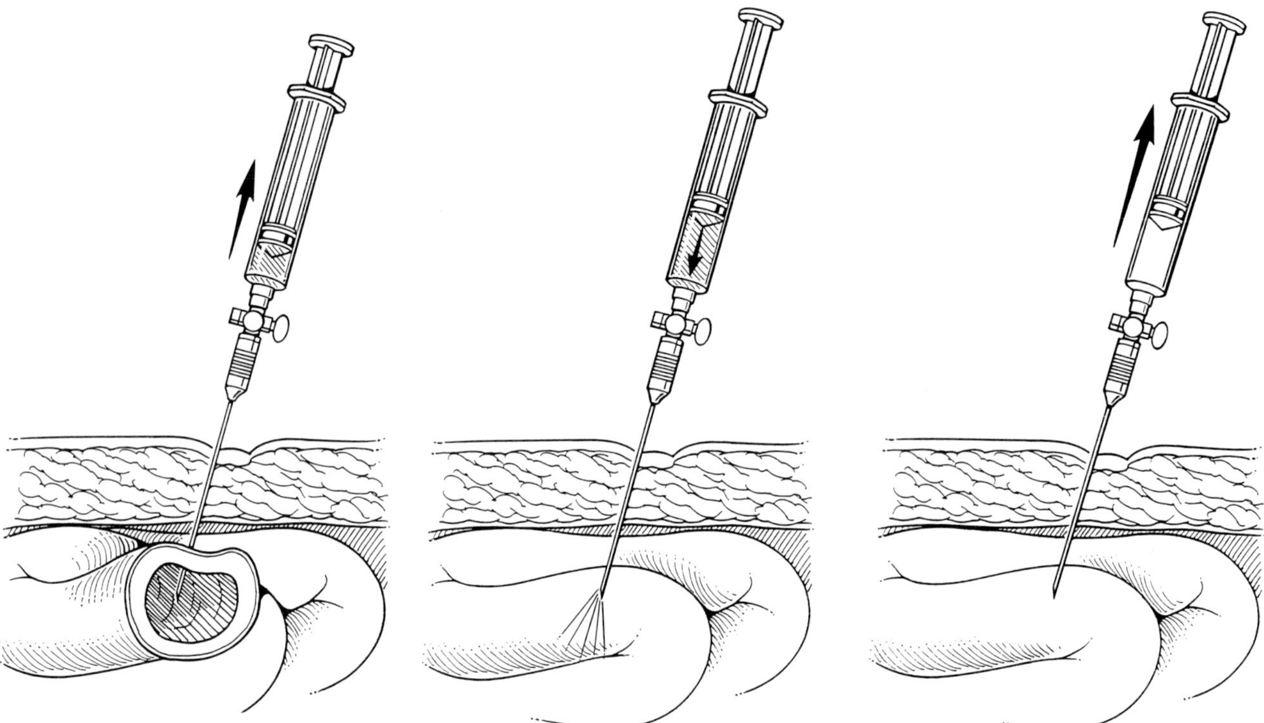

Figure 8-7 Syringe test used to ascertain that bowel or blood vessels are not adherent under the umbilicus prior to trocar insertion. A 10-mL syringe with 5 mL of normal saline is attached to the Veress needle and aspiration verifies the absence of bowel contents of blood.

sions are anticipated or if chromopertubation is necessary.[11] In the obese patient, proper placement of the Veress needle is difficult to achieve. If it is placed below, instead of within, the umbilicus at 45 degrees to the abdominal wall, it can dissect the preperitoneal space. It is preferable to insert the needle and trocar in the umbilicus and at 90 degrees using towel clips for traction and abdominal wall elevation (Figure 8-9).[6]

TABLE 8-3. Tests to Confirm the Proper Position of the Veress Needle

1. Injection and aspiration of fluid through the Veress needle
2. Loss of liver dullness early in insufflation
3. Hanging drop test
4. An unimpeded arc of rotation of the needle to detect anterior abdominal wall adhesions
5. Sound of air entering Veress needle with elevation of the abdominal wall
6. Free flow of gas through the Veress needle
7. Observation of the fluctuation of pressure gauge needle with inspiratory and expiratory diaphragmatic motions

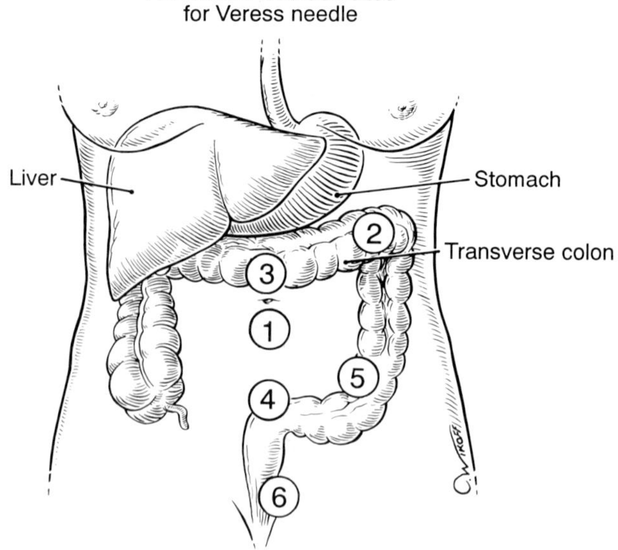

Figure 8-8 Alternative sites of Veress needle insertion. 1, Infra or intraumbilical; 2, left upper quadrant, mid-clavicular; 3, supraumbilical; 4, midline suprapubic; 5, left lower quadrant, McBurney's point; 6, transcervical through the uterine fundus or transvaginal through the posterior fornix into the abdominal cavity.

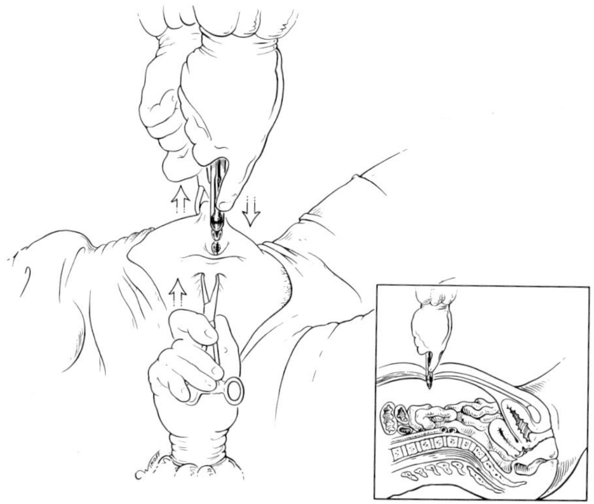

Figure 8-9 Insertion of trocar. Countertraction is applied by lifting the abdominal wall using two towel clips placed 4- to 5-cm lateral to the umbilicus; the surgeon inserts the trocar at a 90-degree angle into the abdomen by palming it and using the index finger as a guard against sudden entry into the abdomen.

Establishment of Pneumoperitoneum

The establishment of a pneumoperitoneum is essential to ensure proper laparoscopic observation and adequate exposure to perform intraperitoneal manipulation for endoscopic surgery. Unless the surgeon is confident about the proper position of the Veress needle, the high flow is not used.

The difference between the operating pressure of the insufflator and the pressure within the abdomen initially should be no greater than 5 mm Hg. If higher pressures are recorded, the surgeon should suspect that the needle is placed improperly. This may result from a needle tip in the omentum, which can be dislodged by gently elevating and shaking the lower abdominal wall. If this maneuver fails, the needle hub should be gently manipulated in a different direction because its distal hole could impinge against the anterior abdominal wall. If neither of these relieves the increased recorded pressure, the Veress needle should be removed and reinserted. Occasionally, while passing through the different layers of the abdomen, tissue lodges in the tip, obstructing the opening. Whenever the Veress needle is withdrawn because of high pressures, check its patency.

After 1 L CO_2 has been insufflated, the surgeon should percuss the right costal margin to check for loss of liver dullness. If liver dullness is detected, the Veress needle is positioned improperly. It should be withdrawn and reinserted. After insufflation of more than 1 L CO_2, accumulation of the gas in a hollow viscus or the preperitoneal space may lead to a loss in liver dullness, giving the surgeon a false sense of security.

Although most insufflators have gauges indicating the volume of gas insufflated, the surgeon should use palpable abdominal distention and the pressure reading rather than the volume because they more accurately reflect adequate pneumoperitoneum. After introduction of the trocars, the intra-abdominal pressure should be preset between 12 to 16 mm Hg during the operative procedure. Higher pressure for long periods can cause subcutaneous emphysema and should be avoided.

Introduction of the Laparoscopic Trocar

During controlled entry, the primary trocar is inserted directly at 90 degrees. Dull trocars, which require increased force during insertion, multiple insertions, and excessive instrumental manipulation, are associated with an increased risk. Insertion of a disposable shielded trocar in the presence of a pneumoperitoneum requires half the force needed for a reusable sharp trocar; however, the disposable trocar shield does not prevent injury completely.[12] The pneumoperitoneum may reduce the proximity of the abdominal wall to the spine and the potential for damage to bowel and vessels,[13] but whether this is associated with a lower incidence of trocar-related injuries has not been proven. Using these new devices can inflict injury because of the unexpected ease of their insertion. Numerous mesenteric, bowel, and vascular injuries have been reported with disposable trocars.

Insertion Techniques

The surgeon should not deviate from standard procedure for trocar insertion without good cause. In a program for laparoscopic sterilization, Soderstrom and Butler[14] demonstrated that the complication rate was reduced tenfold by a consistent operating format.

The trocar is inserted with the patient in a horizontal position. Premature Trendelenburg position not only fails to prevent visceral injury even in the presence of significant adhesions, but as the small bowel is displaced into the upper abdomen, the vessels are more exposed and may be at a higher risk for injury. Altering the patient's position can affect the surgeon's view of important landmarks such as the sacral promontory and aortic bifurcation (Figure 8-3).

The major anatomic landmarks include the umbilicus, located at the level of L-3 and L-4, and the abdominal aorta, which bifurcates between L-4 and L-5 (see Figure 8-6). As noted earlier, we believe that the 90-degree angle of insertion is safer for all patients regardless of their weight, remembering the following parameters. The surgeon must elevate the abdominal wall with two towel clips, noting the thickness of the wall at the umbilicus, and must maintain adequate control of the laparoscopic trocar as it penetrates each layer of the anterior abdominal wall (Figure 8-9). The surgeon must maintain adequate control of the laparoscopic trocar as it penetrates each layer of the anterior abdominal wall. Successful and safe insertion depends on (1) an adequate skin incision, (2) the trocar's working condition (disposable trocars should be checked to be sure they are not locked), (3) their proper orientation, and (4) control over the instrument's force and depth of insertion.

The trocar and its sleeve are held with the index finger extended to the point of maximal planned penetration to prevent the sharp trocar tip from thrusting too deeply and causing intra-abdominal injury. The remaining fingers grasp the trumpet valve or the insufflation valve. The trocar itself is palmed. The dominant hand is used for this procedure. The trocar is rotated in a semicircular fashion with its long axis while controlled, firm, downward pressure is applied (Figure 8-9). As the trocar is advanced, the operator will sense when the fascia has been traversed; the force is reduced as the trocar is advanced slowly to enter the peritoneum. The correct placement of the trocar is confirmed by the free escape of CO_2. Disposable bullet tip trocars are preferable (Ethicon; see Figure 8-9). A disposable shielded trocar has been introduced recently and provides two advantages: a safety shield that snaps into position after the peritoneum is entered and a freshly sharpened instrument for each operation.

Direct Trocar Insertion

Direct insertion of the laparoscopic trocar without creating a pneumoperitoneum initially reduces the number of "blind" procedures, saving operative time and potential complications. Direct insertion has been reported to be a safe alternative to Veress needle insertion[15–21] although only one study prospectively compared the two methods.[15] Nezhat and colleagues[15] reported the results from a randomized, prospectively controlled study com- paring the ease of use and safety of Veress needle insertion and establishment of a pneumoperitoneum with direct insertion of the conventional reusable trocar and direct insertion of the disposable shielded trocar in 200 patients. Minor complications of 22%, 6%, and 0% were observed, respectively. Although the study showed fewer complications with direct insertion of the trocar, no differences were noted in the ease of insertion or the frequency of multiple attempts (Tables 8-4 and 8-5).[15] As with all trocar insertions, the surgeon must hold the instrument properly, with the patient in a supine position at the height of the surgeon's waist or slightly below.

TABLE 8-4. Comparison of Veress Needle and Direct Trocar Insertion

	Veress Needle (n = 100)	Direct Trocar Insertion (n = 100)
Complications	22	3
Two insertions required	20	20
Failed insertions	3	6

Direct trocar insertion is accomplished by elevating the abdominal wall either manually or with towel clips applied close to the umbilicus. After the trocar is inserted into the peritoneal cavity, the laparoscope is introduced to verify correct intraperitoneal placement. Pneumoperitoneum is created with high flow insufflation. At the Center for Special Pelvic Surgery (CSPS), direct trocar insertion is used except in patients who have had multiple laparotomies. Since 1989, more than 3000 direct trocar insertions have been performed without major complications.

Open Laparoscopy

In 1971, Hasson introduced the concept of open laparoscopy to eliminate risks associated with

TABLE 8-5. Comparison of Reusable and Disposable Trocars

	Reusable (n = 50)	Disposable (n = 50)
Complications	3	0
Two insertions required	10	10
Failed insertions	4	2

"blind" introduction of the Veress needle and laparoscopic trocar.[22] This technique involves direct trocar insertion through a small skin incision, without prior pneumoperitoneum, using specially designed equipment consisting of a cannula and trumpet valve fitted with a cone-shaped stainless steel sleeve and a blunt obturator protruding 1 cm from the tip of the cannula. The cone sleeve seals the peritoneal and fascial gap.

A small transverse, curved, or vertical incision is made at the umbilicus. Two Allis clamps, a knife handle with small blade, a straight scissors, a tissue forceps with teeth, a right angle skin hook, four S-shaped retractors, a needle-holder, two curved Kocher clamps, and four small curved hemostats are needed. As the incision is made, Allis clamps or a self-retaining retractor are used to provide adequate exposure. Once the fascia is cut, a 1-cm incision is made in the peritoneum, to avoid injury to the intestine. One suture of 0 polyglactin (Ethicon) is passed through each peritoneal edge and fascia and tagged. The corklike cannula carrying the blunt obturator is inserted through the opening into the peritoneal cavity. The obturator is withdrawn and CO_2 is insufflated through the cannula, which is inserted as deep as required to prevent leakage. The previously placed sutures are used to fix the trocar sleeve so that the laparoscope can move freely within the abdominal cavity. At the end of the procedure, the abdominal wall is closed using the previously placed sutures. This method was designed to eliminate "blind" placement of the Veress needle and sharp laparoscopic trocar, errors in the creation of a pneumoperitoneum, and the complication of an umbilical hernia.

Open laparoscopy usually takes about 5 to 10 minutes longer than closed laparoscopy performed by operators of comparable expertise. In more than 1000 consecutive operations performed by Hasson and colleagues,[23] the frequency of minor wound infection was 0.6% and small bowel injury was 0.1%. In a review of laparoscopic complications, the open technique reduced failed procedures, inappropriate gas insufflation, gas embolism, bladder and pelvic kidney puncture, major vessel injury, and postoperative herniations.[24] With experience and proper technique, surgeons seldom encounter difficulties with either method.

In a survey conducted by Penfield,[25] intestinal laceration was the most serious complication of open laparoscopy, and most complications occurred during the early use of this technique. In 10,840 open laparoscopies performed by 18 board certified obstetricians/gynecologists, six bowel lacerations were reported, four were recognized and repaired, and two were not suspected until several days postoperatively. To minimize the risk of bowel laceration, use a focus spotlight, work with an experienced assistant, make a vertical incision to facilitate exposure, grasp and elevate the fascia with small Kocher clamps, and cut between the clamps. The gynecologist who performs open laparoscopy only in special situations will find that the procedure is slow and cumbersome because of difficulty in exposing and identifying each layer of the abdominal wall.

Accessory Trocars

Accessory cannulas are needed through which various instruments can be introduced into the abdomen for manipulation and operative procedures. Placement sites depend on the patient's anatomy, the contemplated procedure and surgeon's preference. For diagnostic purposes, an incision generally is made 4 to 5 cm above the symphysis pubis in the midline. This area, delineated by the two umbilical ligaments and the bladder dome, is safe and usually avascular. For operative laparoscopy, two accessory trocar sleeves (5 mm) are placed 4 to 5 cm above the symphysis pubis at the outer border of the rectus muscle, 3 to 4 cm below the iliac crest, 2 to 3 cm lateral to the deep inferior epigastric vessels.

These accessory trocars are inserted under direct vision to minimize the risk of intra-abdominal visceral and vascular injury, to clear the uterine fundus, and to provide free access to the posterior cul-de-sac. Vascularization of the lower abdomen is provided mostly by two vessels; one is the deep inferior epigastric originating from the external iliac artery and the second is the superficial epigastric, a branch of the femoral artery. Transillumination helps to identify the superficial vessels but they are difficult to see in obese patients. The deep inferior epigastric vessels run lateral to the umbilical ligaments (Figure 8-10) and in most cases are seen intraperitoneally and identified easily. These vessels branch from the external iliac artery, pass the round ligament, proceed to the anterior abdominal wall, and are seen above the peritoneum. To avoid injuring these vessels, the trocar is inserted medial or lateral to the umbilical ligaments by viewing the underside of the abdomen wall laparoscopically (Figure 8-11). Despite these precautions, aberrant vascular branches occasionally are traumatized and the operator must be able to manage this type of injury.

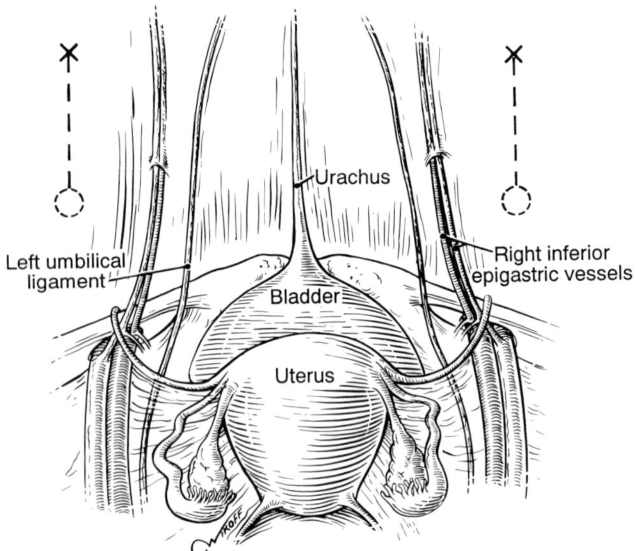

Figure 8-10 Location of deep inferior epigastric vessels, which run lateral to the umbilical ligaments.

To reduce the chance of trauma to the abdominal structures, the proposed site for the secondary puncture is indented by applying abdominal pressure with the index finger and observing the peritoneal surface with the laparoscope. This maneuver is particularly important in a patient with evidence of abdominal wall adhesions and helps ensure safe access.

The trocar is held with the index finger extended on the sheath to control the depth of penetration. The trocar and sheath are inserted through the skin, fat, and fascia, and further advancement is controlled under laparoscopic view (see Figure 8-11). The trocar is aimed toward the hollow of the sacrum because if it is aimed laterally, it may slide down the pelvic side wall without being seen through the laparoscope, resulting in injury to the iliac vessels. The accessory trocars must never be inserted without clear laparoscopic observation of their indentation on the abdominal wall. When insertion of the trocars is viewed directly from the monitor, the surgeon should be sure the camera has not been rotated so that it shows the wrong view of the pelvis. Most laparoscopic procedures do not require more than two accessory trocars but occasionally two additional ones are needed. Other sites of entry include the midpoint between the symphysis pubis and the umbilicus and McBurney's point.

Some lower quadrant sleeves are too long to allow free access to the pelvic structures and tend to slip out of the peritoneal cavity. The presence of trap valves can interfere with the efficient instrument exchange, prevent the introduction and removal of suture material, and prevent removal of tissue. Several new accessory trocar sleeves either screw in or have an umbrella to secure them to the abdominal wall.

High-Risk Patients

Special considerations are required for the obese patient. Because Veress needle and trocar insertions are almost vertical, the distance between the

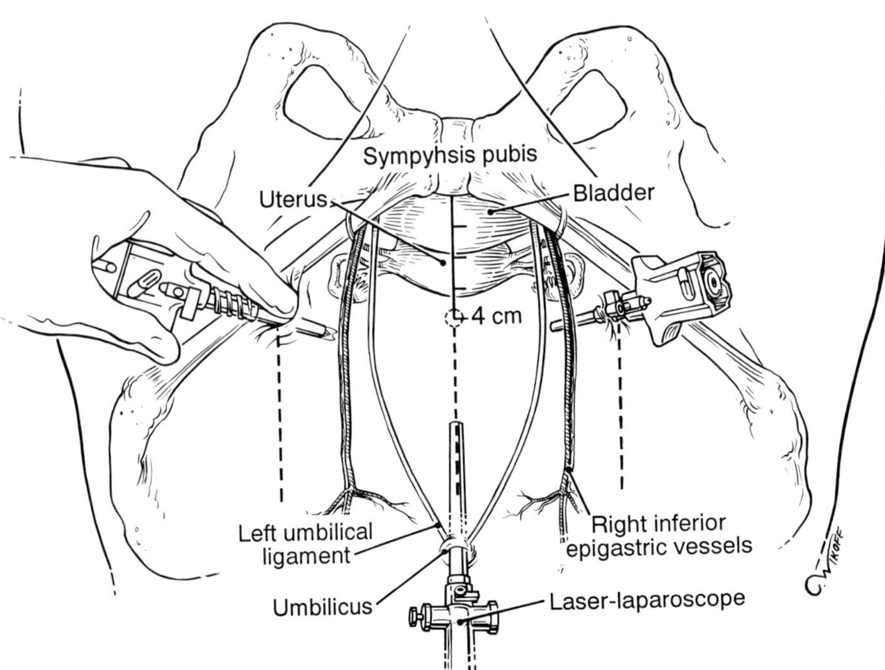

Figure 8-11 Accessory trocars are placed under direct observation to avoid injury to the inferior epigastric vessels and any organs that may be adherent to the pelvic side wall or to the anterior abdominal wall. The trocar is inserted lateral to the left umbilical ligament, avoiding inferior epigastric vessels, which are invariably lateral to umbilical ligaments.

sacral promontory and trocar is relatively small and there is no room for an uncontrolled entry. In thin patients, the distance between the anterior abdominal wall and sacral promontory is often small. It is safer to overdistend the abdomen with CO_2 before trocar insertion. The force required to introduce the trocar is less than anticipated because the fascia is thin and offers little resistance.[24]

Bowel distention secondary to obstruction is a relative contraindication to laparoscopy. This condition may be iatrogenic, resulting from placement of the Veress needle within the bowel lumen. The filling pressure of the small bowel may be the same as that of the abdominal cavity because of the former's large capacity. Therefore, the surgeon may be unaware of this complication. Once an "apparent" pneumoperitoneum is created and the Veress needle is removed, the trocar may lacerate the distended bowel.

Patients with Previous Laparotomy

In women who have had previous laparotomies, the operative laparoscopist must be aware of potentially altered underlying intra-abdominal anatomy during trocar insertion. Inflexible adhesive bridging between the intestine and abdominal wall can nullify any protection from trocar injury usually afforded by elevating the abdominal wall, creating pneumoperitoneum, Trendelenburg positioning, and reliable bowel mobility. In some women, injury inevitably will occur to vasculature of the adherent omentum or directly to the bowel wall. Patients at the highest risk are those who have undergone previous major abdominal surgery, such as bowel resection or exploratory laparotomy for abdominal trauma or ovarian carcinoma.[7] Patients with prior uncomplicated abdominal surgery are at low risk.

In a prospective study at CSPS, the relationship between bowel and omental adhesions and injury to these organs during operative laparoscopy in 360 women who had previously undergone a variety of abdominal operations was evaluated (unpublished data; Tables 8-6, 8-7, and 8-8). The following observations were made:

1. Patients with prior midline incisions have more adhesions than those with prior Pfannenstiel.
2. Patients with multiple prior incisions do not have more adhesions than those with a single prior incision.
3. Patients with prior midline or Pfannenstiel incisions for gynecologic surgery have more adhesions than those having undergone obstetric surgery.
4. Patients with prior midline incisions for obstetric surgery do not have more adhesions than those with a prior Pfannenstiel incision for obstetric surgery.

TABLE 8-6. Patients by Type and Number of Incisions

Incision Type	No. of Incisions						Total No. of Patients
	1×	2×	3×	4×	5×	6×	
PFL	180	51	19	4	4	0	258
MLB	55	18	9	4	0	1	87
MLA	10	2	1	2	0	0	15

PFL, Pfannenstiel; MLB, midline below umbilicus; MLA, midline above umbilicus

The following conditions are associated with severe adhesions:

1. Generalized peritonitis
2. Bowel resection after bowel obstruction
3. Oncologic procedure with omentectomy
4. Previous radiation and intraperitoneal chemotherapy
5. Previous adhesions

During insertion of the primary trocar and entry into the abdominal cavity, injury occurred in 21 (6%) instances (Table 8-9). Of these, six involved the small bowel. Only one patient had a single

TABLE 8-7. Incidence of Adhesions After Previous Laparotomy

Type of Incision	No.	%	Omental (%)	Bowel (%)
PFL	258	72	23	4
MLB	87	24	46	9
MLA	15	4	40	27
Total	360	100		

PFL, Pfannenstiel; MLB, midline below umbilicus; MLA, midline above umbilicus

TABLE 8-8. Patients by Clinical Indication and Incision Type

Incision Type	Gynecologic	Obstetric
PFL	186	43
MLB/MLA	73	12
Total	259	55

PFL, Pfannenstiel; MLB, midline below umbilicus; MLA, midline above umbilicus

incision; the remaining five had multiple incisions and complicated surgical histories. With the exception of 32 patients in whom open laparoscopy was performed, closed technique with prior establishment of pneumoperitoneum was used. The use of open laparoscopy was based on the patients' surgical history (bowel resection, bowel obstruction, ovarian cancer surgery) and our preoperative judgment. Two small bowel injuries occurred during open laparoscopy. In these two patients, the small bowel was attached to the anterior abdominal wall, directly under the umbilicus. The bowel was entered during incision of the fascia that was attached directly to the bowel.

The attachment of the bowel and omentum to the abdominal wall is primarily distal to the umbilicus (Figure 8-12A). If the insertion of the trocar is more vertical than oblique, the possibility of bowel injury is very low, especially if a disposable trocar with a shield is used. However, in patients who have had previous complicated abdominal operations (bowel resection, bowel obstruction, etc.), the bowel may be attached quite near the umbilicus (Figure 8-12B).

In a subsequent, separate study, the safety of direct trocar insertion was evaluated in 246 consecutive patients, with previous uncomplicated Pfannenstiel or midline incisions. All patients underwent bowel preparation and understood that laparotomy was possible. Trocar insertion was almost at a 90-degree angle, while the surgeon and the assistant elevated the abdominal wall, lateral to the umbilicus (see Figure 8-9). Fifty patients had omental adhesions, and 34 had bowel adhesions to the anterior abdominal wall. There were no small bowel injuries. Five omental injuries occurred; in one, the injury was associated with bleeding and was managed laparoscopically.

TABLE 8-9. Incidence of Injury—21/360 (6%)

Type of Injury	Omental Hematoma (Closed Technique)		Omental Bleeding (Closed Technique)		Small Bowel Injury (Closed - 6; open - 2)	
	Single	Multiple	Single	Multiple	Single	Multiple
Number	1	5	7	2	1	5
Percent	0.3	1.4	1.9	0.6	0.3	1.4

Based on the two studies, it is concluded that the incidence of subumbilical bowel adhesions and subsequent bowel injury is related more closely to the indication for previous laparotomy than the type or number of previous laparotomies. The incidence of bowel injuries during insertion of the primary trocar is very low. Closed technique, with or without prior establishment of pneumoperitoneum, may be used in most instances without increasing the chance of bowel injury.

Several procedures have been described to assess the anterior abdominal wall for intestinal adhesions. DeCherney[26] advocates using a small-gauge needle laparoscope 2 to 3 mm in diameter. The needle scope is inserted instead of the Veress needle, under direct vision through the umbilical, preperitoneal, and immediately subperitoneal structures. The Veress needle is inserted intra-abdominally and insufflation proceeds under direct observation.

Exploring the periumbilical area with an 18-gauge needle attached to a syringe after establishing the pneumoperitoneum (Figure 8-13) has been suggested. Should adhesions be detected by these techniques, the options include open laparoscopy or alternative sites of abdominal entry. The primary trocar can be inserted in the midline between the xiphoid and the pubic symphysis, providing care is taken to remain at least 5 cm below xiphoid and 5 cm above the pubic symphysis (see Figure 8-8).[14] Although the above techniques can help detect periumbilical adhesions, they are not definitive and are time consuming.

Based on the above observations, the following approach is recommended:

1. Every patient with previous laparotomy should be allocated to noncomplicated and complicated groups.
2. One-day or 3-day bowel preparation is administered based on the patient's history. All patients must understand that bowel injury is possible and must consent to conversion of the procedure to laparotomy.
3. In the noncomplicated group, open or closed techniques are used. If the closed technique is used, a disposable trocar with a bullet shield is

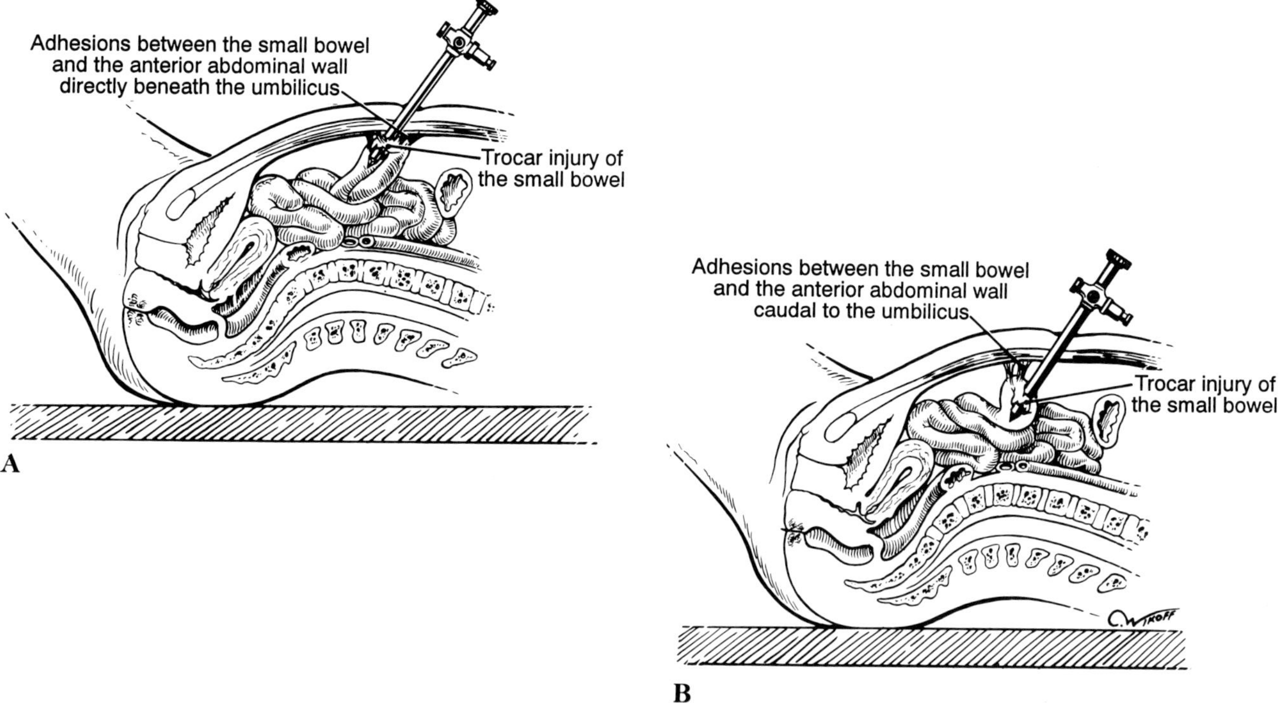

Figure 8-12 Attachment of the bowel to the anterior abdominal wall. A, The bowel is attached directly under the umbilicus. B, The attachment is below and distal to the umbilicus.

preferable. Trocar entry must be controlled and placement angle should be vertical rather than oblique (Figure 8-14). Either previous establishment of pneumoperitoneum by Veress needle or direct trocar insertion can be used, depending on the surgeon's experience and preference. If Veress needle is used, the subumbilical area may be searched for bowel adhesions, before trocar insertion (see Figure 8-12). If there is any suspicion of adhesions, other locations (see Figure 8-8) are explored until a safe area is detected and the trocar is inserted.

4. For patients in the complicated group, a technique called mapping the abdomen is advised. After insertion of the laparoscope, the abdominal wall with adherent bowel or omentum is explored. If the adhesions are severe and no clear space for accessory trocar insertion is seen, the abdominal wall is observed through the laparoscope and gentle, external compression is performed marking areas that seem to be free of adhesions. Before inserting the trocar, we simulate its track with a 21-gauge spinal needle. If this identifies a clear path, the trocar is introduced next to the needle, or the needle is removed and the trocar is introduced.

An advantage to first inserting the 21-gauge needle is its small diameter. Injury incurred during its insertion usually does not require repair. As the needle's placement is seen, there is little risk of missing a visceral injury. The insertion of the needle through the skin of the abdominal wall is quite easy. No force is required, so the surgeon can control the needle precisely and prevent any deviation from the preset course.

Previous operative reports are evaluated to ascertain the probability of adhesions and their location. In patients at risk for significant adhesions, pneumoperitoneum is created by inserting the Veress needle subumbilically or left subcostally in a midclavicular line after aspirating with a syringe to rule out bowel entry. The abdomen is insufflated with CO_2. The area is explored using a 20-gauge needle to inject saline (see Figure 8-13). If no fluid is aspirated (the conditions are favorable), a 5-mm trocar is inserted and a 4-mm laparoscope placed to observe the peritoneal cavity (see Figure 8-14). If there is no intestinal injury, the 5-mm trocar is replaced with the 10-mm trocar. If intestinal entry occurs, the 5-mm trocar is left in place, and a safe area is found to insert the 10-mm trocar and laparoscope. The loops of injured bowel are mobilized and repaired laparo-

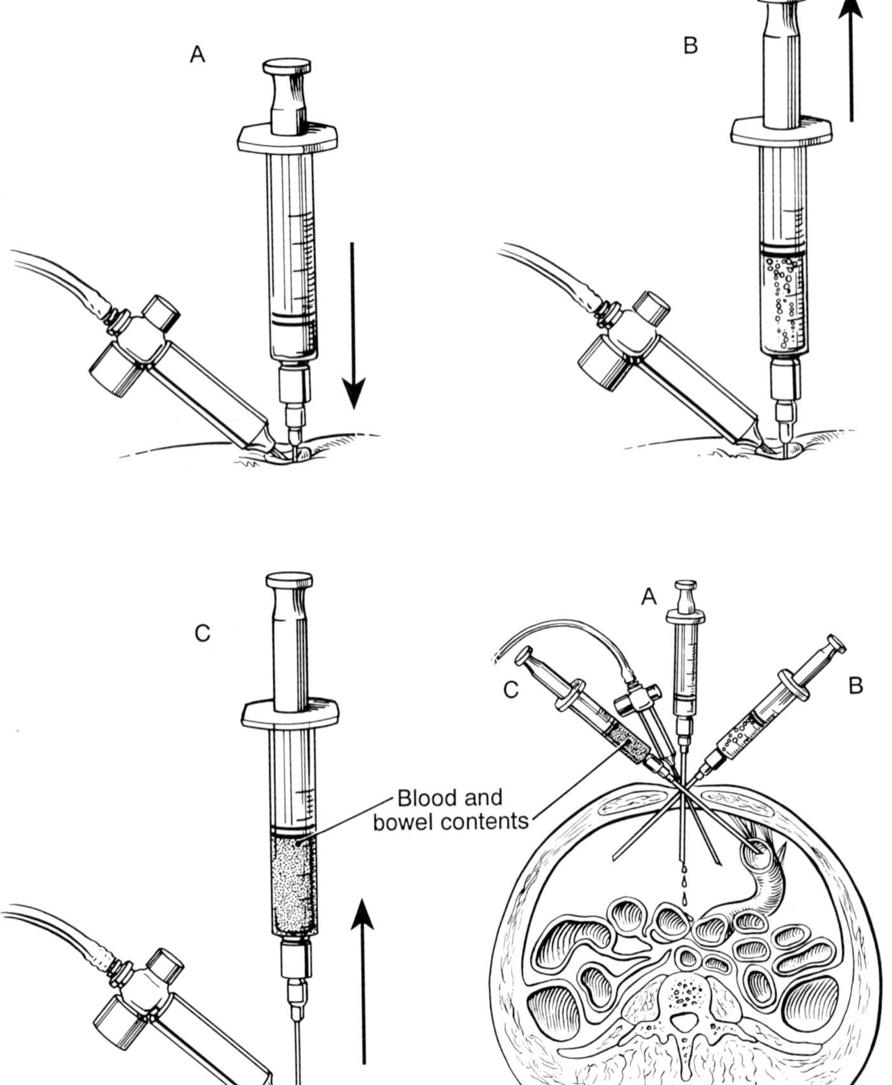

Figure 8-13 Mapping the abdomen using an 18-gauge spinal needle around the Veress needle. A 20-gauge needle is inserted under negative pressure at several cardinal points of a 20-mm circle around the umbilicus. If blood or bowel content is aspirated instead of CO_2 gas at any of these points, alternate sites for trocar insertion should be chosen.

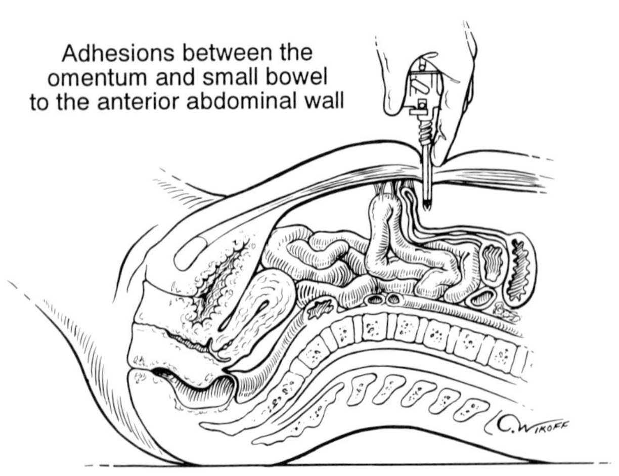

Figure 8-14 Trocar insertion in a patient with bowel adhesions from a previous laparotomy.

scopically or through a minilaparotomy.[3] Since adopting this approach, no bowel injuries have been observed resulting from trocar insertion in more than 700 patients with different types of laparotomy incisions for different indications.

Most, but not all, injuries related to trocar insertion occur during the blind insertion of the primary trocar. In patients with severe omental or bowel adhesions, even though the secondary trocars are introduced under direct observation, bowel injury may result. The procedure can be difficult and may be dangerous. Introduction of the ancillary trocar requires some force from the surgeon, which may cause minute deviation from the intended track of insertion. Even with modifications and safeguards, trocars can puncture the viscera, causing substantial injury.

Pelvic Exploration

The initial phase of laparoscopy is to explore the pelvis, assess the extent of disease, document it with photographs or video recordings, and identify anatomic landmarks. Laparoscopy offers a panoramic view, or an almost microscopic inspection. The characteristics of the bladder, ureters, colon, rectum, uterosacral ligaments and major blood vessels are noted (Figure 8-15). The ovaries are examined on all surfaces and the appendix inspected for endometriosis. The upper abdomen, including the abdominal walls, liver, gallbladder, and diaphragm, is examined for abnormality that could contribute to the patient's symptoms. As the laparoscope is turned toward the left, the intestine is evaluated, and the laparoscope is returned to view the pelvic cavity. The omentum and intestines are evaluated for disease and to confirm that these organs were not injured during insertion of Veress needle and trocar. This organized survey of the pelvis enables the gynecologist to plan the operative procedure, helps in the description for the operative report, and serves as a reference for ascertaining future treatment.

After the posterior cul-de-sac is filled with irrigation fluid, the right adnexa is assessed. The fimbria are lifted, and the posterior aspect of the ovary and ovarian fossa is evaluated. The ureter can be seen and its direction is traced from the pelvic brim to the bladder. The uterus is sharply anteverted and the uterosacral ligaments, posterior cul-de-sac, and rectum are examined. The patient is placed into a 30-degree Trendelenburg position to allow the surgeon to push the small bowel into the upper abdomen to aid in viewing the posterior cul-de-sac (Figure 8-16). The rectosigmoid colon and its folds are evaluated and by pushing the rectosigmoid colon laterally, the left and right pararectal areas are examined. The left ovary and tube are evaluated. In the presence of extensive adhesions, this technique is modified. The gynecologist ascertains the approximate location of the normal structures, assesses the type of adhesions, plans the procedure, and decides whether the procedure is to be performed by laparoscopy or laparotomy. This decision depends on the abnormali-

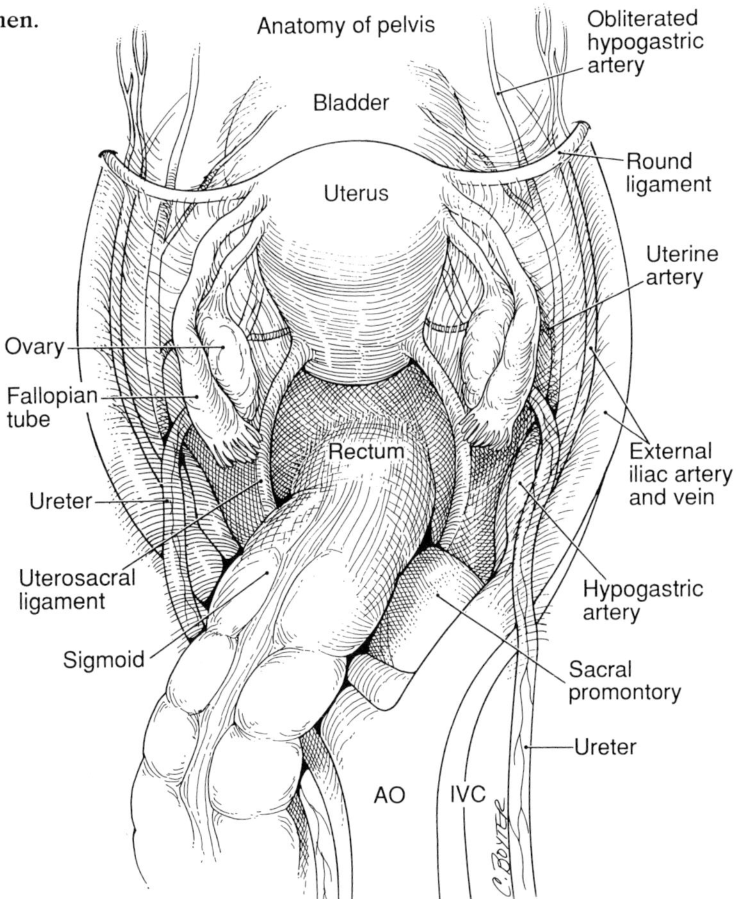

Figure 8-15 Panoramic view of the lower abdomen.

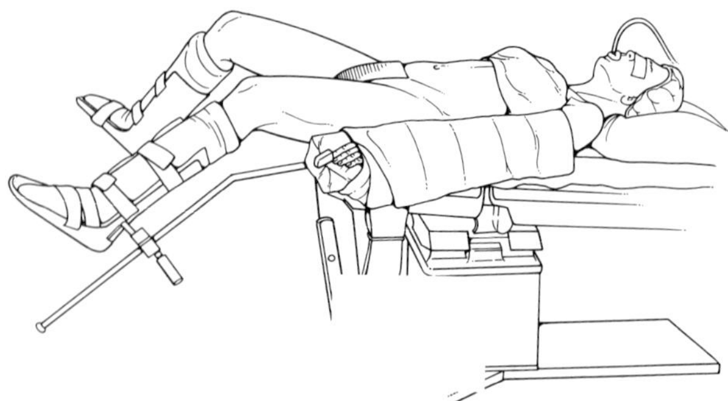

Figure 8-16 The patient is placed in a 30-degree Trendelenburg position.

ties, the time needed to correct them, and the surgeon's experience.

Conclusion of the Procedure

Chromopertubation is performed in all infertility patients intraoperatively. The patient's position is changed from Trendelenburg to horizontal, to allow fluid from the upper abdomen to collect in the pelvic cavity. The entire peritoneal cavity is irrigated copiously with isotonic fluid, usually lactated Ringer's, and inspected for blood clots, pieces of adhesions, cyst wall, endometriosis implants, or bleeding. Bleeding points are identified and coagulated with bipolar forceps. Because the intra-abdominal pressure created by the pneumoperitoneum can tamponade bleeding from small vessels, the gas temporarily is evacuated and the operative sites are reinspected for bleeding before reinsufflating the abdominal cavity. The presence of clear irrigating fluid confirms adequate hemostasis. The procedure is terminated by evacuating the CO_2 from the abdomen.

Release of Pneumoperitoneum

The CO_2 used to distend the abdomen must be evacuated to reduce postoperative shoulder pain caused by gas trapped under the diaphragm. The patient is put in a straight, supine position as the gas is allowed to escape from the umbilical and suprapubic trocars. The suprapubic trocars are removed under low pneumoperitoneal pressure, allowing the detection of possible inferior epigastric vessel injury resulting from trocar insertion. The umbilical trocar is removed and the incision is inspected for bleeding.

Except for patients in whom Interceed (Ethicon) is applied, 300 to 400 mL of lactated Ringer's is left in the abdominal cavity to aid in displacing the gas, and possibly decreasing postoperative adhesion formation.[27] Since this procedure has been instituted, the prevalence of postoperative shoulder pain has decreased. The trocar incisions are closed using Steristrips or an inverted subcutaneous 3-0 polyglactin (Ethicon) suture. Incisions made for trocars larger than 5 mm are closed in layers, especially in older or very thin women, because failure to close the fascia has been associated with small bowel strangulation and hernia.

Postoperative Care and Instructions

Patients should be provided with instructions preoperatively to prepare them for their postoperative experience. The gynecologist sees the patient in the outpatient extended recovery room to explain the operative findings and the expected postoperative course. Before discharge, the patients are given prescriptions for pain medications (usually Tylenol with codeine) as indicated, and routine postoperative instructions. Outpatient nurses or office nurses should contact the patient 1 or 2 days after surgery to answer additional questions and monitor the patient's recovery.

If a patient develops significant pain, fever, or bowel or bladder symptoms, she must be evaluated promptly. Patients are routinely seen 1 to 6 weeks later. Most women return to normal activity within a week. The time required for full recovery, between 1 to 3 weeks, depends on the extent of the pelvic surgery.

Common Postoperative Problems

Nausea and vomiting most likely are related to intra-abdominal CO_2 and the narcotics frequently used perioperatively. Usually, these symptoms respond to parenteral antiemetic medication, but patients occasionally are admitted overnight for continued care. Shoulder pain referred from the collection of CO_2 under the diaphragm is the most frequent complaint and generally resolves within

48 hours. Resting on the abdomen with pillows under it is helpful. Elevating the lower pelvis also will alleviate this pain.

Occasionally a patient will develop hypotension unrelated to blood loss; these patients are cured promptly after a bolus of intravenous fluid is given.

Postoperative incisional pain usually is mild and is managed using a heating pad and analgesics although patients who undergo extensive intra-abdominal procedures can have severe visceral pain. Narcotic or nonsteroidal anti-inflammatory agents are needed in addition to a heating pad. Persistent pain for more than 2 hours requires that the patient be examined.

When large amounts of isotonic fluid are left in the abdomen, the patient tends to drain pinkish fluid through the abdominal puncture wounds, but it resolves within 24 to 48 hours. Reassurance will allay the patient's concern.

Concluding Remarks

To become proficient with operative laparoscopy, the surgeon must understand the learning curve and begin with simple procedures and gradually advance to more complicated ones. It is important to remember that complications can happen while performing the simplest procedures.

The primary steps of any procedure are exposure (by identifying the anatomy and pathology), traction, countertraction, and action (cutting, vaporization, hemostasis, or suturing).

Single Accessory Site

Examples of single accessory site procedures include tubal sterilization, aspiration of an ovarian cyst, or mild peritubal and periovarian adhesiolysis. The suction-irrigator probe is placed through a suprapubic trocar site.

Two Accessory Sites

Examples of two accessory site procedures include lysing peritubal and periovarian adhesions, performing salpingectomy, removing an ectopic pregnancy, or excising moderate pelvic endometriosis. The suction-irrigator and one additional instrument are placed. Traction is required for these procedures. The surgeon uses the suction-irrigator for manipulation and smoke evacuation. Bipolar forceps may replace the grasping instruments if necessary to achieve hemostasis.

Three Accessory Sites

For procedures requiring traction, hemostasis, and suturing almost simultaneously, three sites are necessary. Examples are salpingo-oophorectomy, hysterectomy, repair of an ovarian or uterine defect, lysis of extensive abdominal or pelvic adhesions, myomectomy, cystectomy, etc. During oophorectomy, the surgeon grasps the infundibulopelvic ligament with forceps for traction. The assistant holds the grasping forceps and the surgeon uses the bipolar electrocoagulator to desiccate the infundibulopelvic ligament. Then, the forceps are removed and held by an assistant. The surgeon uses the suction-irrigator probe and while suctioning the plume, the CO_2 laser or any other cutting device is used for excision. During reconstructive surgery, the operator can give the videolaparoscope to the assistant, freeing the former's hands for applying traction and suturing. An assistant can maintain traction with the grasping forceps as the surgeon uses the needle-driver. As with other techniques, surgeons modify procedures as they gain experience. Operative laparoscopy enables the physician to perform complex, delicate procedures through small incisions, thus minimizing the patient's discomfort, morbidity, expense, and duration of convalescence.[28] Laparoscopy is a technique to access the patient's diseased organs and affords the opportunity to remove disease and reconstruct damaged organs depending on the surgeon's training and extent of the disease. Gynecologists trained to correct pelvic abnormalities by laparotomy can learn to treat most conditions laparoscopically.

References

1. Ott DO. Die Beleuchtung der Bauchhohle (Ventroskopie) als Methode bei vaginaler Coeliotomie. *Abl Gynäkol.* 1902;231:817.
2. Palmer R. La coelioscopie gynecologique, ses possibilités et ses indications actuelles. *Sem Hop Paris.* 1954;30:4441.
3. Nezhat CR, Nezhat FR, Silfen SL. Videolaseroscopy: the CO_2 laser for advanced operative laparoscopy. *Obstet Gynecol Clin North Am.* 1991;18:585.
4. Nezhat C, Nezhat F, Pennington E. Laparoscopic treatment of infiltrative rectosigmoid colon and rectovaginal septum endometriosis by the technique of videolaseroscopy and the CO_2 laser. *Br J Obstet Gynaecol.* 1992;99:664.

5. East MC, Steele PRM. Laparoscopic incisions at the lower umbilical verge. *Br Med J.* 1988;296:753.
6. Loffer FD, Pent D. Laparoscopy in the obese patient. *Am J Obstet Gynecol.* 1976;125:104.
7. Hurd WH, Bude RO, DeLancey JOL, Gauvin JM, Aisen AM. Abdominal wall characterization with magnetic resonance imaging and computed tomography: The effect of obesity on the laparoscopic approach. *J Reprod Med* 1991;36:473–476.
8. Neely MR, McWilliams R, Makhlouf HA. Laparoscopy: routine pneumoperitoneum via the posterior fornix. *Obstet Gynecol.* 1975; 45:459.
9. Wolfe WM, Pasic R. Transuterine insertion of Veress needle in laparoscopy. *Obstet Gynecol.* 1990;75:456.
10. Morgan HR. Laparoscopy: induction of pneumoperitoneum via transfundal puncture. *Obstet Gynecol.* 1979;54:260.
11. Awadalla SG. Letter to the editor. *Obstet Gynecol.* 1990;76:314.
12. Corson SL, Batzer FR, Gocial B, Maislin G. Measurement of the force necessary for laparoscopic entry. *J Reprod Med.* 1989; 34:282.
13. Phillips JM. *Laparoscopy.* Baltimore: Williams & Wilkins; 1977:220–246.
14. Soderstrom RM, Butler JC. A critical evaluation of complications in laparoscopy. *J Reprod Med.* 1973;10:245.
15. Nezhat FR, Silfen SL, Evans D, Nezhat C. Comparison of direct insertion of disposable and standard reusable laparoscopic trocars and previous pneumoperitoneum with Veress needle. *Obstet Gynecol.* 1991;78: 148–150.
16. Borgatta L, Gruss L, Barad D, Kaali SG. Direct trocar insertion versus Veress needle use for laparoscopic sterilization. *J Reprod Med.* 1990;35:891.
17. Jarrett JC. Laparoscopy: direct trocar insertion without pneumoperitoneum. *Obstet Gynecol.* 1990;75:725.
18. Kaali SG, Bartfai G. Direct insertion of the laparoscopic trocar after an earlier laparotomy. *J Reprod Med.* 1988;33:739.
19. Saidi MH. Direct laparoscopy without prior pneumoperitoneum. *J Reprod Med.* 1986; 31:684.
20. Copeland C, Wing R, Hulka JF. Direct trocar insertion at laparoscopy: an evaluation. *Obstet Gynecol.* 1983;62:655.
21. Dingfelder JR. Direct laparoscopic trocar insertion without prior pneumoperitoneum. *J Reprod Med.* 1978;21:45.
22. Hasson HM. A modified instrument and method for laparoscopy. *Am J Obstet Gynecol.* 1971;110:886.
23. Hasson HM. Open laparoscopy versus closed laparoscopy: a comparison of complication rates. *Adv Plan Parent.* 1978;13:41.
24. Gomel V, Taylor PJ, Yuzpe AA, Rioux JE. The technique of endoscopy. In: *Laparoscopy and Hysteroscopy in Gynecologic Practice.* Chicago: Yearbook Medical Publishers; 1986:32.
25. Penfield AJ. How to prevent complications of open laparoscopy. *J Reprod Med.* 1985; 30:660.
26. DeCherney AH. Laparoscopy with unexpected viscous penetration. In: Nichols DH, ed. *Clinical Problems, Injuries and Complication of Gynecologic Surgery.* Baltimore: Williams & Wilkins; 1988.
27. Pagidas K, Tulandi T. Effects of Ringer's lactate, Interceed (TC7) and Gore-Tex Surgical Membrane on postsurgical adhesion formation. *Fertil Steril.* 1992;57:199.
28. Luciano AA, Lowney J, Jacobs SL. Endoscopic treatment of endometriosis-associated infertility: therapeutic, economic and social benefits. *J Reprod Med.* 1992;37:573.

9

Laparoscopic Adhesiolysis

Peritoneal adhesions can cause bowel obstruction, pelvic pain, and infertility.[1–3] Caspi and associates reported an inverse relationship between the severity of pelvic adhesions and pregnancy rates.[2] Following adhesiolysis, pregnancy rates vary according to the extent of adnexal damage and, to a lesser degree, the severity of the adhesions.[2–5]

A major detriment to the success of fertility-promoting operations is postoperative adhesion formation. Gynecologic surgeons should understand the mechanism of adhesion formation, use optimal techniques for adhesiolysis, and apply agents or devices to reduce postoperative adhesions. This chapter reviews the pathophysiology of adhesion formation as well as operative techniques and adjuvants used in the prevention and management of pelvic adhesions.

Adhesion Formation

Normal fibrinolytic activity usually prevents fibrinous attachments (fibrinous exudate) for 72 to 96 hours following injury. Mesothelial repair occurs within 5 days of trauma. A single cell layer of mesothelium covers the injured raw area, replacing the fibrinous exudate. However, if the fibrinolytic activity of the peritoneum is suppressed, fibroblasts will migrate, proliferate, and form fibrous adhesions with collagen deposition and vascular proliferation.[1] The factors that suppress fibrinolytic activity and promote formation of postoperative adhesions are listed in Table 9-1.

Formation of Postoperative Adhesions

Microsurgery presupposes the use of magnification, gentle handling of tissues and constant irrigation, meticulous hemostasis, the use of microsurgical instruments, fine nonreactive sutures, and precise approximation of tissue. Fertility-promoting operations performed by laparotomy frequently are followed by reformation of adhesions[6] and the development of new adhesions even when proper microsurgical techniques are applied.[7] Adhesion reformation is found at 37% to 72% of surgical sites[6,7] and 51% of patients develop new adhesions after reproductive surgery by laparotomy.[7]

In several animal and clinical studies, comparisons were made of postoperative adhesion formation after fertility-promoting procedures by laparoscopy and laparotomy. With few exceptions, operative laparoscopy resulted in fewer reformed and new adhesions.[4,8–10] These results are consistent with the observations made a century ago by Von Dembrowski[11] and by Franz,[12] and later confirmed by Ellis.[13] They reported that uncomplicated peritoneal injuries, such as those likely to occur at operative laparoscopy, heal without adhesion formation (Table 9-2).

The Value of Adjuvants

Although microsurgical techniques and operative laparoscopy can reduce the formation of adhe-

TABLE 9-1. Predisposing Factors

Ischemia
Drying of serosal surfaces
Excessive suturing
Omental patches
Traction of peritoneum
Blood clots retained in peritoneal cavity
Prolonged operations
Adnexal trauma
Infection

sions, the benefit derived from various adjuvants remains unclear, despite their widespread use. The most commonly used pharmacologic agents are listed in Table 9-3, but, with few exceptions, they lack the efficacy and safety required for general acceptance.

Steroids and antihistamines are used infrequently because of their questionable efficacy and potential adverse effects such as delayed wound healing and risk of dehiscence.[14] Hyskon, a high-molecular weight dextran is absorbed from the peritoneal cavity over a period of 7 to 10 days. Its osmotic effect draws fluid into the peritoneal cavity to float mobile peritoneal organs, reducing adherence between intraperitoneal structures. Although studies in animals[15] and patients[15,16] have demonstrated reduced postoperative adhesions, inconsistent results suggest limited efficacy. In addition, there have been reports of allergic reactions,[17,18] infections, and complications of fluid overload.

Methods using adhesion barrier membranes may be more promising because they separate peritoneal surfaces and prevent fibrous bands from binding different structures. Two such materials are Interceed (Johnson & Johnson, Arlington, TX), an absorbable fabric of oxidized regenerated cellulose, and Gore-Tex (W.L. Gore and Associates, Inc., Flagstaff, AZ), a nonabsorbable, nonreactive surgical membrane. The latter has been used to repair and reconstruct the pericardium and peritoneum.[19]

In two multicenter studies[20,21] involving 134 and 63 patients, respectively, Interceed was placed on one of the two pelvic sidewalls, which had been treated for comparable disease, at the conclusion of the operation. At second-look laparoscopy, approximately twice (51% versus 24%) as many Interceed-treated sidewalls were free of adhesions compared to untreated sidewalls.[20,21] These observations were extended to four studies[22–25] involving randomly wrapping one of two ovaries with Interceed in a total of 168 patients, also being treated for comparable disease. Again, approximately twice as many ovaries were adhesion free at second-look laparoscopy when Interceed was used.[22–25]

Animal studies have failed to predict the consistent efficacious behavior of Interceed in these six controlled clinical studies since, in animals, Interceed miscellaneously increased,[26] decreased,[27–30] or did not alter[31] adhesion formation. Although a number of animal studies have shown that Gore-Tex Surgical Membrane reduces the formation of adhesions,[30–32] only two small controlled studies have evaluated its effectiveness in gynecologic surgery. In the first of these,[33] patients ($n = 27$) undergoing myomectomy were randomized to have Gore-Tex Surgical Membrane sutured over the closed uterine incisions. At second-look laparoscopy, adhesions were found in 12 out of 27 (44.4%) of the Gore-Tex treated sites and in 25 out of 27 (92.6%) of the control sites. A second study[34] ($n = 29$) compared the effectiveness of Gore-Tex and Interceed when placed on the pelvic sidewall after adhesiolysis. Although no

TABLE 9-2. Historical Perspective

Author	Year	Contribution
Von Dembrowski T[11]	1898	Peritoneal defects in dogs heal mostly without adhesions.
Franz K[12]	1902	
DeRenzi and Boeri[36]	1903	Ischemia is a major etiologic factor in adhesion formation.
Thomas J[37]	1950	Oversewing serosal defects increases rather than decreases adhesion formation.
Ellis H[13]	1971	Excision of parietal peritoneum from rats healed without adhesion formation in 52 of 58 experiments. But "meticulous" repair of peritoneal defects resulted in fibrous adhesions in 16 of 19 experiments.
Ryan et al.[38]	1971	The combination of tissue drying and bleeding is a major promoter of adhesion formation.
Luciano et al.[8]	1989	Postoperative adhesion formation and reformation occur more frequently when surgery is performed by laparotomy than by laparoscopy.

TABLE 9-3. Adjuvants to Prevent Adhesions

Adjuvant	Mechanism of Action
1. Corticosteroids-Antihistamines	Inhibit fibroblast migration, stabilize lysosomal membranes, decrease vascular permeability, and antagonize the effects of histamine
2. Antibiotics	Reduce the risk of infections
3. Nonsteroidal anti-inflammatory	Decrease foreign body reaction
4. Dextran 70 (Hyskon)	Effect hydroflotation of peritoneal organs by drawing fluid into the peritoneal cavity and reducing adherence between peritoneal structures
5. Adhesion barriers	Separate opposing peritoneal surfaces

control group was employed, the study concluded that both barriers were effective in reducing the reformation of adhesions to the pelvic sidewall after reconstructive surgery.

From these studies, it seems that barrier methods using either the absorbable Interceed or the nonabsorbable Gore-Tex are safe and effective in the prevention and reduction of postoperative adhesions. Some patients may be predisposed to such problems, but there is no substitute for careful surgical technique.

Laparoscopic Adhesiolysis

To adequately perform laparoscopic adhesiolysis, three or four abdominal punctures are required—the infraumbilical incision for the operative laparoscope and two to three lower, lateral suprapubic punctures, about 4 cm below the level of the iliac crests (Figure 9-1).

Through the lateral trocar, on the side of the assistant, an atraumatic grasping forceps is inserted to hold the adhesion or involved organ, stretch it, and identify its boundaries and avascular planes. The opposite trocar, on the side of the surgeon, is used for microscissors or the suction-irrigator probe. The latter can serve as a manipulator or backstop when the laser is used (Figure 9-2).

Adhesions should be cut close to the affected organ at both ends and removed from the abdomen if possible. Vascular adhesions are coagulated with lasers or microelectrodes. When scissors are used, filmy and avascular adhesions are stretched and then cut (Figures 9-3 and 9-4, see also Plates 48 and 49). Thick, vascular adhesions must be coagulated before being cut (Figures 9-5 and 9-6, see also Plates 50 and 51).

Bowel adhesions are severed first, followed by periovarian adhesions and peritubal adhesions. This approach allows for progressive exposure of the pelvic structures. Once the intestines are freed from adjacent structures, they can be pushed cephalad. Adherent ovaries are freed from the pelvic sidewall, broad ligament, tubes, and uterus. Grasping forceps are essential for applying traction to the ovary, tube, intestines, or abdominal wall so that a plane of dissection can be identified.

Bleeding areas are coagulated with the laser or bipolar electrocoagulator to maintain a clear field. Whenever possible, either the adhesions or ovarian ligaments should be grasped instead of the ovarian cortex to minimize trauma. Once the ovaries are lifted from the cul-de-sac and mobilized, all peritubal adhesions are removed.

Adhesions can be coagulated effectively and incised with CO_2 laser, superpulse (40 W), ultrapulse (20 to 80 W and 25 to 200 millijoules), fiber laser (15 to 25 W) or microelectrode (15 to 20 W cutting mode). When there are dense adhesions among different organs (bowel, uterus, ovaries, pelvic sidewall, and anterior abdominal wall), hydrodissection with the suction-irrigator probe is useful in creating tissue planes before dissection.

Because an intestinal injury can occur during enterolysis (Figure 9-7A), patients who have a history of previous laparotomies or have severe endometriosis should undergo a bowel preparation. Enterorrhaphy can be accomplished with a one-layer closure of 0 polyglactin (Vicryl, Ethicon) (Figure 9-7B) or an Endoloop (Figure 9-8). Details for repairing an intestinal perforation are found in Chapter 20.

Once the pelvic structures are freed and hemostasis is achieved, the cul-de-sac is filled with lactated Ringer's and the adnexae are allowed to float in the clear fluid (Figure 9-9).[35] Filmy adhesions that are difficult to identify on the surface of the ovary become visible as they float from the ovarian cortex. These adhesions are grasped with the forceps, cut, and removed from their attachments, using laparoscopic microscissors. These adhesions are filmy and avascular so that coagulation is not required.

Agglutinated fimbrial folds are caused by fine avascular adhesions. As the fimbrial folds float and disperse in the fluid, the adhesions become visi-

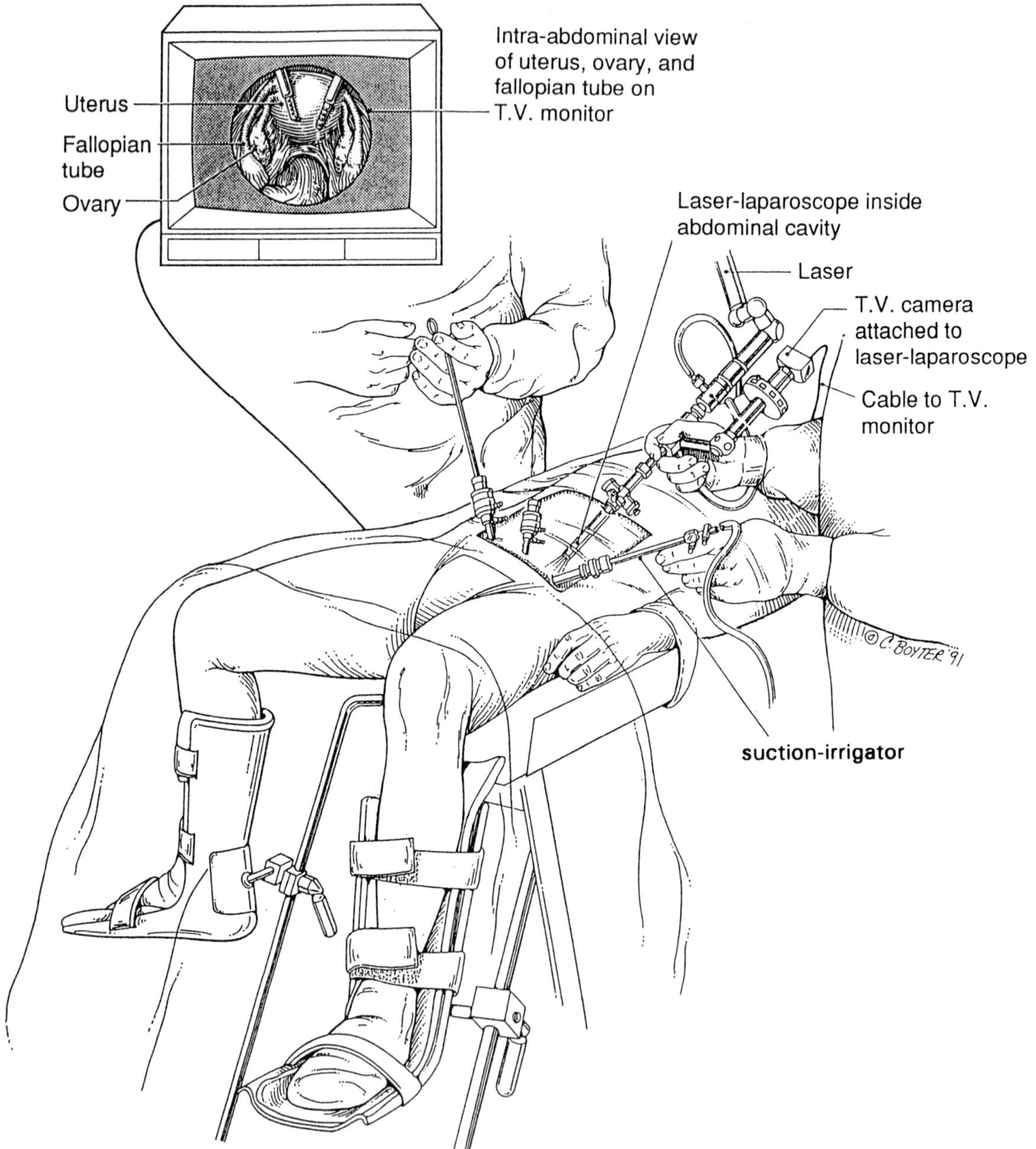

Figure 9-1. Suprapubic punctures are made to introduce the suction irrigator probe and grasping forceps.

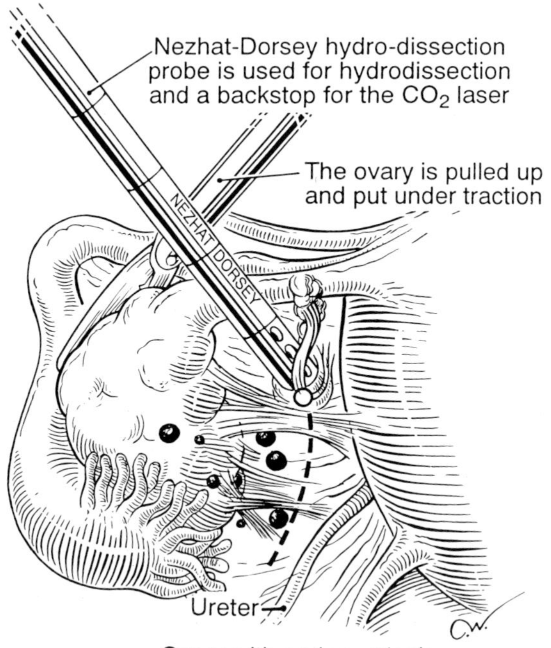

Figure 9-2. Ovariolysis using the CO_2 laser. The left ovary adherent to the pelvic sidewall is grasped and put under traction. The suction-irrigator is used for a backstop and the adhesions are lysed using the CO_2 laser.

ble; they are grasped, stretched, and sharply cut with fine scissors or ultrapulse laser. The laser beam (other than ultrapulse) delivered through the laparoscope is at least 1 mm in diameter and it is too wide for these narrow bands of adhesions. Thermal damage can occur with electrosurgery and the fiber laser (Nd:YAG, KTP, or argon). For delicate microscopic procedures of fimbriolysis and salpingo-ovariolysis, the microscissors or ultrapulse laser is preferable.

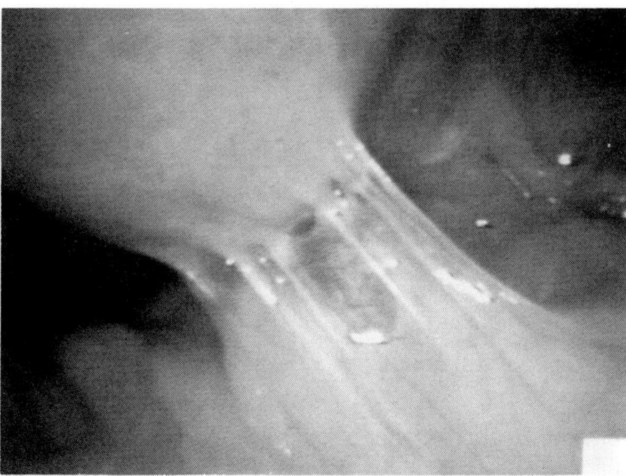

Figure 9-3. Avascular adhesions between the uterus and omentum are put under stretch before dissection with scissors (see Plate 48).

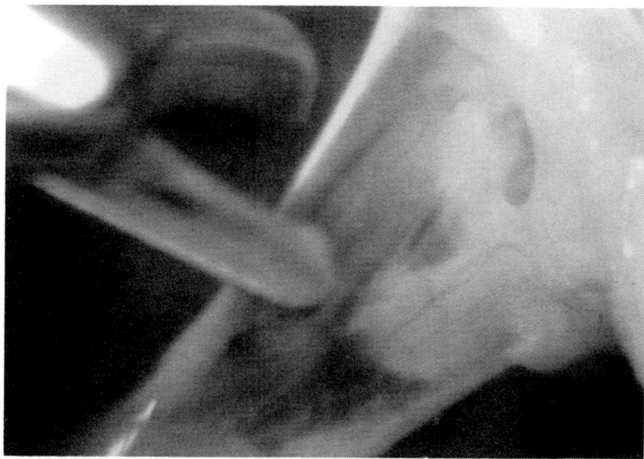

Figure 9-4. Avascular adhesions are dissected with scissors (see Plate 49).

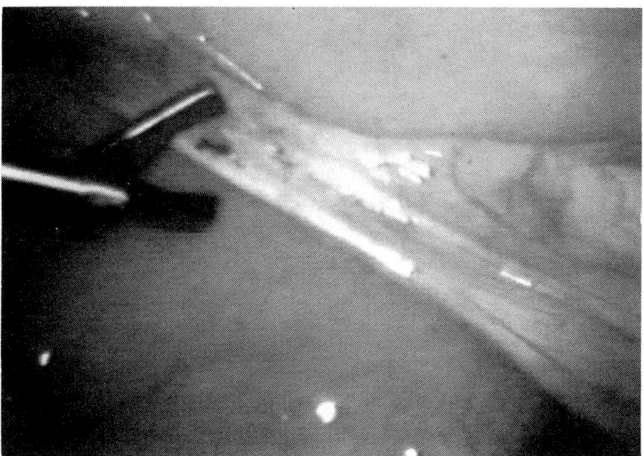

Figure 9-5. Thick, vascular adhesions are coagulated before dissection (see Plate 50).

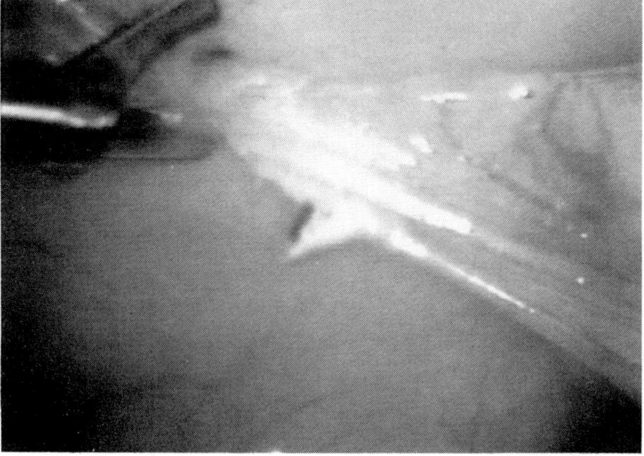

Figure 9-6. A coagulated vascular adhesion is lysed with scissors (see Plate 51).

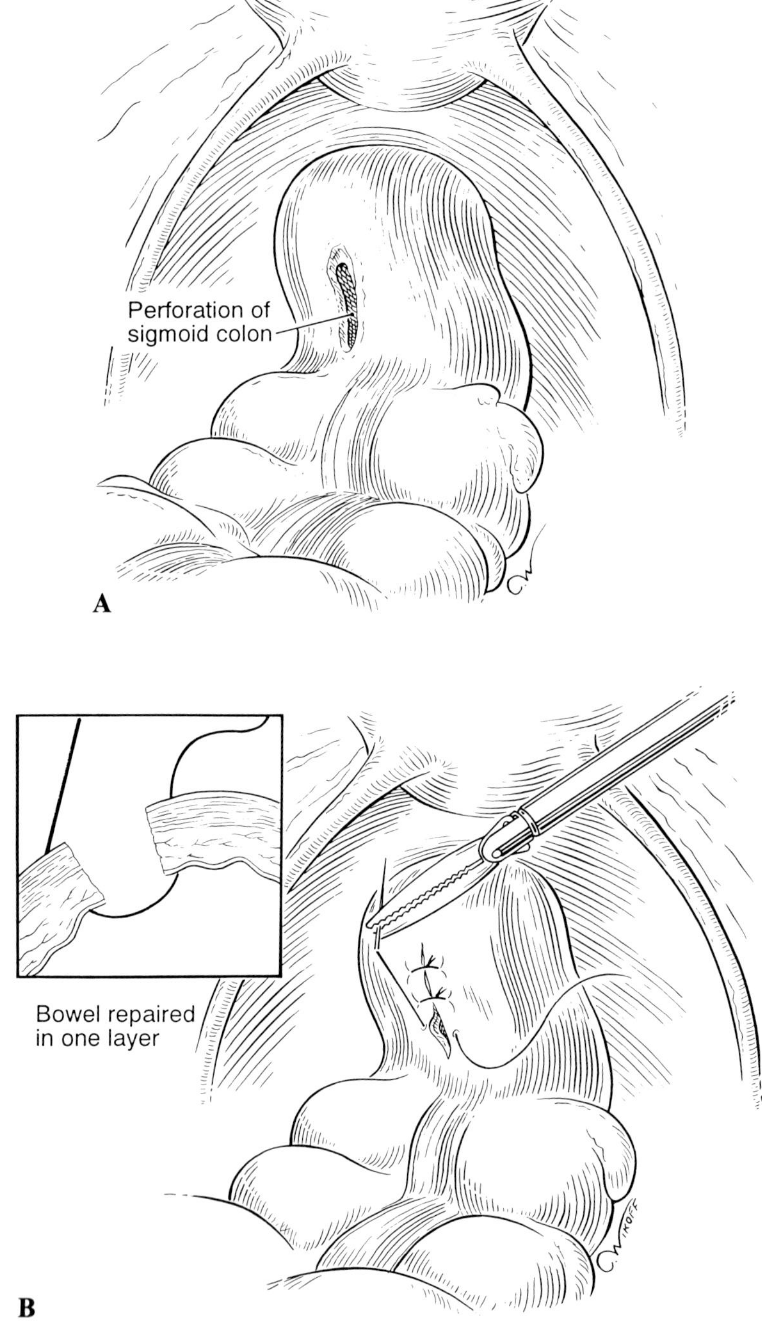

Figure 9-7. A, A rectosigmoid colon injury during adhesiolysis or removal of endometriosis. B, Injury is repaired in one layer using 5–0 (Tevdek). Inset shows a full thickness one-layer repair.

Figure 9-8. A and B, Repair of bowel injury using Endoloop. C, The repair is examined under water. Air bubbles indicate an incomplete closure (inset).

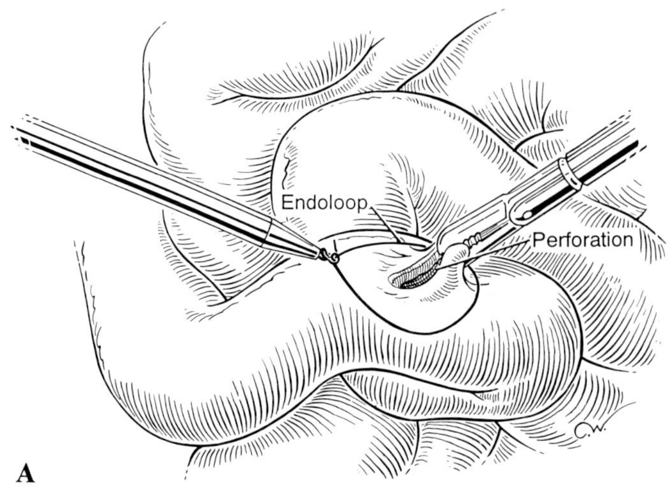

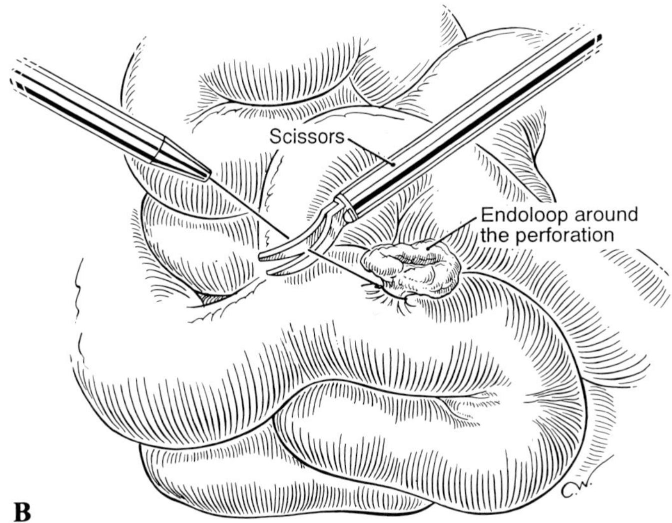

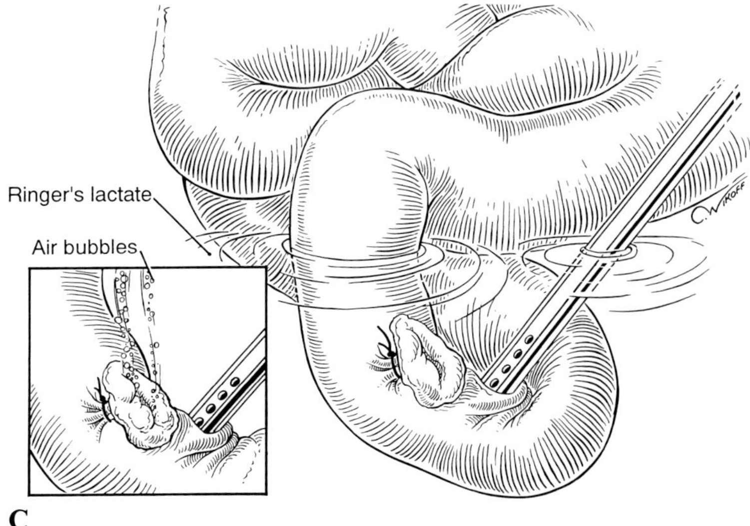

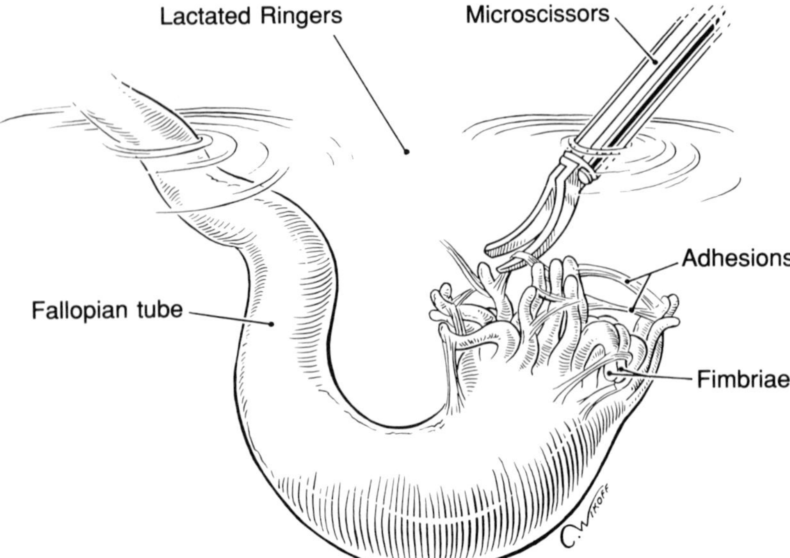

Figure 9-9. Hydroflotation of the tube and fimbria to detect and remove filmy adhesions.

Conclusion

Significant progress has been made toward understanding the pathophysiology of postoperative adhesion development, but adjuvants and microsurgery have not eliminated them. Operative laparoscopy may be more effective than laparotomy in reducing postoperative adhesions and should be the initial step in their management.

References

1. diZerega GSD, Holtz G. Cause and prevention of postsurgical pelvic adhesions. In: Osofsky H, ed. *Advances in Clinical Obstetrics and Gynecology*. Baltimore: Williams & Wilkins; 1982:277–289.
2. Caspi E, Halperin Y, Bukovski I. The importance of periadnexal adhesions in tubal reconstruction surgery for infertility. *Fertil Steril*. 1979;31:296.
3. Hulka JF. Adnexal adhesions: a prognostic staging and classification system based on a five year survey of fertility surgery results at Chapel Hill, North Carolina. *Am J Obstet Gynecol*. 1982;144:141.
4. Nezhat C, Metzger MD, Nezhat F, et al. Adhesion formation following reproductive surgery by videolaseroscopy. *Fertil Steril*. 1990;53:1008.
5. Donnez J, Casanas-Roux F. Prognostic factors of fimbrial surgery. *Fertil Steril*. 1986;45:778.
6. Trimbos-Kemper TCM, Trimbos JB, van Hall EV. Adhesion formation after tubal surgery: results of the 8 day laparoscopy in 188 patients. *Fertil Steril*. 1985;43:395.
7. Gomel V, McComb P. Microsurgery in gynecology. In: Silver JS, ed. *Microsurgery*. Baltimore: Williams & Wilkins; 1979:143.
8. Luciano AA, Maier DB, Koch El, et al. A comparative study of postoperative adhesions following laser surgery by laparoscopy versus laparotomy in the rabbit model. *Obstet Gynecol*. 1989;74:220.
9. Operative Laparoscopy Study Group. Postoperative adhesion development after operative laparoscopy: evaluation at early second-look procedures. *Fertil Steril*. 1991;55:700.
10. Lundorff P, Hahlin M, Kallfelt B, et al. Adhesion formation after laparoscopic surgery in tubal pregnancy: a randomized trial versus laparotomy. *Fertil Steril*. 1991;55:911.
11. Von Dembowski T. Über die urasachen der peritonealein adhäseonen nach chirurgischen mit Rücksicht auf die Frage des Ileus nach Laparotomien. *Arch Klin Chir*. 1888; 37:745.
12. Franz K. Über die Bedeutung der Branchorfe in der Bauchhöhle. *Z Geburtshilfe Gynaköl*. 1902;47:64.
13. Ellis H. The cause and prevention of postoperative intraperitoneal adhesions. *Surg Gynecol Obstet*. 1971;133:497.
14. Jansen BPS. Failure of intraperitoneal adjuncts to improve the outcome of pelvic operations in young women. *Am J Obstet Gynecol*. 1983;153:363.

15. Luciano AA, Hauser KS, Benda J. Evaluation of commonly used adjuvants in the prevention of postoperative adhesions. *Am J Obstet Gynecol.* 1983;146:88.
16. Rosenberg SM, Board JA. High-molecular-weight dextran in human fertility surgery. *Am J Obstet Gynecol.* 1984;148:380.
17. diZerega GS, Hodger GD. Reduction of postoperative pelvic adhesions with intraperitoneal 32% dextran 70: a prospective randomized clinical trial. *Fertil Steril.* 1983;40:612.
18. Borten M, Seibert CP, Taymor ML. Recurrent anaphylactic reaction to intraperitoneal dextran 75 used for prevention of postsurgical adhesions.*Obstet Gynecol.* 1983;61:755.
19. Minale C, Nikol S, Hollweg, G, et al. Clinical experience with expanded polytetrafluoroethylene Gore-Tex surgical membrane for pericardial closure: a study of 110 cases. *J Cardiac Surg.* 1988;3:193.
20. Azziz R and the INTERCEED Barrier Study Group. Microsurgery alone or with INTERCEED Absorbable Adhesion Barrier for pelvic sidewall adhesion reformation. *Surg Gynecol Obstet.* 1993;177:135.
21. Sekiba K and the Obstetrics and Gynecology Adhesion Prevention Committee. Use of Interceed (TC7) absorbable adhesion barrier to reduce postoperative adhesion reformation in infertility and endometriosis surgery. *Obstet Gynecol.* 1992;79:518.
22. Franklin RR, Malinak LR, Larsson B, et al. Reduction of ovarian adhesions by the use of Interceed. *Fertil Steril Prog Suppl.* 1993; 31S, and submitted for publication.
23. Keckstein J, Karageorgieva E, Roth R, et al. Reduction of postoperative adhesion formation after laparoscopic ovarian cystectomy. *Int J Gyn Obstet.* 1994;46 (suppl 1):9.
24. Van Geldorp H. Interceed absorbable adhesion barrier reduces the formation of postsurgical adhesion after ovarian surgery. *Fertil Steril Prog Suppl.* 1994; p. 273.
25. Larsson B, Berg AA, Bryman I, et al. (1995) The efficacy of Interceed Absorbable Adhesion Barrier (TC7) for prevention of reformation postoperative adhesions on ovaries, fallopian tubes, and fimbriae in microsurgical operation for fertility. *Fertil Steril.* (in press.)
26. Haney AF, Doty E. Murine peritoneal injury and de novo adhesion formation caused by oxidized-regenerated cellulose (Interceed* [TC7]) but not expanded polytetrafluoroethylene (Gore-Tex* Surgical membrane) *Fertil Steril.* 1992;57:202.
27. Diamond MP, Linsky CB, Cunningham T, et al. A model for sidewall adhesions in the rabbit: reduction by an absorbable barrier. *Microsurg.* 1987;8:197.
28. Linsky CB, Diamond MP, Cunningham T, et al. Adhesion reduction in the rabbit uterine horn model using an absorbable barrier–TC7. *J Reprod Med.* 1987;32:17.
29. Steinleitner A, Lopez G, Suarez M, et al. An evaluation of Flowgel as an intraperitoneal barrier material for the prevention of postsurgical adhesion reformation. *Fertil Steril.* 1992;57:305.
30. Montz FJ, Monk BJ, Lacy SM. Effectiveness of two barriers at inhibiting post-radical pelvic surgery adhesions. *Gyn Oncol.* 1993;48: 247.
31. Pagidas K, Tulandi T. Effects of Ringer's lactate, Interceed (TC7), and Gore-Tex surgical membrane on PST surgical adhesion formation. *Fertil Steril.* 1992;57:199.
32. Boyers SP, Diamond MP, DeCherney AH. Reduction of postoperative pelvis adhesions in the rabbit with Gore-Tex surgical membrane. *Fertil Steril.* 1988;49:1066.
33. Tulandi T, Rowe G, Rock J, et al. Effects of expanded polytetraflouroethylene Gore-Tex Surgical Membrane on postmyomectomy adhesion. *Fertil Steril Prog Suppl.* 1994; p. 266.
34. Haney AF, Hesla J, Hurst BS, et al. Prevention of pelvic sidewall adhesion reformation using surgical barriers: expanded polytetraflouroethylene (Gore-Tex® Surgical Membrane) is superior to oxidized regenerated cellulose (Interceed® TC7). *Feril Steril Prog Suppl.* 1994; p. 265.
35. Nezhat F, Winer WK, Nezhat C. Fimbrioscopy and salpingoscopy in patients with minimal to moderate pelvic endometriosis. *Obstet Gynecol.* 1990;75:15.
36. DeRenzi E, Boeri G. Das Hetz als Schutzorgan. *Bed klin Wochenschr.* 1903;40:773.
37. Thomas JW. Continued hyaluronidase on formation of intraperitoneal adhesion in rat. *Proc Soc Exp Biol Med.* 1950;74:497.
38. Ryan GB, Groberty J, Majno G. Postoperative peritoneal adhesions. A study of the mechanisms. *Am J Pathol* 1971;675:117.

10

Ectopic Pregnancy

A tubal pregnancy represents certain demise of the gestation, a threat to the woman's life, and a subsequent successful pregnancy in less than 50% of patients. Until 1970, more than 80% of ectopic pregnancies were diagnosed after rupture. With the excellent resolution from transvaginal sonography (TVS), the high sensitivity of radioimmunoassay of beta subunit human chorionic gonadotropin (βhCG), and the increased vigilance of the clinician, more than 80% of ectopic pregnancies can be detected before rupture. Although earlier diagnosis has resulted in decreased maternal mortality and morbidity, the number of hospitalizations for this condition increased from 17,800 in 1970 to 52,200 in 1980, representing a nearly threefold rise.[1,2] Ranging in frequency from 1 in 250 to 1 in 87 live births, ectopic pregnancy has emerged as one of the leading causes of maternal death, accounting for 10% of all maternal mortalities.[3] In 1986, the Centers for Disease Control and Prevention reported 36 maternal deaths attributable to tubal pregnancy, accounting for 13.2% of all maternal deaths in the United States.

The risk of ectopic pregnancy is higher in nonwhite (all races other than white, including black, Asian, and American Indian) women (relative risk is 1.6); it increases three to four times in women between the ages of 35 and 44 compared to those from 15 to 24.[4] About 61% of women subsequently will conceive, but only 38% of them will deliver a living infant. The others will either have a spontaneous abortion or suffer a repeated ectopic gestation.[5,6]

About 95% of ectopic pregnancies occur in the ampulla where fertilization occurs, but they can occur elsewhere in the tube, cervix, ovary, or abdominal cavity (Figures 10-1 through 10-5). A higher risk of ovarian implantation exists in women who conceive while using intrauterine contraceptive devices.[7]

The recent increase in ectopic pregnancy has been attributed to a greater incidence of sexually transmitted disease, previous tubal operations (either reconstruction or sterilization), delayed childbearing, and more successful clinical detection. The major risk factors for this life-threatening condition are listed in Table 10-1. Theoretically, any condition that prevents or retards migration of the fertilized ovum to the uterine cavity could predispose a woman to an ectopic gestation.

Diagnosis

The first step is to establish the presence of a pregnancy, which can be detected as early as 10 days following ovulation using the newer, more sensitive serum assays for βhCG. Once pregnancy has been diagnosed, the serum βhCG titer and the change in titers over the subsequent days become important, especially if the patient is at risk. During the first 5 weeks of a normal gestation, βhCG levels double every 1.5 days, and every 3.5 days at 7 or more weeks of gestation.[8] However, in ectopic pregnancy, one third of patients show a normal serum βhCG pattern. In the others, βhCG levels do not double every 2 to 3 days, but plateau or decline over time.[9] An abnormal βhCG pattern is consistent with an ectopic gestation or threatened, inevitable, or tubal abortion. Besides being associated with lower titers and slower increases in the serum concentration of βhCG than normal pregnancies, ectopics are associated with slower de-

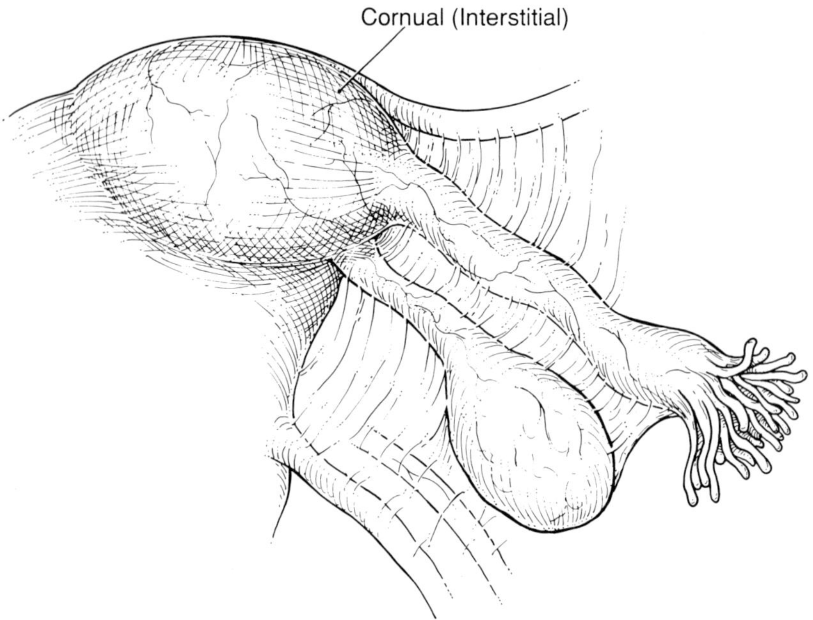

Figure 10-1. Cornual (interstitial) pregnancy.

clines in serum βhCG titers than spontaneous abortions.

Less than 25% of ectopic pregnancies have βhCG concentrations of 6000 mIU/mL or greater at initial evaluation.[10] Pregnancies that demonstrate less than a 66% increase in βhCG levels during a 48-hour period are either ectopic or aborting pregnancies.[11] However, in early pregnancy, 64% of women with a tubal gestation can have a normal doubling of serum βhCG levels.[12] Thus, a normal rise in βhCG levels does not reliably differentiate an ectopic from an intrauterine pregnancy.

A single progesterone assay is predictive of an abnormal pregnancy but not specific for an ectopic pregnancy.[13] A single serum progesterone value of 25 ng/mL or more is strongly indicative of a normal intrauterine pregnancy. A serum proges-

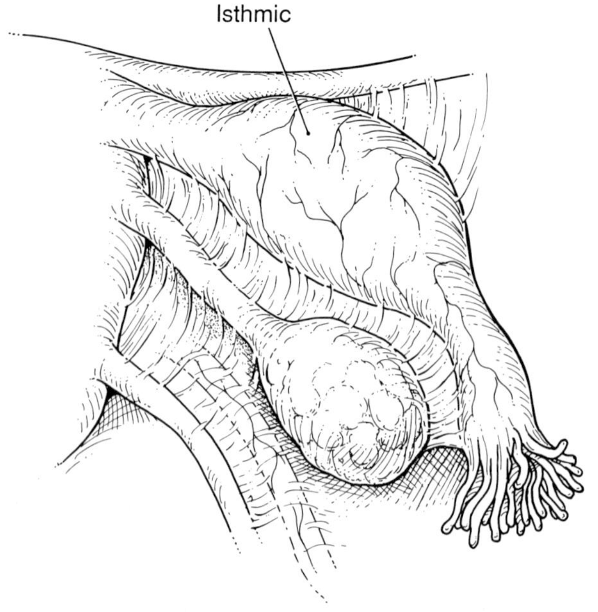

Figure 10-2. Isthmic pregnancy.

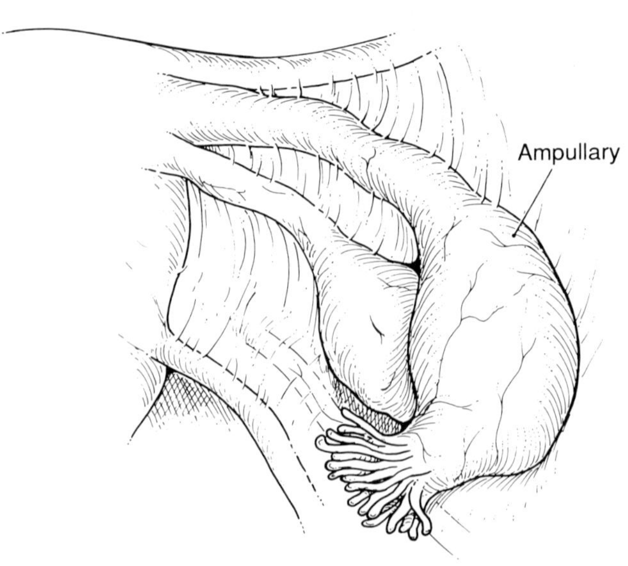

Figure 10-3. Ampullary pregnancy.

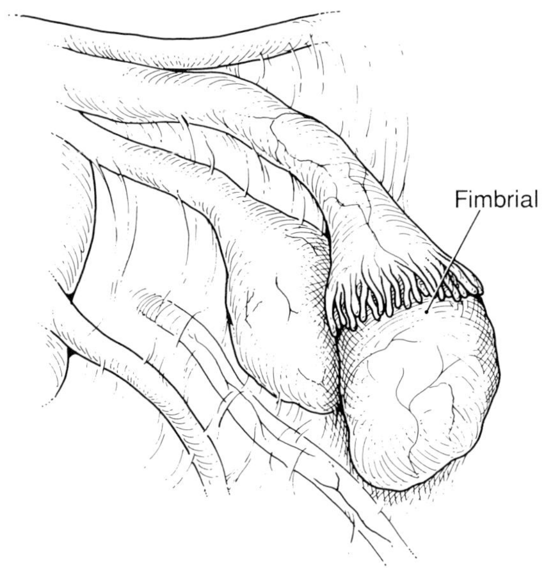

Figure 10-4. Fimbrial pregnancy.

TABLE 10-1. Major Contributing Factors and Associated Relative Risks for Ectopic Pregnancy

Risk Factors	Relative Risk, %
Current use of intrauterine devices	11.9
Use of clomiphene citrate	10.0
Prior tubal surgery	5.6
Pelvic inflammatory disease	4.0
Infertility	2.9
Induced abortion	2.5
Adhesions	2.4
Abdominal surgery	2.3
T-shaped uterus	2.0
Myomata	1.7
Progestin-only contraceptives	1.6

Source: Marchbanks PA, Annegers JF, Coulam CB, et al.[7]

terone value of 15 ng/mL or less suggests an abnormal pregnancy, ectopic or threatened abortion.[14]

Symptoms

The usual pregnancy symptoms, including nausea, vomiting, breast fullness, fatigue, and interruption of the normal menstrual pattern also occur with ectopic pregnancy. Other more typical symptoms of ectopic pregnancy include lower abdominal pain of varying intensity and abnormal uterine bleeding ranging from spotting to heavy bleeding. The presence of shoulder pain suggests possible rupture with intraperitoneal blood flowing toward the diaphragm, causing nerve irritation. About one third of patients with ruptured ectopic pregnancies experience syncope as a result of hypotension caused by hypovolemia.

Physical Findings

Signs of ectopic pregnancy (Table 10-2) include lower abdominal tenderness with or without rebound, usually more severe on the affected side. There may be tenderness on cervical motion. The

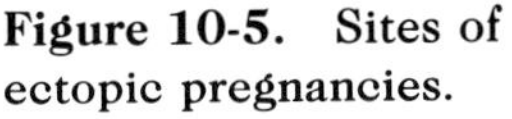
Figure 10-5. Sites of ectopic pregnancies.

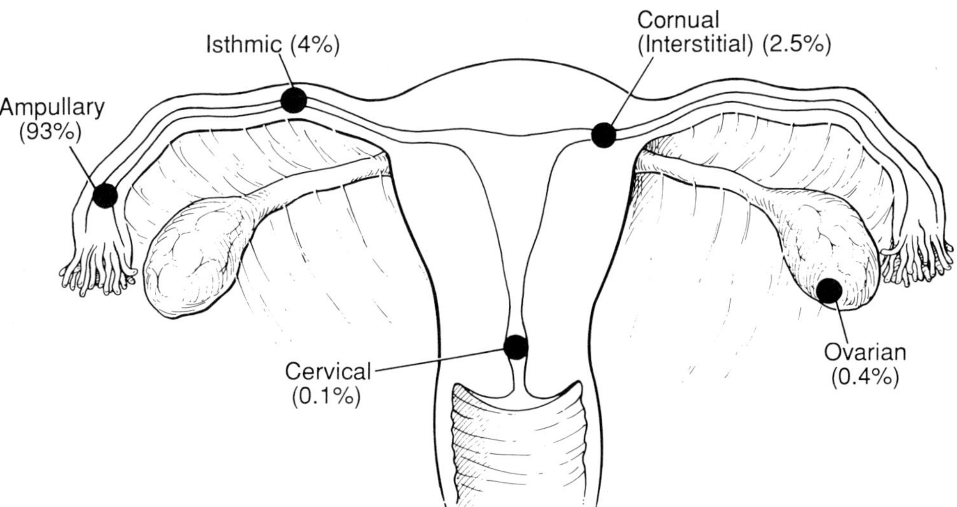

TABLE 10-2. Symptoms and Signs Suggestive of Tubal Pregnancy

1. Nausea, breast fullness, fatigue, interruption of menses
2. Lower abdominal pain, heavy cramping, shoulder pain
3. Uterine bleeding, spotting
4. Pelvic tenderness, enlarged, soft uterus
5. Adnexal mass, tenderness
6. Positive pregnancy test
7. Serum levels of βhCG of <6000 mIU/L at 6 wks
8. Less than 66% increase in βhCG titers in 48 h
9. Positive culdocentesis (83%)
10. Absence of gestational sac in the uterus by TVS
11. Gestational sac outside the uterus by TVS

uterus usually is enlarged slightly and soft. An adnexal mass is palpated in 50% of patients. Culdocentesis revealing nonclotting blood can be found even with unruptured ectopics.[15]

Ectopic pregnancy can be detected early and more precisely with a combination of TVS and measurement of serum βhCG levels. Kadar and colleagues[16] introduced two concepts to aid in the diagnosis of ectopic pregnancy, namely, the appearance of an intrauterine gestational sac seen by abdominal ultrasound with a serum βhCG level of 6000 to 6500 mIU/mL and the doubling of βhCG levels every 48 hours. When the serum βhCG level is above 6500 mIU/mL, the absence of an intrauterine sac strongly suggests an ectopic pregnancy. The presence of an apparent intrauterine sac with βhCG levels below 6000 mIU/mL suggests an ectopic pregnancy, missed or spontaneous abortion. Using these criteria, 15% of normal uterine pregnancies would fall in the ectopic category and 13% of the ectopic pregnancies would be missed. More accurate diagnostic results can be obtained with the high-frequency vaginal transducers capable of detecting a normal gestational sac in 98% of women after the fifth week of pregnancy, when βhCG levels are greater than 1025 mIU/mL.[17]

Treatment

Since 1970, a conservative approach to unruptured ectopic pregnancy has been advocated to preserve tubal function (Table 10-3). Several surgical procedures have been performed successfully,[18] including linear salpingostomy, "milking" the pregnancy from the distal ampulla, and partial salpingectomy followed by anastomosis. Postoperative viable births or repeat ectopic pregnancies are similar between salpingectomy with or without ipsilateral oophorectomy, and salpingostomy.[19]

In 321 tubal pregnancies treated conservatively by laparoscopy, it was reported that 15 (4.7%) required subsequent laparotomy or second laparoscopic procedure because βhCG levels failed to return to normal.[20]

The contemporary surgical approach in hemodynamically stable patients is operative laparoscopy, which yields postoperative pregnancy rates comparable to those reported following laparotomy.[19–24] Vermesh and coworkers[21] pro-

TABLE 10-3. Comparative Results of Conservative Surgery for Ectopic Pregnancy by Laparotomy Versus Laparoscopy

Authors	No. Cases	% Intrauterine Pregnancy	% Ectopic Pregnancy
Laparotomy			
DeCherney, Kase[19]	49	40	12
Stromme[22]	45	71	15
Timonen et al.[23]	240	38	16
Vermesh et al.[21]*	30	42	16
Total	364	47.75	14.75
Laparoscopy			
Pouly et al.[20]	118	64	22
DeCherney, Diamond[18]	79	62	16
Vermesh et al.[21]*	30	50	6
Total	227	58.67	14.67

* Controlled and prospectively randomized to laparotomy and laparoscopy.

spectively randomized patients with unruptured ectopic pregnancy to either laparoscopy or laparotomy, and subsequently analyzed pregnancy rates, tubal patency by hysterosalpingogram, postoperative morbidity, length of hospital stay, duration of convalescence and hospital cost. The authors found that although the two surgical procedures were similarly safe and effective, the laparoscopic approach was more cost effective and required a shorter recovery period. It has been suggested that the laparoscopic approach results in improved fertility rates because of reduced adhesion formation.[25] Subsequent controlled animal[26] and clinical studies[27] confirmed the impression that laparoscopic surgery was associated with reductions of both new adhesion formation and reformation of preexisting adhesions. A comparative analysis of adhesion formation following laparoscopic surgery and laparotomy for the treatment of ectopic pregnancy has been conducted.[28] Tubal healing and the extent of pelvic adhesions were assessed at repeat laparoscopy within 15 weeks of the initial operation. Although tubal patency did not differ between the two groups, patients who had been treated by laparotomy developed more adhesions. Brumsted and colleagues[29] reported shorter convalescence (8.7 ± 7.8 days versus 25.7 ± 16.2 days, $P<.01$) and reduced postoperative analgesia requirements (0.84 ± 2.3 versus 4.64 ± 2.9 doses; $P<.01$) in the laparoscopy group compared to the laparotomy group.

When possible, endoscopy is the preferred surgical option. With adequate practice and surgical experience in operative endoscopy, and with proper instruments, most patients with ectopic pregnancies can be treated successfully by laparoscopy regardless of the gestation's size or location, number of gestations, or the presence of tubal rupture.[30] Following a nonstimulated menstrual cycle, three separate gestational sacs were identified in one woman at initial operative laparoscopy, one in the right tube and two in the left tube.[31] Because of delayed childbearing and the expanded use of assisted reproductive technology, multiple ectopic pregnancies may become more prevalent. Therefore, it is important that at the initial exploratory procedure, the surgeon examine the whole length of both fallopian tubes after the obvious ectopic pregnancy has been identified and treated to avoid missing another ectopic pregnancy.

In the surgical management of a tubal gestation, the gynecologist must consider the patient's desire for further childbearing. In all instances, the patient is informed of the possibility of laparotomy with salpingectomy or a need for more extirpative procedures because of uncontrollable bleeding or unexpected findings. If neither tube can be saved, the uterus and at least one ovary should be preserved to retain the possibility of in vitro fertilization.[32]

Laparoscopic Approach

At laparoscopy, the location, the size, and the nature of the tubal pregnancy are ascertained. Ruptured tubal pregnancies can be treated successfully endoscopically if the bleeding has ceased or can be arrested adequately. Once bleeding is controlled, the products of conception and blood clots are removed. A 10-mm suction instrument will cleanse the abdominal cavity quickly. Forced irrigation with lactated Ringer's solution will dislodge clots and trophoblastic tissue from the serosa of the peritoneal organs with minimal trauma to these structures.

For unruptured tubal pregnancies, the tube is identified and mobilized. To minimize bleeding, a 5- to 7-mL diluted solution containing 20 U Pitressin in 100 mL of normal saline is injected with a 20-gauge spinal or laparoscopic needle in the mesosalpinx just below the ectopic pregnancy and over the antimesenteric surface of the tubal segment containing the gestational products (Figure 10-6). The needle must not be within a blood vessel because intravascular injection of vasopressin solution can precipitate acute arterial hypertension, bradycardia, and even death.[30]

Using a laser, microelectrode, or scissors, a linear incision is made on the antimesenteric surface extending 1 to 2 cm over the thinnest portion of the tube containing the pregnancy. The pregnancy usually protrudes through the incision and slowly slips out of the tube; it may be teased gently out using hydrodissection or laparoscopic forceps (Figures 10-7 and 10-8). Sometimes, more forceful irrigation in the tube's opening can dislodge the gestation from its implantation. As the pregnancy is pulled out or extrudes from the tube, some of the products of conception can adhere to the implantation site by a ligamentous structure containing blood vessels (Figure 10-9). Using the electrocoagulator this structure should be coagulated before removing the tissue. Oozing from the tube is common but usually ceases spontaneously. Occasionally, coagulation is necessary with either a defocused laser beam or with the electrocoagulator. Depending on the size, the products of conception are removed through either a 5- or 10-mm trocar sleeve (Figure 10-10).

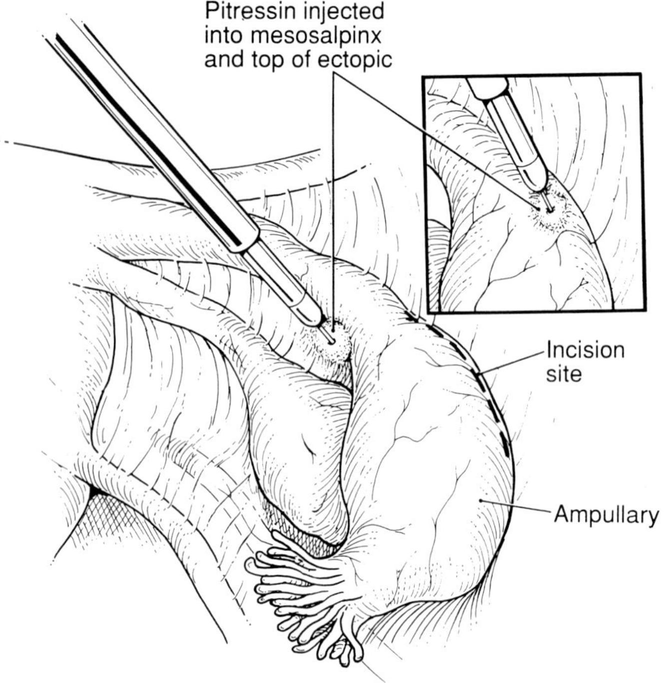

Figure 10-6. Injection of vasopressin into the mesosalpinx; inset shows tubal injection.

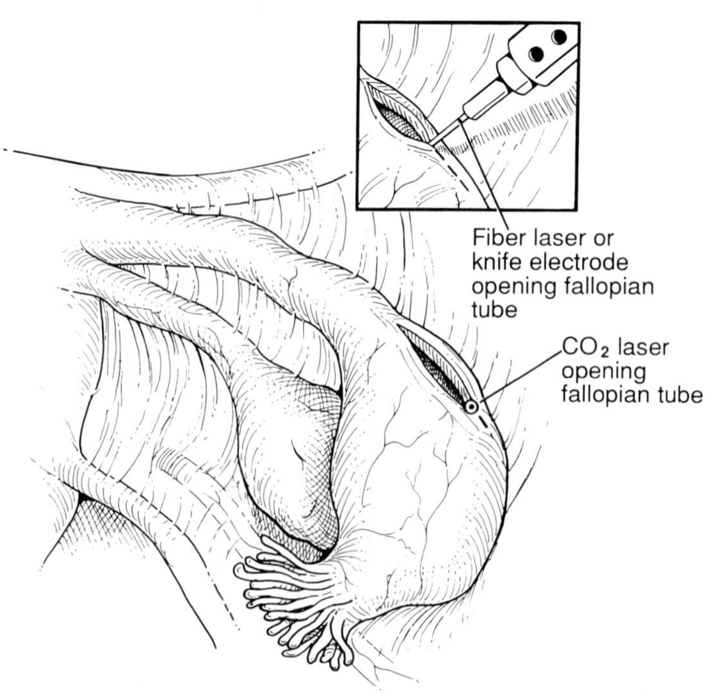

Figure 10-7. Salpingostomy is made with CO_2 laser, fiber laser, or knife electrode (*inset*).

Figure 10-8. Hydrodissection is performed to dislodge the ectopic pregnancy.

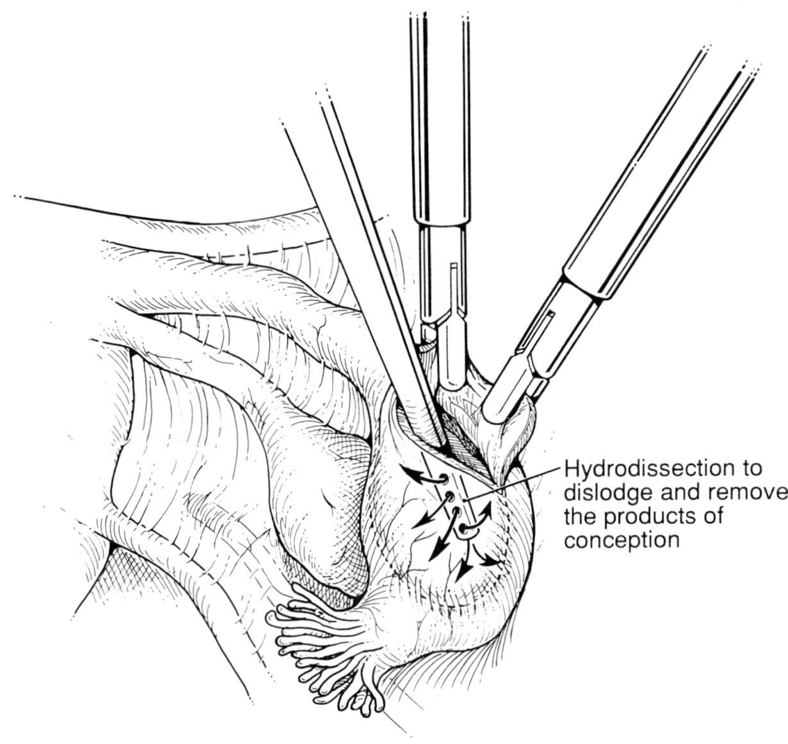

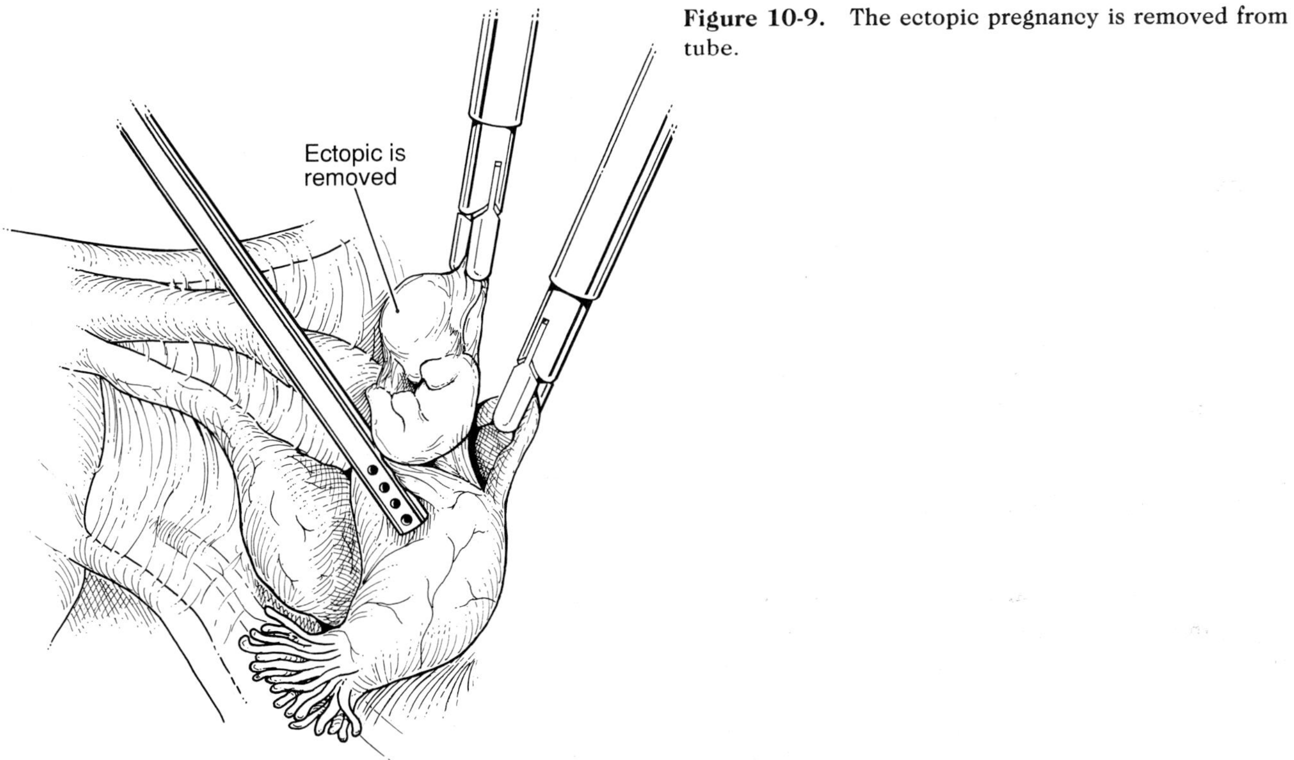

Figure 10-9. The ectopic pregnancy is removed from tube.

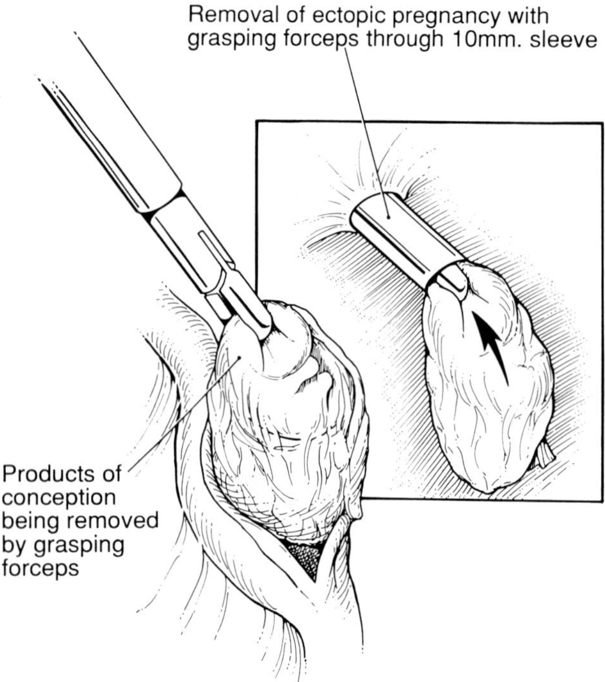

Figure 10-10. The ectopic pregnancy is removed completely and pulled into the 10-mm trocar sleeve (*inset*).

Resection of the tubal segment containing the gestation is preferable to salpingostomy for an isthmic pregnancy or a ruptured tube, or if hemostasis is difficult to obtain. Segmental tubal resection is performed with bipolar electrosurgery, fiber lasers (KTP, argon, or Nd:YAG), CO_2 laser, sutures, or stapling devices.

Bloodless segmental tubal resection is achieved by grasping the proximal and distal boundaries of the tubal segment containing the gestation with the Kleppinger forceps and thoroughly coagulating them from the antimesenteric surface to the mesosalpinx. The segment is cut with laparoscopic scissors or laser, with little risk of bleeding. The mesosalpinx under the pregnancy is coagulated, with particular attention given to the arcuate anastomosing branches of the ovarian and uterine vessels.[33] Following coagulation, the mesosalpinx is cut (Figures 10-11 and 10-12). Similarly, total salpingectomy is performed by progressively coagulating and cutting the mesosalpinx, beginning with the proximal isthmic portion, progressing to the fimbriated end of the tube. It is separated from the uterus using bipolar coagulation and scissors or laser (Figures 10-13, 10-14, and 10-15). The isolated segment containing the ectopic pregnancy is removed intact or in sectioned parts through the 10-mm trocar sleeve. The products of conception can be placed in a plastic bag (Endopouch, Ethicon) and removed (Figure 10-16). A multifire stapling device for salpingectomy requires a 12-mm trocar. Alternatively, one or two Endoloops (Ethicon) can be applied around the salpinx and the tube cut and removed.

Adhesions or other pathologic processes such as endometriosis can be treated simultaneously during removal of the ectopic pregnancy without significantly prolonging the operation. Occasionally, the patient is admitted overnight to be observed for postoperative bleeding and for emotional support by the infertility team. In one week, the patient returns for a serum βhCG to ascertain resolution of the tubal gestation. The βhCG level should be either undetectable or very low. If it is above 20 mIU/mL, a repeat blood test is ordered 1 to 2 weeks later when the βhCG should be undetectable.[34]

Interstitial Pregnancy

This type of pregnancy is associated with an increased risk of traumatic rupture, hemorrhagic shock, and a twofold increase in maternal mortality over other tubal pregnancies. Delayed diagnosis and increased vascularity of this area where the uterine and ovarian vessels join account for these increased risks. Two percent to 4% of ectopic gestations are interstitial (cornual; see Figure 10-1). The anatomy of this region accommodates the growing gestation, accounting for its late onset of symptoms and occasional reports of term interstitial pregnancies.

The traditional management for interstitial or cornual pregnancy is salpingectomy with or without cornual resection, and in some cases, hysterectomy. However, in properly selected women, more conservative and less radical approaches may be used if the diagnosis is made early and the patient is stable. Interstitial pregnancy should be suspected in women with an enlarged asymmetrical uterus and an eccentrically placed gestational sac on TVS. Differential diagnoses include ovarian and abdominal pregnancy or a pregnancy in one horn of a bicornuate uterus. The diagnosis can be confirmed by laparoscopy. Treatment involves immediate laparotomy or a combined laparoscopic and hysteroscopic approach in appropriately selected patients.

At laparoscopy, the interstitial pregnancy is recognized as a cornual bulge stretching the myometrium and serosal surface (see Figure 10-1). If

Figures 10-11 and 12. Segmental resection of an isthmic ectopic pregnancy is performed by coagulating the proximal and distal boundaries of the gestation.

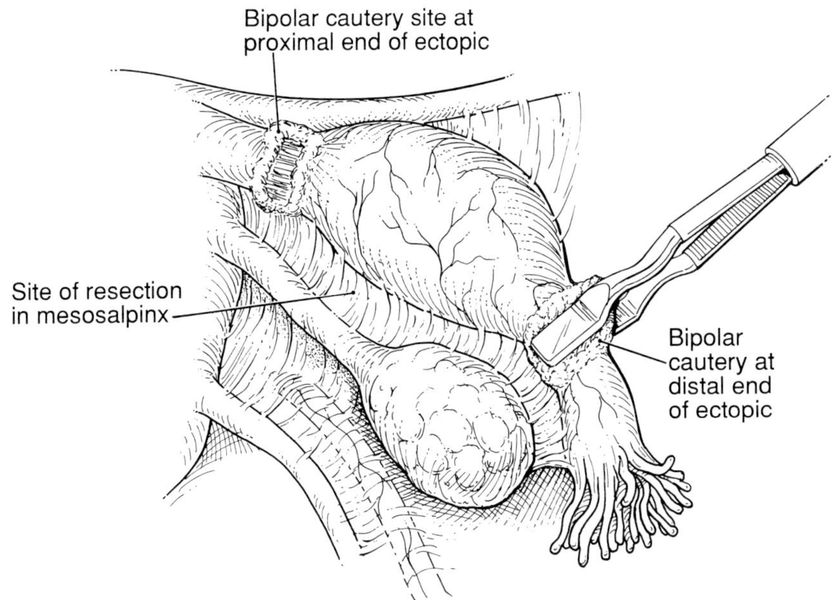

Figure 10–11

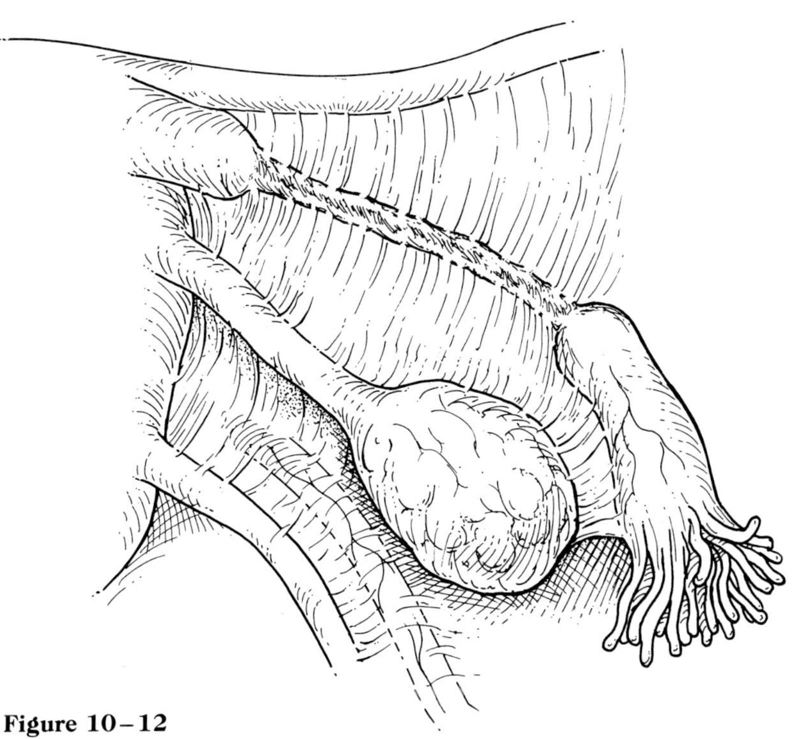

Figure 10–12

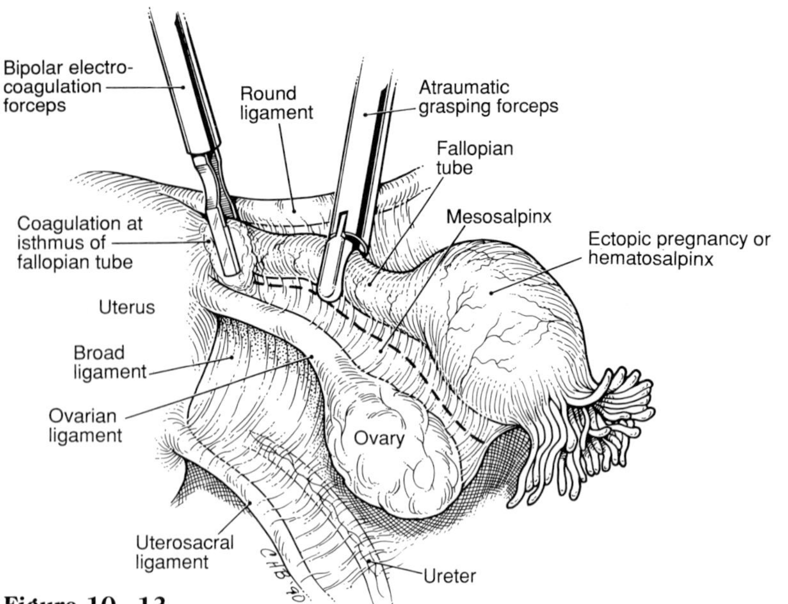

Figure 10–13

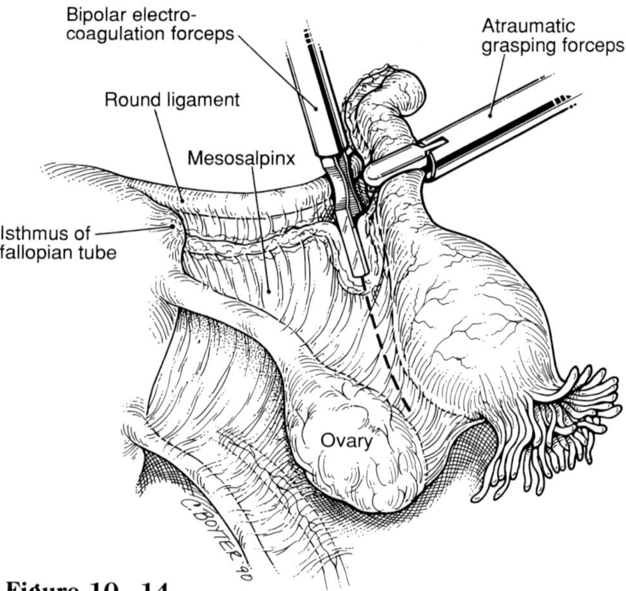

Figure 10–14

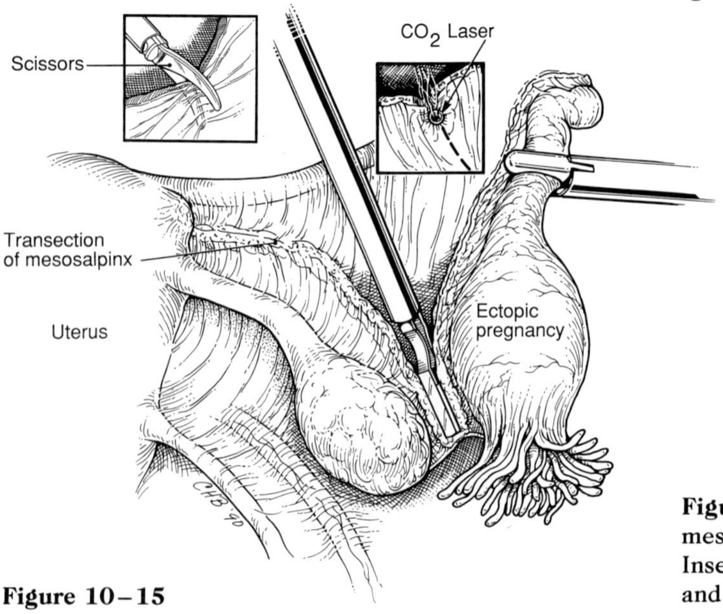

Figure 10–15

Figures 10-13, 14, and 15. Coagulation of the mesosalpinx is performed for complete salpingectomy. Insets show transection of mesosalpinx with scissors and CO_2 laser.

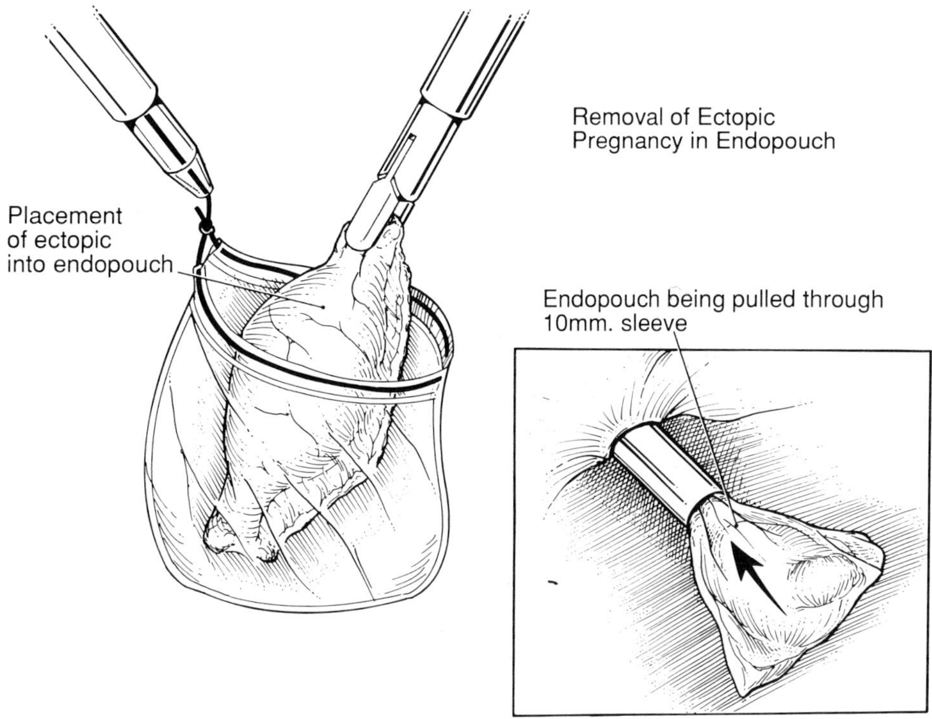

Figure 10-16. Ectopic pregnancy placed in Endopouch. Inset shows removal through 10-mm trocar sleeve.

the overlying myometrium is thick and intact, it is best to attempt removal of the pregnancy by hysteroscopy. A diagnostic laparoscopy should be performed to identify the location of and accessibility to the cornual gestation. If the pregnancy is accessible by hysteroscopy, it may be suctioned or resected using forceps, scissors, or electrosurgery under hysteroscopic control.[35] For larger pregnancies, it may be better and faster to perform a gentle curettage of the dilated interstitial-cornual pregnancy under laparoscopic control to avoid uterine perforation. To ascertain complete removal of the products of conception, hysteroscopic control of the curetted cornu and the interstitial area should be done.

When the pregnancy has eroded through the cornual myometrium, it may be more prudent to perform a laparotomy to evacuate the pregnancy. In properly selected patients, a laparoscopic approach may be considered after appropriate counseling of the patient and if the surgeon is prepared to perform an immediate laparotomy. The cornu is very vascular and profuse bleeding can occur quickly.

Nonsurgical Management of Ectopic Pregnancy

Other approaches to tubal pregnancy include either expectant management or the use of methotrexate (MTX). Because some tubal pregnancies terminate in tubal abortions or complete reabsorption, selected patients can be monitored by obtaining repeated levels of βhCG until tubal abortion or reabsorption occurs as indicated by falling hormone levels.[36] This alternative may preserve tubal function and fertility although tubal occlusion can result from retained ectopic pregnancy.[37] The use of MTX to destroy an ectopic pregnancy has been advocated for women with a cornual pregnancy, an incomplete resolution of surgically treated ectopic gestation, or residual trophoblastic tissue. Patients who are a poor surgery risk because of induced ovarian hyperstimulation syndrome or who are suspected of having extensive intraperitoneal abdominal adhesions can be treated medically[38,39]—if they are hemodynamically stable. In one study, patients were treated with MTX 1 mg/kg intravenously and leucovorin 0.1 mg/kg intramuscularly every other day for 4 days. Patients were admitted to the hospital and monitored during therapy with serum levels of aspartate aminotransferase, lactic dehydrogenase, βhCG, progesterone, and with complete blood and platelet counts.[38] Given the protracted course of such a regimen, the associated delayed resolution of the ectopic gestation, and potential adverse effects and expense involved, systemic chemotherapy is not an attractive alternative.

However, the injection of MTX into the gestational sac under ultrasound guidance or at laparoscopy is feasible and 17 of 25 patients were treated successfully with this technique.[40] Seven patients required additional systemic injections and one patient experienced tubal rupture 3 days after the initial injection. The tubal injection consisted of 10 to 20 mL adrenaline 1 : 80,000 dilution injected into the mesosalpinx with a 22-gauge needle, followed by 100 mg MTX injected into the tubal gestation. Leucovorin 15 mg was given orally 30 hours after the administration of MTX. Subsequent systemic MTX injections were given intramuscularly, 50 mg every 2 to 4 days, according to the level of serum βhCG. The relative efficacy of MTX and prostaglandin sulprostone has been compared.[38] The drug was administered into the gestational sac and intramuscularly on days 3, 5, and 7 after the day of diagnosis and local treatment in 21 patients with an unruptured tubal pregnancy. Both therapies were equally effective in 21 patients studied. However, 34% of patients underwent either laparotomy or laparoscopy for ruptured ectopic pregnancy or a persistent rise in the βhCG levels despite treatment. A single intramuscular injection of MTX (50 mg/m^2) without citrovorum rescue was successfully used in 29 of 30 consecutive patients with unruptured ectopic pregnancies. Six patients experienced an increase in abdominal pain and two were hospitalized for overnight observation.[41] This single-dose regimen administered on an outpatient basis decreases expenses and minimizes side effects associated with the treatment of ectopic pregnancies of 5 cm or less in diameter.

References

1. Rubin GL, Peterson HB, Dorfman SF, et al. Ectopic pregnancy in the United States: 1970 through 1978. *JAMA*. 1983;249:1725.
2. Ectopic pregnancy—United States. 1981–83. *MMWR*. 1986;35:289.
3. Schneider J, Berger CJ, Cattell C. Maternal mortality due to ectopic pregnancy: a review of 102 deaths. *Obstet Gynecol*. 1977;49:557.
4. Ectopic pregnancy—United States, 1986. *MMWR*. 1989;38:1.
5. Schoen JA, Nowak RJ. Repeat ectopic pregnancy: a 16-year clinical survey. *Obstet Gynecol*. 1975;45:542.
6. Sandvei R, Bergsio P, Ulstein M, et al. Repeat ectopic pregnancy—a twenty-year hospital survey. *Acta Obset Gynecol Scand*. 1987;66:607.
7. Marchbanks PA, Annegers JF, Coulam CB, et al. Risk factors for ectopic pregnancy: a population based study. *JAMA*. 1988;259: 1823.
8. Fritz MA, Guo SM. Doubling time of hCG in early normal pregnancy: relationship to hCG concentration and gestational age. Fertil Steril. 1987;47:584.
9. Kadar N, Romero R. Serial human chorionic gonadotropin measurements in ectopic pregnancy. *Am J Obstet Gynecol*. 1988; 158:1239.
10. Dause K, Mundy D, Graves W, et al. Ectopic pregnancy. What to do during the 20-day window. *J Reprod Med*. 1989;34:162.
11. Kadar N, Caldwell BV, Romero R. A method of screening for ectopic pregnancy and its indications. *Obstet Gynecol*. 1981;58:162.
12. Shephard RW, Patton PE, Novy MJ, Burry KA. Serial beta-hCG measurements in the early detection of ectopic pregnancy. *Obstet Gynecol*. 1990;75:417.
13. Gelder MS, Boots LR, Younger JB. Use of a single random serum progesterone value as a diagnostic aid for ectopic pregnancy. *Fertil Steril*. 1991;55:497.
14. Hubinont CJ, Thomas C, Schwers JF. Luteal function in ectopic pregnancy. *Am J Obstet Gynecol*. 1987;156:669.
15. Vermesh M, Graczykowski JW, Sauer MV. Reevaluation of the role of culdocentesis in the management of ectopic pregnancy. *Am J Obstet Gynecol*. 1990;162:411.
16. Kadar N, DeVore G, Romero R. Discriminatory hCG zone: its use in the sonographic evaluation for ectopic pregnancy. *Obstet Gynecol*. 1981;58:156.
17. Goldstein SR, Snyder JR, Watson C, et al. Very early pregnancy detection with endovaginal ultrasound. *Obstet Gynecol*. 1988; 72:200.
18. DeCherney AH, Diamond MP. Laparoscopic salpingostomy for ectopic pregnancy. *Obstet Gynecol*. 1987;70:948.
19. DeCherney AH, Kase N. The conservative surgical management of unruptured ectopic pregnancy. *Obstet Gynecol*. 1979;54:451.
20. Pouly JL, Mahnes H, Mage G, et al. Conservative laparoscopic treatment of 321 ectopic pregnancies. *Fertil Steril*. 1986;46:1093.
21. Vermesh M, Silva PD, Rosen GF, et al. Management of unruptured ectopic gestation by linear salpingostomy: a prospective, randomized clinical trial of laparoscopy versus laparotomy. *Obstet Gynecol*. 1989;73:400.
22. Stromme WB. Conservative surgery for ec-

topic pregnancy. a 20-year review. *Obstet Gynecol.* 1973;41:215.

23. Timonen S, Nieminen U. Tubal pregnancy choice of operative method of treatment. *Acta Obstet Gynecol Scand.* 1967;46:327.
24. Lundorff P, Thornburn J, Lindblom B. Fertility outcome after conservative surgical treatment of ectopic pregnancy evaluated in a randomized trial. *Fertil Steril.* 1992;57:998.
25. Bruhat MA, Manhes H, Mage G, et al. Treatment of ectopic pregnancy by means of laparoscopy. *Fertil Steril.* 1980;33:411.
26. Luciano AA, Maier DB, Koch EI, et al. A comparative study of postoperative adhesions following laser surgery by laparoscopy versus laparotomy in the rabbit model. *Obstet Gynecol.* 1989;74:220.
27. Nezhat C, Metzger MD, Nezhat F, et al. Adhesions reformation after reproductive surgery by videolaseroscopy. *Fertil Steril.* 1990; 53:1008.
28. Lundorff P, Hahlin M, Kallfelt B, et al. Adhesion formation after laparoscopic surgery in tubal pregnancy: a randomized trial versus laparotomy. *Fertil Steril.* 1991;55:911.
29. Brumsted J, Kessler C, Gibson C, et al. A comparison of laparoscopy and laparotomy for the treatment of ectopic pregnancy. *Obstet Gynecol.* 1988;71:889.
30. Nezhat C, Nezhat F. Conservative management of ectopic gestation. *Fertil Steril.* 1990 53:382. Letter.
31. Frishman GN, Steinhoff MM, Luciano AA. Triplet tubal pregnancy treated by outpatient laparoscopic salpingostomy. *Fertil Steril.* 1990;54:934.
32. Luciano AA. Ectopic pregnancy. In: Quilligan EJ, Zuspan FP, eds. *Current Therapy in Obstetrics and Gynecology.* Philadelphia: WB Saunders; 1990:226.
33. Nezhat F, Winer W, Nezhat C. Salpingectomy via laparoscopy: a new surgical approach. *J Laparoendosc Surg.* 1991;1:91.
34. Jafri SZH, Longinsky JS, Bouffard JA, et al. Sonographic detection of interstitial pregnancy. *J Clin Ultrasound.* 1987;15:253.
35. Meyer WR, Mitchell DE. Hysteroscopic removal of an interstitial ectopic gestation: a case report. *J Reprod Med.* 1989;34:929.
36. Kamreava MM, Taymor M, Berger MJ, et al. Disappearance of human chorionic gonadotropin following removal of ectopic pregnancy. *Obstet Gynecol.* 1983;62:486.
37. Tulandi T, Ferenczy A, Berger E. Tubal occlusion as a result of retained ectopic pregnancy: a case report. *Am J Obstet Gynecol.* 1988;158:1116.
38. Fernandez H, Baton C, Lelaidier C, et al. Conservative management of ectopic pregnancy: prospective randomized clinical trial of methotrexate versus prostaglandin sulprostone by combined transvaginal and systemic administration. *Fertil Steril.* 1991; 55:746.
39. Ory SJ, Villanueva AL, Sand PK, et al. Conservative treatment of ectopic pregnancy with methotrexate. *Am J Obstet Gynecol.* 1986;154:1299.
40. Kooi S, Kock H CLV. Treatment of tubal pregnancy by local injection of methotrexate after adrenaline injection into the mesosalpinx: a report of 25 patients. *Fertil Steril.* 1990;54:580.
41. Stovall TG, Ling FW, Gray LA. Single doses methotrexate for treatment of ectopic pregnancy. *Obstet Gynecol.* 1991;77:754.

11

Laparoscopic Treatment of Endometriosis

Endometriosis is a progressive, often debilitating disease, affecting 10% to 15% of women during their reproductive years,[1,2] and accounts for 25% of laparotomies performed by gynecologists. Among gynecologic disorders, endometriosis is surpassed in frequency only by leiomyomas.[3]

Patients with endometriosis may present with different clinical complaints and at various stages of disease. Treatment depends on the age of the patient, the extent of disease, severity of symptoms, and desire for fertility. Intervention usually is indicated for pain, infertility, or impaired function of the bladder, ureter, or intestine. Medical and surgical management are available.

This chapter focuses on surgical therapy for management of pelvic pain and infertility associated with endometriosis by laparoscopy and laparotomy. The pros and cons of each method are presented with emphasis on the technical aspects.

Historical Perspectives

Rokitansky described pelvic endometriosis of the fallopian tubes, ovaries, and uterus in 1860.[4] Before 1960, therapy involved hysterectomy and bilateral salpingo-oophorectomy.[5] Conservative operations to relieve pain and preserve fertility have been modified significantly since its introduction. Recognizing the negative impact of surgical trauma and postoperative adhesions on success rates, microsurgical techniques were developed and applied with improved results.[6] Nevertheless, recurrences were not eliminated,[7] and the search for a better solution continued. The development of operative laparoscopy enabled definitive treatment following diagnosis. Whether laparotomy or operative laparoscopy is more effective for the treatment of advanced endometriosis is not clear. Both reduce implants, relieve dysmenorrhea and pelvic pain, and improve fertility potential.[8–12] However, unlike radical surgery, conservative operations seldom are curative.[13,14]

Surgical Approach

The goals of conservative surgical procedures are to remove all implants, resect adhesions, relieve pain, reduce the risk of disease recurrence and postoperative adhesion formation, and restore involved organs to a normal anatomic and physiologic condition. For the infertile patient, restoration of the normal tubo-ovarian relationship is essential to enhance fertility. These goals may be achieved using various surgical instruments (scalpel, scissors, lasers, or electrodes), and a variety of techniques (laparoscopy, laparotomy, or combined endoscopy and minilaparotomy).

Since 1980, surgical instruments and techniques with varying degrees of efficacy have been introduced including lasers, video cameras, monitors, electric generators, hydrodissection, microelectrodes, microsurgery, and operative laparoscopy.[15] When optimally used, these instruments are effective and safe for treating endometriosis. There are definite advantages to using a high-powered CO_2 laser (especially the Ultrapulse 5000 L) as a long knife through the operative channel of the laparoscope. Because this laser does not penetrate water, it can be used with hydrodissection[16] to selectively treat sensitive areas such as the bowel, bladder, ureters, and blood vessels. Unlike other instruments, the CO_2 laser beam does not obstruct the surgeon's vision during dissection.

Known advantages of operative laparoscopy include faster patient recovery and reduced cost.[17] In addition, as surgeons become more skilled, pregnancy rates following operative laparoscopy should improve and surpass those following laparotomy.

Laparoscopy or Laparotomy

Comparing results from endoscopy and laparotomy is difficult because the outcome is determined by many factors.[18] In contrast, animal experiments can be randomized and properly controlled. Three studies compared postoperative adhesion formation and re-formation following a standardized laser injury and laser adhesiolysis by both surgical approaches.[19–21] Laparoscopy caused fewer postoperative adhesions compared to laparotomy. Following microsurgical salpingoplasty or adhesiolysis by laparotomy, adhesion recurrence rates were 40% to 72%[22–26] and de novo adhesions occurred in over 50% of patients.[22] However, when comparable operations are performed laparoscopically, recurrence of postoperative adhesions appears less frequent,[27] and de novo adhesion formation is either absent or less than 20%.[28] Lundorff and colleagues[25] evaluated adhesion formation following laparoscopy and laparotomy in patients treated for ectopic pregnancy. The authors stratified 105 women with tubal pregnancy by age and risk factors and prospectively randomized them to surgery by laparoscopy or laparotomy. Second-look laparoscopy revealed significantly more adhesions in the laparotomy group.[25]

Data from animal[19–21] and clinical studies[22–26] suggest that laparoscopic surgery is more effective for adhesiolysis, causes fewer de novo adhesions than laparotomy, and reduces impairment of the tubo-ovarian function.[25] The efficacy of laparotomy or laparoscopy has not been evaluated for restoring fertility or reducing symptoms of pelvic pain. However, it has been reported that pain relief and pregnancy rates after operative laparoscopy are comparable to or better than those following laparotomy[7–12,17,18,25,29–32] for endometriosis (mild to severe), hydrosalpinges, and ectopic pregnancy.

Gomel described the therapeutic efficacy of laparoscopic adhesiolysis in 1975.[33] In a follow-up publication, he stated that "in trained hands, laparoscopic salpingo-ovariolysis is a low-risk procedure associated with a surprisingly good success rate."[34] In his series of 92 patients with moderate to severe adnexal adhesive disease, the intrauterine pregnancy rate was 62%.[34] Subsequent studies confirmed that the results of laparoscopy were better than those obtained by laparotomy, especially for severe endometriosis.[11,12,18,29–32] Even extensive endometriosis can be treated more effectively at laparoscopy and with better results than at laparotomy.[9,10]

As evidenced by most studies summarized in Table 11-1 which are neither prospective nor controlled, comparison is difficult. Fayez and Collazo noted better pregnancy rates following laparoscopy (58%) than after laparotomy (36%).[30] Chong and colleagues[35] assessed the relative efficacy of CO_2 laser surgery by laparoscopy versus laparotomy in treating infertile patients with severe endometriosis; the mean rAFS scores were 59 (laparoscopy) and 58 (laparotomy) with similar pregnancy

TABLE 11-1. Number of Patients (N) and Pregnancy Rates (%) Following Conservative Surgery for Endometriosis by Laparotomy or Laparoscopy

	Minimal		Mild		Moderate and Severe	
Laparotomy	N	%	N	%	N	%
Buttram[103]	69	82.6	92	58.7	84	45.2
Rock et al.[104]	45	62.2	88	54.5	81	48.2
Rantala et al.[105]	44	59.1	39	56.4	46	39.1
Gordts et al.[106]	20	40.0	99	42.4	57	35.1
Chong et al.[35]	0		0		13	53.8
Fayez et al.[30]	0		0		42	35.7
Adamson et al.[11]					52	34.6
Total	178	66.9	318	52.2	375	41.3
Laparoscopy						
Feste[107]	47	51.1	6	66.7	5	40.0
Martin[8]	27	25.9	19	15.8	4	25.0
Nezhat et al.[9]	24	75.0	51	62.8	27	44.4
Olive et al.[18]	59	39.0	48	45.8	20	50.0
Nezhat et al.[10]	39	71.8	86	69.8	118	67.8
Chong et al.[35]	0		0		11	54.5
Fayez et al.[30]	0		0		44	50.0
Adamson et al.[11]	0		0		48	37.5
Luciano et al.[17]	0	0	36	61	60	60.0
Total	196	51.0	210	57.6	337	55.5

*No patients with severe endometriosis were included in this study.

rates (see Table 11-1).[35] In two other studies, CO_2 laser laparoscopy was compared to laparotomy as a treatment for all stages of endometriosis associated with infertility.[11,12] Operative laparoscopy was found to be safe and effective for all stages of endometriosis.

Only if the results with laparoscopy are equal to or better than laparotomy should the endoscopic approach be considered.[9,10,35] The reduced hospital cost and recovery period obtained with the laparoscopic approach cannot compensate for failure to achieve optimal treatment.

Radical Surgery

Hysterectomy and bilateral salpingo-oophorectomy are indicated for patients with severe symptoms who have not responded to medical or conservative surgical treatment and who are not interested in pregnancy. Fibrosis obliterates tissue planes and sometimes causes suspicion of malignancy because of extensive involvement of the intestinal and urinary tracts. In advanced disease, the ovaries may be encased and densely adherent to the pelvic sidewall. Ovarian dissection entails risk of injury to the ureter, major blood vessels, and bowel. A retroperitoneal approach can isolate the ureter throughout its course to ensure complete removal of ovarian tissue and avoid ovarian remnant syndrome.[36] Bilateral oophorectomy must be performed to eliminate the estrogen that sustains and stimulates the ectopic endometrium.[37] Although conserving one ovary has resulted in reasonable cure rates,[14,38,39] failure rates of 13% and 40% at 3 and 5 years, respectively, have been reported after laparotomy when ovarian function is preserved.[40] Consequently, in patients who do not desire fertility and whose complaints justify definitive surgical treatment, concomitant removal of both ovaries is recommended as the best chance for relief, particularly if ovarian disease is severe.

Hormone Replacement

Following hysterectomy and bilateral salpingo-oophorectomy, patients often require hormone replacement therapy to relieve menopausal symptoms. Administering the minimal effective dose of estrogen is associated with only a small risk of recurrence.[41–43] In a retrospective study of 85 women with endometriosis, Henderson and coworkers[42] reported a recurrence rate of 1.1% in women receiving estrogen replacement. In contrast, 25% of women with comparable disease and residual ovarian tissue required additional surgery.

Hormone replacement therapy should begin postoperatively. Patients with residual disease may benefit from receiving progestins for 3 to 6 months, followed by combined estrogen and progestin for an additional 9 months. A single intramuscular injection of 100 mg medroxyprogesterone acetate (Depo-Provera) administered on the second postoperative day can suppress hot flashes for up to 12 weeks and, with the hypoestrogenemia following castration, cause regression of residual implants.[44] Similar effects may be achieved with oral medroxyprogesterone acetate (20 to 30 mg/d) for 3 to 6 months postoperatively.[45] Subsequently, combined estrogen and progestin may be administered for up to 12 months after surgery.[43,46] These patients are treated with conjugated estrogen (0.625 mg) or Estrace (1.0 mg daily) and medroxyprogesterone acetate (2.5 mg or 5.0 mg daily) to minimize the risk of recurrence and prevent menopausal symptoms. Estrogen-progestin therapy is continued for the first postoperative year to induce further regression of residual disease. Women who are treated with estrogen only are protected against bone loss and cardiovascular disease and have a lower risk of recurrence of endometriosis. The use of estradiol pellets (25 to 50 mg) and testosterone (75 mg) administered subcutaneously every 4 to 6 months has been reported with good results.[47]

Chetkowski and colleagues[48] have suggested that there are varying degrees of responsiveness of the various organs to blood estradiol levels. Although the precise serum concentration of estrogen required to prevent growth of endometriosis has not been ascertained, it seems that the serum concentration of estradiol required to induce growth and proliferation of endometriosis is significantly higher (greater than 50 pg/mL) than that required to stabilize bone mineral density (20 to 50 pg/mL) and prevent osteoporosis.[41,48] Transdermal estrogen may be substituted (50 μg semiweekly) if circulating levels of estradiol are kept between 40 and 70 pg/mL to maximize therapeutic effects and minimize the risk of symptom recurrence.[43]

Conservative Surgery

Conservative surgery is indicated for women who desire pregnancy and whose disease is responsible for their symptoms of pain or infertility. Although seldom curative, surgery improves the likelihood of pregnancy and offers at least temporary pain relief. Approximately 25% of patients undergoing conservative operations will require a subsequent operation because of recurrence of endometriosis or progression of residual (microscopic) disease.[49] The rate of repeat surgical intervention is related directly to the extent of disease and the ability to conceive postoperatively. Of those who achieve pregnancy after the initial operation, only 10% require another operation.[40,49] Conservative operations are cytoreductive and recurrence of symptoms most likely is caused by the progression of existing, microscopic disease that was not seen during surgery.[50–52]

Appearances of Endometriosis

Complete removal of the endometriotic implants is difficult because of their variability in appearance and visibility. Powder burn lesions represent foci of inactive disease containing stroma and glands embedded in hemosiderin deposits (Figure 11-1, see also Plate 53).[53] These lesions are more common in older women and may not cause pain or infertility.[54] When implants involve the uterosacral ligaments, they are palpable as tender nodularities and may cause dysmenorrhea and dyspareunia (see Figure 11-1). Atypical and nonpigmented lesions, seen as clear vesicles, pink vascular patterns, white scarred lesions, red lesions, yellow-brown patches, and peritoneal windows (Table 11-2; Figures 11-2 and 11-3, see also Plates 54 and 55) represent active endometriosis and secrete prostaglandin in the peritoneal fluid.[55]

The depth of endometrial implants may be related to the level of disease activity and symptoms. Cornille and coworkers[56] reported that cellular activity of endometriosis was greater for both superficial and deep implants (58% and 68%, respectively) than for intermediate implants (25%). They postulated that early lesions result from proliferation of retrograde menstrual tissue and present as superficial implants. These lesions progress to an intermediate depth where they either become inactive or progress and infiltrate deeper layers, usually more than 5 mm (see Figures 11-1 through 11-3). Implants continue their biologic activity and proliferate, being stimulated by circulating steroid hormones because they are no longer de-

TABLE 11-2. Histologic Confirmation of Endometriosis by Its Appearance at Laparoscopy

Clinical Appearance of Endometriosis	Histologic Confirmation Rate of Endometriosis (%)
Typical—dark, black	90[53,101]
White—opacified	81[102]
	91[101]
Red, flamelike	75[102]
	81[101]
Glandular lesions	67[102]
Subovarian adhesions	50[102]
Intraovarian cysts	48[60]
Yellow-brown patches	47[102]
Circular peritoneal defects	45[102]
	33[101]
Hemosiderin lesions	33[101]
Normal peritoneum	13–25[50–52]

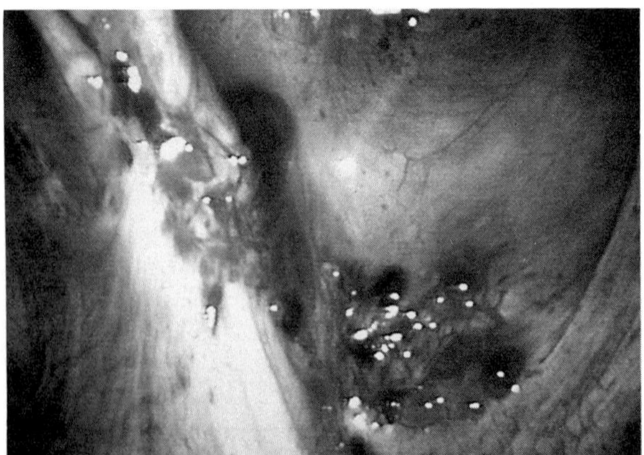

Figure 11-1 Powder burn lesions represent foci of inactive disease containing "burned out" stroma and glands embedded in hemosiderin deposits (see Plate 53).

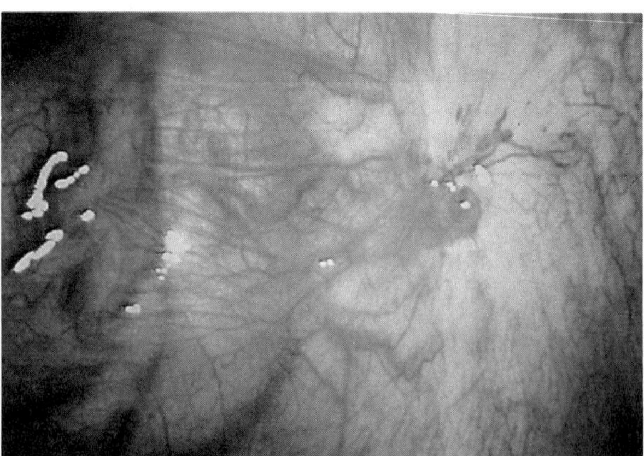

Figure 11-2 Atypical and nonpigmented lesions, seen as clear vesicles, pink vascular patterns, white scarred lesions, red lesions, yellow-brown patches, and peritoneal windows, represent active endometriosis (see Plate 54).

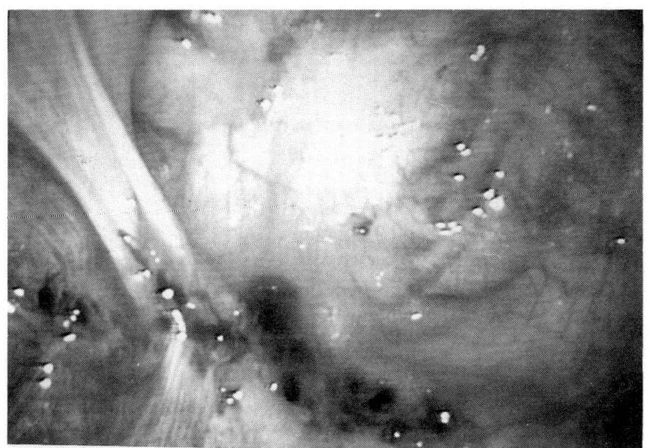

Figure 11-3 These lesions progress to an intermediate depth, become inactive, or infiltrate deeper (usually more than 5 mm) (see Plate 55).

pendent on the steroids present in the peritoneal fluid.[55,57]

Microscopic endometriosis may be overlooked during surgical exploration but is identified by light and electron microscopy in normal-appearing peritoneum. This finding has been noted in patients with visible endometriosis in other areas of the pelvis,[50,51] and in patients with unexplained infertility in whom no endometriosis was seen at laparoscopy.[52,58] Microscopic presentation may preclude total resection, but two techniques can enhance visual detection.[59] Near-contact laparoscopy magnifies the peritoneal area. In our series of 20 women with pelvic endometriosis, biopsy specimens were taken from peritoneum that appeared normal. The histologic studies of this tissue revealed only one case of microscopic endometriosis and an additional two cases were suspicious for endometriosis.[51] The second technique for improved detection of microscopic endometriosis is "painting" the peritoneum and broad ligament with blood or serosanguinous fluid to render atypical lesions more evident.[59] Performing retroperitoneal hydrodissection of the anterior cul-de-sac posterior broad ligaments, and pelvic sidewall sometimes facilitates the identification of lesions.

The peritoneum must be examined from different angles and at different degrees of illumination to see vesicles or whitish lesions. The peritoneal folds must be stretched and searched for small, atypical lesions. Although the resolution of cameras has improved, it is still not comparable to direct vision through the laparoscope. Reinspection of the peritoneal cavity for endometrial implants should be performed by direct vision to ensure identification of all foci.

Normal-appearing ovaries can contain endometriosis under an apparently normal cortex. By inserting a needle deep in the stroma and aspirating the ovary, Candiani and coworkers[60] identified small endometriomas in 48% of otherwise normal-appearing or slightly enlarged ovaries. They suggested that preoperative ultrasonographic evaluation is useful to screen for small subcortical ovarian cysts, which should be explored surgically with needle aspiration.[60]

The diagnosis of endometriosis is missed in at least 7% of patients and understaged in as many as 50%.[53] A careful examination of the pelvis is essential to diagnose and stage endometriosis, to be aware of the various appearances of endometriosis, including its presence as microscopic implants on visually normal peritoneal surfaces, or as small, deep endometriomas within slightly enlarged but otherwise normal ovaries (see Table 11-2).

Treatment of Endometrial Implants

Diagnostic Laparoscopy

Initially, the surgeon must first explore the pelvic cavity and assess the extent of disease, preferably with photographs or video recordings. The surgeon identifies anomalies or distortions of the pelvic organs. The location and boundaries of the bladder, ureter, colon, rectum, pelvic gutters, uterosacral ligaments, and major blood vessels are noted. All pelvic organs are inspected thoroughly. The upper abdominal organs, abdominal walls, liver, and diaphragm should be evaluated for endometriosis or any other abnormality that may contribute to the patient's symptoms. The omentum and the small bowel are evaluated for disease and to ensure that they were not injured during Veress needle or trocar insertion.

A rectovaginal examination is performed to evaluate deep retroperitoneal endometriosis found in the lower pelvis to search for involvement of the rectovaginal septum, uterosacral ligament, lower colon, and pararectal area. However, deep retroperitoneal endometriosis is rare without a connection to the surface peritoneum.

An implant that has penetrated retroperitoneally several centimeters is called an "iceberg" lesion. It can be detected laparoscopically by palpating areas of the pelvis and bowel with the suction-irrigator probe. In 15% of patients who have endometriosis, the appendix is involved and should be examined.[61]

With the forceps or probe, the endometriotic implants are examined to gauge size, depth, and proximity to normal pelvic structures. The diagnostic laparoscopy is extended to an operative procedure if the patient has been advised of this possibility.

Operative Laparoscopy

The operative procedure begins by lysing adhesions between the bowel and pelvic organs to adequately expose the pelvic cavity. The ovaries are dissected from the cul-de-sac or pelvic sidewall, and the tubes are freed from adhesions and chromotubated. Endometrial implants and endometriomas are resected or vaporized, and if the patient has significant central pelvic pain, uterosacral nerve ablation or presacral nerve resection is performed.

Lysis of Bowel Adhesions

Bowel adhesions vary in thickness, vascularity, and cohesiveness. Some adhesions are stretched without tearing the tissue, excised with laser or electrosurgery at the points of attachment to the pelvic organs, and removed. Dense adhesions are excised either with scissors or the ultrapulse CO_2 laser. The latter has a more controlled penetration than electrosurgery or fiber lasers. The structures are separated with forceps and a cleavage plane is formed. Hydrodissection is useful to identify and develop the dissection plane, using laser or dissecting scissors.

Peritoneal Implants

When treating peritoneal endometriosis, the implants should be destroyed in the most effective and least traumatic manner to minimize postoperative adhesions. Although different modalities have been used, we believe hydrodissection and high-power superpulse or ultrapulse CO_2 laser are the best choices for endometriosis treatment.[16] Because the CO_2 laser does not penetrate water, a fluid backstop (hydrodissection) allows the surgeon to work on selected tissue with a greater safety margin than would otherwise be available (Figure 11-4).[16] A small opening is made in the retroperitoneum using the laser or scissors, and lactated Ringer's is injected beneath the lesion to provide a protective cushion of fluid between the lesion to be excised and the underlying ureter or blood vessels. The fluid under the implant absorbs the CO_2 laser energy, buffering the underlying tissue.[16] For retroperitoneal disease, the lesion is picked up with grasping forceps, pulled medially and removed using sharp or blunt dissection.

Superficial peritoneal endometriosis is vaporized with the laser, coagulated with monopolar or bipolar electrode, or excised. Implants less than 2 mm are coagulated, vaporized, or excised. As lesions exceed 3 mm, vaporization or excision is needed. For lesions greater than 5 mm, deep vaporization or excisional techniques are used (Figures 11-5 through 11-8, see also Plates 56 through 59). Superficial implants on the pelvic sidewall are ablated with the CO_2 laser (3500 to 5500 W/cm^2). Low-power densities inflict greater damage and cause more charring, yet high-power densities penetrate too deeply and injure underlying normal structures or cause unnecessary bleeding. Firing in a continuous mode will ablate the lesion from the surface to its base, where the peritoneal fat should appear as unpigmented and soft, rather than fibrotic like endometriosis or scars. To suction the laser plume and irrigate the lesion base, the suction-irrigator is placed next to or behind the lesion, removing char and identifying any vascular structure within the operative field. If carbon is allowed to accumulate, the field is obscured. In either situation, carbon can be mistaken for endometriosis. Therefore if vaporization is chosen, it is important to copiously irrigate and remove the charred areas to confirm complete removal of the lesion and to avoid confusing endometriosis with a carbon deposit (see Figure 11-5). When used in the superpulse/ultrapulse mode, the CO_2 laser achieves more rapid vaporization and decreased carbonization.

Resection of Ovarian Endometriosis

The ovaries are a common site for endometriosis. Endometrial implants or endometriomas less than 2 cm in diameter are coagulated, laser ablated, or excised using scissors, biopsy forceps, lasers, or electrodes. For successful eradication, all visible lesions and scars must be removed from the ovarian surface. Entrapment of oocytes within the luteinized ovarian follicle, as reported in experimental animal models, must be avoided.[62] Endometriomas more than 2 cm diameter must be resected thoroughly to prevent recurrence. Draining the endometrioma or partial resection of its wall is inadequate because the endometrial tissue lining the cyst is likely to remain functional and can cause the symptoms to recur.[63] However, photocoagulation of the cyst wall has been equally therapeutic and occasionally less difficult.[30,64,65] Brosens and Puttemansi[64] recommend performing

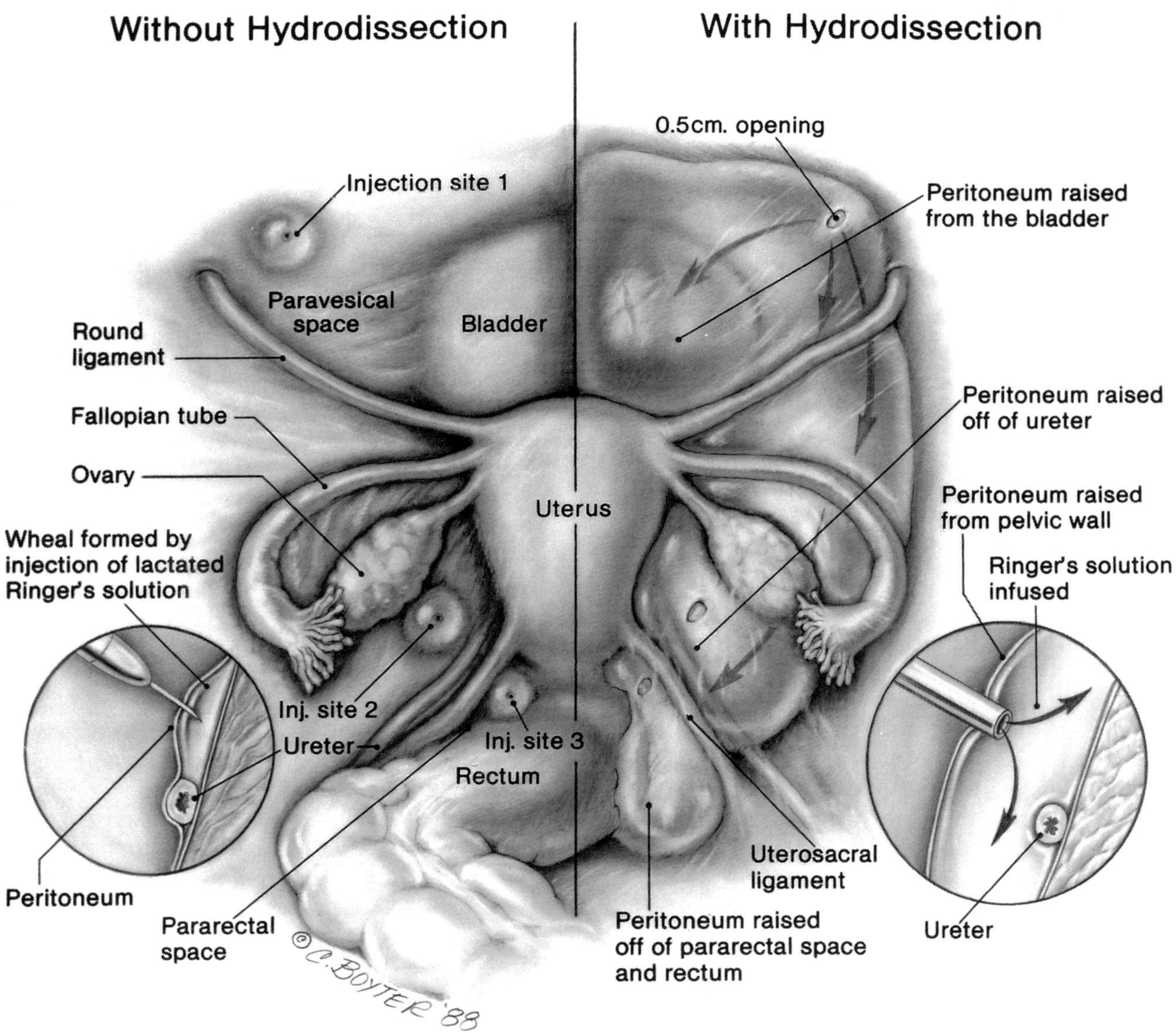

Figure 11-4 Hydrodissection protects the retroperitoneal structures such as the bladder, ureter, or blood vessels from the CO_2 laser.

ovarian cystoscopy and biopsy of the cyst wall before ablating the cyst. By using a double optic laparoscope, which involves the passage of a smaller operative endoscope through the channel of the main laparoscope, the ovarian cyst is punctured, drained, the fluid sent for cytology, and the lining inspected. Any suspicious area is biopsied and sent for frozen section. Once it has been ascertained that the cyst is not malignant, its wall is ablated to a depth of 3 to 4 mm, using a laser or an electrocoagulator introduced through the operative channel of the second laparoscope. This procedure is analogous to endometrial ablation and has been reported to be successful with no recurrence on follow-up ultrasound or second-look laparoscopy.

For endometriomas over 2 cm in diameter, the cyst is punctured with the 5-mm trocar and aspirated with the suction-irrigator probe. Using high-pressure irrigation, at 500 to 800 mm Hg, the cyst is irrigated, causing it to expand, and aspirated several times.[66] This procedure allows examination of the cyst wall. Following the repeated expansion and shrinkage with irrigation and suction, the cyst wall should separate from the surrounding ovarian stroma. If it does not, 5 to 20 mL of lactated Ringer's is injected between the stroma and

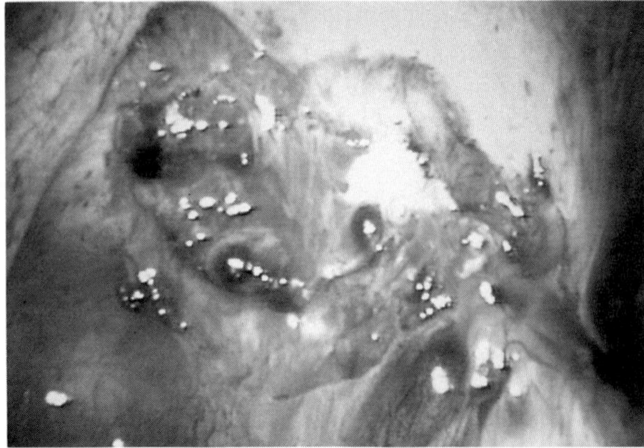

Figure 11-5 Superficial peritoneal endometriosis is vaporized with laser, coagulated with monopolar or bipolar current, or excised (see Plate 56).

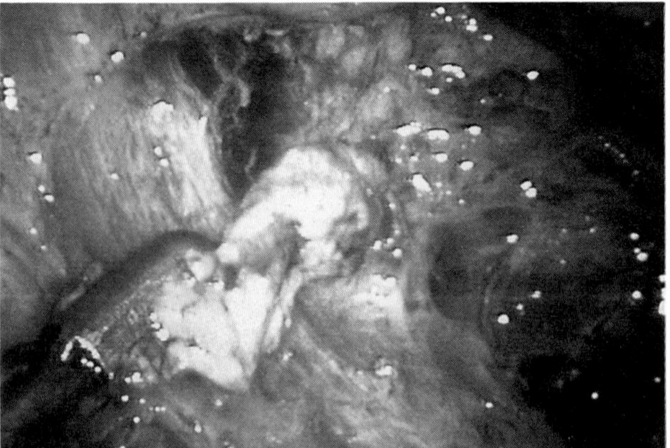

Figure 11-7 A wide dissection is necessary to be able to remove the entire lesion (see Plate 58).

cyst wall.[66] The cyst wall is removed by grasping its base with laparoscopic forceps and peeling it from the ovarian stroma. If unsuccessful, the wall is separated from the ovarian cortex with forceps at the puncture site. A cleavage plane is created by pulling the two forceps apart and by cutting between the structures with laser or needle electrode. The laser or electrosurgery minimizes bleeding because the blood vessels supplying the endometrioma are usually small enough to be cut and coagulated simultaneously.[66] Another method involves hydrodissection of the plane between the cyst wall and the ovarian stroma.[16,32] These techniques can be applied successfully to completely remove the cyst wall, which should be sent for histologic evaluation to rule out malignancy. If the entire cyst cannot be separated from the ovary, the adherent sections are ablated or coagulated.[63–66] When the entire cyst wall is ablated, representative biopsies are taken for histologic diagnosis.

Cyst wall closure is not necessary, according to animal experiments[67] and clinical experience.[68] For large defects that result from resecting endometriomas larger than 5 cm, the edges of the ovarian cortex are approximated with a single suture placed within the ovarian stroma. The knot is tied inside the ovary, so that no part of the suture penetrates the ovarian cortex or is exposed to the ovarian surface so as to minimize adhesion formation. Fibrin sealant has been described to atraumatically approximate the edges of large ovarian defects, without adhesion formation.[69]

Although rare, some patients present with localized symptoms and severe involvement of one ovary with disease and adhesions while the oppo-

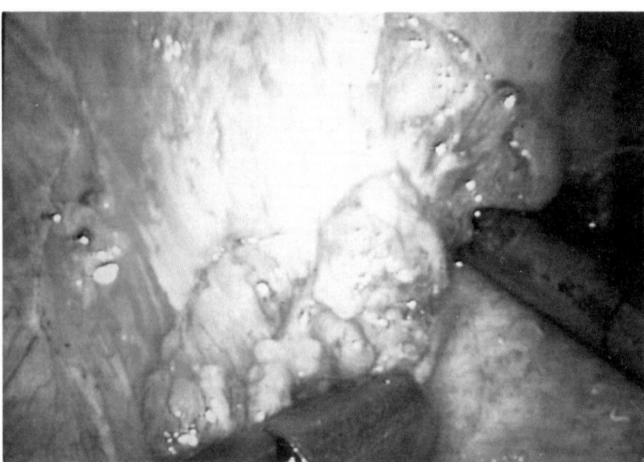

Figure 11-6 After an incision is made around the lesion, it is elevated with a grasping forceps and either cut or vaporized with CO_2 laser (see Plate 57).

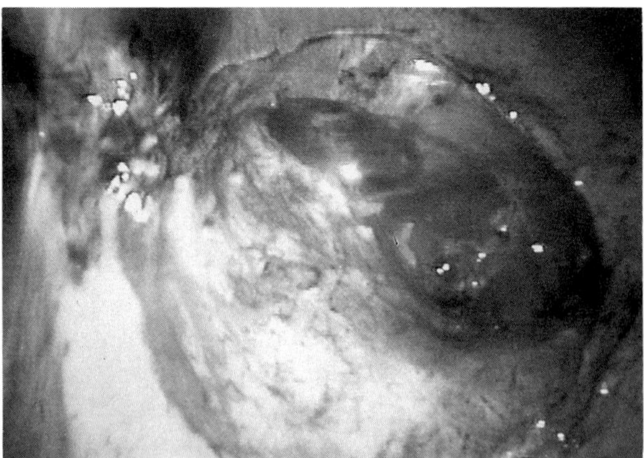

Figure 11-8 Posterior cul-de-sac and right uterosacral ligament after the fibrotic lesion is removed (see Plate 59).

site ovary is normal, requiring unilateral salpingo-oophorectomy. By removing the diseased ovary, the risk of disease recurrence is minimized, and the fertility potential is improved by limiting ovulation to the healthy side.

Genitourinary Endometriosis

Ureteral involvement has been reported in 1% to 11% of women diagnosed with endometriosis.[70] Endometriosis of the urinary tract tends to be superficial but can be invasive and cause complete ureteral obstruction.

Decreased bladder capacity and stability unresponsive to conventional therapy may result from endometriosis. Goldstein and Brodman[71] report one case of bladder endometriosis, which they monitored cystometrically over a 4-year period. They found that decreased bladder capacity and bladder instability, unresponsive to conventional parasympatholytic therapy, were corrected following surgical destruction of superficial bladder endometriosis. When bladder symptoms recurred 2 years later, a course of danazol again reversed bladder instability. Clinicians should consider a diagnosis of endometriosis in cases of refractory and unexplained urinary complaints.

If urinary tract endometriosis is suspected, a complete preoperative evaluation is performed, including an intravenous pyelogram, ultrasound of the kidneys, and routine blood and urine work-up. In selected cases of recurrent hematuria, cystoscopy is indicated.

Superficial implants over the ureter generally are treated by a variation of hydrodissection. Approximately 20 to 30 mL of lactated Ringer's is injected subperitoneally on the lateral pelvic wall; this elevates the peritoneum and backs it with a bed of fluid. The CO_2 laser is used to create a 0.5-cm opening on this elevation. The opening in the peritoneum is made anteriorly and laterally, close to the corresponding round ligament. The hydrodissection probe is inserted into the opening and approximately 100 mL of lactated Ringer's is injected under 300 mm Hg pressure into the retroperitoneal space along the course of the ureter (see Figure 11-4). The fluid surrounds the ureter, moves it posteriorly, and allows superficial CO_2 laser dissection or vaporization of the area.

After creating a fluid shelf, a superpulse or ultrapulse CO_2 laser (20 to 80 W) is used to vaporize or excise the lesion with a circumference of 1 to 2 cm. When the lesions are large, or excision is preferred, a circular line with a 1- to 2-cm margin is made around the lesion. The peritoneum is held with an atraumatic grasping forceps and peeled away with the help of the CO_2 laser and the suction-irrigation probe. If the endometrial implant is embedded and has formed scarring down to the subperitoneal connective tissue, hydrodissection allows fluid to tunnel beneath the lesion, often separating scar tissue. The lesion then can be treated safely. After vaporization or excision of these lesions, the area is irrigated and washed to remove all charcoal and verify that endometriosis has been treated properly. In over 500 consecutive procedures (275 bladder, 250 ureter), there have been no major complications involving bladder or ureter injury.[15] Two patients who were unable to void immediately after surgery had an indwelling catheter placed. It was removed the day after surgery and they were able to void spontaneously. Four patients who had bladder endometriosis experienced minimal hematuria that resolved several hours postoperatively. Following hydrodissection of the broad ligaments and the pelvic sidewall, about 5% of the patients developed swelling of the external genitalia, most likely from the penetration of water through the inguinal canal to the labia majora. This swelling resolved in most cases within 1 to 2 hours without sequelae.

Ureteral Obstruction

The incidence of ureteral obstruction by endometriosis is low, and conventional therapy previously consisted of laparotomy and resection of the obstructed segment of the ureter. Laparoscopic ureteroureterostomy was performed in 1990 by Nezhat and colleagues on a 36-year-old woman with long-term ureteral obstruction caused by endometriosis.[72] The condition was diagnosed previously at laparoscopy. The patient refused conventional laparotomy and had a nephrostomy tube for 4 years. At laparoscopy, a 3- to 4-cm fibrotic nodule over the left ureter was seen approximately 4 cm above the bladder, distorting the course of the ureter (Figure 11-9, see also Plate 59). This corresponded to the level of obstruction seen on radioimaging techniques. Under laparoscopic observation, an attempt to place a retrograde catheter was unsuccessful, so the nodule was excised using videolaseroscopy and hydrodissection. The left retroperitoneal space was entered at the pelvic brim. After treating all associated endometriosis, fibrosis, or adhesions, the ureter was dissected with the CO_2 laser (Figure 11-10). The nodule involved the entire thickness of the ureter; a partial resection was done (Figure 11-11).

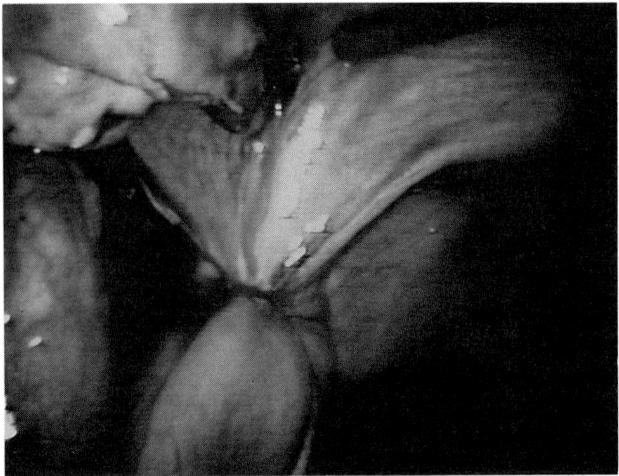

Figure 11-9 At laparoscopy, a 3- to 4-cm fibrotic nodule over the left ureter was found approximately 4 cm above the bladder, distorting the course of the ureter (see Plate 60).

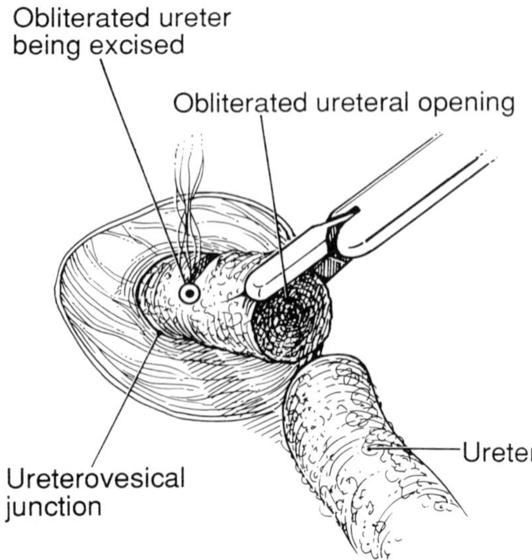

Figure 11-11 During dissection, it was discovered that the nodule involved the entire thickness of the ureter; a partial resection was done.

Under cystoscopic guidance, a 7F ureteral catheter was passed through the ureterovesical junction, at which level the CO_2 laser was used to open the ureter. Indigo carmine was injected into the patient's intravenous line to ensure patency of the proximal ureter. The distal ureter was transected over the stent, and the obstructed portion was removed. The ureteral stent was introduced into the proximal ureter and advanced into the renal pelvis (Figure 11-12A and B). Finally, the edges of the ureter were approximated with sutures. To perform anastomosis, four interrupted 4-0 polydioxanone sutures (PDS) were placed at 6, 12, 9, and 3 o'clock to approximate the proximal and distal ureteral ostia. (Figure 11-13). Estimated blood loss was less than 100 mL and the procedure lasted 117 minutes. The pathology report confirmed severe endometriosis and fibrosis of the resected ureter.

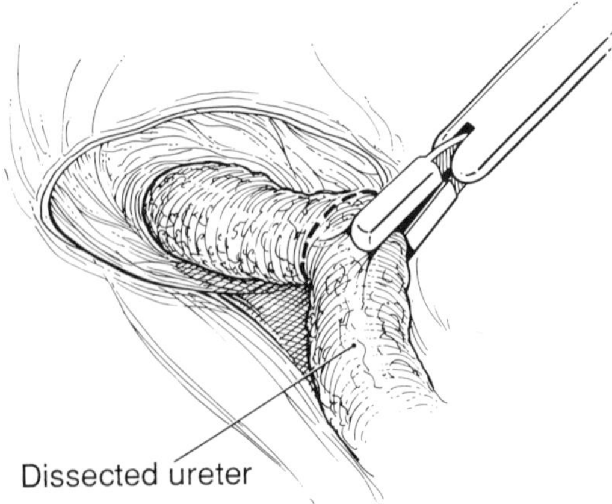

Figure 11-10 After treating all associated endometriosis, fibrosis, or adhesions, the ureter was dissected with the CO_2 laser.

The patient went home the next day. The postoperative course was uncomplicated. An intravenous pyelogram (IVP) confirmed ureteral patency and renal function (Figure 11-14).

Since then we have treated 12 more patients with severe endometriosis of the ureter in which endometriosis and fibrosis caused partial or complete ureteral obstruction. All patients had a known history of endometriosis and underwent different surgical and medical treatments. In four women, the ureteral endometriosis was removed completely without entering the ureteral lumen. In three women, the obstructed ureter required a complete segmental resection. One right and one left ureteroureterostomy and one anastomosis of the left ureter to the bladder (ureteroneocystostomy) were performed using four through-and-through interrupted 4-0 PDS to approximate the edges over the ureteral catheter. In five women, the ureter was involved partially. The severe retroperitoneal and ureteral endometriosis was excised or vaporized cautiously using the CO_2 laser until ureterotomy occurred.

In three women, the ureterotomy was very small and was detected by intravenous injection of indigo carmine. A ureteral stent was left in place and no suture was required. In two patients, the ureterotomy was repaired using 4-0 PDS to overlap the laceration after stent placement. Histological examination of the resected specimen revealed

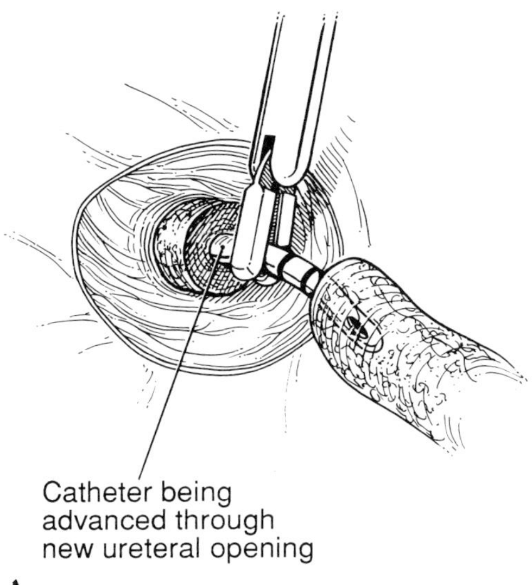

A

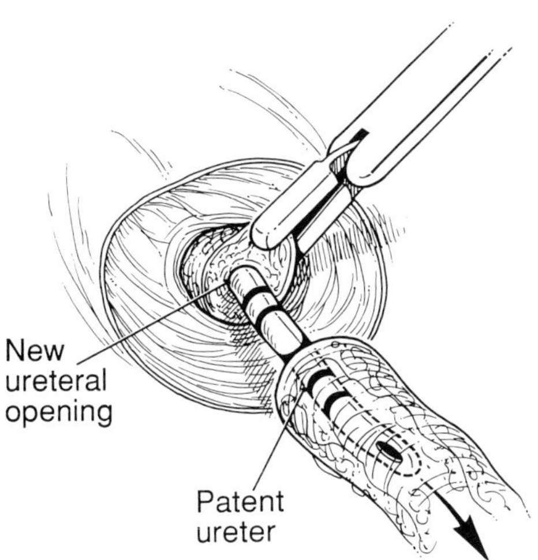

B

Figure 11-12 The ureteral stent was introduced into the proximal ureter and advanced into the renal pelvis.

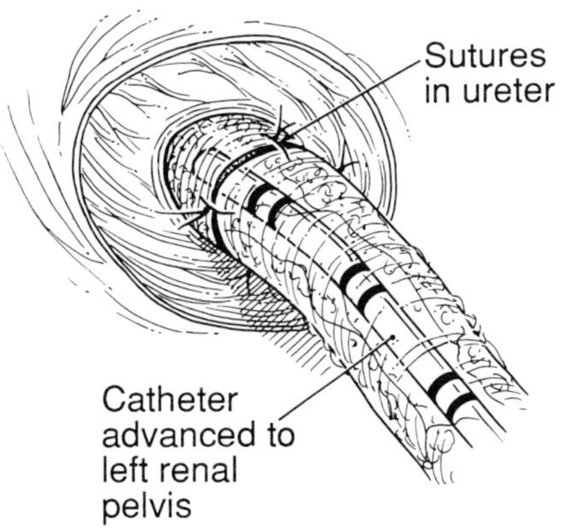

Figure 11-13 To perform anastomosis, four interrupted 4-0 polydioxanone sutures were placed at 6, 12, 9, and 3 o'clock to approximate the proximal and distal ureteral edges.

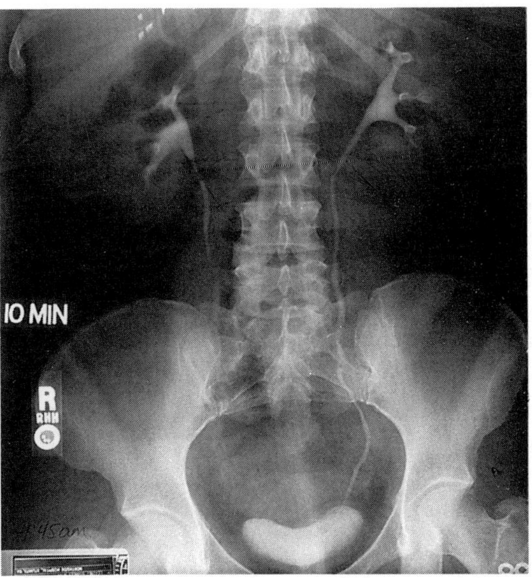

Figure 11-14 An IVP confirmed ureteral patency and renal function.

fibrosis, endometriosis, or both in all women. A rare case of endometriosis with focal severely atypical hyperplasia was found in the specimen of a 46-year-old woman. She had undergone total abdominal hysterectomy and bilateral salpingo-oophorectomy followed by hormonal replacement therapy at another institution. All patients had an uneventful intra- and postoperative course and reported symptomatic relief of their symptoms. Imaging techniques demonstrated patent ureters with a functioning kidney in all patients except for one. She was a 24-year-old woman who had been diagnosed several months earlier with pelvic endometriosis that was treated partially at initial laparoscopy followed by GnRH analog therapy postoperatively. During a second laparoscopy, she was found to have severe left uterosacral, left pelvic sidewall endometriosis and left ureteral endometriosis that had caused complete obstruction of the ureter. Segmental resection and ureteroureterostomy were performed. Intraoperative intravenous injection of indigo carmine did not reveal any leakage from the ureter and raised the question of a nonfunctioning kidney. Postoperative follow-up and imaging revealed a 10–20% functioning kidney. However, the ureter was patent.

In such cases, an external ureteral stent is left in the ureter for at least 4 weeks, at which time it is exchanged cystoscopically for an internal stent. This stent remains in place for approximately 2 months postoperatively. The patient's follow-up should include IVP, ultrasound, or excretion scans.

Bladder Endometriosis

The bladder wall is one of the sites least frequently involved with endometriosis.[71] If the lesions are superficial, hydrodissection and vaporization are adequate for removal. Using hydrodissection, the areolar tissue between the serosa and muscularis beneath the implants is dissected. The lesion is circumcised with the laser and fluid is injected into the resulting defect. The lesion is grasped with forceps and dissected with the laser. Traction allows the small blood vessels supplying the surrounding tissue to be coagulated as the lesion is resected. Frequent irrigation is necessary to remove char, ascertain the depth of vaporization, and ensure that the lesion does not involve the muscularis and the mucosa.

Endometriosis extending to the muscularis but without mucosal involvement can be treated laparoscopically and any residual or deeper lesions may be treated successfully with postoperative hormonal therapy.[71] When endometriosis involves full bladder wall thickness, the lesion is excised and the bladder reconstructed.[73] Four cases of full-thickness bladder endometriosis were treated by excision and a one-layer reconstruction. The exposure seemed to be better than that at laparotomy.[73] Simultaneous cystoscopy is performed and bilateral ureteral catheters are inserted. The bladder dome is held near the midline with the grasping forceps and the endometriotic nodule is excised 5 mm beyond the lesion (Figure 11-15). An incision is made with the CO_2 laser using the suction-irrigation probe as a backstop. The specimen is removed from the abdominal cavity with a long grasping forceps through the operative channel of the laparoscope. The tissue is transferred to a previously placed grasping forceps. The lesion is regrasped and removed with the laparoscope as one unit. CO_2 gas distends the bladder cavity, allowing excellent observation of its interior (Figure 11-16). After again identifying the ureters and examining the bladder mucosa, the bladder is closed with several interrupted 4-0 polydioxanone through-and-through sutures using extracorporeal or intracorporeal knotting (Figure 11-17). Cystoscopy is performed to identify possible leaks. The duration of laparoscopic segmental cystectomy is approximately 35 minutes. Patients are discharged

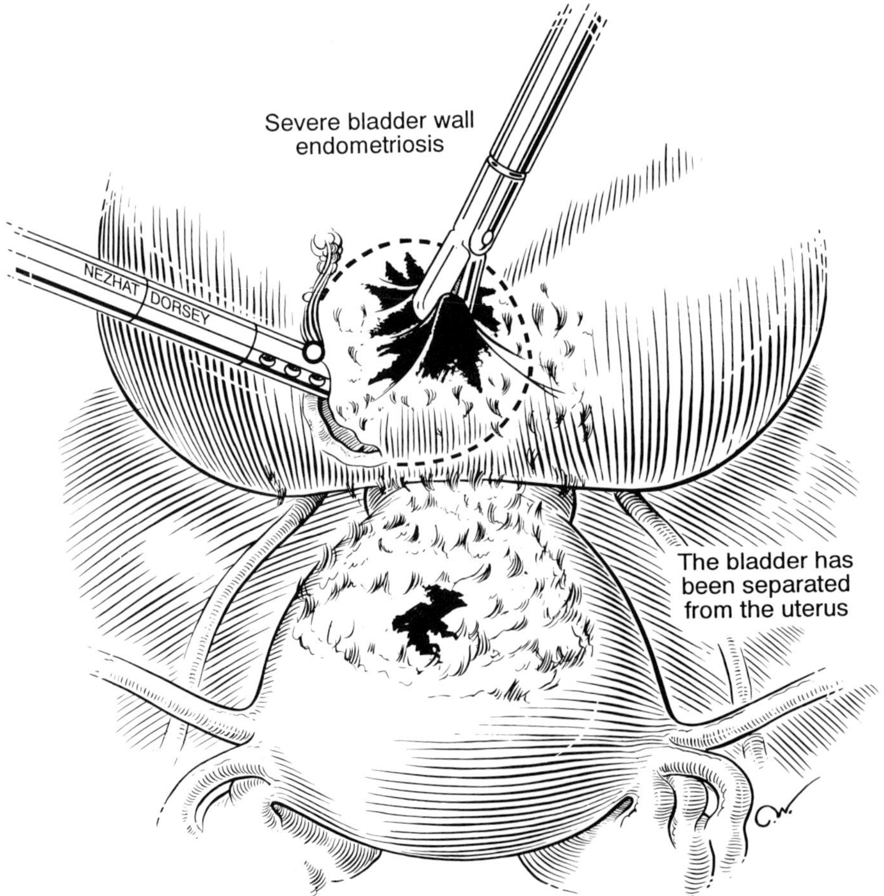

Figure 11-15 The bladder dome is held near the midline with the grasping forceps and the endometriotic nodule is excised 5 mm beyond the lesion.

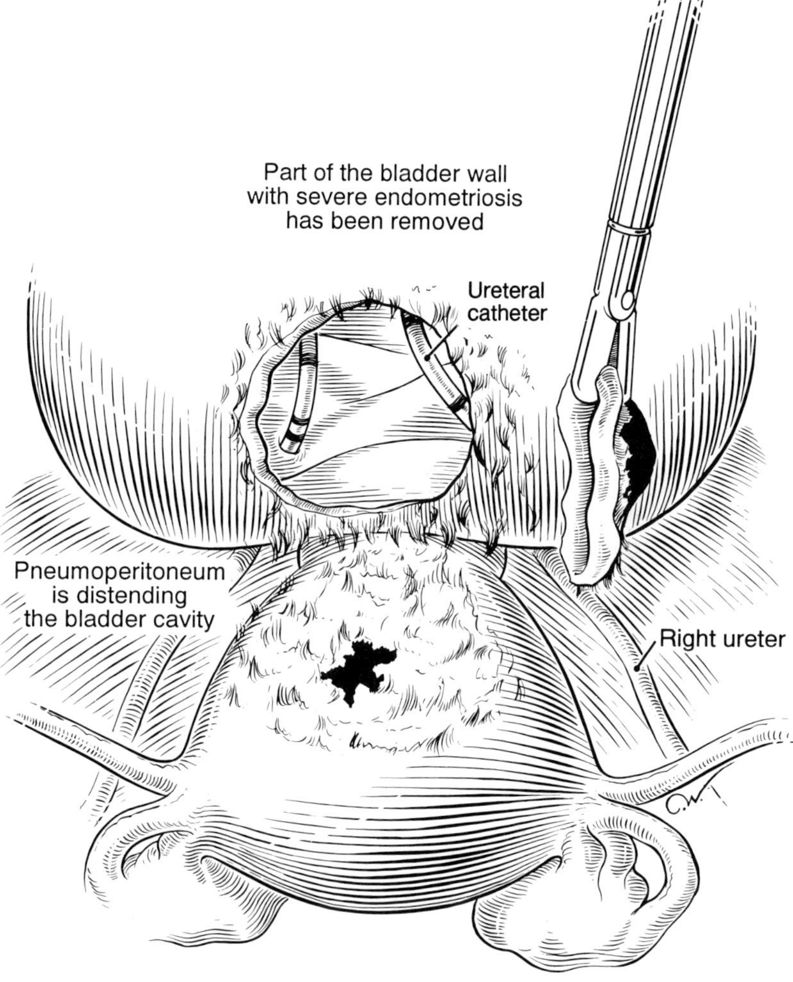

Figure 11-16 The bladder is distended after parts of the bladder wall are removed because of endometriosis involvement.

the following day and instructed to take trimethoprim and sulfamethoxazole for 2 weeks. The Foley catheter is removed 7 to 14 days later and cystograms are done. Blood loss is minimal. In this group of four patients, the pathology report confirmed severe endometriosis and fibrosis of the resected bladder wall. No intraoperative or postoperative complications were noted. Ten to 13 months postoperatively, the women are doing well, with no hematuria at menstruation.

Gastrointestinal Involvement

Gastrointestinal endometriosis was described in 1909 by Sampson,[74] during the histologic examination of resected sigmoid colon, which had been diagnosed intraoperatively as a carcinoma. The gastrointestinal tract is believed to be involved in 3% to 37% of women with endometriosis.[75,76] However, in a specialized practice, the number of patients with bowel involvement could be as high as 50% if patients with serosal and subserosal lesions are included. Endometrial implants may be found between the small intestine and anal canal. The clinical presentation varies from an incidental finding at celiotomy to bowel obstruction.[77]

Severe endometriosis commonly involves the uterosacral ligaments, rectovaginal septum, and rectosigmoid colon with partial or complete posterior cul-de-sac obliteration. Patients can present with lower abdominal pain, back pain, dysmenorrhea, dyspareunia, diarrhea, constipation, and tenesmus, and occasionally rectal bleeding.[15] Symptoms usually occur cyclically at or about the time of menstruation.

Intestinal endometriosis should be suspected in women of childbearing age who present with gastrointestinal symptoms and a history of endometriosis.[61] Proctoscopy and colonoscopy are suggestive, but the lesions usually are not identified before laparoscopy. Although microscopic exami-

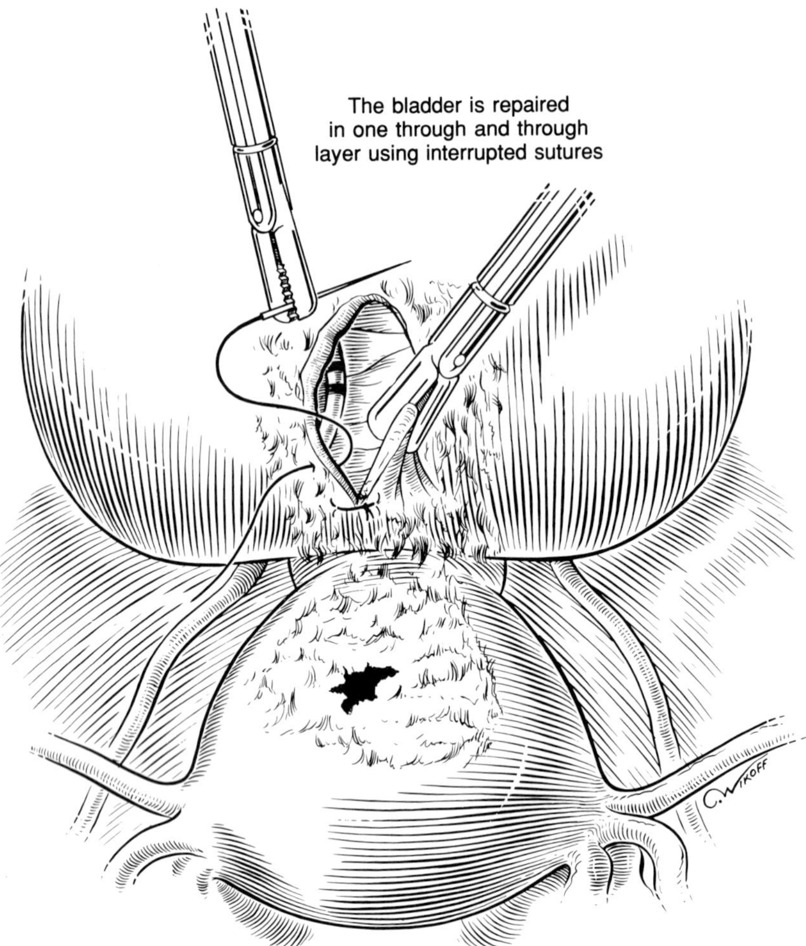

Figure 11-17 The bladder is closed with several interrupted O Vicryl or 4-0 polydioxanone through-and-through sutures using extracorporeal knotting.

nation of the bowel mucosa may reveal endometrial glands, colonoscopic biopsy is usually not diagnostic.[78]

In patients with severe symptoms, medical therapy rarely yields satisfactory long-term results.[75] Surgical intervention is necessary to dissect and resect infiltrating bowel endometriosis. These patients generally undergo laparoscopy after previous surgical or hormonal management fails to relieve their discomfort.[15] Large bowel resection for obstructing endometriosis of the sigmoid colon was reported in 1909 by Mackenrodt.[79] Colonic resection has been shown to be safe with low morbidity, providing satisfactory pain relief and favorable pregnancy rates.[80]

Intestinal endometriosis involves the rectum and sigmoid colon in 76% of cases, the appendix in 18%, and the cecum in 5%.[61] Operative laparoscopy is performed to treat endometrial implants on the intestinal wall, appendix, and rectovaginal space.[15]

Appendiceal Involvement

Appendiceal lesions may be noted by only palpation, so that incidental appendectomy is recommended for patients with severe endometriosis.

Bowel Resection

In cases of severe disease of the bowel wall, resection may be necessary. Laparoscopically assisted anterior rectal wall resection and anastomosis were described in 1991 by Nezhat and coworkers for symptomatic, infiltrative rectosigmoid endometriosis.[81]

Preoperative mechanical and antibiotic bowel preparation is necessary. Three 5-mm suprapubic trocars are placed, one each in the midline and right and left lower quadrants for the insertion of grasping forceps, Endoloop suture applicators, a suction-irrigator probe, and a bipolar electrocoagulator.

The technique includes laparoscopic mobilization of the lower colon, transanal prolapse, resection, and anastomosis.[81,82]

When the lesion involves only the anterior rectal wall near the anal verge, the rectovaginal septum is delineated by simultaneous vaginal and rectal examinations performed by an assistant. The rectum is mobilized along the rectovaginal septum anteriorly to within 2 cm of the anus, using the CO_2 laser and hydrodissection. Mobilization continues along the left and right pararectal spaces by electrodesiccating and dividing branches of the hemorrhoidal artery, and partially posteriorly, as well. When the rectum is mobilized sufficiently, the tumor is prolapsed to the level of the anus, the perineal body is retracted, and an RL30 (Ethicon) multifire stapler is applied across the segment of the anterior rectal wall containing the nodule. Two staple applications may be required to traverse the width of the involved mucosa. The tumor nodule is excised using electrosurgery, and two additional interrupted 2-0 polyglactin sutures are inserted along the staple line. The rectum is returned to the pelvis under direct observation, and closure is confirmed by insufflating the rectum while the cul-de-sac is filled with lactated Ringer's.

In patients with circumferential lesions, the entire rectum is mobilized, the lateral rectal pedicles are electrodesiccated, and the presacral space is entered to the level of the levator ani muscles to be able to mobilize the bowel. The branches of the inferior mesenteric vessels of the bowel segment to be resected are electrodesiccated and cut. The rectum is transected proximal to the lesion, and the proximal limb is prolapsed into the distal limb, using Babcock clamps (Figure 11-18). A 2-0 purse-string suture is inserted to the end of the proximal bowel to secure the opposing anvil of a no. 29 or 33 ILA stapler (Ethicon) (Figure 11-19). The anvil is replaced transanally into the pelvis along with the proximal bowel.

The rectal stump, containing the endometrial lesion, is prolapsed through the anal canal and transected proximal to the lesion using an RL60 linear stapler (Figure 11-20; Ethicon). The resected segment is sent for pathologic diagnosis. The rectal stump is replaced through the anal canal into the pelvis. The ILS stapler is placed into the rectum, and the anvil trocar within the proximal bowel is inserted into the stapling device using the laparoscope. The device is fired, creating an end-to-end anastomosis (see Figure 11-20). A proctoscope is used to examine the anastomosis for structural integrity and bleeding. The pelvis is filled with lactated Ringer's and observed with the

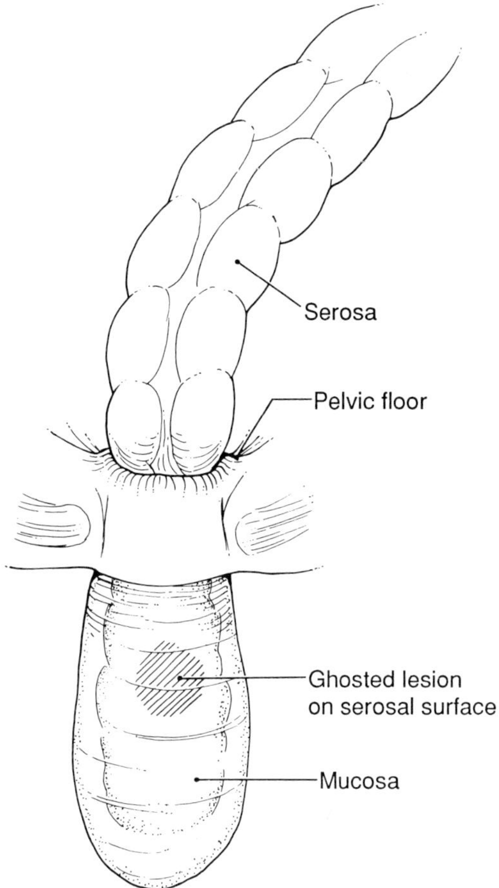

Figure 11-18 In patients with circumferential lesions, the rectum is transected distal to the lesion and the proximal limb is prolapsed into the distal limb.

laparoscope as the rectum is insufflated with air to check for leakage. Air leaks can be corrected using 2-0 polyglactin sutures placed transanally. This technique is identical to resection at laparotomy, with the bipolar electrocoagulator and laser replacing suture and scissors.[83]

Another method utilizes a 60-mm Endostapler (Ethicon) to resect the bowel intra-abdominally. The Endostapler is fired distal to the lesion. The proximal limb of the colon is delivered from the abdomen and exteriorized through a small incision. The lesion is amputated, and the anvil of the stapler is inserted in the lumen following placement of a purse-string suture. At this stage, anastomosis is completed with the stapler gun.

A simplified method to treat severe disease of the anterior wall of the colon eliminates stapling devices.[84] The extent of the lesion is evaluated visually and by palpation, using the tip of the suction-irrigator probe. If the lesion is low enough, an assistant can identify it by performing a rectal ex-

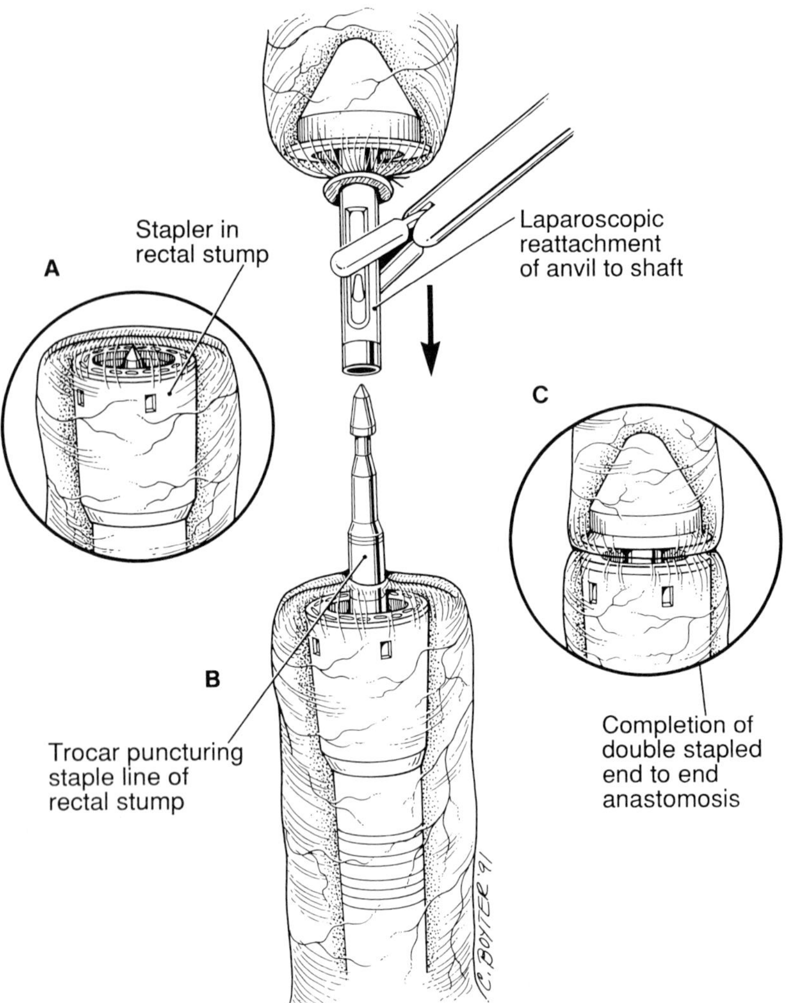

Figure 11-19 A 2-0 polypropylene purse-string suture is placed around the circumference of the proximal limb of the bowel. The ILS stapler is placed into the rectum, and the anvil trocar within the proximal bowel is inserted into the stapling device using the laparoscope. The device is fired, creating an end-to-end anastomosis.

amination. A sigmoidoscope is used to further delineate the lesion and guide the surgeon. After identifying the ureters to avoid inadvertent injury, the lower colon is mobilized in all aspects except posteriorly. Depending on the location of the lesion, the right or left pararectal area is entered using the CO_2 laser and hydrodissection, and the colon is separated from the adjacent organs. Full-thickness excision is carried out, beginning above the area of visible disease. After the normal tissue is identified, the lesion is held at its proximal end with grasping forceps. An incision is made using the CO_2 laser through the bowel serosa and muscularis, and the lumen is entered (Figure 11-21). The lesion is excised entirely from the anterior rectal wall (Figure 11-22). The suction-irrigator probe is used as a backstop for the laser and to evacuate the laser plume. After complete excision of the lesion, the pelvic cavity is irrigated and suctioned. Debris is extracted through the operative channel of the laparoscope using a long grasping forceps, or from the anus using polyp forceps, and submitted for pathology. The bowel is repaired transversely in one layer (Figure 11-23). Two traction sutures are applied to each side of the defect, transforming it to a transverse opening (Figure 11-24). The stay sutures are brought out through the right and left lower quadrant trocar sleeves. The sleeves are removed, then replaced in the peritoneal cavity next to the stay sutures, and the sutures are secured outside the abdomen. The bowel is repaired by placing several interrupted through-and-through sutures in 0.4- to 0.6-cm increments until it is anastomosed completely (Figure 11-25). No. 0 polyglactin or polydioxanone sutures with a straight needle (Ethicon) and extracorporeal knot tying are used. At the end of the procedure, sigmoidoscopy is performed to ensure that the closure is watertight and that there is no bowel stricture.[85]

Figure 11-20 The rectal stump, containing the endometrial lesion, is prolapsed through the anal canal and after applying an RL60 linear stapler, it is transected proximal to the lesion using a sharper electrosurgical knife (Ethicon).

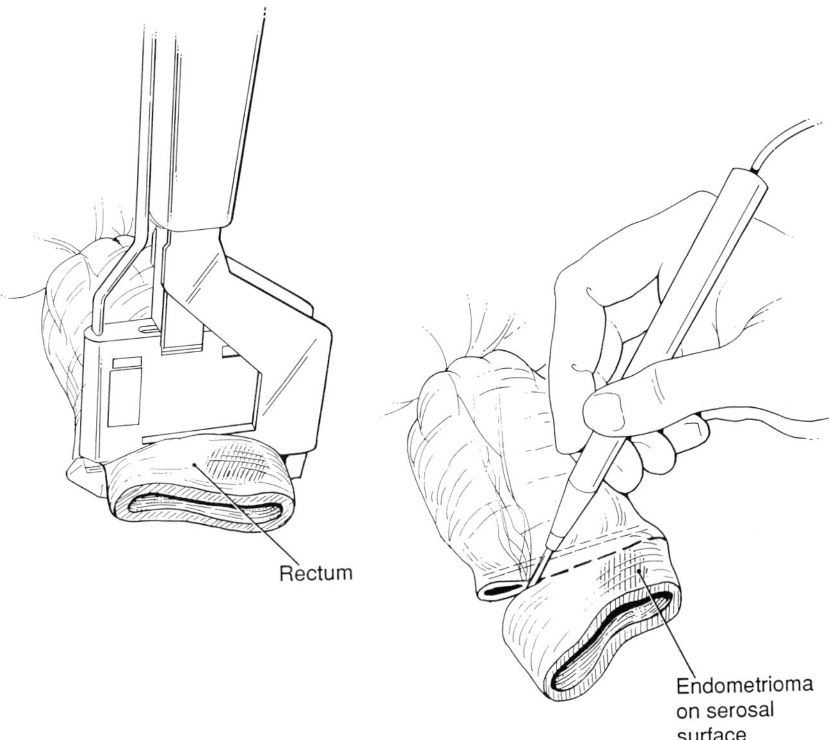

Cul-de-Sac Restoration

Cul-de-sac obliteration, common among patients with severe endometriosis and pain, suggests rectovaginal involvement with deep endometriosis and dense adhesions, and significant distortion of the regional anatomy involving bowel, vaginal apex, posterior cervix, ureter, and major blood vessels.[85] Cul-de-sac restoration requires great surgical expertise and should not be attempted by an inexperienced laparoscopist or a gynecologic surgeon unfamiliar with bowel and urinary tract surgery. Most cases involve the rectum and the rectovaginal septum and do not require bowel resection. To aid in identifying anatomic landmarks and tissues planes, an assistant stands between the patient's legs and performs rectovaginal examination with one hand, while holding the uterus up with a rigid uterine elevator. An uninvolved area

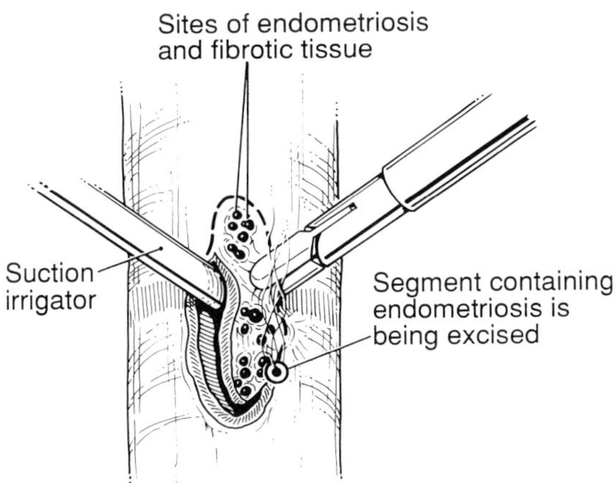

Figure 11-21 An incision is made using the CO_2 laser through the bowel serosa and muscularis, and the lumen is entered.

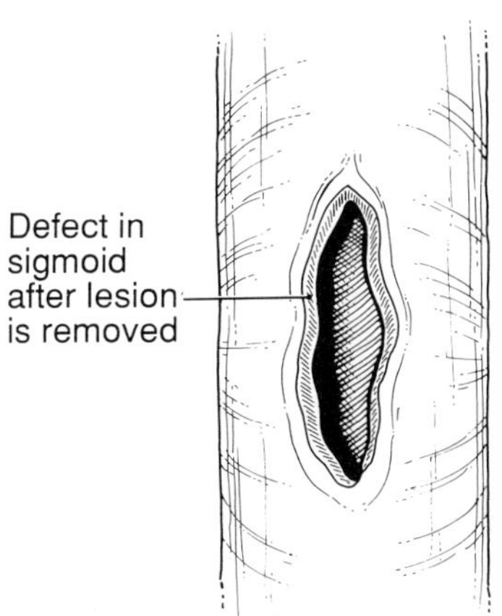

Figure 11-22 The lesion is excised entirely from the anterior rectal wall.

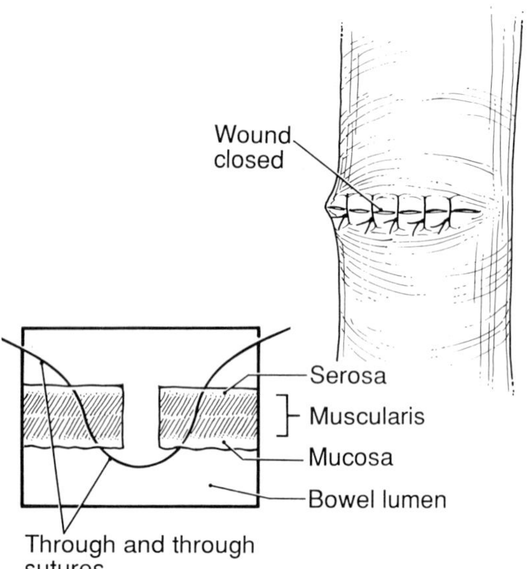

Figure 11-23 The bowel is repaired transversely in one layer.

of peritoneum is identified and injected with 5 to 8 mL of diluted vasopressin (10 U in 100 mL of lactated Ringer's) with an 18-gauge laparoscopic needle. Using the CO_2 laser, scissors, electrocautery knife, or needle, the peritoneum is opened (Figure 11-26). Using high-power CO_2 laser and hydrodissection, the rectum attached to the uterosacral ligaments and the back of the cervix is separated (Figure 11-27). If rectal involvement is more extensive, a sigmoidoscope can be used to guide the surgeon and rule out bowel perforation. After complete separation of the rectum, lesions on the rectum or rectovaginal septum are removed or vaporized (Figure 11-28). The cul-de-sac is filled with irrigation fluid and is observed through the laparoscope while air is introduced into the rectum through the sigmoidoscope. Air bubbles observed in the cul-de-sac fluid indicate perforation. As the assistant guides the surgeon by rectovaginal examination, the rectum is freed from the back of the cervix. Generalized oozing or bleeding is controlled with an injection of 3 to 5 mL diluted vasopressin solution (1 ampule in 100 mL lactated Ringer's), laser, or bipolar electrocoagulator. Bleeding from the stalk vessels caused by dissection or vaporization of the fibrotic uterosacral ligaments and pararectal area is controlled with a bipolar electrocoagulator.

Because the ureters are usually lateral to the uterosacral ligaments, the surgeon should try to stay between them. If the dissection is extended lateral to the uterosacral ligaments, the ipsilateral ureter should be identified by opening the overlying peritoneum and tracing it to the area of the lesion. The ureter, uterine arteries, and veins are exposed. Bipolar forceps or Hemoclips must be available and fully functional to control unexpected bleeding.

For posterior cul-de-sac nodularity and infiltration of endometriosis toward the vagina, dissection and resection of the nodularity continue as an assistant palpates the nodule to ensure its removal.[81] Endometriosis rarely penetrates the mucosa of the colon but commonly involves the serosa, subserosa, and muscularis. When significant portions of both muscularis layers have been excised or vaporized and the mucosa is reached, the bowel wall is reinforced by interrupted 4-0 polydioxanone sutures. The procedure requires maximal coordination between assistant and surgeon.

The bowel can be entered while removing nodular endometrial lesions of the rectosigmoid colon.[31] Endometrial lesions up to 3 cm are resected. The bowel wall is repaired in one layer using interrupted 3-0 silk or 4-0 polydioxanone sutures without sequelae.

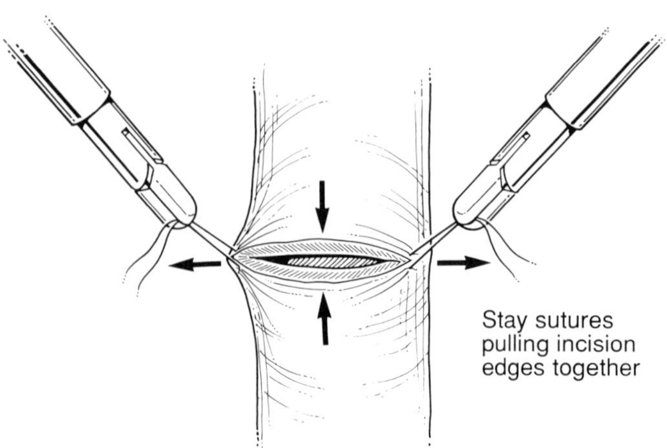

Figure 11-24 Two traction sutures are applied to each side of the defect transforming it to a transverse opening.

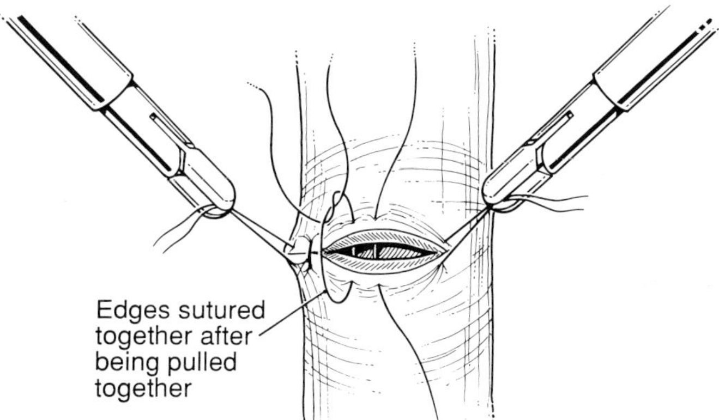

Figure 11-25 The bowel is repaired by placing several interrupted through-and-through sutures in 0.4- to 0.6-cm increments until it is repaired completely.

When the rectovaginal space is dissected and hemostasis is accomplished, the pelvis is filled with lactated Ringer's to observe the cul-de-sac and the area of dissection. This magnifies and clarifies the dissected tissue to help identify residual disease, to verify the intact anatomy of the ureters and bowel, and to coagulate small bleeders. The raw surfaces of the rectum or cul-de-sac are not reperitonealized because several studies have demonstrated that reperitonealization is not necessary and promotes adhesion formation.[67,68,86,87]

This procedure was performed in 185 women, aged 25 to 41 years. Eighty patients had complete posterior cul-de-sac obliteration. All were successfully managed by laparoscopy and discharged within 24 hours except for nine patients with bowel perforation and one with a partial bowel resection who were discharged after 2 to 4 days. The procedures lasted from 55 to 245 minutes. Of 185 patients, 174 were available for follow-up after 1 to 5 years. Moderate to complete pain relief was observed in 162 of 174 patients (93%). Thirteen (8%) required two procedures, and four patients required three procedures. Twelve (7%) had persistent or worse pain after surgery.[88]

In a series of 356 women who underwent lapa-

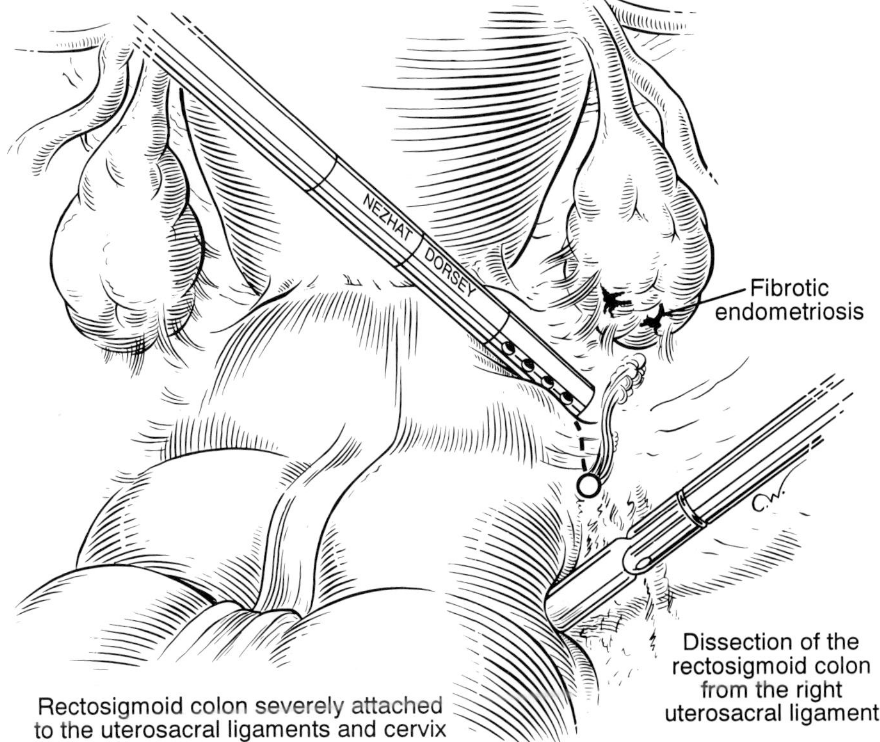

Figure 11-26 To dissect the rectum from the back of the uterus, first make an incision in the right pararectal area in an uninvolved peritoneum with the CO_2 laser.

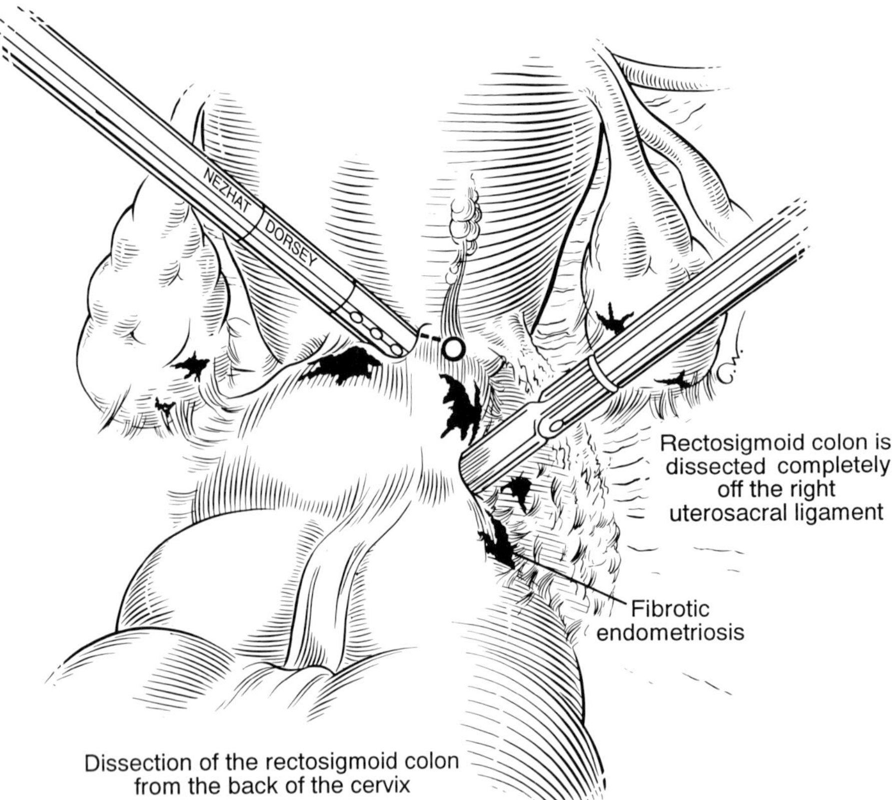

Figure 11-27 Using hydrodissection and CO_2 laser, the rectum is separated from the back of the cervix gradually.

roscopic treatment of bowel endometriosis using different techniques, 2 patients required intraoperative laparotomy early in our experience (CN,FN). The first patient underwent laparotomy for repair of enterotomy after treatment of infiltrative rectal endometriosis. The other patient required laparotomy for anastomosis following an unsuccessful attempt to place a purse-string suture around the patulous rectal ampulla. Significant postoperative complications occurred in 1.7% of patients. Two women developed leaks and pelvic infections. One required a temporary laparoscopic colostomy with subsequent take down and repair, and one was managed by prolonged drainage. One woman had bowel stricture requiring resection and anastomosis by laparotomy. One developed a pelvic abscess and subsequently underwent laparoscopic right salpingo-oophorectomy. One had an immediate rectal prolapse that was reduced without surgical management. Her original bowel symptoms persisted, and she finally had a colectomy.

Minor complications included skin ecchymosis, temporary urinary retention, temporary diarrhea or constipation, and dyschezia.

Diaphragmatic Endometriosis

The diaphragm rarely is a reported site of endometriosis.[89] Women should be asked about pleuritic, shoulder, or upper abdominal pain occurring with menses because they do not make the connection between these distant anatomic landmarks. The laparoscope is an excellent modality to diagnose and possibly treat endometriosis on the diaphragm, which is difficult to reach by laparotomy[90] (Figure 11-29, see also Plate 61).

Before treating diaphragmatic endometriosis by laparotomy or laparoscopy, other options are discussed with the patient because surgery at this location can injure the diaphragm, phrenic nerve, lungs, or heart.

For women interested in preserving their reproductive organs, medical treatment should be administered. If the patient does not desire to preserve her reproductive organs, bilateral oophorectomy may relieve her symptoms and further intervention may not be necessary. However, if she does want to preserve her fertility potential, her symptoms are not responsive to medical therapy, and she requests surgery after discussing all possi-

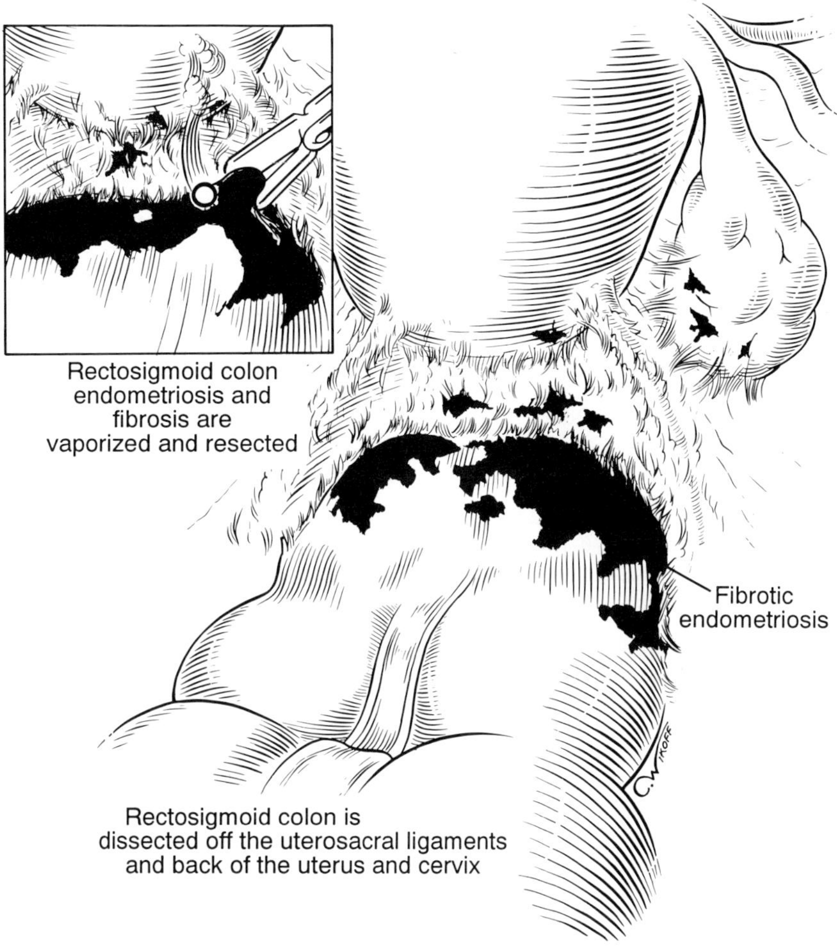

Figure 11-28 After complete separation of the rectum, the endometriosis and fibrosis from the anterior rectum and rectovaginal septum is resected completely or vaporized using high-power CO_2 laser.

ble complications, surgical intervention may be performed.

Most implants are superficial and cause no discomfort. We have found symptomatic diaphragmatic lesions in 8 of 4875 patients. Because many women prefer definitive surgery, including bilateral salpingo-oophorectomy, it is rarely necessary to treat these implants surgically. Others benefit from medical therapy and the chance of recurrence on the diaphragm is low.

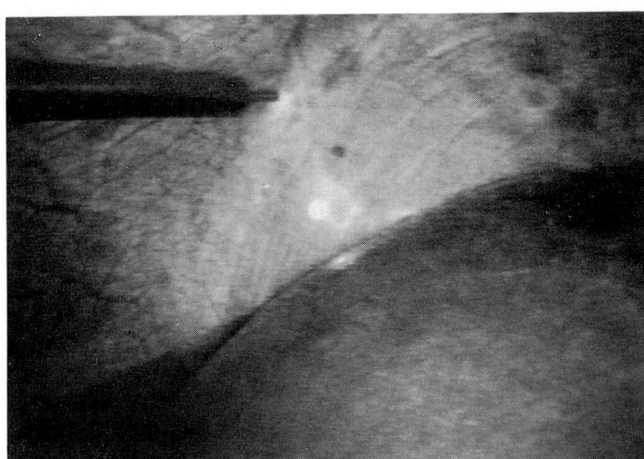

Figure 11-29 Endometriotic lesions on the diaphragm above the liver (see Plate 61).

Endoscopic treatment begins with introducing a 10-mm laparoscope at the umbilical port and placing three additional trocars in the upper quadrant (right or left according to implant location), similar to the arrangement for laparoscopic cholecystectomy. Two grasping forceps are used to push the liver from the operative field and enable better exposure of the diaphragm. Lesions are removed using hydrodissection and vaporization or excision. If a diaphragmatic defect is formed, it is repaired with 4-0 PDS or staples.

Following the procedure, the patient should be evaluated by a cardiopulmonary consultant. The pharynx, larynx, and trachea are examined with a rigid bronchoscope. A flexible scope is introduced to examine the distal trachea and proximal main bronchi.

We have treated symptomatic diaphragmatic endometriosis implants in eight women (CN,FN). In three cases, the lesions were directly over the phrenic nerve or the diaphragmatic vasculature. The lesions were excised in three and vaporization was performed in three others. In one patient, the lesion was treated by combined laser and ultrasound (CUSA, Cavitational Ultrasonographic Surgical Aspirator, Valley Lab, Boulder, CO). In the remaining patient, only a bilateral salpingo-oophorectomy was performed. No intraoperative or postoperative complications were noted. Six patients were without pain 6 to 36 months later. In one woman, the pain returned after one year, and another experienced no significant pain relief. Both responded to hormonal suppressive therapy.

Restoration of Tubo-ovarian Anatomy

Once all lesions are resected or ablated and the adnexa are freed of adhesions, the anatomic relationship between the ovary and ipsilateral tube is evaluated and any distortion caused by adhesions is corrected. The mesosalpinx often adheres to the ovarian cortex along the ampullary segment of the tube. These adhesions cover a significant surface area of the ovarian cortex and may interfere with the ovulatory process at oocyte release.[62] Moreover, the fimbriae frequently are agglutinated, which may inhibit their ability to capture the oocyte. Adhesiolysis along the ovarian surface and mesosalpinx can be accomplished with CO_2 laser, which requires a backstop inserted into the space between the ovary and mesosalpinx. If this space is not accessible, the ovary and tube are grasped with atraumatic forceps, and the plane between them is dissected with laser, electrode, or scissors. However, fimbrial adhesions should be resected only with laparoscopic microscissors under liquid or an ultrapulse CO_2 laser with high millijoules. Adhesiolysis performed in a fluid medium offers a clearer view of the anatomy than is provided with the pneumoperitoneum alone. The pelvis is filled with lactated Ringer's to allow the fimbriae to float freely in the clear fluid away from each other and from the filmy adhesions which, being lighter than the fimbria, float higher and separate from the normal tissue. As they float away from the fimbrial folds, adhesions are grasped with a fine forceps and atraumatically divided with microscissors without bleeding or injury to the normal tissues.[91]

Pain Relief

Besides infertility, the most common complaint of patients with endometriosis is pain, usually in the pelvis, frequently worse at menses, and occasionally during coital activity. The classic symptom triad of infertility, dysmenorrhea, and dyspareunia, although not diagnostic of endometriosis, strongly suggests the disease. Focal or localized pain associated with endometriosis usually responds to removal or destruction of endometriosis and associated adhesions. However, in some women the pain is disproportionate to the extent of the disease or does not improve subsequent to resection of endometriosis and adhesions. For recalcitrant or diffuse pain, interruption of pelvic nerves either by uterosacral resection or presacral neurectomy is advised.[92–94]

Minimizing Recurrence

The surgical treatment of endometriosis involves destroying endometrial implants (coagulation, vaporization, resection) and associated adhesions, and restoring normal anatomy. The anatomic, physiologic, and genetic factors that predispose each patient to developing endometriosis are not altered by the surgical treatment. Therefore, recurrence is unavoidable unless endometrial proliferation, menstruation, or the predominantly estrogenic milieu of the patient is altered. For those who desire pregnancy, an early success will be therapeutic since the 9-month gestational period, besides precluding menstrual flow, results in a predominantly progestational milieu that reduces endometrial proliferation and the extent of disease. Patients not desiring pregnancy have an increased risk of earlier recurrence and may benefit from preventive measures targeted at decreasing known risk factors, such as short length of menstrual cycles, lack of exercise,[95] menorrhagia,[96] and outflow obstruction.[97] Müllerian anomalies that predispose the patient to outflow obstruction should be corrected.[97] Postoperatively, exercise and hormonal therapy (progestational agents or low-dose oral contraceptives) are suggested. For the first 9 months postoperatively, Provera 30 mg daily is prescribed to induce amenorrhea in more than 75% of patients and regression of residual disease.[47,98] Continuous oral contraceptive pills may be prescribed for certain patients. When using the

Provera regimen, the switch to low-dose oral contraceptives, frequently is associated with hypomenorrhea that may be therapeutic. If symptoms recur, medroxyprogesterone acetate therapy or gonadotropin-releasing hormone analog is given to control pain.[46] Second-look laparoscopy may be necessary to treat recurrent or persistent endometriosis.

Future Development

New developments in fiberoptic endoscopes, with diameters of less than 1 mm, may allow the gynecologic surgeon to diagnose and stage the disease in an office setting under local anesthesia, possibly at earlier stages. Further development of laser surgery and photodynamic therapy may make therapeutic microendoscopy possible in an office setting.[99] Manyak and colleagues[100] conducted experiments evaluating photodynamic therapy of endometriosis using rabbit endometrial implants. Following the intravenous injection of dihydroporphyrin ether (DHE), the rabbits were treated with low-energy Argon laser, which is absorbed mainly by the photosensitive chemical concentrated in the endometrial implants but not in the surrounding normal tissues. The selective absorption of the laser energy by the DHE enables the low-power laser energy to destroy only the endometriotic lesions containing DHE, sparing the normal tissue. Because DHE is absorbed by both gross and microscopic disease, a more thorough surgical resection of endometriosis is possible with photodynamic therapy, less invasively and much more safely. The ability to diagnose and treat disease at earlier stages and in an office setting may prevent the progression and invasion of endometriosis, reducing its adverse impact on health, quality of life, and fertility potential.

References

1. Hasson HM. Incidence of endometriosis in diagnostic laparoscopy. *J Reprod Med.* 1976;16:135.
2. Schmidt LC. Endometriosis: a reappraisal of pathogenesis and treatment. *Fertil Steril.* 1985;44:157.
3. Williams TJ, Pratt JHL. Endometriosis in a 1000 consecutive celiotomies: incidence and management. *Am J Obstet Gynecol.* 1977;129:245.
4. Rokitansky C. Ueber Uterusdrusen—Neubildung in uterus and ovarial sarcomen. *Z Gesellschaft Aertz Wein.* 1860;16:755.
5. Williams TJ. Endometriosis. In: Thompson JD, Rock JA, eds. *Te Linde's Gynecology,* 7th ed. Philadelphia: JB Lippincott; 1992:488.
6. Gomel V, McComb P. Microsurgery in gynecology. In: Silver JS, ed. *Microsurgery*. Baltimore: Williams & Wilkins; 1979:143.
7. Cook AS, Rock JA. The role of laparoscopy in the treatment of endometriosis. *Fertil Steril.* 1991;4:663.
8. Martin DC. CO_2 laser laparoscopy for the treatment of endometriosis associated with infertility. *J Reprod Med.* 1985;30:409.
9. Nezhat C, Crowgey S, Nezhat F. Surgical treatment of endometriosis via laser laparoscopy. *Fertil Steril.* 1986;45:778.
10. Nezhat C, Crowgey S, Nezhat F. Videolaseroscopy for the treatment of endometriosis associated with infertility. *Fertil Steril.* 1989;51:123.
11. Adamson DG, Subak LL, Pasta DJ, et al. Comparison of CO_2 laser laparoscopy with laparotomy for the treatment of endometriomata. *Fertil Steril.* 1992;57:965.
12. Adamson DG, Hurd SJ, Pasta DJ, et al. Laparoscopic endometriosis treatment: is it better? *Fertil Steril.* 1993;59:35.
13. Ranney BR. Endometriosis III: complete operations. *Am J Obstet Gynecol.* 1971; 109:1137.
14. Wilson EA. Surgical therapy for endometriosis. *Clin Obstet Gynecol.* 1988;31:857.
15. Nezhat C, Nezhat F, Nezhat CH. Operative laparoscopy (minimally invasive surgery): state of the art. *J Gynecol Surg.* 1992; 8:111.
16. Nezhat C, Nezhat FR. Safe laser endoscopic excision or vaporization of peritoneal endometriosis. *Fertil Steril.* 1989;52:149.
17. Luciano AA, Lowney J, Jacobs SL. Endoscopic treatment of endometriosis-associated infertility: therapeutic, economic and social benefits. *J Reprod Med.* 1992; 37:573.
18. Olive DL, Martin DC. Treatment of endometriosis associated infertility with CO_2 laser laparoscopy: the use of 1- and 2-parameter exponential models. *Fertil Steril.* 1987; 48:18.
19. Filmar S, Gomel V, McComb P. Operative

laparoscopy versus open abdominal surgery: a comparative study on postoperative adhesion formation in the rat model. *Fertil Steril.* 1987;48:486–490.
20. Luciano AA, Maier DB, Nulsen ZC, et al. A comparative study of postoperative adhesion formation following laser surgery by laparoscopy versus laparotomy in the rabbit model. *Obstet Gynecol.* 1989;74:220.
21. Maier DB, Klock A, Nulsen J, et al. Laser laparoscopy vs laparotomy in lysis of dense and incidental pelvic adhesions. *J Reprod Med.* 1992;37:965.
22. Diamond MP, Daniell SF, Feste J, et al. Adhesion reformation and de novo formation after reproductive pelvic surgery. *Fertil Steril.* 1987;47:864.
23. Luciano AA, Moufauino-Oliva M. Comparison of postoperative adhesion formation—laparoscopy versus laparotomy. *Infert Reprod Med Clin North Am.* 1994;5:437.
24. Marana R, Luciano AA, Morendino VE, et al. Reproductive outcome after ovarian surgery: microsurgery versus CO_2 laser. *J Gynecol Surg.* 1991:7:159.
25. Lundorff P, Hahlin M, Kallfelt B, et al. Adhesion formation after laparoscopic surgery in ectopic pregnancy: a randomized trial versus laparotomy. *Fertil Steril.* 1991; 55:91.
26. Trimbos-Kemper TCM, Trimbos JB, van Hall EV. Adhesion formation after tubal surgery: results of the 8 day laparoscopy in 188 patients. *Fertil Steril.* 1985;43:395.
27. Nezhat C, Nezhat F, Metzger DA, et al. Adhesion reformation after reproductive surgery by videolaseroscopy. *Fertil Steril.* 1990;53:1008.
28. Operative Laparoscopy Study Group: Postoperative adhesion development after operative laparoscopy evaluation at early second look procedures. *Fertil Steril.* 1991; 55:700.
29. Donnez J. Carbon dioxide laser laparoscopy in infertile women with endometriosis and women with adnexal adhesions. *Fertil Steril.* 1987;48:190.
30. Fayez JA, Collazo LM. Comparison between laparotomy and operative laparoscopy in the treatment of moderate and severe endometriosis. *Int J Fertil.* 1990;35:272.
31. Nezhat C, Silfen SL, Nezhat F, et al. Surgery for endometriosis. *Curr Opin Obstet Gynecol.* 1991;3:385.
32. Nezhat C, Winer W, Cooper J, et al. Endoscopic infertility surgery. *J Reprod Med.* 1989;34:127.
33. Gomel V. Laparoscopic tubal surgery in infertility. *Obstet Gynecol.* 1975;46:4752.
34. Gomel V. Salpingo-ovariolysis by laparoscopy in infertility. *Fertil Steril.* 1983; 40:607.
35. Chong AP, Luciano AA, O'Shaughnessy AM. Laser laparoscopy versus laparotomy in the treatment of infertility patients with severe endometriosis. *J Gynecol Surg.* 1990;6:179.
36. Nezhat C, Nezhat F. Operative laparoscopy for the management of ovarian remnant syndrome. *Fertil Steril.* 1992;57:1003.
37. Nezhat F, Nezhat C, Silfen SL. Videolaseroscopy for oophorectomy. *Am J Obstet Gynecol.* 1991;165:1323–1330.
38. Betts WJ, Buttram CVJ. A plan for managing endometriosis. *Contemp Ob/Gyn.* 1980;15:121.
39. Ranney BR. Endometriosis: conservative operations. *Am J Obstet Gynecol.* 1970; 107:743.
40. Wheeler JH, Malinak LR. Recurrent endometriosis: incidence, management, and prognosis. *Am J Obstet Gynecol.* 1983; 146:247.
41. Barbieri RL. Hormonal therapy of endometriosis. *Infertil Reprod Med North Am.* 1992;3:187.
42. Henderson AF, Studd JW, Watson N. A retrospective study of estrogen replacement therapy following hysterectomy for the treatment of endometriosis. In: Shaw RW, ed. *Advances in Reproductive Endocrinology* (vol. 1) *Endometriosis.* Carnforth, Lancs, Parthenon; 1989:131.
43. Luciano AA. Hormone replacement therapy in post menopausal women. *Infert Reprod Med Clin North Am.* 1992;3:109.
44. Luciano AA, Manzi D. Treatment options for endometriosis—surgical therapies. *Infert Reprod Med Clin North Am.* 1992; 3:657.
45. Luciano AA, Turksoy RN, Carleo J. Evaluation of oral medroxyprogesterone acetate in the treatment of endometriosis. *Obstet Gynecol.* 1988;72:323.
46. Luciano AA, Roy M, De Souza MJ, et al. Evaluation of low dose estrogen and progestin therapy in postmenopausal women. *J Reprod Med.* 1993;38:207.

47. Greenblatt RB, Nezhat C, Natrajan PK. Update on the male and female climacteric. *J Am Geriatr Soc.* 1979;27:481.
48. Chetkowski RJ, Meldrum DR, Steingold KA, et al. Biological effects of transdermal estradiol. *J Clin Endocrinol Metab.* 1986; 314:1615.
49. Schenken SR, Malinak RL. Reoperation after initial treatment of endometriosis with conservative surgery. *Am J Obstet Gynecol.* 1978;131:416.
50. Murphy AA, Green WR, Bobbie D, et al. Unsuspected endometriosis documented by scanning electron microscopy in visually normal peritoneum. *Fertil Steril.* 1986; 46:522.
51. Nezhat F, Allan JC, Nezhat C, et al. Nonvisualized endometriosis at laparoscopy. *Int J Fertil.* 1991;36:340.
52. Vasquez G, Cornille F, Brosens IA. Peritoneal endometriosis: scanning electron microscopy and histology of minimal pelvic endometriotic lesions. *Fertil Steril.* 1984; 42:696.
53. Martin DC, Hubert GD, Vander-Zwaag R, et al. Laparoscopic appearances of pelvic endometriosis. *Fertil Steril.* 1989;51:63.
54. Redwine DB. Age-related evolution in color appearance of endometriosis. *Fertil Steril.* 1987;48:1062.
55. Vernon MW, Beard JS, Graves K, et al. Classification of endometriotic implants by morphologic appearance and capacity to synthesize prostaglandin. *Fertil Steril.* 1990; 53:984.
56. Cornillie FJ, Ooosterlynck D, Lauweryns JM, et al. Deeply infiltrating pelvic endometriosis: histology and clinical significance. *Fertil Steril.* 1990;53:978.
57. Crain LJ, Luciano AA. Peritoneal fluid evaluation in infertility. *Obstet Gynecol.* 1983; 61:1591.
58. Nisolle M, Paindavene B, Boudon A, et al. Histologic study of peritoneal endometriosis in infertile women. *Fertil Steril.* 1990;53:984.
59. Redwine DB. Peritoneal blood painting: an aid in the diagnosis of endometriosis. *Am J Obstet Gynecol.* 1989;161:865.
60. Candiani GB, Vercelli P, Fedele L. Laparoscopic ovarian puncture to correct staging of endometriosis. *Fertil Steril.* 1990; 53:984.
61. Prystowsky JB, Stryker SJ, Ujiki GT, et al. Gastrointestinal endometriosis: incidence and indications for resection. *Arch Surg.* 1988;7:855–858.
62. Luciano AA, Marana R, Krakta S, et al. Ovarian function after incision of the ovary by scalpel, CO_2 laser and microelectrode. *Fertil Steril.* 1991;56:349.
63. Hasson HM. Laparoscopic management of ovarian cysts. *J Reprod Med.* 1990;25:863.
64. Brosens I, Puttemansi P. Double optic laparoscopy. *Ballieres Clin Obstet Gynecol.* 1989;3:595.
65. Keye WR, Hansen LW, Astin M, et al. Argon laser therapy of endometriosis: a review of 92 consecutive patients. *Fertil Steril.* 1987;47:208.
66. Nezhat F, Nezhat C, Allan CJ, Metzger DA, Sears DL. A clinical and histologic classification of endometriomas: implications for a mechanism of pathogenesis. *J Reprod Med.* 1992;37:771–776.
67. Marana R, Luciano AA, Muzii L, et al. Reproductive outcome after ovarian surgery: suturing versus nonsuturing of the ovarian cortex. *J Gynecol Surg.* 1991;7:155.
68. Nezhat C, Nezhat F. Postoperative adhesion formation after ovarian cystectomy with and without ovarian reconstruction. Abstract O-012, 47th annual meeting of the American Fertility Association, Orlando, FL, October 21–24, 1991.
69. Donnez J, Nisolle M. Laparoscopic management of large ovarian endometrial cyst: use of fibrin sealant. *Surgery.* 1991;7:163.
70. Stanley EK, Utz DC, Dockerty MB. Clinically significant endometriosis of the urinary tract. *Surg Gynecol Obstet.* 1965; 120:491.
71. Goldstein MS, Brodman ML. Cystometric evaluation of vesical endometriosis before and after hormonal or surgical treatment. *Mt Sinai J Med.* 1990;57:109.
72. Nezhat C, Nezhat F, Green B. Laparoscopic treatment of obstructed ureter due to endometriosis by resection and ureteroureterostomy: a case report. *J Urol.* 1992;148:659.
73. Nezhat C, Nezhat F. Laparoscopic segmental bladder resection for endometriosis: a report of two cases. *Obstet Gynecol.* 1993; 81:882.
74. Sampson JA. Intestinal adenomas of endometrial type. *Arch Surg.* 1922;5:217.
75. Jenkinson EL, Brown WH. Endometriosis: a study of 117 cases with special reference to

constricting lesions of the rectum and sigmoid colon. *JAMA.* 1943;122:349.

76. Samper ER, Sagle GW, Hand AM. Colonic endometriosis, its clinical spectrum. *South Med J.* 1984;77:912.
77. Ponka JL, Brush BE, Hodgkinson CP. Colorectal endometriosis. *Dis Colon Rectum.* 1973;16:490.
78. Meyers WC, Kelvin FM, Jones RS. Diagnosis and surgical treatment of colonic endometriosis. *Arch Surg.* 1979;114:169–175.
79. Meyer R. Uber entzundliche heterage Epithelwucherungen in weiblichen Genitalgebiete und uber cine bir in die Wurzel des Mescolon ausgedehnte benigne Wucherung des Darmepithels. *Virchows Arch Pathol Anat.* 1909;195:487.
80. Coronado C, Franklin RR, Lotze EC, et al. Surgical treatment of symptomatic colorectal endometriosis. *Fertil Steril.* 1990;3:411.
81. Nezhat C, Pennington E, Nezhat F, Silfen SL. Laparoscopically assisted anterior rectal wall resection and reanastomosis for deeply infiltrating endometriosis. *Surg Laparosc Endosc.* 1991;1:106–108.
82. Nezhat C, Nezhat F, Pennington E. Laparoscopic proctectomy for infiltrating endometriosis of the rectum. *Fertil Steril.* 1992; 57:1129.
83. Nezhat F, Nezhat C, Pennington E, Ambroze W. Laparoscopic segmental resection for infiltrating endometriosis of the rectosigmoid colon: a preliminary report. *Surg Laparosc Endosc.* 1992;2:212–216.
84. Nezhat C, Nezhat F, Pennington E, Nezhat CH, et al. Laparoscopic disk excision and primary repair of the anterior rectal wall for the treatment of full-thickness bowel endometriosis. *Surg Endosc.* 1994;8:682.
85. Nezhat C, Nezhat F, Ambroze W, Pennington E. Laparoscopic repair of small bowel, colon, and rectal endometriosis: a report of twenty-six cases. *Surg Endosc.* 1993;7: 88–89.
86. Brumsted JR, Deaton J, Lavigne E, et al. Postoperative adhesion formation after ovarian wedge resection with and without ovarian reconstruction in the rabbit. *Fertil Steril.* 1990;53:723.
87. Ellis H. The cause and prevention of postoperative intraperitoneal adhesions. *Surg Gynecol Obstet.* 1971;133:497.
88. Nezhat C, Nezhat F, Pennington E. Laparoscopic treatment of lower colorectal and infiltrative rectovaginal septum endometriosis by the technique of video-laseroscopy. *Br J Obstet Gynaecol.* 1992;99: 664–667.
89. Shiraishi T. Catamenial pneumothorax: report of a case and review of the Japanese and non-Japanese literature. *Thorac Cardiovasc Surg.* 1991;39:304–307.
90. Nezhat F, Nezhat C, Levy JS. Laparoscopic treatment of symptomatic diaphragmatic endometriosis: a case report. *Fertil Steril.* 1992;58:614–616.
91. Nezhat F, Winer WK, Nezhat C. Fimbrioscopy and salpingoscopy in patients with minimal to moderate pelvic endometriosis. *Obstet Gynecol.* 1990;75:15–17.
92. Black WT. Use of presacral sympathectomy in the treatment of dysmenorrhea: a second look after twenty-five years. *Am J Obstet Gynecol.* 1964;89:16.
93. Lee RB, Stone K, Magelssen D, et al. Presacral neurectomy for chronic pelvic pain. *Obstet Gynecol.* 1986;68:517.
94. Tjaden B, Schlaff WD, Kimball A, et al. The efficacy of presacral neurectomy for the relief of midline dysmenorrhea. *Obstet Gynecol.* 1990;76:89.
95. Cramer DW, Wilson E, Stillman RJ, et al. The relation of endometriosis to menstrual characteristics, smoking and exercise. *JAMA.* 1986;255:1904.
96. Sensky TE, Liu DTY. Endometriosis: association with menorrhagia, infertility and oral contraceptives. *Int J Gynecol Obstet.* 1980;17:573.
97. Olive DL, Henderson DY. Endometriosis and mullerian anomalies. *Obstet Gynecol.* 1987;69:412.
98. Moghissi KS, Boyce CR. Management of endometriosis with oral medroxyprogesterone acetate. *Obstet Gynecol.* 1976;47:265.
99. Henzi MR, Corson SL, Moghissi K, et al. Photodynamic therapy of rabbit endometrial implants: a model treatment of endometriosis. *Fertil Steril.* 1989;52:140.
100. Manyak MJ, Nelson LM, Solomon D, Russo A, et al. Photodynamic therapy of rabbit endometrial implants: a model treatment of endometriosis. *Fertil Steril.* 1989;52:140.
101. Stripling MC, Martin DC, Chatman DL, et al. Subtle appearance of pelvic endometriosis. *Fertil Steril.* 1988;49:427.
102. Jansen R, Russell P. Nonpigmented endometriosis: clinical, laparoscopic, and pathological definition. *Am J Obstet Gynecol.* 1986;155:1154.

103. Buttram VC. Surgical treatment of endometriosis in the infertile female: a modified approach. *Fertil Steril.* 1979;32:635–640.
104. Rock JA, Guzick DS, Sengoo C, et al. The conservative surgical treatment of endometriosis: evaluation of pregnancy successes with respect to the extent of disease as categorized using contemporary classification systems. *Fertil Steril.* 1981;35:131.
105. Rantala ML, Kahanpaa KV, Koskimies AL, et al. Fertility prognosis after surgical treatment of pelvic endometriosis. *Acta Obstet Gynecol Scand.* 1983;62:11.
106. Gordts S, Boeck W, Brosens I. Microsurgery of endometriosis in infertile patients. *Fertil Steril.* 1984;42:520.
107. Feste JR. Laser laparoscopy: a new modality. *J Reprod Med.* 1985;30:413.

12

Ovarian Cysts

Almost all persistent ovarian cysts must be treated surgically, and evolving laparoscopic technology has enabled endoscopic management of most of them. Although most are benign, the possibility of malignancy usually requires a laparotomy using a midline incision.

Laparoscopic Management of Adnexal Masses

Although most ovarian cysts can be removed by laparoscopy, its unsafe and inappropriate use should be discouraged. One percent to 2% of women will develop ovarian cancer during their lifetime, and unfortunately, by the time they are detected, two thirds are in stage III or IV with a poor prognosis.[1] A laparoscopist can diagnose advanced ovarian cancer so that immediate laparotomy and appropriate staging are possible. A serious concern is the presumed benign lesion that subsequently proves to be stage I ovarian carcinoma. If the cyst is managed with the assumption that it is benign and spillage of contents occurs during the aspiration or ovarian cystectomy, the stage is upgraded from IA to IC. A laparotomy may be required for optimal surgical therapy, and postoperative radiotherapy or chemotherapy is needed.

The risks associated with spillage of cyst contents[2] have been reevaluated. In a multivariate analysis of stage I epithelial ovarian cancer, the factors that influenced the rate of relapse in 519 patients were the tumor grade, the presence of dense adhesions, and a large volume of ascites. Intraoperative spillage at laparotomy demonstrated no adverse effect on prognosis of stage I ovarian cancer.[3] The survival of women with borderline tumors who were managed initially by cystectomy, with or without spillage, was not decreased, nor was there evidence of development of disseminated disease for an average of 7.5 years after diagnosis.[4] Thus, when patients receive the appropriate operation, the risk of dissemination remains conjectural.

In two large studies, the incidence of ovarian malignancy in patients with a known adnexal mass was between 1.2%[5] and 0.3%.[6] The results of a 1991 survey of the members of the American Association of Gynecologic Laparoscopists (AAGL) indicated that laparoscopic excision of unsuspected, invasive ovarian cancer was uncommon. Only 53 instances were reported among 13,739 laparoscopic ovarian cyst procedures, an incidence of 0.4%.[7] However, a recent survey of gynecologic oncologists[8] found 12 borderline ovarian tumors and 30 invasive ovarian cancers initially managed by laparoscopic excision, and most patients did not have a staging laparotomy for weeks after their cancer was found. These patients did not have careful preoperative screening and appropriate surgical management was delayed. Therefore, the patient must be informed that laparoscopic removal of ovarian cysts is not yet the standard of care because cancer can be encountered and an immediate laparotomy may be necessary. Management of benign-appearing adnexal masses must follow a protocol that includes obtaining cytology of pelvic and cyst fluid, possible frozen section of a biopsy specimen, and removing the mass for histologic examination. Aspirating a cyst and vaporizing or coagulating the capsule are not acceptable alternatives.

TABLE 12-1. CA-125 Levels Correlated With Type of Cyst

					CA-125 Level (U/mL)		Ultrasonographic Characteristics of Cysts							
							Cystic		Semicystic		Solid		Other	
No. of Women	Cyst	No.	Size (cm)	Age Range (y)	Range	Mean	No.	%	No.	%	No.	%	No.	%
360	Endometrioma	162	2–5	16–54	>2–212	45.7	123	68.9	22	22.8	14	7.5	3	0.8
		179	6–10		2–195	28.7	115		54		10		—	
		19	11–25		5–237	48.2	10		6		3		—	
219	Functional	172	2–5	11–47	<2–135	15.7	98	58.0	40	25.1	6	3.7	28	13.2
		45	6–10		<2–53	11.2	28		14		2		1	
		2	11–12		6	6.0	1		1		—		—	
34	Simple	13	2–5	23–47	5–76	7.0	10	76.5	—	8.8	—	5.9	3	8.8
		19	6–10		2–195	31.5	14		3		2		—	
		2	11–12		—	—	2		—	—	—		—	
30	Benign cystic teratoma	16	2–5	17–44	<5–9	7.0	7	43.3	7	36.7	1	13.3	1	6.7
		12	6–10		5–29	14.9	6		3		2		1	
		2	11–14		12	12.0	—		1		1		—	
17	Serous	8	2–5	33–40	14–47	30.5	7	82.4	—	5.9	—	5.9	1	5.9
		7	6–10		10–42	23.7	6		1		—		—	
		2	11–15		47–51	49.0	1		—		1		—	
11	Mucinous	4	2–5	31–35	<5	<5.0	2	54.5	2	45.5	—	—	—	—
		5	6–10		<5–30	10.6	2		3		—		—	
		2	11–25		9–11	10.0	2		—		—		—	
17	Hydrosalpinges	16	5–10	26–45	<5–35	12.8	6	41.2	8	47.1	—	—	2	11.8
		1	11–12		<5	<5.0	1		—		—		—	
46	Miscellaneous	30	2–5	22–45	<5–135	27.4	19	67.4	2	6.5	—	4.3	9	21.7
		15	6–10		<5–10	5.5	11		1		2		1	
		1	11–17		36	36.0	1		—		—		—	

The safe laparoscopic management of ovarian cysts has been described in several reports. Mage and colleagues[5] reported the laparoscopic treatment of 481 women (ages 9 to 88) who had ovarian cysts, including 96 functional cysts, 100 endometriomas, 100 serous cysts, 91 teratomas, 51 mucinous cysts, and 58 paraovarian cysts. Of these women, 19 underwent laparotomy for confirmed or suspected malignancy based only on laparoscopic evaluation; 10 of them were found to be benign. Five ovarian cancers and four borderline tumors were found and managed immediately by laparotomy. Dense pelvic adhesions or cysts larger than 10 cm were the indications for laparotomy in 42 women.

Nezhat and coworkers evaluated 1011 premenopausal women with ovarian cysts laparoscopically and found four ovarian cancers.[6] Preoperative assessment included an initial pelvic examination, vaginal ultrasound, and CA-125 level (Table 12-1).[6] Three of the four unsuspected cancers were found on frozen or permanent section of the cyst wall. One of the malignant tumors was 3 cm and its gross appearance was that of an endometrioma; histologic examination revealed an endometrioid carcinoma (Table 12-2).[6] Preoperative examinations did not detect malignancy.

Preoperative Evaluation

Laparoscopic management of adnexal masses depends on the patient's age, pelvic examination, sonographic images, and serum markers. A large, solid, fixed, or irregular adnexal mass accompanied by ascites is suspicious for malignancy (Table 12-3). Cul-de-sac nodularity, ascites, cystic adnexal structures, and fixed adnexae occur with endometriosis and ovarian malignancy.

TABLE 12-3. Malignant Potential of Ovarian Cyst by Physical Examination

Clinical Findings	Benign	Malignant
Size > 7 cm	++	++
Size < 7 cm	++	++
Unilateral	++++	+
Bilateral	++	++++
Cystic	++++	+
Solid	++	+++
Solid and cystic	+	++++
Mobile	++++	+
Fixed	+	++++
Irregular	+	++++
Smooth	++++	+
Ascites	+	++++
Cul-de-sac nodules	+	+++

+, least probable; ++++, most probable.

Ultrasound

Transvaginal ultrasound scanning (TVS) is the primary imaging modality for evaluating adnexal masses.[9] Cystic, unilocular masses less than 10 cm that are unilateral with regular borders are likely to be benign. Malignant ovarian cysts are associated with irregular borders, size greater than 10 cm, papillae, solid areas, thick septa (greater than 2 mm), ascites, and matted bowel. Using ultrasonographic criteria, accurate prediction of benign masses was made in 96% of patients.[9,10] Nezhat and colleagues found that none of the four malignant cysts in their series had any of the ultrasound criteria for malignancy.[6]

Functional cysts tend to gradually regress or resolve either spontaneously or with hormonal suppressive therapy within 8 weeks. However, persistent cysts that appear to be functional or hemorrhagic on ultrasound should be removed.

TABLE 12-2. Findings at Laparoscopy in Four Women With Ovarian Cancer

	Case 1 Serous Cystadenocarcinoma	Case 2 Endometrioid Low Malignant Potential Tumor	Case 3 Papillary Mucinous Cystadenocarcinoma	Case 4 Clear Cell Carcinoma
Pt. age (y)	44	45	43	33
Stage	IIIC	IA	IIA	IA
Tumor size (cm)	7	3	13	6
Serum CA-125 level (U/mL)	N/A	7	17	2
Ultrasonographic finding	Septated semicystic	Cystic	Septated semicystic	Septated semicystic

Hormonal Suppressive Therapy

Oral contraceptives have been prescribed for some cystic adnexal masses (less than 6 cm) in reproductive-aged women on the assumption that decreasing gonadotropin stimulation to a functional cyst will hasten its resolution. The results of a recent study failed to report any benefit from ovarian suppressive therapy, and the author noted that time was the most important factor in differentiating functional from pathologic cysts.[11] However, the cysts were less than 5 cm, and the study included women who had received ovulation-induction medication. Until further reports confirm these findings, hormonal suppressive therapy is recommended for 6 to 8 weeks. Either danazol (800 mg/d) or oral contraceptive pills with 50 μg estrogen are advised for any cyst suspected of being functional.

CA-125

CA-125 is a tumor-associated antigen used to ascertain the nature of the ovarian cyst (Table 12-4). Levels below 35 U/mL are associated with benign tumors. However, the sensitivity and specificity varies, and the presence of other benign conditions can elevate CA-125 levels. In 80% of premenopausal women, elevated CA-125 levels were associated with pregnancy, endometriosis, fibroids, adenomyosis, cystic teratomas, and acute or chronic salpingitis. More importantly, only 50% of patients with stage I ovarian cancers had elevated CA-125 levels compared to 90% with stage II.[12]

Cyst Aspiration

Cystic fluid may not provide accurate cytologic diagnosis in many patients[13] because 10% to 65% of aspirates have been interpreted as benign when malignancy is present.[6,14,15] In a recent review, the accuracy of transvaginal and transrectal fine needle aspiration and ultrasound-guided puncture of ovarian cysts were associated with disappointing results.[16] This procedure is not indicated for treatment because of the high rate of recurrence.[17–19]

Computed Tomography and Magnetic Resonance Imaging

Computed tomography (CT) and magnetic resonance imaging (MRI) can detect additional anatomic structures and subtle tissue difference. The resolution characteristics of CT depend on differences in x-ray attenuation between calcium, water, fat, and air. Soft tissue differences can be enhanced with intravenous contrast. MRI relies on differences in the hydrogen content of fat and water, magnetic relaxation time, and blood flow, ultimately resulting in additional soft tissue contrast. The role of CT and MRI relative to ultrasound in evaluating an ovarian cyst is evolving. In one study, MRI had a sensitivity of 95% and a specificity of 88% in discriminating malignant from benign lesions, whereas TVS had a 75% sensitivity and 98% specificity.[20] Given the acceptable sensitivity and specificity of ultrasound combined with CA-125, the additional expense of CT and MRI is not justified.

Recommended Approach

Although ovarian neoplasms can occur at any age, the risk of malignancy is highest during prepuberty and menopause. Ovarian activity is associated with a high incidence of functional ovarian cysts and other benign pathologic conditions. These observations, combined with the age differences in the sensitivity and specificity of clinical testing, suggest the following recommendations in evaluating and managing adnexal masses. Malignancy is not the only concern in managing an ovarian cyst. Patients who wish to preserve their reproductive organs should have the least aggressive therapy.

Because the risk of malignancy is relatively low in young women, preoperative evaluation should include a history and physical examination, pelvic ultrasound to evaluate both ovaries (to rule out bilateral endometriomas or teratomas), possible hormonal suppressive therapy, and a blood sample

TABLE 12-4. Sensitivity and Specificity of Diagnostic Tests

	Premenopausal, %		Postmenopausal, %	
	Sensitivity	Specificity	Sensitivity	Specificity
Specialist ultrasound	50	96	78	92
Clinical impression	17	92	68	85
CA-125	50	69	84	92

Source: Modified from Finkler N, Benacerrat B, Lavin F. Comparison of serum CA-125, clinical impression and ultrasound in the preoperative evaluation of ovarian masses. *Obstet Gynecol.* 1988;72:659.

to be held for baseline tumor marker status if the mass subsequently is found to be malignant. In premenopausal women, in addition to ascertaining the characteristics of the adnexal mass, resection of ovarian tissue can cause adhesions and should be minimized (Table 12-5).

In postmenopausal women, with the more frequent use of diagnostic imaging, the incidental finding of adnexal masses will increase. Routine pelvic sonographic screening of asymptomatic postmenopausal women may find early ovarian cancer, but the procedure may not be cost effective. Wolf and colleagues screened 149 asymptomatic women over 50 years of age and discovered cysts in 22 (14.8%) ranging in size from 0.4 to 4.7 cm.[21] Two additional women had septated masses, but no ovarian cancers were detected. In another study, screening 5479 women aged 45 or older revealed 6.1% with abnormal scans.[22] When these scans were repeated 2 to 8 weeks later, only 59% of them were persistently abnormal. Five ovarian cancers were found, two in the first screen and three in the follow-up screen; all were stage I. Thus, about 1000 TVSs were performed to detect one ovarian cancer. These data do not seem to support the view that screening asymptomatic postmenopausal women who have a normal pelvic examination is justified.

Figure 12-1 describes the preoperative evaluation for an ovarian cyst that includes a history, pelvic examination, ultrasound, and serum CA-125. If any combination of these tests suggests malignancy, an abdominal and pelvic CT scan is performed. If the scan indicates malignancy (ascites, omental cake, etc.), the patient undergoes a staging laparotomy or chemotherapy. If the CT scan is negative, a laparoscopy is planned and consent obtained for laparotomy.

Preoperatively, the patient has a mechanical and antibiotic bowel preparation, a chest x-ray, and signs the appropriate consent.

TABLE 12-5. Premenopausal Ovarian Cyst

Preoperative Evaluation	Intraoperative Evaluation
History and physical examination	Diagnostic laparoscopy
Transvaginal ultrasound	Peritoneal washing
Hormonal suppressive therapy, if indicated	Cyst aspiration
Informed consent	Evaluation of the cyst
Draw blood and save for possible tumor marker	Possible frozen section
	Cystectomy or oophorectomy

Intraoperative Considerations

Intraoperative evaluation includes cell washings from the pelvis and upper abdomen to be saved for evaluation should a malignancy be found. The upper abdomen and pelvis are explored and excrescences or suspicious areas are sampled and sent for frozen section.

After the pelvis and upper abdomen have been examined, the cyst contents should be aspirated. Once the capsule is opened, the interior of the capsule is examined and suspicious areas biopsied and sent for frozen section. The entire cyst capsule must be removed to search for an early carcinoma that may elude gross detection.[6] Whether to perform oophorectomy or cystectomy depends on the patient's age and characteristics of the mass.

Ovarian Cystectomy

An ovarian cystectomy removes the cyst intact with minimal trauma to the residual ovarian tissue. Alternatively, the cyst fluid can be drained to minimize spillage and facilitate its removal. Three methods to manage such cysts are drainage, excision and thermal ablation, or coagulation. By excising the cyst, histopathologic examination is more complete and the risk of recurrence is minimized. Aspiration is recommended for functional cysts, which are diagnosed laparoscopically and confirmed by frozen section followed by postoperative hormonal suppressive therapy. Thermal ablation does not destroy the entire cyst wall, and the underlying ovarian cortex can be damaged by the heat. Therefore, excision is preferred.

Cyst Aspiration Before Cystectomy

Many cysts are ruptured during their manipulation despite a delicate technique. The removal of a cyst 10 cm or larger intact is difficult laparoscopically. Aspiration before removal of large cysts is practical and can be accomplished using one of two methods. An 18-gauge laparoscopic needle is passed through the suction irrigator probe while stabilizing the cyst with suction applied over the cyst. The needle is inserted into the cyst and the contents are aspirated (Figure 12-2). The suction irrigator system reduces the spillage by applying suction at the cannula, or the suction-irrigator probe can be inserted into the cyst (see Figure

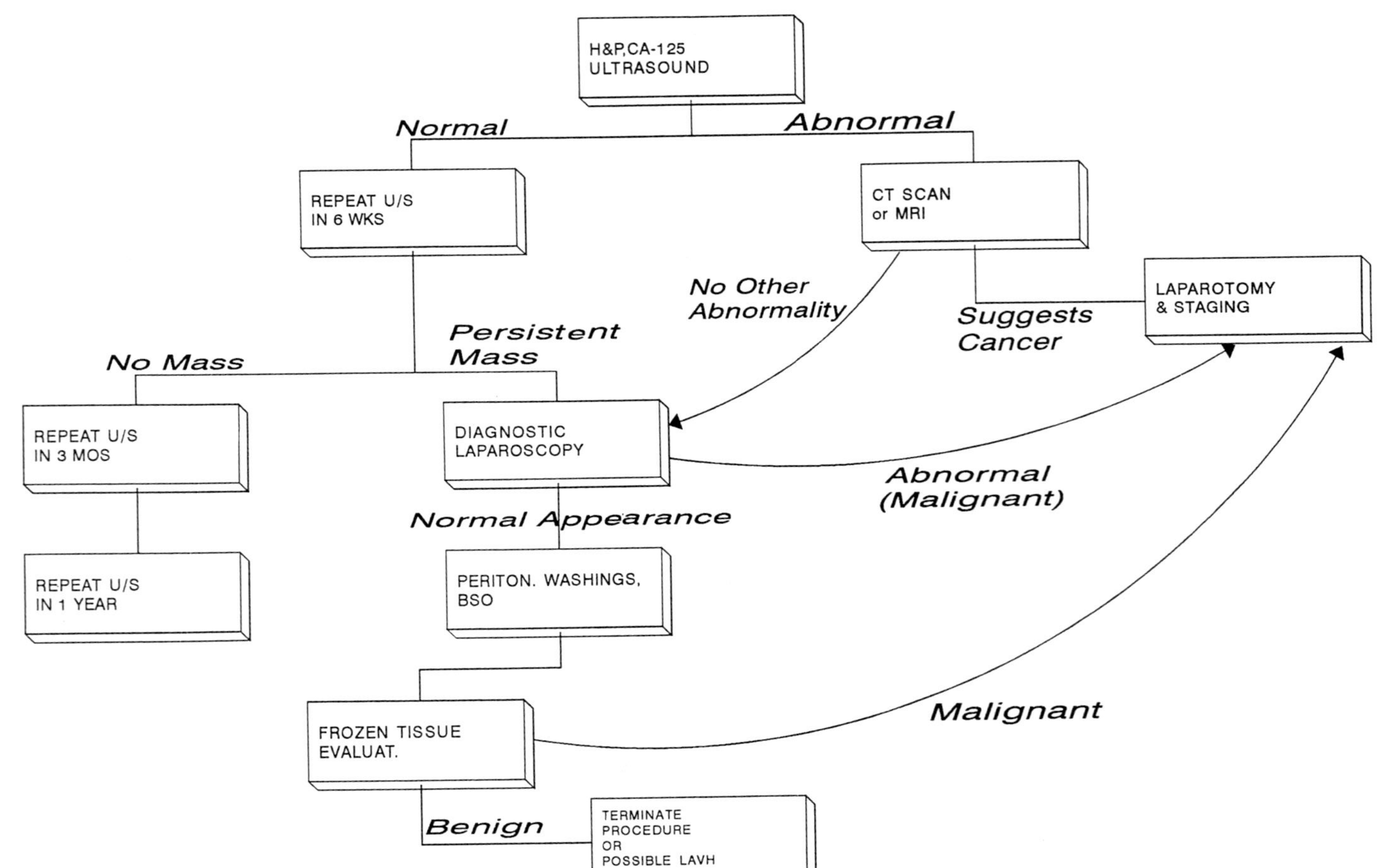

Figure 12-1. Evaluation of the postmenopausal ovarian cyst.

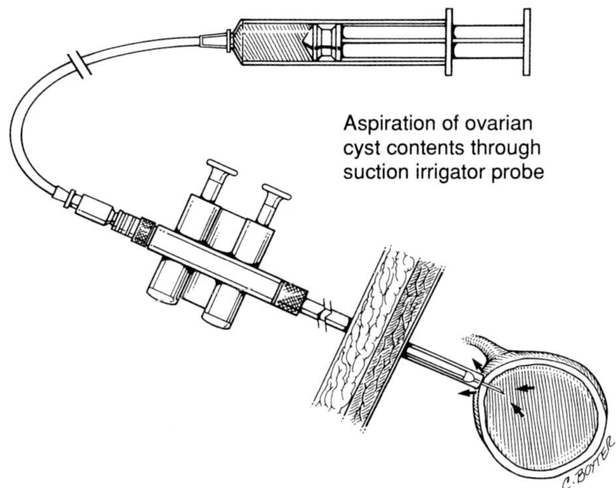

Figure 12-2. For pure cysts larger than 10 cm, an 18-gauge laparoscopic needle is passed through the suction irrigator probe, and while stabilizing the cyst with suction applied over the cyst wall the needle is inserted into the cyst and the contents are aspirated.

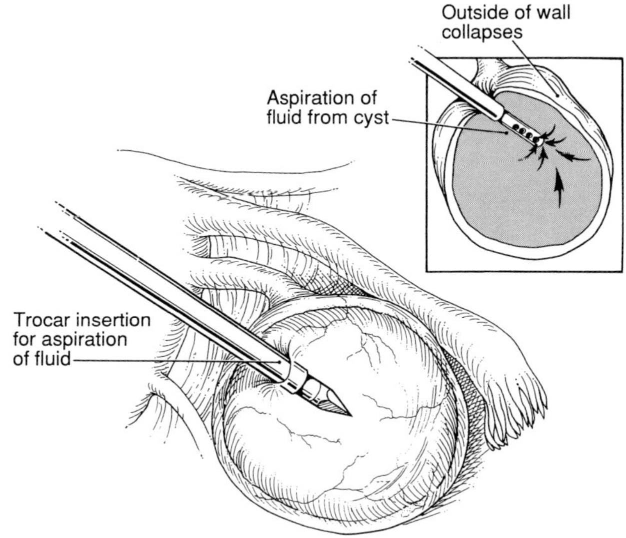

Figure 12-3. The trocar is placed into the cyst, then removed, and the suction-irrigator (*inset*) is inserted.

12-2). Alternatively, a 5-mm trocar and sleeve are introduced through a suprapubic port. The trocar is placed into the cyst, then removed, and the suction-irrigator inserted (Figure 12-3). This method works well for endometriomas and mucinous cystadenomas but is not advisable for benign teratomas, which contain hair.

The aspirate is sent for cytologic examination and the ovary is freed from adhesions to the lateral pelvic wall, uterus, or bowel. The cyst and pelvis are irrigated continuously, especially for benign cystic teratomas, mucinous cystadenomas, or endometriomas. The most dependent portion of the cyst wall is opened and the internal surface is inspected (Figure 12-4). If excrescence or papillae are found, a biopsy specimen is sent for frozen section (see Figure 12-4 *inset*). Dilute vasopressin is injected between the capsule and ovarian cortex to create a plane for hydrodissection and to reduce oozing in the capsule (Figure 12-5). The cap-

Figure 12-4. The most dependent opened portion of the cyst is enlarged and the internal surface is inspected. If excrescences or papillae are found (*inset*), a biopsy is taken and sent for frozen section.

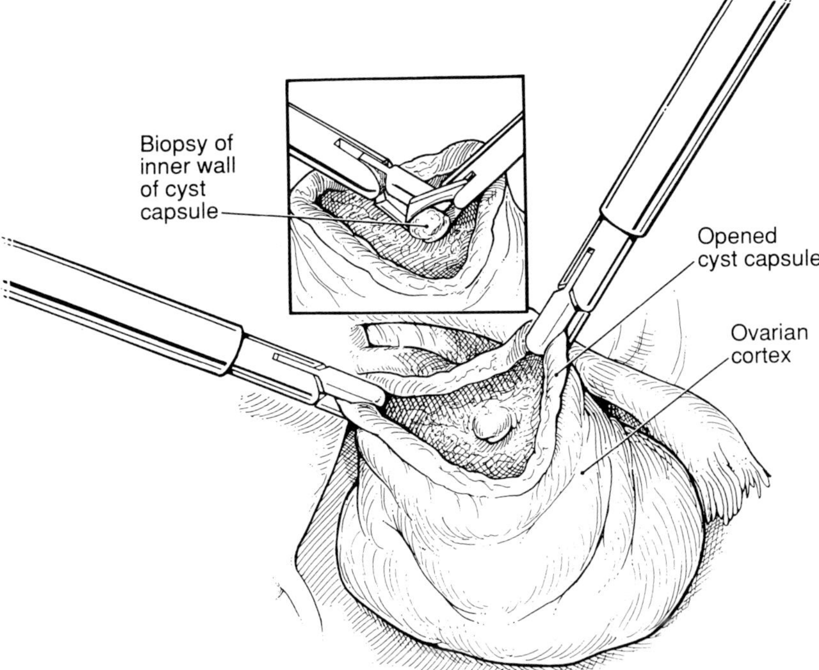

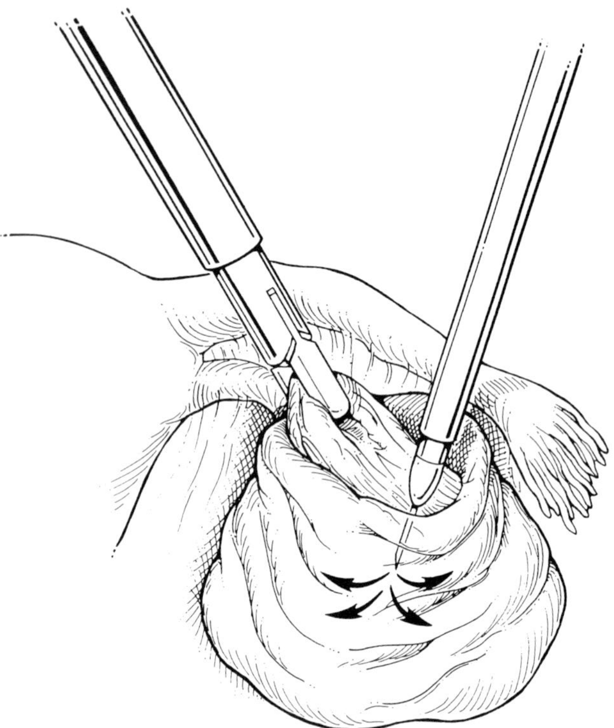

Figure 12-5. Dilute vasopressin is injected (*arrows*) between the capsule and ovarian cortex to create a plane for hydrodissection and to reduce oozing from the capsule bed.

sule is stripped from the ovarian stroma using two grasping forceps and the suction-irrigator probe for traction and countertraction. It is sent for histologic examination (Figure 12-6). The laser can be used at low power (10 to 20 W, continuous) to seal blood vessels at the base of the capsule and at higher powers to vaporize small remnants of capsule. Bipolar forceps also can be used to control bleeding (Figure 12-7).

Sometimes it is difficult to remove the capsule from the ovarian cortex so that injecting dilute vasopressin between the capsule and cortex facilitates the stripping procedure. If the cyst wall cannot be identified clearly, the edge of the ovarian incision can be "freshened" with scissors and the resulting clean edge reveals the different structures. If this does not free the capsule, the base of the cyst is grasped, and traction applied to the cyst with countertraction to the ovary. The entire cyst or portions of the wall may be densely adherent to the ovary, requiring sharp or laser dissection to completely free the cyst wall. Large cysts require partial oophorectomy, using high-power laser or scissors to remove the distorted portion of the ovary, and the remaining cyst wall can be stripped from the ovarian stroma (Figure 12-8).

Teratomas often can be excised intact but

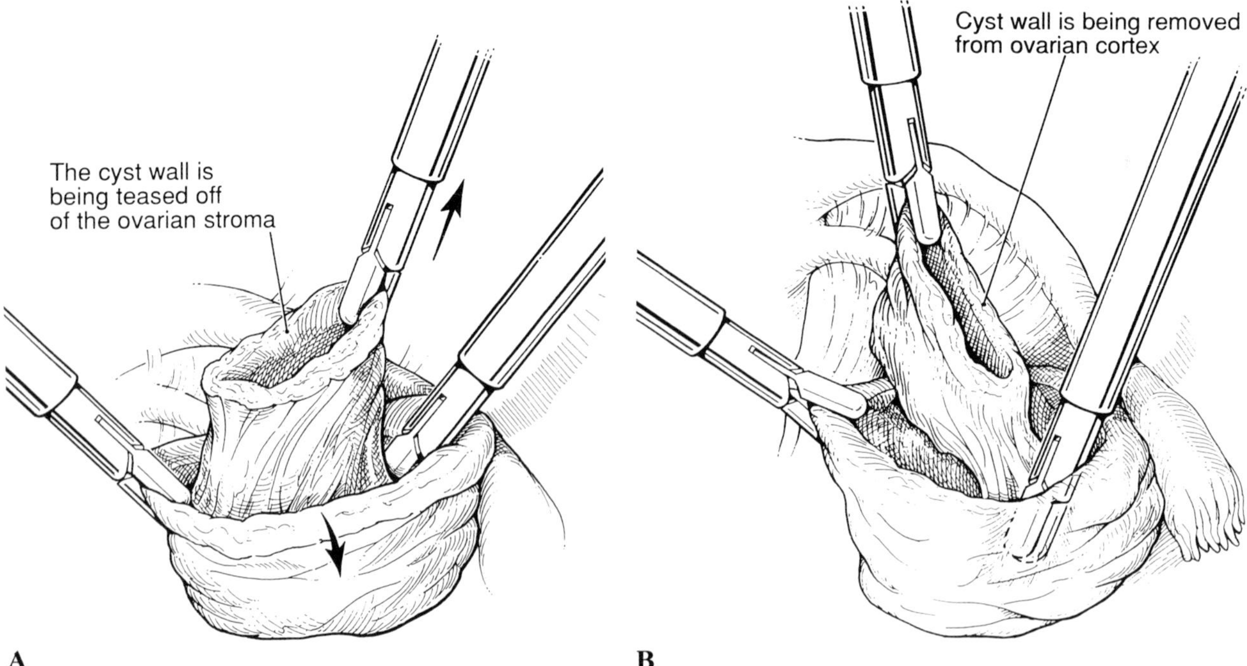

Figure 12-6. The capsule is stripped gradually from the ovarian stroma using two grasping forceps and the suction-irrigator probe for traction and countertraction, then submitted for histologic examination.

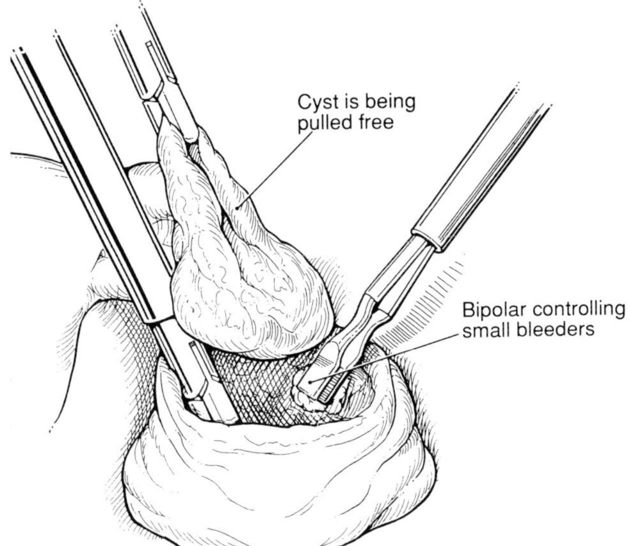

Figure 12-7. Bipolar forceps are used to control bleeding.

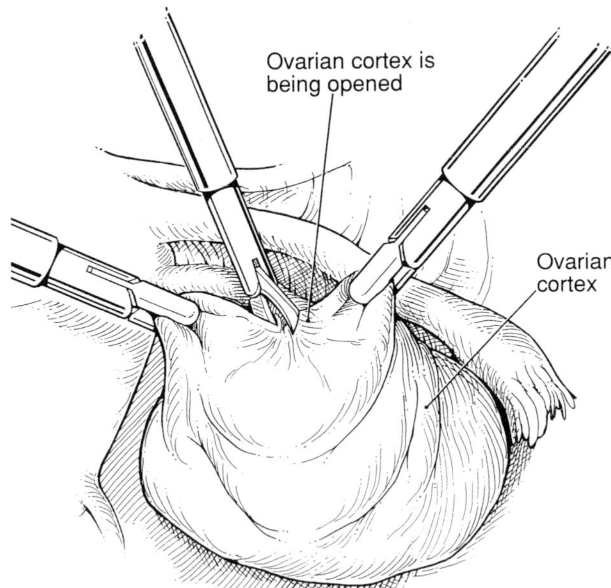

Figure 12-8. Large cysts require partial oophorectomy. Scissors are used to remove the distorted portion of the ovary.

should the cyst rupture, the resulting contamination would be greater than if the cyst were opened and aspirated. An important step is the atraumatic development of the plane between the cyst wall and ovarian tissue, which is accomplished using hydrodissection. An 18- or 20-gauge needle is introduced through an accessory trocar sleeve, or a 7.5-inch spinal needle (American Hydro-Surgical Instruments) is introduced through the abdominal wall into the space between the cyst wall and the ovary (Figure 12-9). The plane is further developed using the suction-irrigator as a blunt probe (Figure 12-10). After the cyst is removed, the base of the capsule is irrigated and coagulation is achieved with either CO_2 laser or bipolar electrocoagulation. The edges of the ovarian cortex can be approximated with a low-power laser (10 to 20 W) or bipolar electrocoagulator (Figure 12-11). A grasping forceps helps to approximate the ovarian edges (Figure 12-12). If the ovarian edges overlap, the defect is left to heal without suturing because adhesions are more likely following the use of suture (Table 12-6).[23] If the edges of the

Figure 12-9 A, An 18- or 20-gauge needle is introduced through an accessory trocar sleeve into the space between the cyst wall and the ovary. B, A plane is developed between the cyst wall and ovarian tissue.

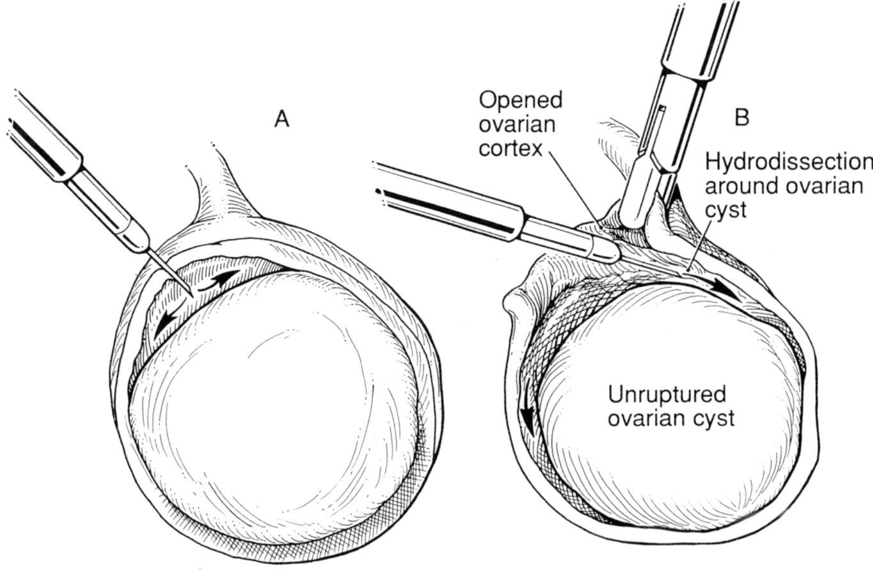

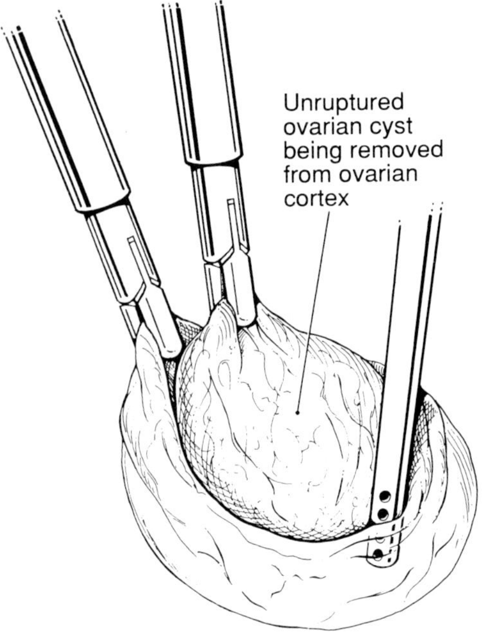

Figure 12-10. Further separation by hydrodissection with the suction-irrigator probe.

ovarian capsule do not spontaneously approximate, low-power laser applied to the inner surface will invert them. In rare instances one or two fine, absorbable monofilament sutures may be needed to approximate the ovarian edges (Figure 12-13). The sutures are placed inside the ovary to decrease formation of adhesions.

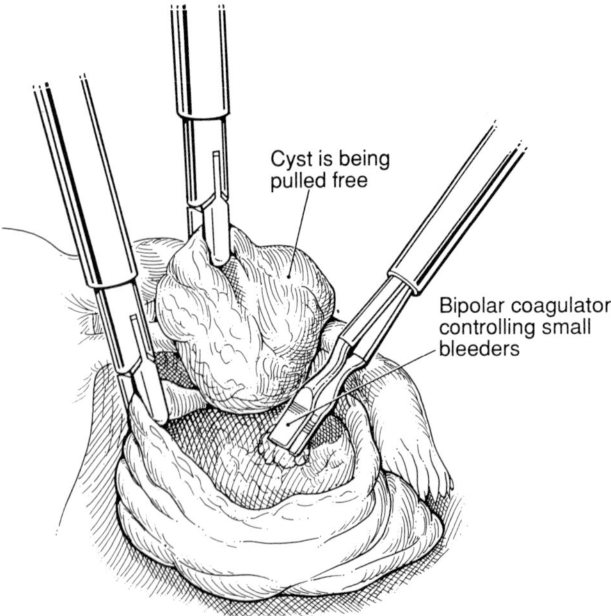

Figure 12-11. Coagulation is achieved with bipolar electrocoagulation.

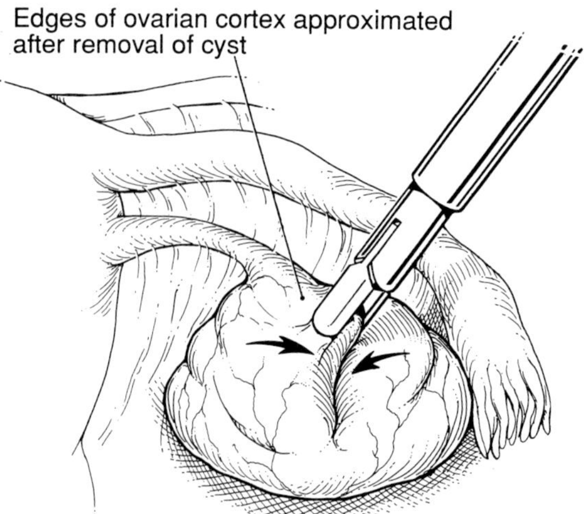

Figure 12-12. A grasping forceps approximates the ovarian edges (*arrows*).

Ovarian endometriosis causes the adhesions between the ovarian surface and the broad ligament. As the ovary enlarges, endometriomas form. In 1921, Sampson[24] noted that the histologic findings in these cysts varied in different portions of the same cyst and noted that luteal membrane and ovarian epithelial tissues are frequently present. Sampson believed that in addition to the local spread of endometriosis by salpingeal reflux, some foci developed from the implantation of endometrioma contents after rupture, suggesting that endometriomas could arise as a result of invasion of functional cysts by surface implants.

Based on the surgical treatment of ovarian endometriomas and correlation of clinical observations to the histologic results, it seems that superficial ovarian endometriosis is similar to endometriosis in extraovarian sites because the formation of superficial cysts is limited in size by fibrosis and scarring. Large endometriomas may develop as a result of secondary involvement of follicular or luteal cysts by surface implants. In 1979, Czernobilsky and Morris[25] described a variety of epithelial characteristics found in ovarian endometriosis.

Nissole-Pochet and colleagues studied the microscopic characteristics of 113 cases of ovarian endometriosis before and after hormonal therapy and were able to identify typical endometrial glandular epithelium and stroma.[26] In 18% of women, the epithelium presented as cyst lining only, and in the others as both flattened endometrial epithelium and typical glandular and stromal structures. Areas with ciliated cells representing oviduct-like epithelium were seen in 47%.

TABLE 12-6. Incidence of Adhesion Formation With and Without Laparoscopic Ovarian Suturing

	Type of Cyst					Adhesions			
Suture	Endometrioma	Benign Cystic Teratoma	Mucinous	Serous	Simple	None	Filmy/Minimal Vascularity	Dense/ Nonvascular	Dense/ Vascular
No	27	4	2	1	2	11	22	2	1
Yes	19	6	0	2	4	5	6	15	5

Martin and Berry[27] examined 41 chocolate cysts and found that 61% were microscopically confirmed endometriomas and 27% were corpora lutea; in 12% no lining was found. Vercellini and coworkers, in evaluating the value of visual diagnosis of endometriomas, confirmed 97.7% of visually diagnosed endometriomas.[28] They used at least two of the following four microscopic patterns to diagnose endometriomas: the presence of endometrial epithelium, endometrial glands or glandlike structures, endometrial stroma, and hemosiderin-laden macrophages. However, the accepted histologic criteria are the presence of both endometrial glands and stroma.[29]

Fayez and Vogel[30] found no endometrial lining in 66 endometriomas from 50 patients. Such findings could be explained by inadequate sampling of the cyst walls for histologic diagnosis. An alternative theory for the development of endometriomas is that endometrial lesions found deep in the ovary could originate from metaplasia of celomic epithelium that lines the cystic epithelial inclusions frequently found in the ovaries.[31,32]

According to Nezhat and colleagues, hemorrhagic ovarian cysts clinically resembling endometriomas can be classified into two major types.[33] Type I endometriomas, or pure endometriomas, are small (1 to 2 cm), contain dark fluid, develop from surface endometriosis, and are difficult to remove surgically (Figure 12-14). Histologic analysis reveals endometrial tissue in all of them (Table 12-7).

Type IIA endometriomas are large, the cyst wall is separated easily from the ovarian tissue, and if endometrial implants are seen, they do not penetrate the cyst wall (Figure 12-15). These hemorrhagic cysts are either follicular or luteal in origin (see Table 12-7).

Types IIB and IIC are endometriomas with features of functional cysts involved deeply with surface endometriosis, with histologic findings of endometriosis in the cyst wall (see Table 12-7). In type IIB, the lining is separated easily from the ovarian capsule and stroma except adjacent to the

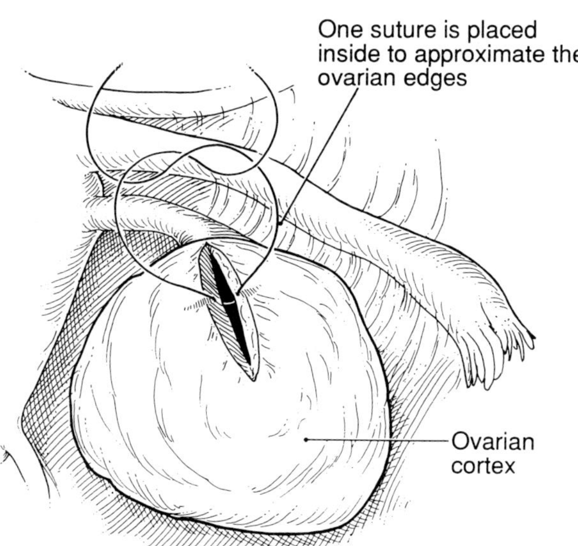

Figure 12-13. Absorbable monofilament suture inside the ovary approximates the ovarian edges.

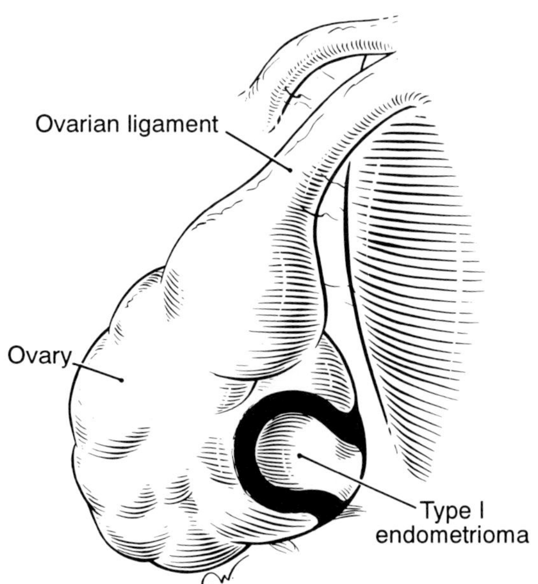

Figure 12-14. Type I endometriomas are small (1 to 2 cm), contain dark fluid, develop from surface endometriosis, and are difficult to remove surgically.

TABLE 12-7. Characteristics of Presumed Endometriomas

Type	No.	Size in cm (mean)	Luteal Lining	Endometrial Lining	No Diagnostic Lining	Adhesions Dense/Filmy	Hemosiderin and/or Fibrosis
I	15	1–2 (1.67)	0	15	0	5/3	15
IIA	57	2–6(3.9)	46	0	9	5/11	6
IIB	46	3–12(5.4)	14	23	9	22/13	35
IIC	98	3–20(7.0)	10	84	4	88/2	88

areas of endometriosis (Figure 12-16). In Type IIC, surface endometrial implants penetrate more deeply into the cyst wall, making excision more difficult (Figure 12-17). The degree of endometrial invasion of the cyst wall forms the basis for differentiating between these two subtypes and is characterized by the progressive difficulty in removing the cyst wall.

Treatment

Buttram[34] suggested the use of danazol (3 months of 800 mg/d or 6 months of 400 mg/d) preoperatively to reduce intraoperative hemorrhage. Ovarian suppression can reduce the size or resolve many follicular and corpus luteum cysts found in the type II group, minimizing damage to normal ovarian tissue intraoperatively. Similar benefits may result from the use of preoperative gonadotropin-releasing hormone (GnRH).

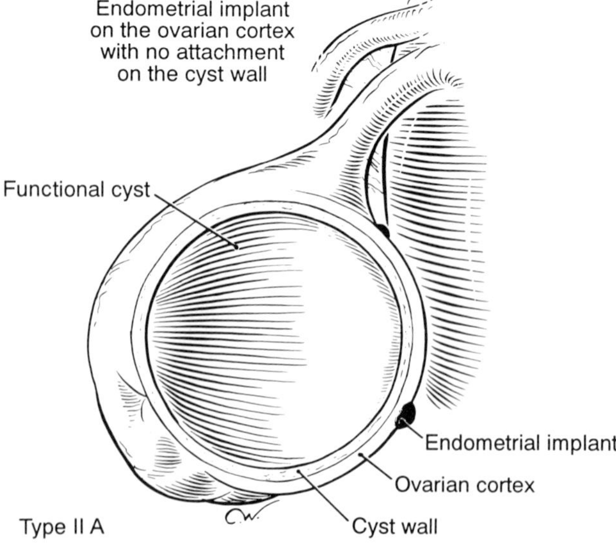

Figure 12-15. Type IIA endometriomas. These are large, and the cyst wall is separated easily from the ovarian tissue. Endometrial implants do not penetrate the cyst wall.

Surgical Therapy

Because the medical management of endometriomas has proven ineffective, either laparotomy or operative laparoscopy is necessary.[28,30,35] The least invasive and the technically simplest approach to endometriomas involves laparoscopic fenestration and removal of "chocolate" fluid without cystectomy or ablation of the cyst wall. However, fenestration and irrigation are associated with a 50% recurrence rate compared to 8% in the group with the capsule removed.[35] Fayez and Vogel advocated a wide opening in the cyst wall to drain its contents because this technique created fewer periadnexal adhesions (27%).[30] When compared to complete resection of endometriomas, stripping of the lining, or vaporization of the lining by CO_2 laser in a continuous mode, adhesions were seen in 100%, 37%, and 30%, respectively. However, persistence of endometrioma was much higher in all groups in which the cyst wall was not removed completely. All recurrent endometriomas were larger than 4 cm. Vercellini and coworkers showed that simple aspiration and washing of the capsule of endometriomas was ineffective.[28] In their series of 33 women, most endometriomas recurred although many patients took GnRH analogs postoperatively. Hasson[36] found no therapeutic value to simple aspiration as he noted recurrence in eight of nine endometriomas treated by fenestration alone.

Surgical Technique

Although small type I endometriomas are difficult to remove intact because of associated fibrosis and adhesions, they can be biopsied, drained, and vaporized using laser or electrosurgery, or removed in pieces. The larger type I lesions (2 to 3 cm) must be removed completely (Figure 12-18).

In type IIA lesions, the periovarian adhesions are lysed, the ovarian cortex is evaluated, and the cyst is aspirated. Superficial implants are vaporized or excised. The cyst is opened and its wall is

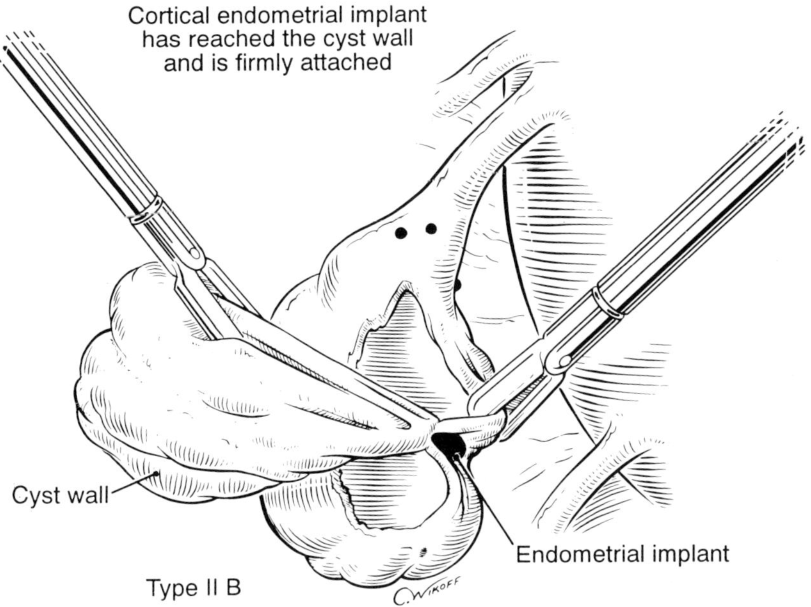

Figure 12-16. Type IIB endometrioma. Lining is separated easily from the ovarian capsule and stroma, except adjacent to the areas of endometriosis.

examined. If it has a yellowish appearance and removal is easy, biopsy is taken for frozen section. Postoperatively, either danazol 800 mg/d or a GnRH analog is used for 6 to 8 weeks.

Types IIB and IIC endometriomas are large, are associated with periovarian adhesions attaching them to the pelvic sidewall and the back of the uterus, and tend to rupture during separation. After mobilizing the ovary, the contents of the cyst are removed with the suction-irrigator probe and the cavity is irrigated. For IIB, an opening is made and the suction-irrigator probe is introduced inside the cystic cavity. By alternating suction and irrigation, the contents are removed. The inside of the cyst is evaluated and the portion of ovarian cortex involved with endometriosis is removed (Figure 12-19). Using the grasping forceps and the suction-irrigator probe, the cyst wall is grasped and separated from the ovarian stroma by traction and countertraction.[33] Hydrodissection facilitates complete removal.[37,38] Small blood vessels from the ovarian bed and bleeding from the ovarian hilum can be controlled with bipolar electrocoagulation.

In type IIC, it is difficult to develop a plane between the cyst wall and the ovarian capsule so that the portion of the ovary attached to the cyst wall is removed until an area is found to develop a

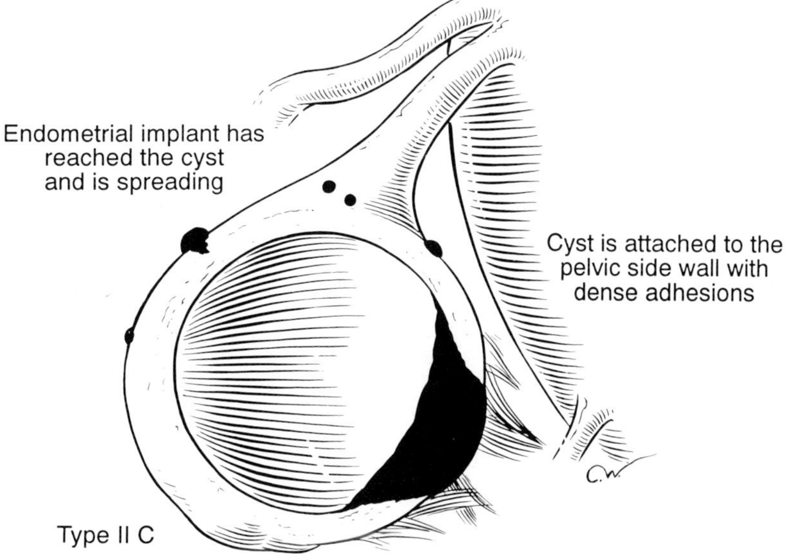

Figure 12-17. Type IIC endometrioma. Surface endometrial implants penetrate into the cyst wall.

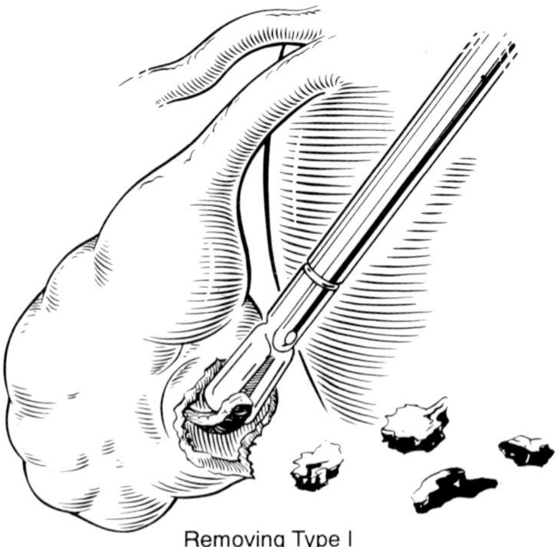

Figure 12-18. A type I endometrioma is difficult to remove and is removed in pieces.

plane. The remainder of the procedure is similar to that used for IIB endometrioma (Figure 12-20).

The redundant ovarian tissue is approximated with low-power laser or electrosurgery to avoid adhesions. Low-power, continuous laser or bipolar coagulation applied to the inside wall of the redundant ovarian capsule causes it to invert, but excessive coagulation of the adjacent ovarian stroma must be avoided. Sutures, if needed, are placed inside the capsule and 4-0 polydioxanone sutures used. Fewer sutures result in fewer adhesions.[23]

The ability to diagnose and treat endometriosis at earlier stages may prevent its progression and invasion, reducing its adverse impact on health, quality of life, and fertility potential.

Benign Cystic Teratomas

These germ cell tumors occur predominantly in young women. Although laparoscopic removal can be technically difficult, it can be performed successfully. Following laparoscopic excision and removal by a posterior colpotomy, normal ovaries and few adhesions were seen at a repeat laparoscopy.[39] If unsuccessful, one should proceed to laparotomy to ensure complete tumor excision. The surgeon should avoid rupturing the cyst. If the cyst is ruptured during excision, it is important to clean the body cavity of all sebaceous material and hair.

The suction-irrigator is placed in the cyst, the contents aspirated, and the cavity copiously irrigated. The interior of the cyst is inspected and its lining is grasped and removed from the ovary. The lining is removed from the pelvis through a 10-mm accessory trocar, the operating channel of the laparoscope, a culdotomy, or in an Endobag. The cyst wall is inspected and sent for frozen section. The pelvis is irrigated with lactated Ringer's solution until all evidence of sebaceous material is removed because incomplete removal of this material can cause peritonitis. During irrigation, the ovarian stroma is inspected to verify hemostasis.

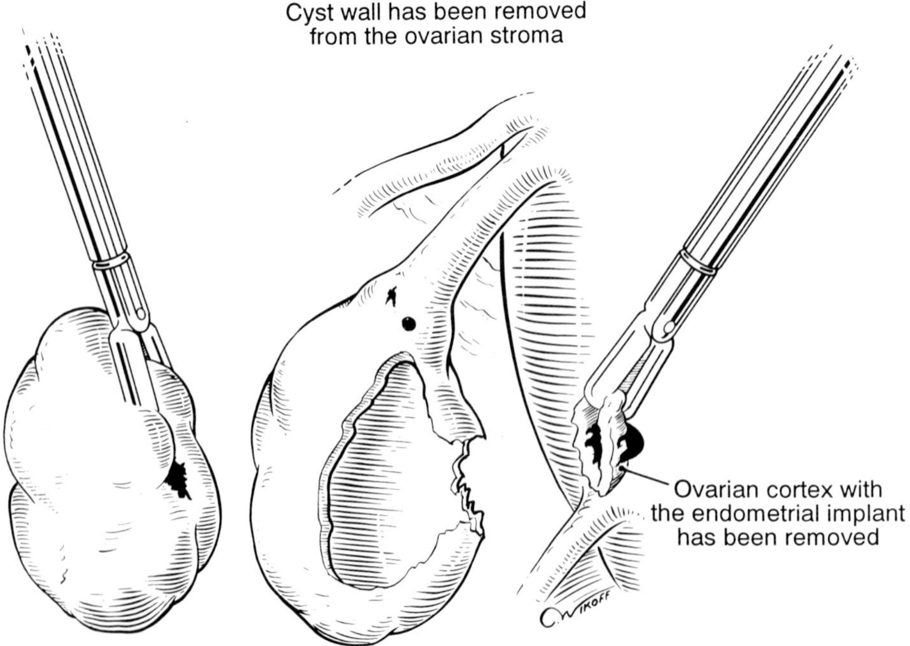

Figure 12-19. Type IIB endometrioma. Portion of ovarian cortex involved with endometriosis is removed.

Figure 12-20. Type IIC endometrioma. Portion of the ovary attached to the cyst wall is removed until a plane is found. The cyst wall is grasped and stripped from the ovarian stroma.

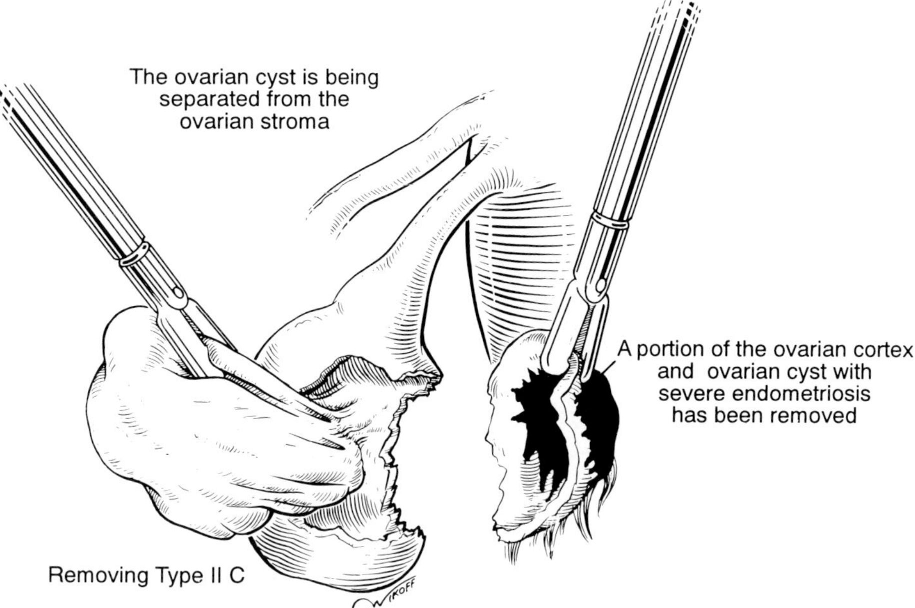

Bleeding points are controlled with a defocused laser or bipolar forceps.

For large teratomas (greater than 8 cm), the ovary can be placed in the cul-de-sac adjacent to a culdotomy incision. Draining the cyst and removing its wall transvaginally minimizes the risk of contamination and maintains a minimally invasive approach. The vagina should be prepared with Betadine before colpotomy or culdotomy.

Oophorectomy/Salpingo-oophorectomy

In postmenopausal women or for those patients in whom the ovary and tube cannnot be conserved, salpingo-oophorectomy is perfomed.

When the cyst wall is benign and the tissue is fragmented, it can be removed through a 5-, 10-, 12- or 30-mm suprapubic port. No tissue should be left in the pelvic cavity or on the abdominal wall. Implantation of ovarian tissue in the abdominal and pelvic cavity resulting in ovarian remnant is possible.[40] Contamination of the anterior abdominal wall should be avoided and if this happens, all tissue must be removed and the incision copiously irrigated and washed. Abdominal wall metastasis has been reported following contamination of the wall during laparoscopy for ovarian cancer.[41]

The tissue can be removed from the abdominal cavity using one of the following techniques:

1. *Containment bags.* Excised tissue is placed into a small, plastic, prepared bag introduced into the pelvis through a 10-mm trocar (Endobag, Ethicon; Figure 12-21). The tissue is placed in the bag and then removed by applying traction to the bag and pulling it through a trocar incision to the anterior abdominal wall by removing the port. The edges of the bag are pulled from the abdomen and the cyst contents aspirated. The deflated cyst is pulled out of the abdomen. The solid mass is morcellated inside the bag and then removed (Figure 12-22). Pulling the bag before the cyst is col-

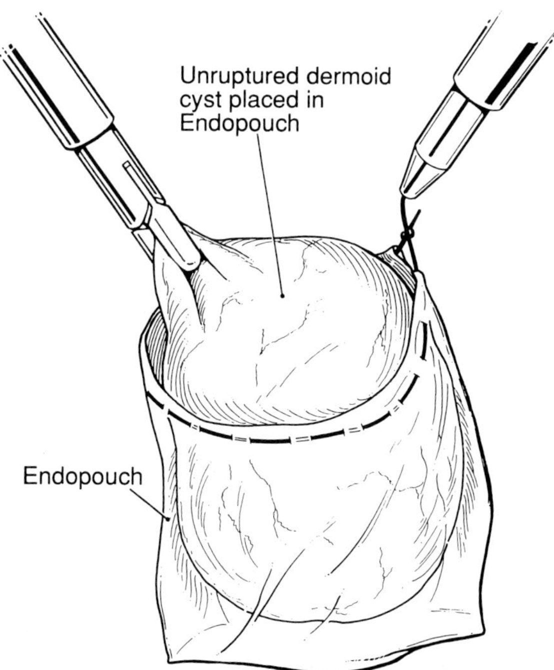

Figure 12-21. Excised tissue is placed into an Endobag.

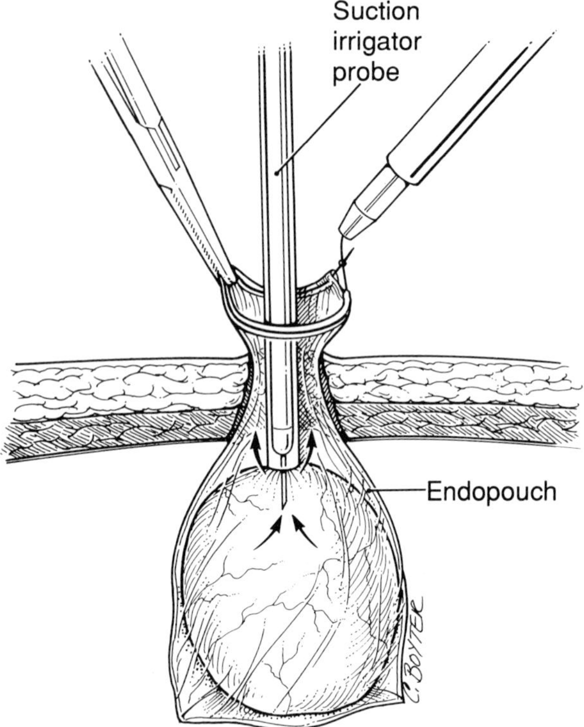

Figure 12-22. The solid mass can be morcellated inside the bag and then removed.

lapsed or morcellated ruptures the bag and contaminates the abdominal cavity or anterior abdominal wall.

2. A *culdotomy* can be used to remove large pieces of solid tissue such as myomas or cystic masses. Large cystic masses are fragile so that it is usually impossible to remove them intact through a culdotomy. The cystic mass should be brought to the incision and drained transvaginally as it is drawn into the vagina (Figure 12-23). After the mass is removed, the pelvic cavity is irrigated and suctioned. The culdotomy can be repaired either vaginally or laparoscopically. Nezhat and colleagues have shown that laparoscopic culdotomy is not associated with significant postoperative adhesions.[42]

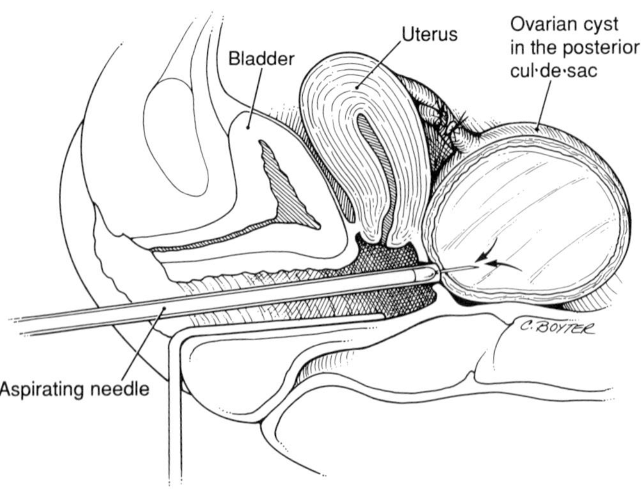

Figure 12-23. The cystic mass is brought to the incision and drained transvaginally as the reduced mass is drawn into the vagina.

3. With an *abdominal incision*, the cystic mass is brought to the surface of the abdominal incision, drained, and extracted similarly to the technique for removal by culdotomy.

References

1. Cancer of the ovary and uterine tube. In: Precis IV. *An Update in Obstetrics and Gynecology*. Washington, DC: American College of Obstetricians and Gynecologists; p 1990:266.
2. Webb MJ, Decker DG, Mussey E, et al. Factors in influencing survival in stage I ovarian cancer. *Am J Obstet Gynecol.* 1973;116:222.
3. Dembo AJ, Davy M, Stenwick AE, et al. Prognostic factors in patients with stage I epithelial ovarian cancer. *Obstet Gynecol.* 1990; 74:263.
4. Lim-Yan S, Cajigas H, Scully R. Ovarian cystectomy for serous borderline tumors. A follow-up study of 35 cases. *Obstet Gynecol.* 1988;72:775.
5. Mage G, Canis M, Manhes H, et al. Laparoscopic management of adnexal cystic masses. *J Gynecol Surg.* 1990;6:71.
6. Nezhat C, Nezhat F, Welander CE, et al. Four ovarian cancers diagnosed during laparoscopic management of 1,011 adnexal masses. *Am J Obstet Gynecol.* 1992;167:790.
7. Hulka JF, Parker WH, Surrey M, et al. Management of ovarian masses: AAGL 1990 survey. *J Reprod Med.* 1992;37:599.
8. Maimon M, Seltzer V, Boyce J. Laparoscopic excision of ovarian neoplasms subsequently found to be malignant. *Obstet Gynecol.* 1991;77:653.
9. Herrmann U, Locher G, Goldhirsch A. Sonographic patterns of malignancy: prediction of malignancy. *Obstet Gynecol.* 1987;69:777.
10. Granberg S, Norstrom A, Wikland M. Comparison of endovaginal ultrasound and cytological evaluations of cystic ovarian tumors. *J Ultrasound Med.* 1991;10:9.
11. Steinkampf MP, Hammond KR, Blackwell

RE. Hormonal treatment of functional ovarian cysts: a randomized, prospective study. *Fertil Steril.* 1990;54:775.

12. Jacobs I, Bast R. The CA-125 tumor associated antigen: a review of the literature. *Hum Reprod.* 1989;4:1.
13. DeCrespigny L, Robinson HP, Daboren RAM, et al. The "simple" cyst: aspirate or operate? *Br J Obstet Gynecol.* 1989;96:1035.
14. Kjellgren RK. Ovarian cyst fenestration via laparoscopy. *J Reprod Med.* 1978;21:16.
15. Trope C. The preoperative diagnosis of malignancy of ovarian cysts. *Neoplasia.* 1981;28:117.
16. Hasson HM. Ovarian surgery. In: JS Sanfilippo, RL Levine, eds. *Operative Gynecological Endoscopy.* New York: Springer-Verlag; 1989:86.
17. Kleppinger RK. Ovarian cyst fenestration via laparoscopy. *J Reprod Med.* 1978;21:16.
18. Larsen JF, Pedersen OD, Gregerson E. Ovarian cyst fenestration via the laparoscope. *Acta Obstet Gynecol Scand.* 1986;65:529.
19. Marana R, Muzii L, Caruana P, et al. Laparoscopic management of adnexal cystic masses: excision versus aspiration (in press).
20. Scoutt L, McCarthy SM, Lange R, et al. Evaluation of ovarian masses on MRI with ultrasound correlation. *Radiology.* 1990;177:242.
21. Wolf Sl, Gosnik BB, Feldesman MR, et al. Prevalence of simple adnexal cysts in postmenopausal women. *Radiology.* 1991; 180:65.
22. Campbell S, Goessens L, Goswamy R, et al. Real-time ultrasonography for the determination of ovarian morphology and volume. A possible early screening test for ovarian cancer. *Lancet.* 1982;1:415.
23. Nezhat C, Nezhat F. Postoperative adhesion formation after ovarian cystectomy with and without ovarian reconstruction. Presented at the 47th Annual Meeting of the American Fertility Society, Orlando, FL, October 21–24, 1991.
24. Sampson JA. Perforating hemorrhagic (chocolate) cysts of the ovary. *Arch Surg.* 1921;3:245.
25. Czernobilsky B, Morris WJ. A histologic study of ovarian endometriosis with emphasis on hyperplastic and atypical changes. *Obstet Gynecol.* 1979;53:318.
26. Nissole-Pochet M, Casanas-Roux F, Donnez J. Histologic study of ovarian endometriosis after hormonal therapy. *Fertil Steril.* 1988; 49:423.
27. Martin DC, Berry JD. Histology of chocolate cysts. *J Gynecol Surg.* 1990;6:43.
28. Vercellini P, Vendola N, Bocciolone L, et al. Reliability of the visual diagnosis of ovarian endometriosis. *Fertil Steril.* 1991;56:1198.
29. Sternberg SS, ed. *Histology for Pathologists.* New York: Raven Press; 1992;513.
30. Fayez JA, Vogel MF. Comparison of different treatment methods of endometriomas by laparoscopy. *Obstet Gynecol.* 1991;78:660.
31. Blaustein A, Kantius M, Kaganowicz A, et al. Inclusions in ovaries of females aged 1–30 years. *Int J Gynecol Pathol.* 1982;1:145.
32. Kerner H, Gaton E, Czernobilsky B. Unusual ovarian, tubal and pelvic mesothelial inclusions in patients with endometriosis. *Histopathology.* 1981;5:277.
33. Nezhat F, Nezhat C, Allan CJ, et al. A clinical and histologic classification of endometriomas: implications for a mechanism of pathogenesis. *J Reprod Med.* 1992;37:771.
34. Buttram VC. Use of danazol in conservative surgery. *J Reprod Med.* 1990;35:82.
35. Nezhat C, Winer WK, Nezhat F. Is endoscopic treatment of endometriosis and endometrioma associated with better results than laparotomy? *Am J Gynecol Health.* 1988; 2:78.
36. Hasson HM. Laparoscopic management of ovarian cysts. *J Reprod Med.* 1990;25:863.
37. Nezhat C, Silfen SL, Nezhat F, et al. Surgery for endometriosis. *Curr Opin Obstet Gynecol.* 1991;3:385.
38. Nezhat C, Nezhat F. Safe laser excision or vaporization of peritoneal endometriosis. *Fertil Steril.* 1989;52:1:149.
39. Nezhat C, Winer W, Nezhat F. Laparoscopic removal of dermoid cysts. *Obstet Gynecol.* 1989;73:278.
40. Nezhat C, Nezhat F. Operative laparoscopy for the management of ovarian remnant syndrome. *Fertil Steril.* 1992;57:1003.
41. Gleeson NC, Nicosia SV, Mark JE, et al. Abdominal wall metastases from ovarian cancer after laparoscopy. *Am J Obstet Gynecol.* 1993;169:522.
42. Nezhat F, Brill AI, Nezhat CH, et al. Adhesion formation after endoscopic posterior colpotomy. *J Reprod Med.* 1993;38:534.

13

Ovarian Surgery

Most ovarian abnormalities can be managed laparoscopically and often a laparoscopic examination of the adnexa will enable the gynecologist to decide if laparotomy is indicated.

Mobilization

It is often difficult to immobilize the ovary because of its smooth surface and firm texture. The uterine-ovarian ligament can be grasped to lift and rotate the ovary or the ovary can be wedged against the pelvic sidewall using the flattened edges of the opened or closed forceps. Sometimes Morgagni peritubal cysts can be used as a handle or the uterus can be manipulated under the ovary to provide a shelf (Figure 13-1). Overly aggressive manipulation can cause lacerations in the capsule, follicles, or cysts and result in bleeding.

Ovarian Biopsies

A punch biopsy specimen of a lesion from the antimesenteric border of the ovary may be sufficient for most purposes. Palmer biopsy forceps can take tissue without penetrating the vascular medulla[1] although small wedge resection yields the best histologic features of the ovarian stroma and cortex. Alternatively, tissue can be obtained using toothed forceps and laparoscopic scissors or the laser (Figure 13-2). Bleeding is controlled with bipolar electrocoagulation; sutures should not be used so as to minimize postoperative adhesions.[2]

Oophorectomy

In 1984, Semm[3] reported his experience with a laparoscopic approach to oophorectomy and salpingo-oophorectomy. Since then, several authors have described the efficacy and safety of the procedures using different techniques.[4–8] Laparoscopy may encourage ovarian conservation during hysterectomy and more conservative management of pain caused by adnexal disease. If necessary, oophorectomy can be performed laparoscopically with a short hospital stay and recovery period at a later date.

The indications for oophorectomy are:

1. Persistent localized pain despite previous lysis of adhesions or ablation of endometriosis
2. Residual ovary syndrome
3. Dysgenetic gonads
4. Ovarian cysts greater than 5 cm with ovarian damage, or when spillage of cystic contents increases the likelihood of complications (cystic teratomas, mucinous cystadenomas, malignancy)
5. Tubo-ovarian abscess
6. Prophylactic therapy for advanced breast cancer
7. Early ovarian cancer in young women (stage I)

General Principles

A uterine manipulator should be inserted for traction and countertraction to aid in the exposure and manipulation of the ovary. The pelvis and es-

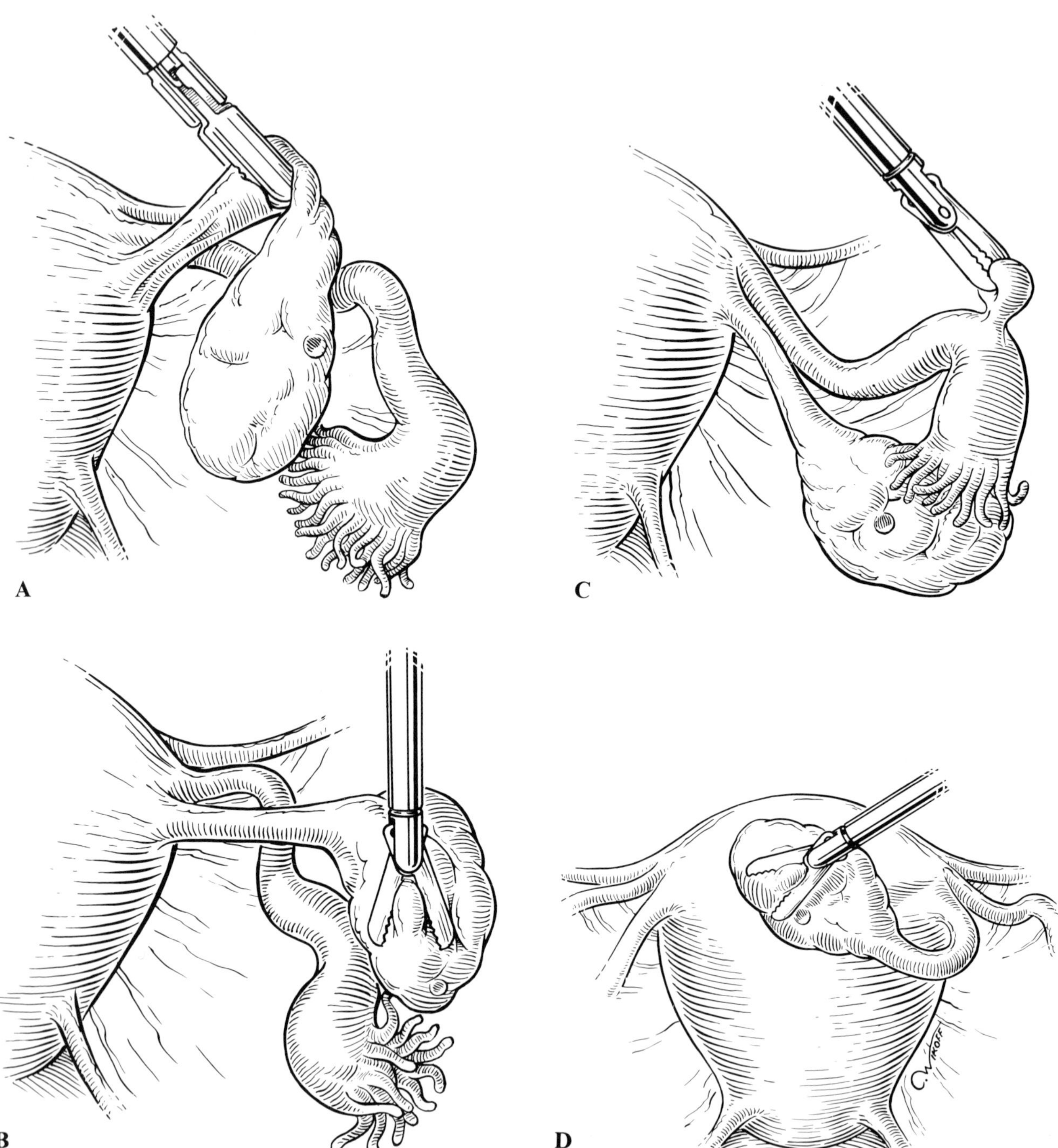

Figure 13-1. Different methods of immobilizing the ovary. A, Grasping the utero-ovarian ligament. B, Wedging the ovary against the pelvic sidewall. C, Grasping tubal or ovarian inclusion cysts. D, Using the uterus as a platform.

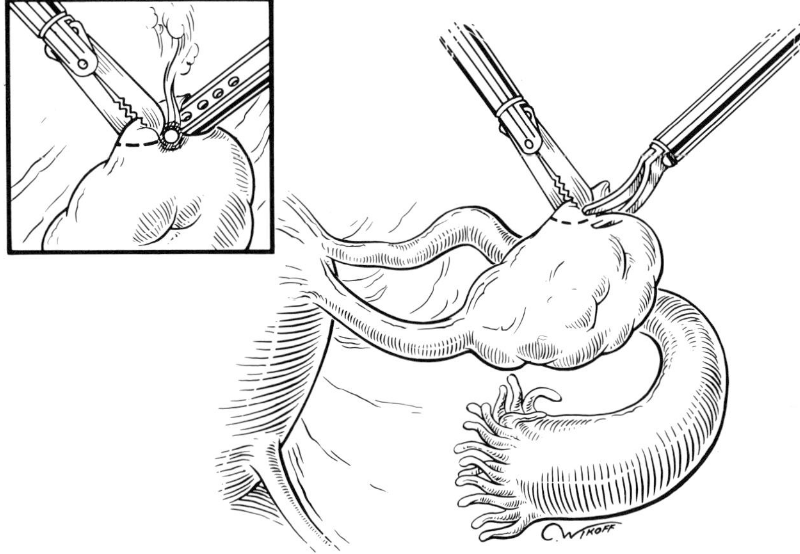

Figure 13-2. Small wedge biopsy of the ovary using scissors or CO_2 laser (*inset*).

pecially the adnexa should be inspected to plan the surgical approach. Before starting the procedure, it is important to observe the course of the ureter as it crosses the external iliac artery near the bifurcation of the common iliac artery at the pelvic brim. The left ureter can be more difficult to find because it is often covered by the base of the sigmoid mesocolon. If the ureter cannot be seen through the intact peritoneum, it must be identified by retroperitoneal dissection. If the patient does not have a uterus, it is essential to insert a vaginal probe or sponge stick so that the surgeon can maintain orientation, particularly with procedures involving extensive adhesions. When anatomic landmarks are distorted by adhesions, endometriosis, or prior surgical extirpation, begin the procedure at the most normal area and work toward the more distorted parts of the operative field. The entire ovary must be removed to prevent ovarian remnant syndrome or tumor development in a dysgenetic gonad. At the conclusion, the operative field is inspected and clots are removed with a suction-irrigator or grasping forceps. Pedicles are inspected under water and with decreased pneumoperitoneum,[9] and any bleeding can be controlled with bipolar electrocoagulation.

Management of the Infundibulopelvic Ligament

Three techniques have been described for managing the infundibulopelvic ligament—bipolar electrodesiccation, suture ligation with pretied suture, and automatic stapling. Patient cost for the linear stapler is approximately $600 and $48 for each pretied ligature. There is no extra charge for bipolar electrocoagulation.

A bipolar forceps is preferable for hemostasis of the infundibulopelvic ligament.[4] Endoloop sutures cannot be applied in the presence of adhesions that distort the anatomy, and it is difficult to place Endoloop sutures on large pedicles such as the mesovarium and infundibulopelvic ligament, even if the anatomy is normal. Once applied, the slipknot can loosen under the tension of the large pedicle, increasing the risk of intraoperative hemorrhage, or a piece of the ovary may be left in the pedicle, predisposing the patient to ovarian remnant syndrome.[10]

Aside from cost, the stapling device has several other drawbacks. It must be introduced though a 12-mm trocar, which can injure the inferior epigastric artery and predispose the patient to a postoperative hernia. The instrument is bulky and the operator must note its proximity to the ureter, bowel, and bladder. However, a major advantage of this instrument is its speed, especially for the beginner endoscopist.

Adequate desiccation of tissue with bipolar forceps by monitoring the flow of electrons on an ammeter has been suggested before transecting the pedicles. Excessive desiccation creates friable tissue, increases thermal damage, and allows the tissue to adhere to the forceps. A self-limiting bipolar electrocoagulator (Valley Lab Force II series generator, Boulder, CO) provides controlled desiccation without charring the adjacent tissue. In this mode, the power peaks at 100 ohms instead of 300 to 500 ohms in typical generators. The power will then "roll off" to provide the desired surgical effect without excess drying, blanching, or tissue destruction.

The mechanism of closure of large blood vessels

with high-frequency electrocoagulation was described by Sigel and Dunn.[11] Electrocoagulation begins with shrinkage of the vessel wall resulting from the denaturation of tissue proteins combined with the melting of the carbohydrate tissue components and the dehydration of tissue fluids. The resulting coagulum formed by this melting and fusion of the vessel wall obliterates the lumen. The most successful closures are characterized by low levels of heating ending before char is formed, which preserve the inherent fibrillar structure of the connective tissue. Too much heating destroys the inherent fibrillar structure, forming a more amorphous coagulum, poorly penetrated by fibroblasts and capillaries, and characterized by an inflammatory-type reorganization and healing process that results in unsuccessful or weak closures. Further heating during electrocoagulation causes complete disintegration of the amorphous coagulum and carbonization.[11,12] Ammeters or flowmeters measure only the flow of current in relation to the tissue resistance and have no value in ensuring hemostasis.

Pedicles should be reinspected after the intra-abdominal pressure has been lowered[9] because they can bleed again at the termination of a procedure once the hemostatic effects of the elevated abdominal pressures are lost.

Oophorectomy

The technique for oophorectomy is similar to salpingo-oophorectomy except that the tube must be protected from thermal damage. The procedure begins at the utero-ovarian ligament (Figure 13-3). The pedicles are desiccated and cut.[4] The mesovarium is coagulated and cut into 2-cm bites, working from the uterine side to the fimbria until the ovary is removed (see Figures 13-3B-D.) This latter step may jeopardize the fallopian tube if the mesovarium is desiccated excessively. In some circumstances it may be preferable to sharply incise the individual leaves of the mesovarium if the distance between the tube and ovary is small. The underlying vascular tissue can be coagulated and divided to allow excision of the remaining ovary.

Salpingo-oophorectomy

An ovary and tube minimally involved with adhesions or endometriosis can be approached either from the infundibulopelvic or utero-ovarian ligament. Filmy adhesions limiting the mobility of the ovary are lysed. Ovarian cysts are aspirated and deflated, making removal of the ovary easier. The adnexa can be removed by beginning with the infundibulopelvic ligament. This approach is preferable if the uterus is to be removed or significant disease is found in the uterine-ovarian ligament, in patients with prior hysterectomy, or if hemostasis of the ovarian vessels is necessary. The procedure begins with ureteral identification through the peritoneum as it enters the pelvic brim and travels parallel to the infundibulopelvic ligament.

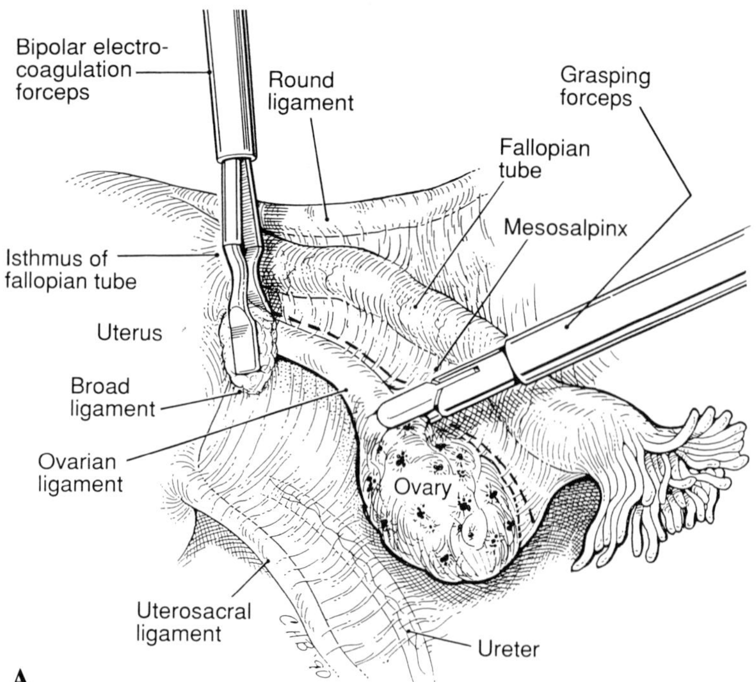

Figure 13-3. Oophorectomy by desiccating and cutting the mesovarium. The procedure starts from the utero-ovarian ligament and continues toward the fimbria.

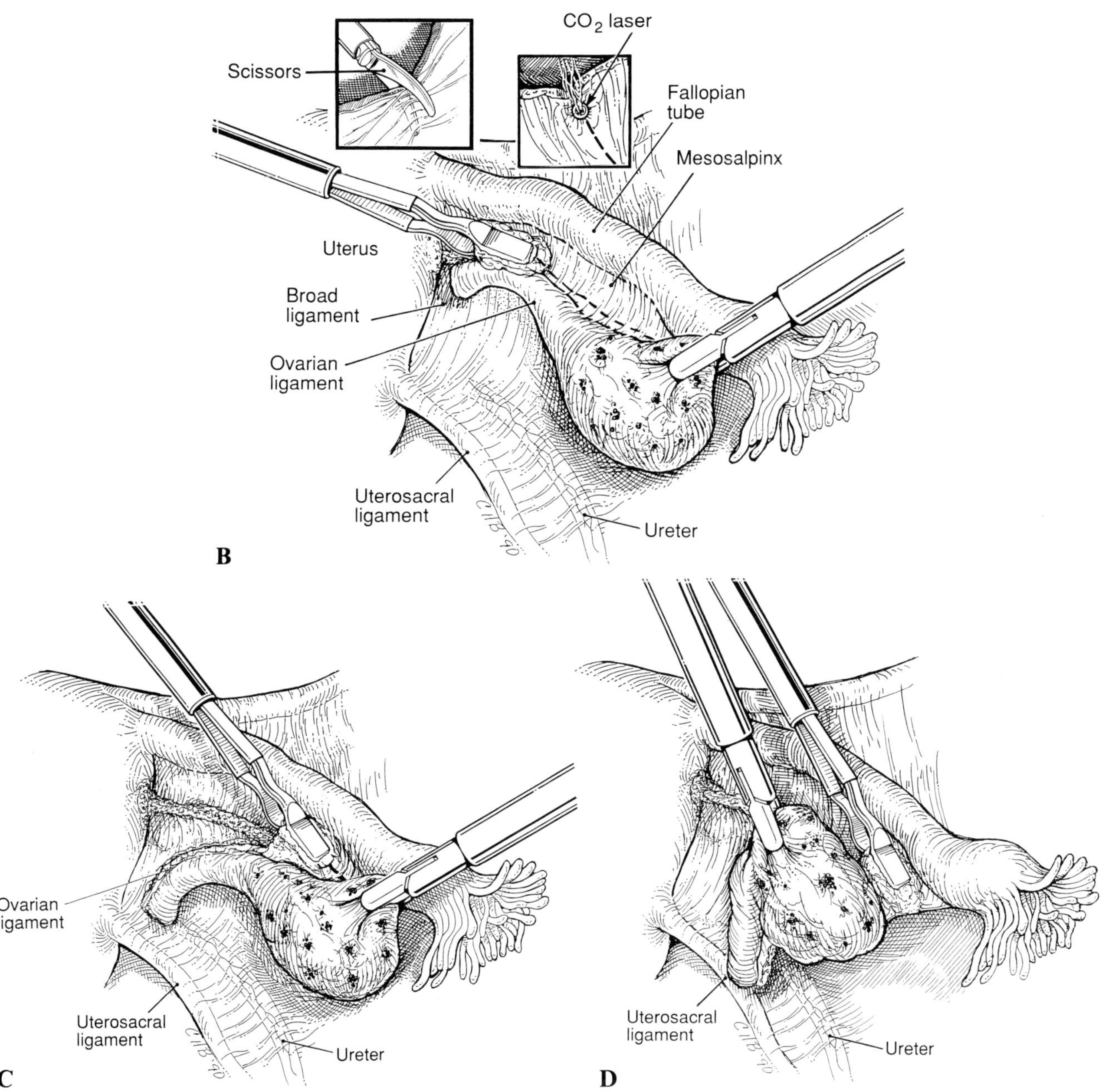

Figure 13–3 *(continued)*

The isthmic portion of the tube and ovarian ligament are desiccated and cut (Figure 13-4). The ovary is held with a grasping forceps and the infundibulopelvic ligament is put under traction by pulling it up and medially. The infundibulopelvic ligament is desiccated with bipolar forceps and cut with a laser or scissors in 1- to 2-cm increments working from lateral to medial until the adnexae are removed (Figures 13-5 through 13-8). It is important to use traction on the tube and ovary to avoid excessive coagulation and damage to the lateral pelvic sidewall.

Salpingo-oophorectomy Using a Stapling Device

The laparoscopic linear stapling device used during gynecologic procedures has been modified from the stapling device used for bowel resection. This instrument is introduced through a 12-mm trocar sleeve. The trocar site used to introduce the stapler is modified depending on adnexal disease. The trocar is introduced between the symphysis pubis and umbilicus lateral to the rectus muscle and inferior epigastric vessels, although injury to inferior epigastric vessels is possible. At the end of

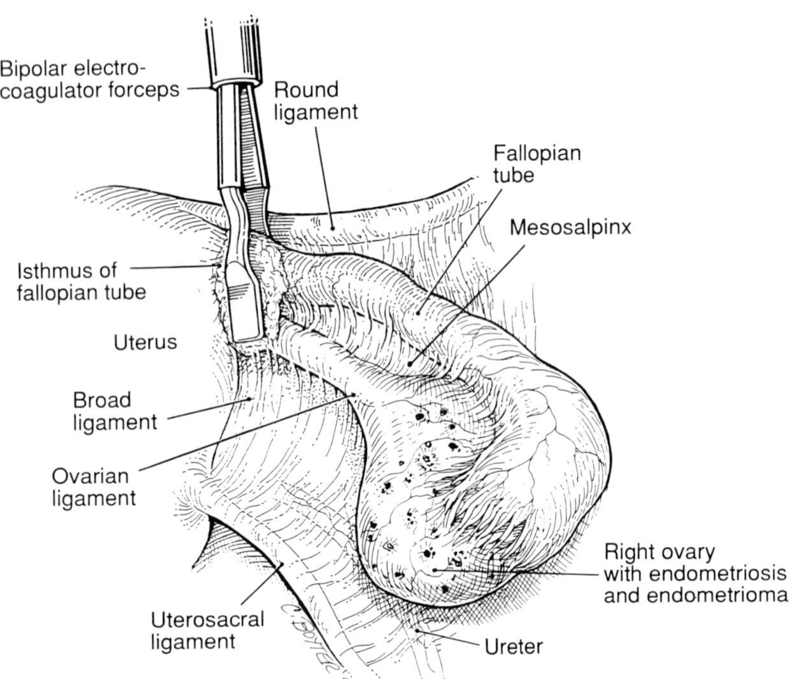

Figure 13-4. The procedure of salpingo-oophorectomy is begun by electrodesiccation and transection of the utero-ovarian ligament and isthmic portion of the fallopian tube.

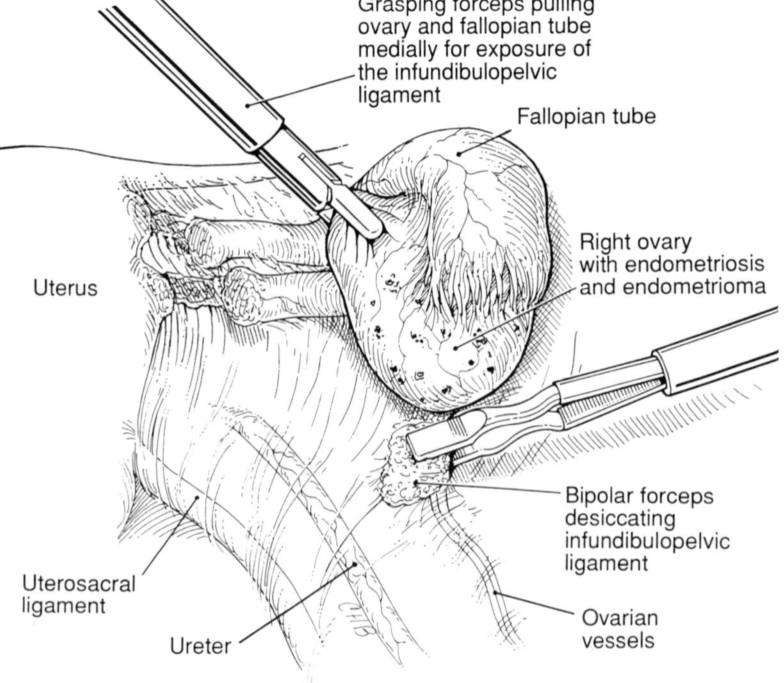

Figure 13-5. After identification of the ureter, using bipolar electrocoagulator, the infundibulopelvic ligament is desiccated while applying gentle traction to the adnexa.

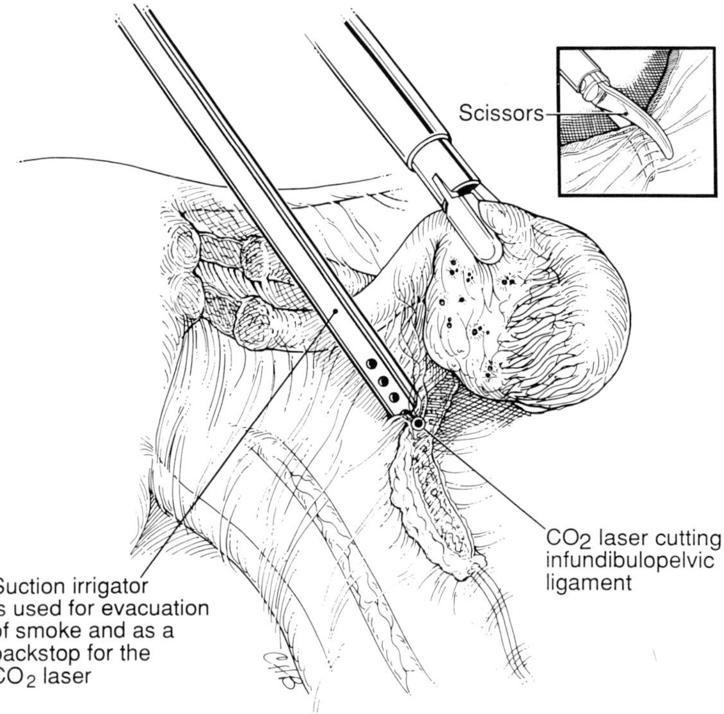

Figure 13-6. Laser or scissors (*inset*) are used to cut the coagulated infundibulopelvic ligament.

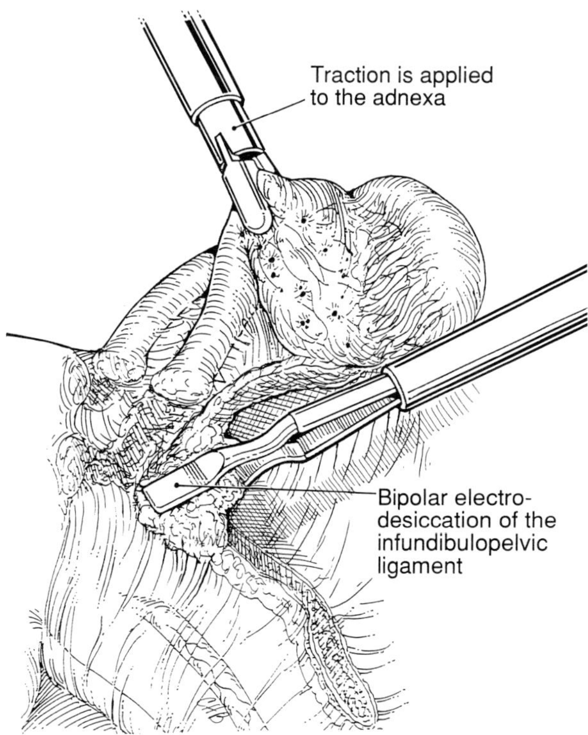

Figure 13-7. Desiccation and cutting of the infundibulopelvic ligament continues in 1- to 2-cm increments until it is completely removed.

the procedure, the fascia must be closed to prevent a hernia.

After introducing the stapler, the adnexa is grasped with laparoscopic forceps and retracted medially and caudally to stretch and outline the

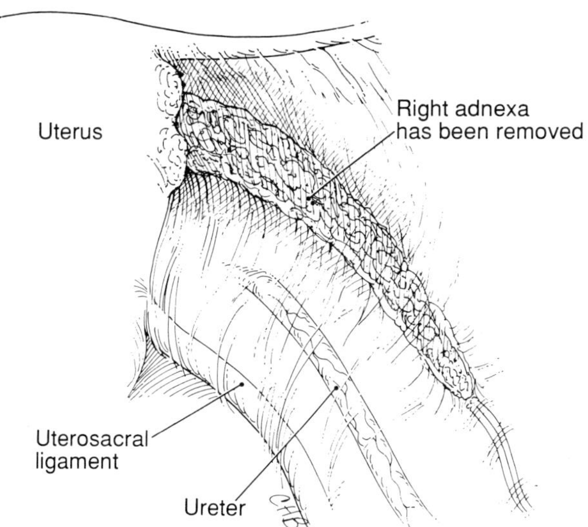

Figure 13-8. A view of the pelvic sidewall after the adnexa is removed with bipolar electrodesiccation.

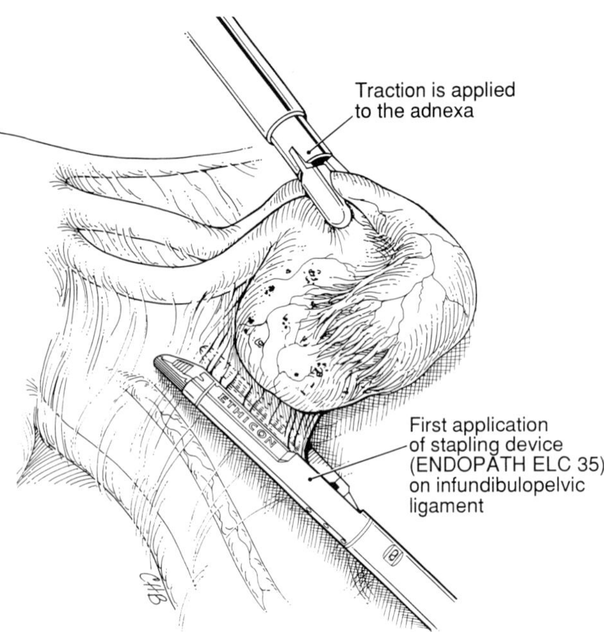

Figure 13-9. A right salpingo-oophorectomy is performed using a stapling device. The tube and ovary are under traction as the Endopath ELC 35 is applied across the infundibulopelvic ligament.

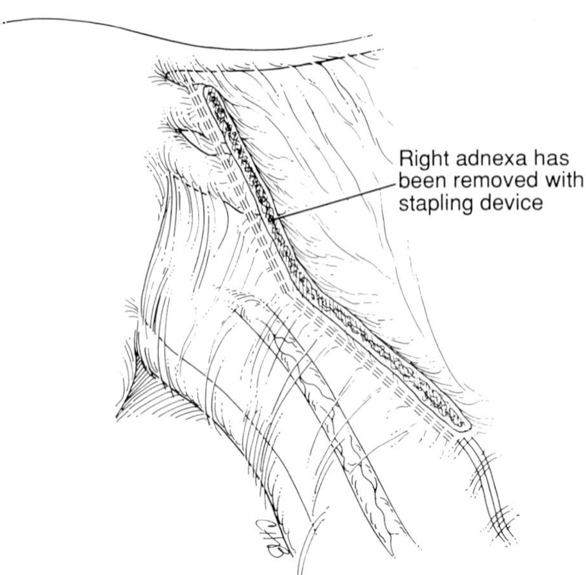

Figure 13-11. The pelvic sidewall is seen after adnexectomy with a stapling device.

infundibulopelvic ligament. The ligament is grasped and secured with the stapler (Figures 13-9 and 13-10). The stapler should not be fired until the contained tissue is identified and the ureter's safety is assured. Once transected, the staple line is examined for placement and hemostasis (Figure 13-11). Usually between one and two stapler applications are required for each adnexa.

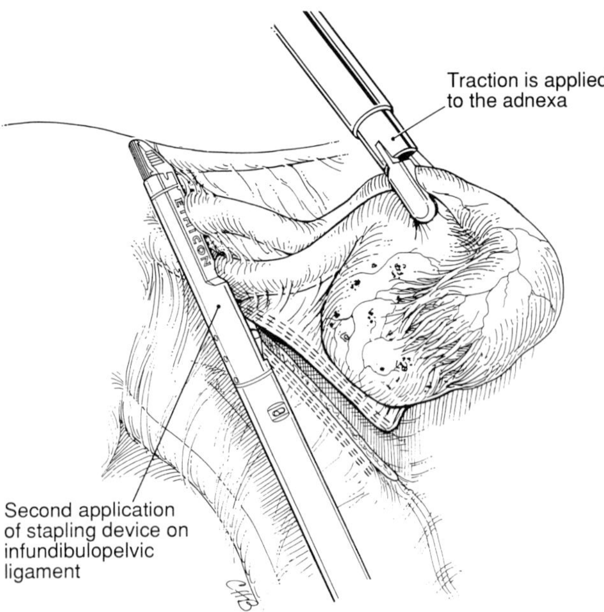

Figure 13-10. In most cases, the second application is necessary for complete removal of the adnexa.

Oophorectomy and Salpingo-oophorectomy by Endoligature

Pretied Endoloop suture can be used to perform oophorectomy and salpingo-oophorectomy.[13]

Oophorectomy. Periovarian adhesions are lysed and the ovary is freed. If a cyst is present, it is aspirated so that manipulation will be easier. The mesovarium and ovarian ligament are electrodesiccated and dissected to facilitate placement of the Endoligature (Figure 13-12).

The Endoloop (0 polydioxanone or polyglactin suture, Ethicon) is introduced into the abdominal cavity through the mid-suprapubic trocar sleeve. Using forceps, the ovary is pulled through the Endoloop (see Figure 13-12). Atraumatic forceps are used to assist in placement. The suture is pushed into the mesovarium while a knot pusher is used on the opposite side to place the slipknot at the most lateral position on the mesosalpinx and mesovarium. The suture is tightened as the ovary is pulled toward the midline and the tube is retracted with the atraumatic forceps. A second, and if necessary, a third Endoloop is placed, each successively closer to the pelvic wall so that the me-

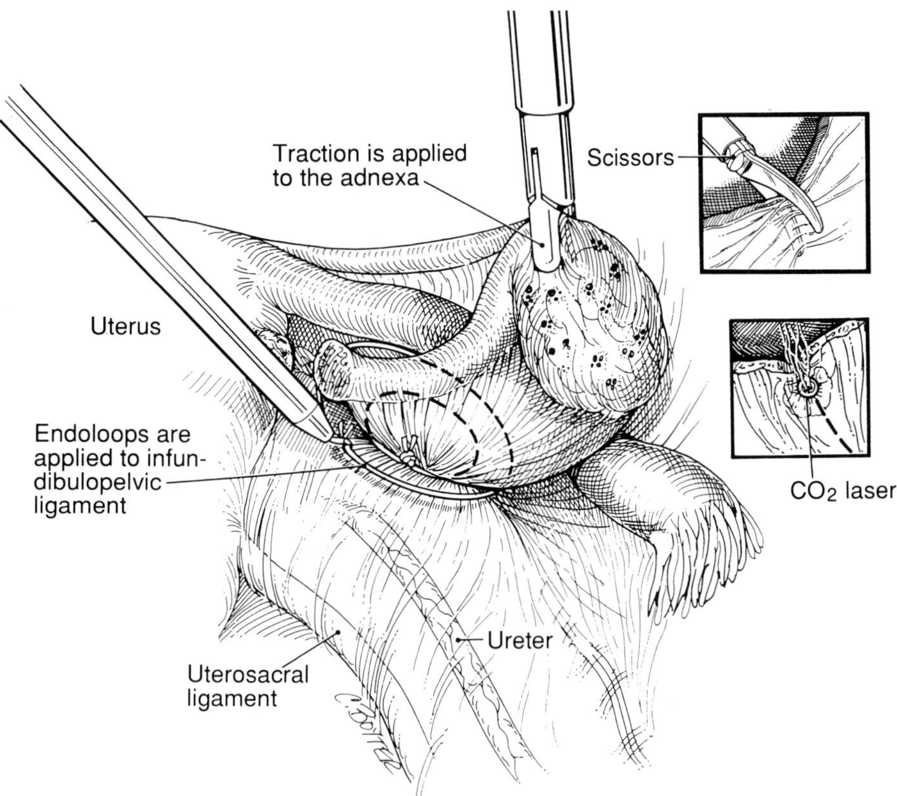

Figure 13-12. Simple oophorectomy with pretied Endoloop. After the ovarian ligament is electrodesiccated and cut, two Endoloop sutures are passed over the ovary and mesovarium and tied beyond the ovarian tissue.

sovarian pedicle will be long. The mesovarium is transected with scissors. The pedicle is evaluated to confirm that the sutures are placed beyond any ovarian tissue to avoid ovarian remnant syndrome (Figure 13-13).

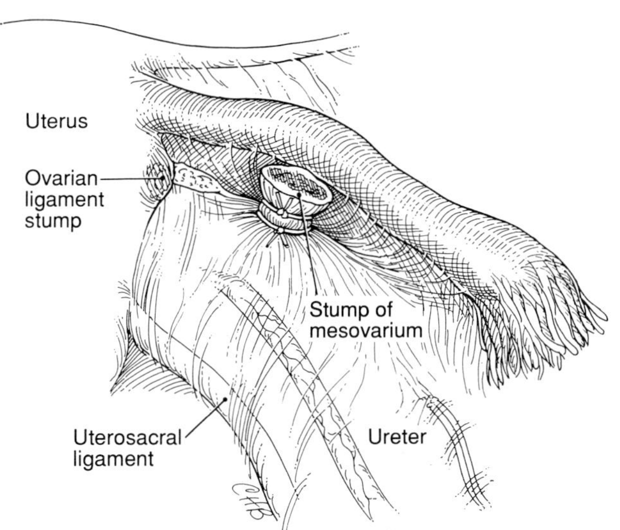

Figure 13-13. The right ovary is removed. An adequate stump should be left to avoid slippage of the ligature.

Salpingo-oophorectomy. After the ovarian ligament and tubal isthmus have been electrocoagulated and cut, an Endoloop is placed over the adnexa. The ovary and tube are grasped with forceps and pulled contralaterally. Simultaneously, the atraumatic forceps are used to push the Endoloop laterally, ensuring that the ligature is placed as far lateral as possible on the infundibulopelvic ligament. One or two additional sutures are placed progressively closer to the pelvic wall (at least 1 cm below the infundibulopelvic ligament) so that the pedicle will be long enough to prevent the sutures from slipping (Figure 13-14). The adnexal pedicle is transected with scissors. The ureters are evaluated at the pelvic brim to confirm that they are not damaged (Figure 13-15).

Dysgenetic Gonads

Individuals with XY gonadal dysgenesis require gonadectomy to protect them from developing gonadoblastoma. These gonads present as streaks, and the boundaries between the gonadal tissue and the mesovarium are not always clear. Because there is a chance that some of the dysgenetic gonadal tissue can be missed, the peritoneal borders must be kept wide.

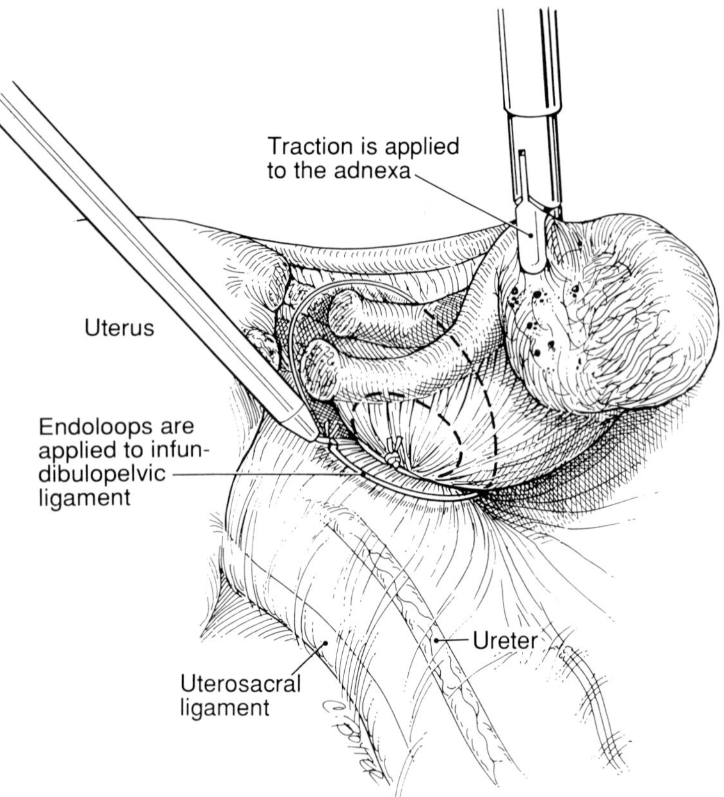

Figure 13-14. Right salpingo-oophorectomy using a pretied Endoligature. After the ovarian ligament and tubouterine junction are electrodesiccated and cut, the Endoloop is passed over the tube, ovary, and infundibulopelvic ligament, and tied. One to two additional sutures may be necessary.

The laparoscopic procedure for removing a dysgenetic gonad is similar to removing an ovary densely adherent to the pelvic sidewall.[14,15] Both the utero-ovarian and infundibulopelvic ligaments are desiccated and cut. The mesovarium above and below is incised with scissors or the CO_2 laser with hydrodissection (Figure 13-16). The loose areolar tissue immediately below the gonad is dissected from the gonad.

Adnexectomy in the Presence of Adhesions

Adhesions between the ovary and pelvic sidewall, broad ligament, and bowel must be lysed with the

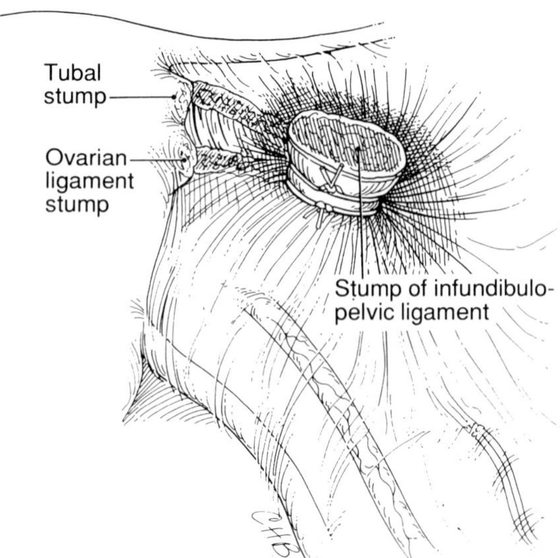

Figure 13-15. A view of the pelvic sidewall after removal of the right adnexa with Endoloop ligature.

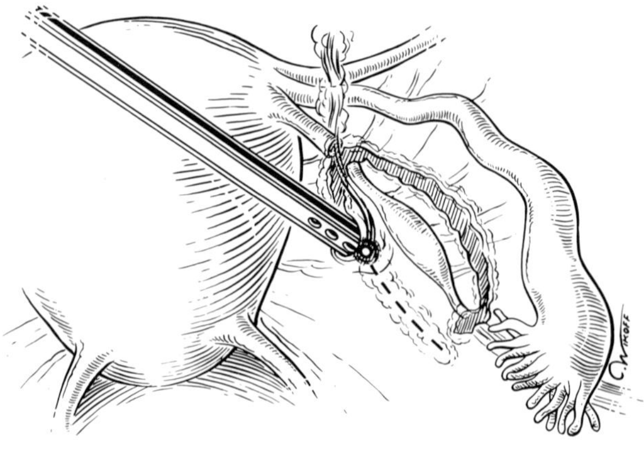

Figure 13-16. Excision of a streak ovary or dysgenetic gonad. The utero-ovarian and infundibulopelvic ligaments are coagulated and cut. The mesovarium is incised to free the tissue.

CO_2 laser or scissors until the ovary is freed. The ovary is grasped with a toothed forceps and pulled up. It is put on stretch to create a plane between the ovary and peritoneum. To avoid injury to ureters, blood vessels, or other underlying structures, the retroperitoneal area is entered and hydrodissection performed.[16] Using the suction-irrigator probe as a backstop, the adhesions are lysed close to the ovary. Removal of ovarian tissue may require excision of the peritoneum attached to the ovary.

The ovary may be enlarged, adherent to the pelvic sidewall and broad ligament, or contain endometriomas, so that the surgeon may need to enter the retroperitoneal space (Figure 13-17). In this case, the ovary is removed by retroperitoneal dissection. After hydrodissection is performed, an incision is made between the round and infundibulopelvic ligaments medial to the pelvic sidewall (Figure 13-18). Blunt dissection, hydrodissection, and sharp dissection with the CO_2 laser or other cutting modality are used to lyse adhesions and to separate the adnexa and peritoneum, ureter, and blood vessels (Figure 13-19). Hemostasis is achieved with bipolar forceps. After dissecting the pelvic sidewall, the remaining infundibulopelvic ligament, ovarian ligament, and proximal portion of the tube are coagulated and cut (Figure 13-20). The ureter is dissected from the ovary and the adnexa removed (Figure 13-21).

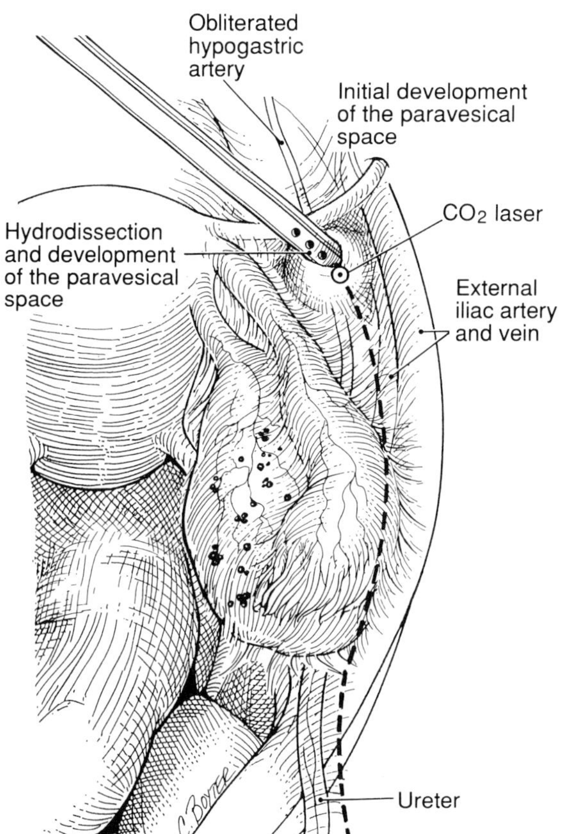

Figure 13-18. Oophorectomy by retroperitoneal dissection. An incision is made with the CO_2 laser between the round ligament and infundibulopelvic ligament. Hydrodissection and the suction-irrigator probe are used as backstops for the laser.

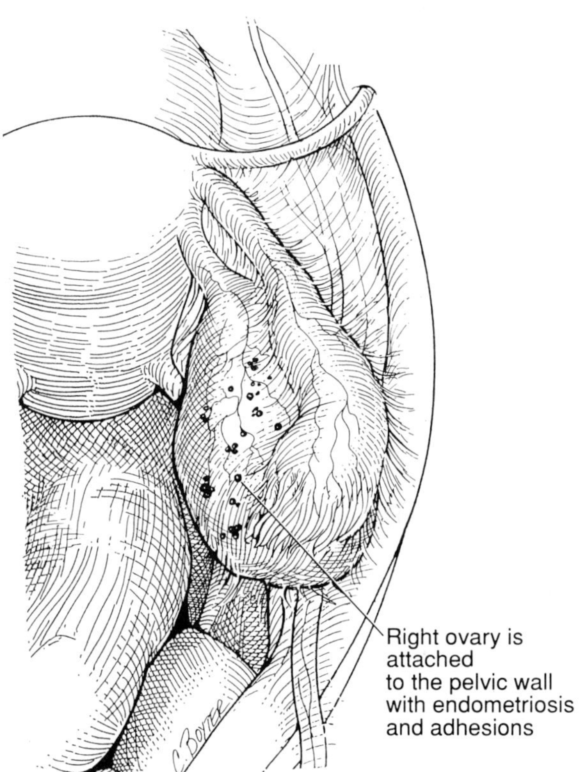

Figure 13-17. A large right endometrioma is attached to the pelvic sidewall and ureter with fibrosis and adhesions.

Residual Ovary

In patients with a previous hysterectomy, many of the usual landmarks in the pelvis are absent and extensive adhesions may involve the left ovary and descending colon. Lysis of adhesions should be performed cautiously to avoid damaging the bowel. If the ureter cannot be identified, it is necessary to open the retroperitoneal space. A sponge stick placed in the vagina may aid in orientation.

The ovary often is adherent to the vaginal cuff and should be dissected using scissors or the laser. The ureter is proximal to the lateral margins of the vaginal cuff and its position may be altered by previous surgery. No ovarian fragments should remain in the pelvic sidewall or vaginal cuff.

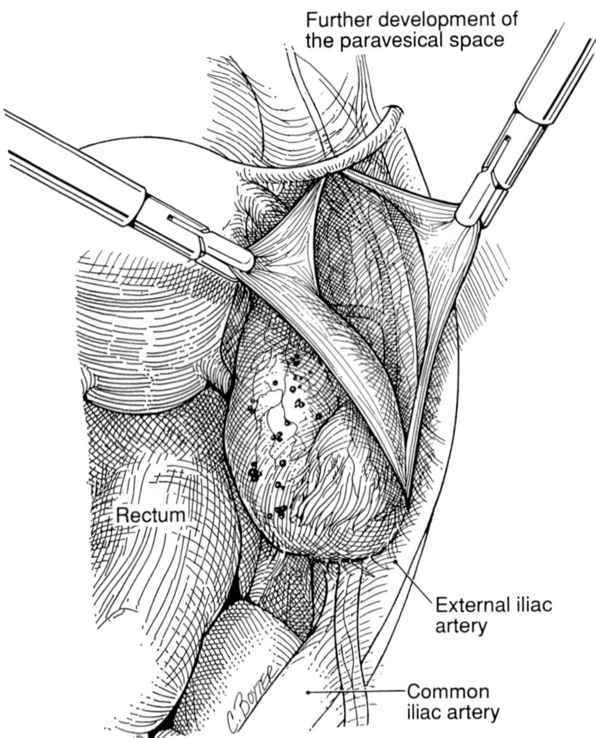

Figure 13-19. The peritoneum attached to the ovary is dissected medially from the retroperitoneal ureter and major pelvic sidewall vessels.

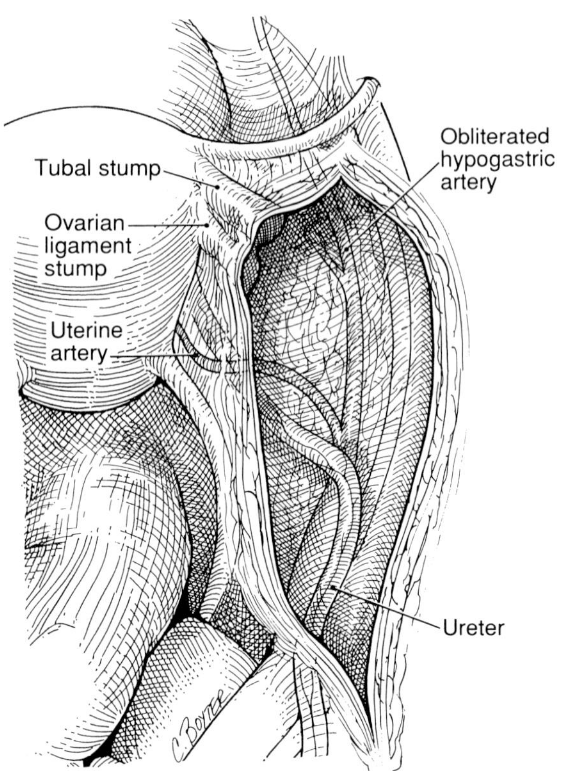

Figure 13-21. The pelvic sidewall after the right adnexa is removed with retroperitoneal dissection. The ureter and major retroperitoneal vessels can be seen.

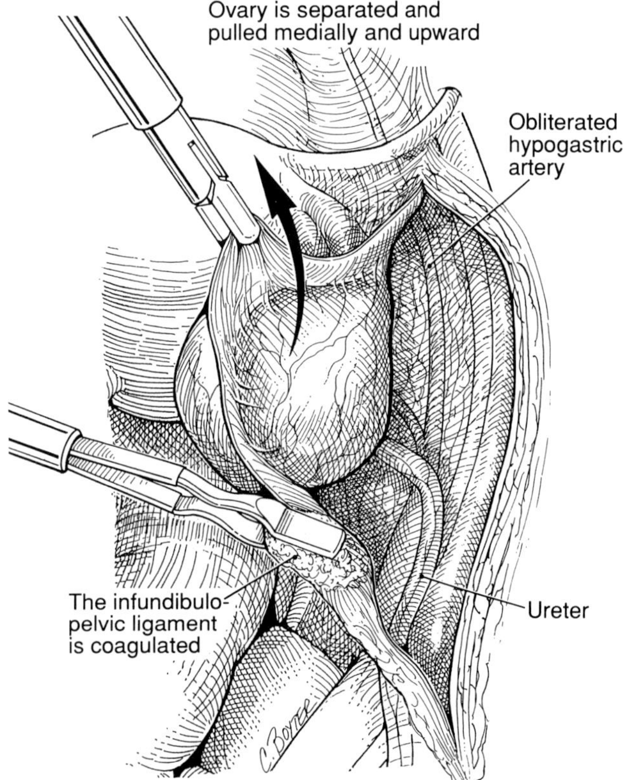

Figure 13-20. The adnexa is under traction and the infundibulopelvic ligament is electrodesiccated.

The ovary is held with a grasping forceps, put on stretch, and the infundibulopelvic ligament is desiccated and transected in 1- to 2-cm increments until the ovary is removed. Depending on the pelvic anatomy, it may be preferable to begin the oophorectomy from the infundibulopelvic ligament to better define anatomic relationships.

The ovary is removed through an abdominal incision as described. If the ovary is large, it may be cut into pieces. Colpotomy can be performed if the ovary is greater than 5 cm. However, colpotomy remote from hysterectomy is technically difficult and associated with significant risks if the bladder and rectosigmoid colon are adherent to the vaginal cuff.

Tissue Removal

Removal of the ovary can be difficult if it is more than 5 cm in size. It can be removed through a 10-mm trocar sleeve placed in a suprapubic puncture, pulling the sleeve and forceps together and bringing the tissue to the incision. A Kelly or Kocher clamp is used to grasp the tissue to remove it from the abdomen. Alternatively, a long clamp is inserted through the accessory trocar incision and the tissue is grasped under direct observation and pulled from the abdomen through the trocar incision. The tube and ovary can be divided with scissors, a morcellator, or laser and removed through trocar sleeves, if fragmentation is not contraindicated because of the characteristics of the cyst. If an open laparoscopy is performed, the ovary can be removed through the umbilical incision, enlarging it if necessary. After the ovary is removed, the pelvic cavity is irrigated and the pelvis examined to ensure hemostasis.

For endometriomas and other cysts larger than 5 cm, the tissue is removed by posterior colpotomy. The cul-de-sac is identified by placing a sponge stick in the vagina and applying pressure to the posterior fornix between the uterosacral ligaments. An incision is made between the uterosacral ligaments with laser or unipolar knife electrode. Once the incision extends to the sponge stick, the ovary is brought to the incision and grasped vaginally with an Allis clamp. If a cyst is present, it is deflated using a large-bore needle or trocar while traction is applied to the ovary. As the ovary collapses, it is pulled into the vagina intact with minimal spillage of its contents. The colpotomy is closed vaginally or laparoscopically using two to three sutures. Removal of the ovary and vaginal closure of the colpotomy are facilitated by placing the patient's legs in the position for a vaginal hysterectomy.

If it is necessary to avoid spillage of the cyst contents, the ovary is removed in a specially designed laparoscopic bag (Endopouch, Ethicon).[17] The bag is removed through a posterior colpotomy incision or an extended suprapubic incision. When the ovary is large and cystic, the bag is brought to the suprapubic incision or posterior colpotomy, the cyst is drained, and the deflated, contained cyst is pulled from the abdominal cavity.

TABLE 13-2. Frequency of Adhesions Following Wedge Resection by Laparotomy

Authors	No. of Patients	Percent With Adhesions
Stein[46]	6	67%
Buttram, Vaquero[42]	40	100%
Weinstein, Polishuk[47]	19	42%
Adashi et al.[30]	7	100%
Toaff et al.[48]	7	100%
Portuondo et al.[49]	12	92%
Total	91	85%

Ovarian Wedge Resection

Stein and Leventhal[19] described the enlarged polycystic ovaries with the clinical features of menstrual aberrations, obesity, and hyperandrogenism. Although polycystic ovarian disease (PCOD) has variable manifestations, its hallmark is chronic anovulation. It was believed that the enlarged ovaries caused the condition, so ovarian wedge resection was advocated. Because ovulation-inducing agents were unavailable, ovarian wedge resection represented a major breakthrough with ovulation and pregnancy rates of 80% and 50%, respectively. However, many patients who were initially ovulatory reverted to their previous anovulatory state after several months.[20] Although most had apparently normal ovulatory cycles, only 50% conceived (Table 13-1) because postoperative adhesions developed in many women (Table 13-2).

The availability of ovulation-inducing medications in the 1960s and 1970s [clomiphene citrate (CC) and human menopausal gonadotropins (hMG)] offered a nonsurgical approach to the treatment of anovulatory infertility that was safer

TABLE 13-1. Results of Bilateral Ovarian Wedge Resection by Laparotomy

Authors	No. of Patients	Medical Failure	Percent Ovulation	Percent Conception
Goldzieher, Green[41]	219	yes/no	85%	67%
Buttram, Vaquero[42]	173	no	62%	43%
Adashi et al.[30]	90	yes/no	64%	48%
Lunde[43]	92	yes	80%	58%
Hjortrup et al.[44]	29	no	86%	77%
Ronnberg et al.[45]	23	yes	61%	22%

TABLE 13-3. Results of Wedge Resection/Ovarian Drilling by Laparoscopy

Authors	No. of Patients	Failure	Percent Medical Ovulation	Percent Conception
Campo et al.[22]	12	yes	45%	41%
Gjonaess[20]	62	no	92%	69%
Aakvag[23]	58	no	72%	—
Greenblatt, Casper[50]	6	no	82%	50%
Daniell, Miller[27]	85	yes	71%	56%
Kojima[21]	12	yes	83%	58%
Armar et al.[51]	21	yes	81%	50%
Keckstein et al.[26]	19 (CO_2)	yes	72%	44%
	11 (YAG)	yes	73%	27%
Kovacs et al.[25]	10	yes	70%	30%

than ovarian wedge resection. As a result, ovarian wedge resection rarely was performed. CC therapy does not induce ovulation in all women. The alternative, hMG, is expensive, requires intensive monitoring, and can cause ovarian hyperstimulation.

Some endoscopic surgeons have performed the ovarian wedge resection laparoscopically.[21] Others reduced ovarian volume with multiple biopsies,[20,22] by coagulating with monopolar current,[23–25] by creating craters on the ovarian surface with lasers,[26,27] or by puncturing the small cysts on the ovarian surface.[28] Laparoscopic ovarian drilling appears to be associated with comparable rates of ovulation and conception (Table 13-3). Regardless of the method used to decrease thecal-like ovarian stroma, hormonal changes observed with the laparoscopic procedures are similar to those observed following ovarian wedge resection by laparotomy.[29,30] A disappointing finding is that the risk of postoperative adhesions is high (average 30%) in women undergoing ovarian drilling (Table 13-4).

Theoretically, wedge resection and ovarian drilling work by reducing the androgen production in the ovarian stroma. Appropriate patients are women who fail to ovulate after 3 to 4 months on CC and who do not respond to hMG.

TABLE 13-4. Frequency of Postoperative Adhesions Following Laparoscopic Ovarian Drilling

Authors	No. of Patients	Percent With Adhesions
Portuondo et al.[49]	24	0%
Greenblatt, Casper[50]	6	100%
Gurgan et al.[52]	17	82%
Dabirashrafi et al.[53]	43	16%
Total	90	30%

The procedure is performed using a 10-mm videolaparoscope coupled to a CO_2 laser. A 5-mm second puncture is placed suprapubically in the midline and is used for a suction-irrigator or grasping instrument. Associated pelvic abnormalities are corrected before ovarian coagulation. Each ovary is fixed in the anterior cul-de-sac or held by the utero-ovarian ligament during treatment. The ultrapulse (40 to 80 W, 25 to 200 millijoules) or superpulse (25 to 40 W) CO_2 laser is used. All visible subcapsular follicles are vaporized and drained, and randomly placed 2- to 4-mm diameter craters are made in the ovarian stroma (Figure 13-22). Each ovary is treated symmetrically, and cysts are vaporized. The ovaries are irrigated and hemostasis is obtained with bipolar forceps.

The KTP, YAG, or Argon laser can be used as well.[26,27] However, a third trocar is required for fiber introduction. The fiber can be threaded

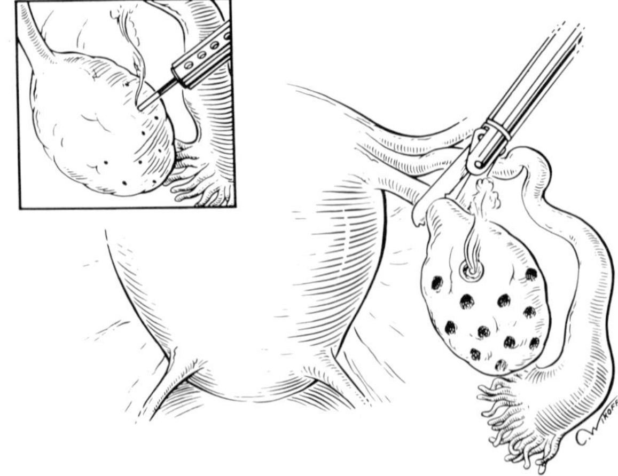

Figure 13-22. Procedure for ovarian drilling for PCOD. While grasping the ovarian ligament and holding the ovary, multiple surface crates are created by the CO_2 laser, fiber laser, or needle electrode.

through the central channel of a special 5-mm dual-channel suction-irrigation probe. By using the dual-channel probe, it is possible to suction the smoke from vaporization at the site of occurrence. Holes are drilled in the ovary in a manner similar to that described for the CO_2 laser.

Ovarian coagulation has been presented using unipolar punch biopsy forceps[28] or a needle electrode.[22–24] The power setting for the monopolar current is 20 to 30 W, in a cutting mode to minimize thermal damage; the power is activated just before touching the ovary. The ovary is penetrated in approximately 10 to 15 sites at a depth of 3 to 5 mm.

Ovarian Torsion

Adnexal torsion is a surgical emergency. When diagnosed early, the adnexa can be unwound. However, the diagnosis often is delayed because of the inconsistent presenting symptoms and signs and intermittent pain. When the diagnosis is delayed, the adnexa becomes congested, ischemic, hemorrhagic, and necrotic. Gynecologists have been taught to remove tissue that has undergone torsion and ischemia because of the risk of thrombotic embolism arising from the ovarian vein.

Way[31] first reported successful conservative management of adnexal torsion. The affected structure was straightened to assess the viability, and even ovaries that appeared infarcted at laparotomy regained normal color after untwisting. No complications related to the procedure were reported. Because adnexal torsion produces no pathognomonic clinical findings, laparoscopy can be used for diagnosis and treatment. Prompt laparoscopic examination is essential because delay is associated with gangrene.

The causes of ovarian or adnexal torsion include parovarian cysts, functional and pathologic ovarian cysts, ovarian hyperstimulation, ectopic pregnancy, adhesions, and congenital malformation.[32,33] The ischemic structures are straightened gently with atraumatic forceps to avoid additional adnexal damage. In women with ovarian hyperstimulation, the functional cysts should be drained before untwisting.[34] The abnormalities contributing to torsion should be treated. It may be necessary to shorten the utero-ovarian ligament if its length may have contributed to ovarian torsion. A running suture of monofilament material is placed along the length of the utero-ovarian ligament (Figure 13-23) and tied to shorten it, limiting ovarian mobility.

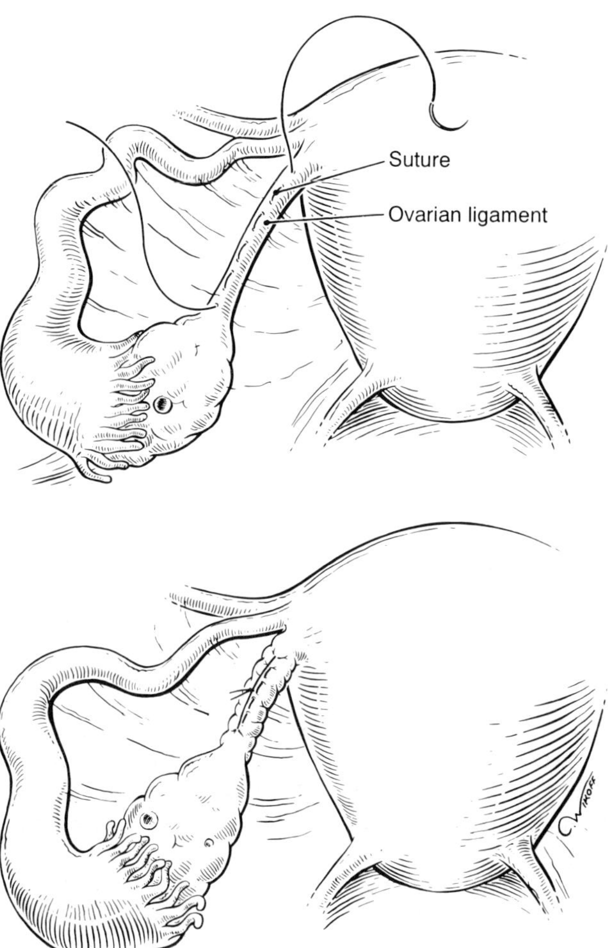

Figure 13-23. Ovarian suspension. A monofilament suture is placed along the length of the utero-ovarian ligament and tied.

In a report of 35 cases, Mage and colleagues noted that 21 women showed no gross evidence of ischemia or mild changes with immediate and complete recovery within 10 minutes of untwisting.[32] In eight, the tube or ovary was dark red or black, but partial recovery was apparent after the pedicle was untwisted. Six had gangrenous adnexa that required salpingectomy or oophorectomy. The first two groups were managed conservatively; the latter group underwent excision of the involved organ(s). The postoperative course in all patients was uneventful. Six of the eight women in the intermediate group underwent a second-look laparoscopy that showed complete recovery.

Ovarian Remnant Syndrome

In premenopausal women who had bilateral oophorectomy, a small piece of functional ovarian tissue can respond to hormonal stimulation with growth, cystic degeneration, or hemorrhage and produce pain.[35–37] Ovarian remnants remain because of dense adhesions and distorted anatomic relationships, which invariably worsen with subsequent operations. It is not unusual for these patients to have had previous attempts to excise an ovarian remnant. Removal of the ovarian tissue is preferred, although the reported incidence of complications with laparotomy ranges from 16% to 30%.[38] The challenge and complications are related directly to the presence of extensive pelvic and abdominal adhesions from multiple previous operations, endometriosis, pelvic inflammatory disease, or ovarian cysts.

Diagnosis is based on history and localization of pelvic pain. Although some patients have cystic adnexal structures or ill-defined fixed masses, others have normal pelvic findings. Vaginal ultrasound helps to locate the ovarian remnant. Low or borderline follicle-stimulating hormone levels in patients with documented bilateral oophorectomy are consistent with the presence of active ovarian tissue.[35] Hormonal suppression with oral contraceptives or gonadotropin-releasing hormone agonist provides no relief in most patients.[10] CC or hMG may be used to increase ovarian remnant size to confirm the diagnosis preoperatively or to aid in locating the tissue intraoperatively.[39]

Most reviews of ovarian remnant syndrome consider laparoscopy to be ineffective in the management because of the presence of dense pelvic adhesions.[36–38] However, the absence of complications in a series of 22 patients attests to the feasibility of the laparoscopic approach.[10] Attention should be focused on prevention. Factors associated with ovarian remnant syndrome include the use of Endoloops for laparoscopic oophorectomy, multiple surgical procedures with incomplete removal of pelvic organs, densely adherent ovaries, and multiple ovarian cystectomies for functional cysts.[10] When pretied sutures are used for the infundibulopelvic ligament, it is important that they be placed below the ovarian tissue. Electrodesiccation and transection of the infundibulopelvic ligament or the application of clips are preferred. When the ovary is densely adherent to the pelvic sidewall, retroperitoneal hydrodissection, meticulous adhesiolysis, and removal of the peritoneum underlying the ovary are essential in performing a laparoscopic oophorectomy (see Figure 13-20). The need for restraint in managing functional cysts is underscored by the fact that some patients in our series had only a corpus luteum resected at first laparotomy.

Procedure Guidelines

A preoperative bowel preparation of Go-LYTELY, enemas, and oral metronidazole are indicated. Anterior abdominal wall adhesions are probable following multiple laparotomies, and an open laparoscopy or mapping technique[40] should be used. After all instruments are inserted, intra-abdominal adhesions are lysed and the ovarian remnants dissected.

The anatomy of the retroperitoneal space is identified when the ovarian remnant is adherent to the lateral pelvic wall. The space beneath the peritoneum is injected with lactated Ringer's solution and the peritoneum is opened to the infundibulopelvic ligament or its remnant. Adhesions are lysed until the course of the major pelvic blood vessels and the ureter can be traced and, if necessary, dissected. The ovarian blood supply is desiccated with bipolar forceps and the ovarian tissue is excised and submitted for histologic examination.

When the remnant is adherent to the bowel, adhesions are lysed using hydrodissection and the CO_2 laser or other cutting modality. Ovarian tissue embedded in the muscularis of the bowel is removed superficially, skinning the mucosa beneath it. The serosa and muscularis layers are imbricated with one to three interrupted 4-0 polydioxanone sutures in one layer. All remnant ovary should be removed. When the lesion is embedded in the bowel or bladder muscularis, or when the ureter is involved or possibly obstructed, resection and repair of affected structures are necessary.

References

1. Yuzpe AA, Rioux JE. The value of laparoscopic ovarian biopsy. *J Reprod Med.* 1975;15:57.
2. Nezhat C, Nezhat F. Postoperative adhesion formation after ovarian cystectomy with and without ovarian reconstruction. Annual Meeting of the American Fertility Society, Orlando, FL, October 21, 1991.
3. Semm K. Course of endoscopic abdominal surgery. In: Friedrich E, ed. *Operative Manual for Endoscopic Abdominal Surgery.* Chicago: Year Book Medical Publishers; 1984:180.
4. Nezhat F, Nezhat C, Silfen SL. Videolaseroscopy for oophorectomy. *Am J Obstet Gynecol.* 1991;165:1323.
5. Silva PD, Juffel ME, Beguin EA. Open laparoscopy simplifies instrumentation required

for laparoscopic oophorectomy and salpingo-oophorectomy. *Obstet Gynecol.* 1991; 77:482.
6. Perry CP, Upchurch JC. Pelviscopic adnexectomy. *Am J Obstet Gynecol.* 1990;162:79.
7. Nezhat C, Nezhat F, Silfen SL. Laparoscopic hysterectomy and bilateral salpingo-oophorectomy using multifire GIA surgical stapler. *J Gynecol Surg.* 1990;6:287.
8. Daniell JF, Jurtz BR, Lee JY. Laparoscopic oophorectomy: comparative study of ligatures, bipolar coagulation and automatic stapling devices. *Obstet Gynecol.* 1992;80:325.
9. Nezhat C, Nezhat F, Winer W. Salpingectomy via laparoscopy: a new surgical approach. *J Laparosc Surg.* 1991;1:91.
10. Nezhat C, Nezhat F. Operative laparoscopy for the management of ovarian remnant syndrome. *Fertil Steril.* 1992;57:1003.
11. Sigel B, Dunn MR. The mechanism of blood vessel closure by high frequency electrocoagulation. *Surg Gynecol Obstet.* 1965; October: 823.
12. Nezhat C, Nezhat F. Laparoscopic electrosurgical oophorectomy: risk of using "blanching" as the end point. *Am J Obstet Gynecol.* 1992;167;1151. Letter.
13. Semm K. Color atlas. *Operative Manual for Endoscopic Abdominal Surgery.* Chicago: Year Book Medical Publishers; 1984: 334–346.
14. Droesch K, Droesch J, Chumas J, et al. Laparoscopic gonadectomy for gonadal dysgenesis. *Fertil Steril.* 1990;53:360.
15. Seifer DB. Laparoscopic adnexectomy in a prepubertal Turner mosaic female with isodicentric Y. *Hum Reprod.* 1991;6:566.
16. Nezhat C, Nezhat F. Safe laser excision or vaporization of peritoneal endometriosis. *Fertil Steril.* 1989;52;149.
17. Nezhat C, Nezhat F, Welander CE, et al. Four ovarian cancers diagnosed during laparoscopic management of 1,011 adnexal masses. *Am J Obstet Gynecol.* 1992;167:790.
18. Nezhat F, Brill AI, Nezhat CH, et al. Adhesion formation after endoscopic posterior colpotomy. *J Reprod Med.* 1993;38:534.
19. Stein IF, Leventhal ML. Amenorrhea associated with bilateral polycystic ovaries. *Am J Obstet Gynecol.* 1935;29:181.
20. Gjonnaess H. Polycystic ovarian syndrome treated by ovarian electrocautery through the laparoscope. *Fertil Steril.* 1984;41:20.
21. Kojima E. Ovarian wedge resection with contact Nd:YAG laser irradiation used laparoscopically. *J Reprod Med.* 1989;34:444.
22. Campo S, Garcia N, Caruso A, et al. Effect of celioscopy ovarian resection in patients with polycystic ovaries. *Gynecol Obstet Invest.* 1983;15:213.
23. Aakvaag A. Hormonal response to electrocautery of the ovary in patients with polycystic ovarian disease. *Br J Obstet Gynecol.* 1985;92:1258.
24. Casper RF, Greenblatt EM. Laparoscopic ovarian cautery for induction of ovulation in women with polycystic ovary disease. *Semin Reprod Endocrinol.* 1990;8:209.
25. Kovacs G, Buckler H, Bangah M, et al. Treatment of anovulation due to polycystic ovarian syndrome by laparoscopic ovarian electrocautery. *Br J Obstet Gynecol.* 1991; 98:30.
26. Keckstein G, Rossmanith W, Spatzier K, et al. The effect of laparoscopic treatment of polycystic ovarian disease by CO_2 laser or Nd-YAG laser. *Surg Endosc.* 1990;4:103.
27. Daniell JF, Miller W. Polycystic ovaries treated by laparoscopic laser vaporization. *Fertil Steril.* 1989;51:232.
28. Sumioki H, Utsunomyiya T, Matsuoka K, et al. The effect of laparoscopic multiple punch resection of the ovary on the hypothalamo-pituitary axis in polycystic ovary syndrome. *Fertil Steril.* 1988;50:567.
29. Judd HL, Rigg LA, Anderson DC, et al. The effects of ovarian wedge resection on circulating gonadotropin and ovarian steroid levels in patients with polycystic ovarian syndrome. *J Clin Endocrinol Metab.* 1976;43:347.
30. Adashi EY, Rock JA, Guzick D, et al. Fertility following bilateral ovarian wedge resection: a critical analysis of 90 consecutive cases of the polycystic ovary syndrome. *Fertil Steril.* 1981;36:320.
31. Way S. Ovarian cystectomy of twisted cysts. *Lancet.* 1946;2:47.
32. Mage G, Canis M, Manhes H, et al. Laparoscopic management of adnexal torsion. *J Reprod Med.* 1989;34:520.
33. Wagaman R, Williams RS. Conservative therapy of adnexal torsion. *J Reprod Med.* 1990;35:833.
34. Ben-Rafael Z, Bider D, Mashiach S. Laparoscopic unwinding of twisted ischemic hemorrhagic adnexum after in vitro fertilization. *Fertil Steril.* 1990;53:569.

35. Steege JF. Ovarian remnant syndrome. *Obstet Gynecol.* 1987;70:64.
36. Petit PD, Lee RA. Ovarian remnant syndrome: diagnostic dilemma and surgical challenge. *Obstet Gynecol.* 1988;71:580.
37. Webb MJ. Ovarian remnant syndrome. *Aust N Z J Obstet Gynecol.* 1989;29:433.
38. Price FV, Edwards R, Buschsbaum HJ. Ovarian remnant syndrome: difficulties in diagnosis and management. *Obstet Gynecol Surv.* 1990;45:151.
39. Kaminski PF, Sorosky JI, Mandell MJ, et al. Clomiphene citrate stimulation as an adjunct in locating ovarian tissue in ovarian remnant syndrome. *Obstet Gynecol.* 1990;76:924.
40. Nezhat C, Nezhat F, Silfen SL. Videolaseroscopy: the CO_2 laser for advanced operative laparoscopy. *Obstet Gynecol Clin North Am.* 1991;18:585.
41. Goldzieher JW, Green JA. The polycystic ovary. Clinical and histological features. *J Clin Endocrinol Metab.* 1962;22:325.
42. Buttram VC, Vaquero C. Post-ovarian wedge resection adhesive disease. *Fertil Steril.* 1975;26:874.
43. Lunde O. Polycystic ovarian syndrome; a retrospective study of the therapeutic effect of ovarian wedge resection after unsuccessful treatment with clomiphene citrate. *Ann Chir Gynecol.* 1982;71:330.
44. Hjortrup A, Kehlet H, Lockwood K, et al. Long term clinical effects of ovarian wedge resection in polycystic ovarian syndrome. *Acta Obstet Gynecol Scand.* 1983;62:55.
45. Ronnberg L, Ylostalo P, Ruokonen A. Hormonal parameters and conception rate during 5 different types of treatment of polycystic ovarian syndrome. *Int J Gynecol Obstet.* 1985;23:177.
46. Stein IF. Wedge resection of the ovaries: the Stein Leventhal syndrome. In: Greenblatt RB, ed. *Ovulation.* Philadelphia: JB Lippincott; 1966:150–157.
47. Weinstein D, Polishuk WZ. The role of wedge resection of the ovary as a cause for mechanical sterility. *Surg Gynecol Obstet.* 1975; 141:417.
48. Toaff R, Toaff ME, Peyser MR. Infertility following wedge resection of the ovaries. *Am J Obstet Gynecol.* 1976;124:92–96.
49. Portuondo JA, Melchor JC, Neyro JL, et al. Periovarian adhesions following ovarian wedge resection or laparoscopic biopsy. *Endoscopy.* 1984;16:143.
50. Greenblatt E, Casper RF. Endocrine changes after laparoscopic ovarian cautery in polycystic ovary syndrome. *Am J Obstet Gynecol.* 1987;156:279.
51. Armar NA, McGarrigle HHG, Honour J, et al. Laparoscopic ovarian diathermy in the management of ovulatory infertility in women with polycystic ovaries: endocrine changes and clinical outcome. *Fertil Steril.* 1990;53:45.
52. Gurgan T, Kisnisci H, Yarali H, et al. Evaluation of adhesion formation after laparoscopic treatment of polycystic ovarian disease. *Fertil Steril.* 1991;56:1176.
53. Dabirashrafi H, Mohamad K, Behjatnia Y, et al. Adhesion formation after ovarian electrocauterization on patients with polycystic ovarian syndrome. *Fertil Steril.* 1991; 55:1200.

14

Tubal Surgery

Primary tubal disease is a relatively frequent cause of infertility, affecting up to 20% of women who have difficulty conceiving. The most common predisposing factors are pelvic inflammatory disease (PID), previous pelvic surgery, ruptured appendix, and endometriosis. The prevalence of some of these etiologic factors has increased over the past decade.[1]

Traditionally, distal tubal obstruction has been managed by laparotomy and microsurgical techniques with pregnancy rates of 20% to 30% 2 years postoperatively.[2] Although laparoscopy for tubal infertility has been a significant factor in reducing medical costs, hospitalization, and recuperation, the technique has not resulted in a significant increase in pregnancy rates.[3] For some women with severe tubal damage, in vitro fertilization (IVF) offers a better chance for term pregnancy (72.3%) compared to surgery (27.3%).[4] Fimbrioplasty and lysis of peritubal and periovarian adhesions have been associated with good pregnancy rates.[5] In these patients, IVF is appropriate when pregnancy is not achieved postoperatively after a few years.

This chapter reviews the use of laparoscopy for managing acute PID and for tubal reconstruction in the infertile woman.

MANAGEMENT OF ACUTE PELVIC INFLAMMATORY DISEASE

Pelvic inflammatory disease usually results from sexually transmitted diseases caused by chlamydia or gonococcus infection, an intrauterine device (IUD), or postpartum endometritis. PID has four primary sequelae: infertility, ectopic pregnancy, chronic pelvic pain, and recurrent upper genital tract infection. The degree of tubal damage and pelvic adhesions often depends on the severity of the infection, the number of PID episodes, and etiology. Severe peritonitis is associated with a 17% risk of infertility compared to 3% for mild infection. With each successive episode of PID, the risk of infertility doubles. Despite its typically mild presentation, chlamydial PID results in a threefold increase in infertility compared to gonococcal PID. The risk of ectopic pregnancy is 6 to 10 times higher in women who have had PID. In addition, chronic pelvic pain has been shown to occur in 15% to 18% of patients after PID, usually because of adhesions. Up to 20% to 25% of patients will have at least one recurrent infection because damaged fallopian tubes are more susceptible to infection.[6]

Laparoscopy is being used increasingly in patients suspected of having PID to make a precise diagnosis and thereby avoid the potential sequelae. Prompt surgical confirmation of the diagnosis is possible with laparoscopy. A tubo-ovarian abscess (TOA) can be drained, reducing the risk of serious morbidity associated with rupture.

Diagnosis. The clinical diagnosis of PID is difficult because of the wide variation in symptoms and signs. Many women with PID report subtle, vague, or mild symptoms that are not specific, such as dyspareunia, postcoital spotting, or abnormal uterine bleeding. In these situations, a bimanual examination may demonstrate cervical motion or adnexal tenderness.

Tubo-ovarian abscess is a severe sequela and

TABLE 14-1. Differential Diagnosis of Pelvic Inflammatory Disease

Endometriosis
Ruptured ovarian cyst
Appendicitis
Torsion of adnexa
Gastroenteritis
Urinary tract infection

occurs in as many as 34% of patients hospitalized with PID. Symptomatic or subclinical infections can progress rapidly into a TOA[7] and these abscesses can rupture, resulting in severe peritonitis.

It should be noted that even in the presence of "classic" symptoms and signs of PID (lower abdominal pain, cervical motion tenderness, adnexal tenderness, elevated white cell count, fever or mass on ultrasound), other causes are possible and may require different management (Table 14–1). Several studies indicate that clinical diagnosis is accurate in only 65% of patients.[8–10] The routine use of laparoscopy to diagnose acute salpingitis is widespread in Europe.[11]

Treatment. The treatment objectives are to cure the initial infection and prevent sequelae. The management of a mild infection involves outpatient treatment with broad-spectrum antibiotics effective against both penicillin-resistant gonococcus and chlamydia (Table 14–2). Droegmueller recommends hospitalizing women suspected to have mild PID so that intravenous antibiotics may be administered.[12] The generally accepted criteria for admission are listed in Table 14–3.

Treatment of tubo-ovarian abscess. In the past, the accepted treatment for a TOA was a total abdominal hysterectomy with bilateral salpingo-oophorectomy regardless of the patient's age. The risk from a ruptured abscess was minimized and

TABLE 14-3. Indications for Hospital Admission for Pelvic Inflammatory Disease

Uncertain diagnosis
Suspected pelvic abscess
Pregnant patient
Adolescent patient
Concomitant severe illness
Inability to follow or tolerate outpatient regimen
Desires future fertility
Failure to respond to outpatient therapy

Source: Centers for Disease Control, 1989 STD Treatment Guidelines. *MMWR.* 1989;38(suppl 31S).

the chance for cure was excellent. At present, surgical intervention is used only to treat a TOA when medical management is ineffective.

Laparoscopy for TOA. The laparoscopic procedure for managing pelvic abscesses has been described by several authors.[7,11,13] Once TOA is diagnosed laparoscopically, two 5-mm trocars are placed suprapubically through which a suction-irrigator probe and grasping forceps are inserted. The pelvis, upper abdomen, and pelvic gutters should be examined for free or loculated purulent material, and the course of both ureters should be identified. Such collections are dispersed gently with the suction-irrigator. Purulent fluid is aspirated from the pelvis, and cultures are taken from the aspirated fluid and the inflammatory exudate. If necessary, the suction-irrigator is used to mobilize the omentum, small bowel, rectosigmoid, and tubo-ovarian adhesions bluntly until the abscess cavity is localized (Figure 14–1). After the abscess cavity is drained, the suction-irrigator is used to separate the bowel and omentum completely from the reproductive organs and to lyse tubo-ovarian adhesions using a combination of blunt lysis and hydrodissection. Electrosurgery, laser surgery, and scissors are not helpful in treat-

TABLE 14-2. Treatment of Outpatient and Inpatient Pelvic Inflammatory Disease

Outpatient

Cefoxitin 2 g IM + probenecid 1 g PO bid × 10-14 d Ceftriaxone 250 mg IM	} doxycycline 100 mg or tetracycline 500 mg qid × 10-14 d

Inpatient

Cefoxitin 2 g IV q6h or cefotetan 2 g IV q6h plus doxycycline 100 mg q12h
Clindamycin 900 mg IV q8h plus gentamycin, loading dose followed by 1.5 mg/kg IV q8h
Continue inpatient regimen for at least 48 h after clinical improvement.
Continue doxycycline 100 mg PO bid for 10-14 d after discharge.

Source: Centers for Disease Control and Prevention, 1990.

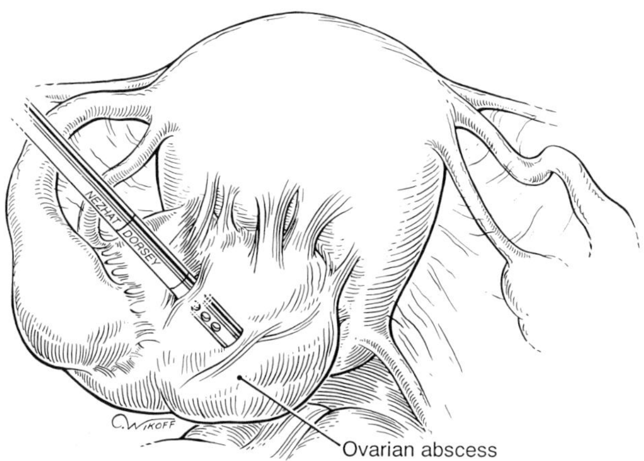

Figure 14-1 Suction-irrigator probe is used for blunt dissection and drainage of abscess cavity.

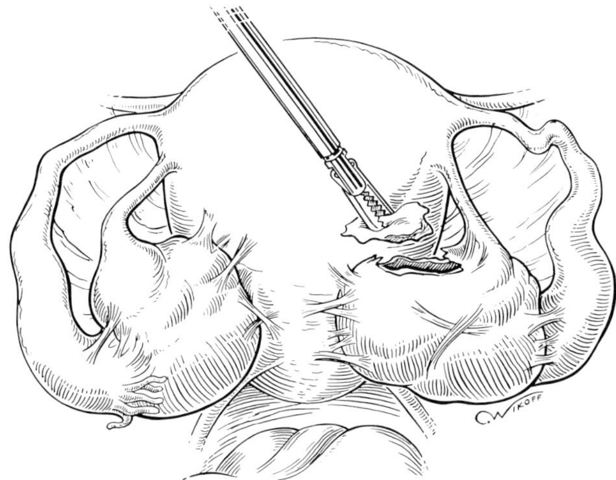

Figure 14-3 Abscess cavity is removed in pieces from attached organs.

ing acute pelvic abscesses. Adhesions caused by acute PID are soft and can be disrupted by gentle blunt dissection and hydrodissection. Hydrodissection is performed by placing the tip of the suction-irrigator against the interface between the tissue. The pressure of the fluid spray and the gentle force of the instrument create a plane for dissection (Figure 14–2). The 5-mm graspers provide traction and countertraction, improving observation of the affected area. After the abscess has been mobilized, its walls are removed in sections using the 5-mm graspers (Figure 14–3). Although technically arduous, meticulous dissection of the abscess from surrounding structures is critical for surgical success. The infection may involve the ovulation site. Once the ovary is mobilized, rents or holes in the ovary are irrigated copiously. Suture is not required to repair the ovary. The graspers are inserted into the tubal ostium to spread it and free agglutinated fimbriae. Chromopertubation is not indicated because edema in the interstitial tissue of the tube occludes the lumen.

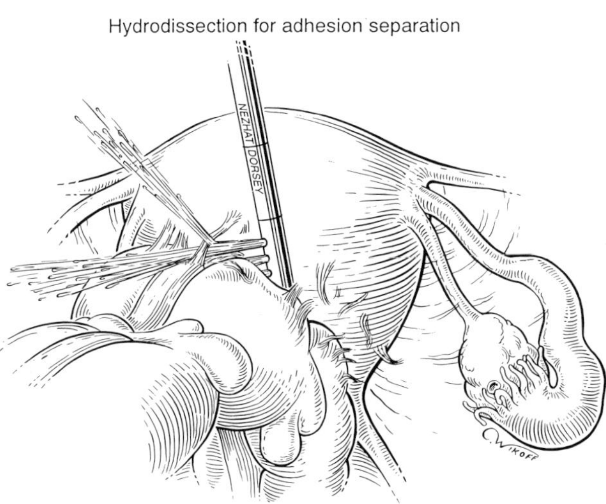

Figure 14-2 Hydrodissection is used to separate the planes for dissection in the presence of acute infection and adhesions.

At the end of the procedure, the peritoneal cavity is irrigated with lactated Ringer's until the effluent is clear. The upper abdomen also is irrigated, and the remainder of the irrigation fluid is aspirated with the patient in a reverse Trendelenburg position. Between 300 and 400 mL of irrigation fluid are left in the pelvis to separate these organs during the early healing phase.

In contrast to the easily lysed adhesion associated with acute PID and abscess formation, chronic TOAs have dense walls. The bowel often adheres to pelvic organs and can be dissected with difficulty; the adnexa appear as a dense mass, making it difficult to distinguish between the pyosalpinx and ovary. Adhesiolysis is technically difficult and associated with a high risk of complications.[11] Hydrodissection and gentle blunt dissection decrease the potential for intestinal or ureteral injury (Figure 14-4); the laser and electrosurgery should be used sparingly.

Henry-Suchet and colleagues presented data on 50 patients with TOA and noted clinical improvement in 90% within 5 days of combined treatment with laparoscopic abscess drainage and antibiotics.[11] Eight patients required laparotomy for removal of some or all reproductive organs at a later date. Second-look laparoscopy revealed bilateral adhesions with tubal obstruction in only 16% of patients. Similar results were found in other studies.[13,14]

TABLE 14-4. Principles of Tubal Surgery

Magnification
Meticulous hemostasis
Prevention of tissue desiccation
Complete excision of pathologic tissue
Prevention of tissue ischemia/thermal damage
Avoidance or minimal use of sutures
Gentle/atraumatic handling of tissues
Adhesion-preventing regimens/devices

Mecke and coworkers reported data on 66 patients with pelvic abscesses.[14] Twenty-five required laparotomy, whereas the remainder underwent operative laparoscopy. The procedure was based on age, clinical presentation, and operative findings. The abscesses involving both adnexa and adnexal masses in older women were managed by laparotomy. In women over 40, fertility is less often a consideration. In these patients, TOAs are associated more often with ovarian cancer and systemic illness such as diabetes rather than with sexually transmitted disease.[15]

Laparoscopic Tubal Reconstruction

The successful outcome of tuboplasty depends on the extent of adnexal disease and the degree of postoperative adhesion formation. The adhesions can be filmy, dense, and vascular and involve the tubes and ovaries. Tubal abnormality and other pelvic disease (ie, endometriosis, fibroids) also affect the outcome. The principles of laparoscopic tuboplasty are listed in Table 14–4.

Magnification. Prior to the refinements in laparoscopy, most tubal operations were aided by an operating microscope or with magnifying loupes. These reduced tissue trauma and increased the detection of abnormalities. Magnification, which enabled the use of microsurgical instruments and fine, nonreactive sutures, was an improvement over macrosurgical techniques. The development of videolaparoscopy helped integrate minimally invasive surgery. The combination of the laparoscope and the video monitor make it possible to perform tubal microsurgery using laparoscopic instruments.

Handling fallopian tubes. The serosa of the fallopian tube is delicate and easily traumatized, especially when graspers are used to apply traction. Although laparoscopic Babcock clamps allow atraumatic manipulation of the tube, it is still possible to tear the mesosalpinx and lacerate vessels. It is preferable to use a manipulating probe, a closed grasper, or the suction-irrigator to position the tube and apply traction (Figure 14–5). If necessary, the tubal serosa should be held behind the fimbria on the antimesenteric aspect using atraumatic grasping forceps.

The fimbria are very vascular and bleed with little provocation. The bleeding is difficult to localize precisely and frequent attempts to achieve hemostasis may damage tubes. Unless a large vessel is torn, most bleeding will stop spontaneously. An injection of 3 to 5 mL of dilute Pitressin in the mesosalpinx can be used to decrease bleeding. The removal of any large clots is vital to prevent adhesion formation (Table 14–5).

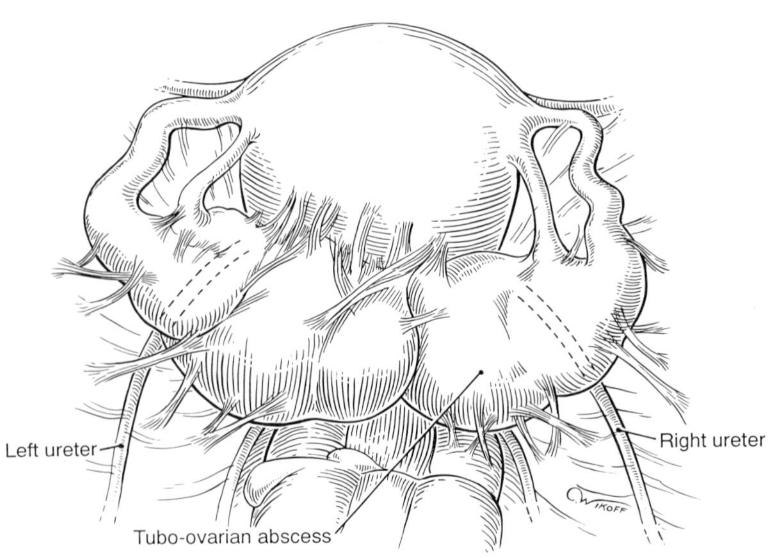

Figure 14-4 Positions of ureters are noted in the presence of bilateral TOAs.

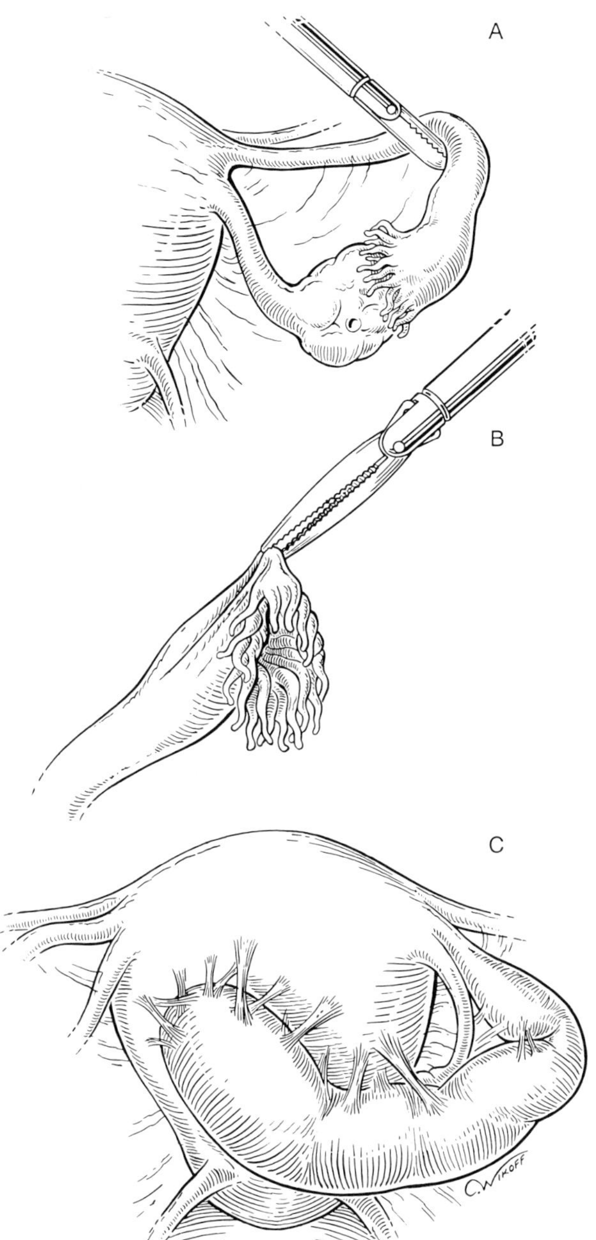

Figure 14-5 Methods are shown for positioning the fallopian tube for surgical procedures. A, Use blunt probe to pin the tube against the sidewall. B, Grasp an adhesion or peritubal cyst. C, Use the uterus as a shelf, which is useful particularly for large hydrosalpinges.

Use of sutures. Although use of sutures in the pelvis increases the risk of adhesions, in certain circumstances the judicious use of suture can improve the operative outcome. For example, during neosalpingostomy, if the defocused laser is unsuccessful in flaring back the tubes, or if the tubal mucosa is thick, a monofilament suture is recommended (ie, 4–0 PDS or similar type).

TABLE 14-5. Factors Associated With Increased Risk of Adhesion Formation

Ischemia
Reperitonealization
Sutures
Peritoneal/omental grafts
Tissue drying
Blood clots
Infection
Tissue necrosis
Tissue abrasion

Use of prophylactic antibiotics. Surgical trauma can predispose a patient with a patent salpingitis to a recurrence. Therefore, prophylactic antibiotics are recommended for any woman having reconstructive tubal surgery.

Distal Tubal Occlusion

A hydrosalpinx is caused by distal tubal occlusion and is characterized by a dilated tube filled with clear fluid. It is usually a consequence of infectious salpingitis and is associated with intrinsic tubal disease. Distal tubal obstruction also can be caused by ruptured appendix, adhesions from previous pelvic surgery, or endometriosis, all of which result in extrinsic disease and do not significantly affect the delicate tubal mucosa.

The pregnancy outcome following tuboplasty is related to many variables that reflect the severity of preexisting disease. Only a small percentage of patients achieve intrauterine pregnancy. Boer-Meisel and colleagues[16] and Schlaff and coworkers[17] analyzed several factors and found that the best pregnancy rates (77% and 80%) correlated with a normal endosalpinx and the absence of adhesions. In contrast, pregnancy rates approached zero when there were numerous dense adhesions, fixed adhesions, and a thick tubal wall. No clear pattern was associated with the risk for ectopic pregnancy. Several scoring systems have been proposed to predict the probability of conception (Table 14–6).[18,19]

To date, no randomized study has been published comparing the relative efficacy of tuboplasty by laparotomy, microsurgery, and laparoscopy (Table 14–7).[20–53] However, several studies comparing conventional surgery and microsurgery show a clear advantage to the latter.[2] The few published series suggest that pregnancy after laparoscopic tuboplasty may be comparable to that following microsurgery (Table 14–8).[54–63] Studies comparing the CO_2 laser to electrosurgery have

TABLE 14-6. Classifications of Tubal Disease

Rock et al., 1978[18]

Mild (80% pregnancy rate)
- Absent or small hydrosalpinx < 15 mm diameter
- Inverted fimbria easily recognized when patency achieved
- No significant peritubal or periovarian adhesions
- Preoperative hysterogram reveals a rugal pattern

Moderate (31% pregnancy rate)
- Hydrosalpinx 15–30 mm diameter
- Fragments of fimbria not readily identified
- Periovarian or peritubular adhesions without fixation, minimal cul-de-sac adhesions

Severe (16% pregnancy rate)
- Large hydrosalpinx > 30 mm diameter
- No fimbria
- Dense pelvic or adnexal adhesions with fixation of the ovary and tube to either the broad ligament, pelvic sidewall, omentum and/or bowel
- Obliteration of the cul-de-sac
- Frozen pelvis (adhesion formation so dense that limits of organs are difficult to define)

Boer-Meisel et al., 1986 (modified)[16]

Four questions	Four answers	Factor score
1. Is the tube wall thin?	yes	1
	no	2
2. Is the gross condition of the endosalpinx normal?	yes	1
	no	2 or 3
3. Are there many adhesions?	yes	3
	no	1 or 2
4. Are the adhesions fixed?	yes	3
	no	1 or 2

Four “yes” answers—good prognosis (77% conception rate); three “yes” answers—intermediate prognosis (21% conception rate); two “yes” answers—poor prognosis (3% conception rate).

Mage et al., 1986[19]

Factors	Scoring
Tubal patency	Partial occlusion—2; total occlusion—5
Tubal mucosa (HSG)	Normal folds—0; decreased folds—5; no folds or honeycomb—10
Tubal wall (direct exam)	Normal—0; thin —5; thick or rigid—10

Grade I, 2–5 (58.8% pregnancy rate); grade II, 7–10 (36.6% pregnancy rate); grade III, 12–15 (9.5% pregnancy rate); grade IV, 12–15 (0% pregnancy rate).

not shown a clear advantage to either method (Table 14–9).

However, the CO_2 laser can be used through the operative channel of the laparoscope as a long knife, thus avoiding another incision in the abdomen.[63]

Fimbrioplasty. Tubal phimosis can be caused by fimbrial agglutination or by adhesions that bind the fimbriated end to the ovary or cover the distal end. Intrinsic and extrinsic tubal disease affects fimbria. The goal of fimbrioplasty is to expose the fimbria to restore normal function. This is accomplished by lysing any periadnexal adhesions so that the tube is freely mobile. Chromopertubation will distend the tube, or if the tube is patent, allow observation of the ostia. The tube is immobilized either using the uterus as a shelf or by steadying its position with a blunt probe. If adhesions cover the ostia, they are incised with scissors and separated using the CO_2 laser, microscissors, fiber laser, or fine electrode tip (Figure 14–6). To deagglutinate the fimbria, a closed 3-mm forceps is inserted into the fallopian tube through the phimotic opening. The jaws of the forceps are opened within the tube; the open forceps are withdrawn. This procedure is repeated until satisfactory

TABLE 14-7. Results of Macrosurgery and Microsurgery for Tuboplasty

	N	Pregnancies	Ectopic	Follow-up
Macrosurgery				
Palmer, 1960[20]	51	35%	22.2%	
Mulligan, 1966[21]	66	30%	30%	
Garcia, 1968[22]	25	28%		
Crane, 1968[23]	34	26%	22.2%	
O'Brien, 1969[24]	83	29%	8.3%	
Young, 1970[25]	114	32.5%	16.7%	2 y
Grant, 1971[26]	217	22%	10.6%	
Lamb, 1972[27]	48	15%	42.9%	
Umezaki, 1974[28]	52	23%	17%	
Comninos, 1977[29]	30	43%	15.4%	
Rock, 1978[18]	87	28%	20.8%	
Siegler, 1979[30]	26	35%	55.6%	
Spadoni, 1980[31]	7	43%	0	
DeCherney, 1981[32]	9	22.2%		
Wallach, 1983[33]	24	20.8%		
Fayez, 1982[5]	128	35.9%		
Total	1001	28.4%		
Microsurgery				
Swolin, 1975[34]	33	46%	40%	
Marik, 1977[35]	52	23%		
Salat-Baroux, 1979[36]	42	33%	7.1%	
Siegler, 1979[30]	32	47%	26.7%	
Betz, 1980[37]	27	26%	42.9%	
Gomel, 1980[38]	72	29%		
DeCherney, 1981[32]	72	42%	13.3%	
Frantzen, 1982[39]	85	14.1%		
Hulka, 1982[40]	61	9.8%		
Fayez, 1982[5]	73	50.6%		
Verhoeven, 1983[41]	115	29%	9.4%	
Bellina, 1983[42]	56	48.2%	4.4%	
Tulandi, 1984[43]	68	28%	26.3%	
Russell, 1986[44]	72	58%	14.3%	
Donnez, 1986[45]	83	38.5%	19%	4 y
Kitchin, 1986[46]	103	38.8%	35%	
Mage, 1986[19]	76	35.5%	25.9%	
Daniell, 1986[47]	48	21%	10%	
Carey, 1987[48]	87	24%	13%	> 18 mo
Jacobs, 1988[49]	161	32%	18%	5 y
Williams, 1988[50]	69	42%	41.4%	
Schlaff, 1990[17]	95	27%	26.9%	> 2 y
Audibert, 1991[51]	211	40.8%	24%	2 y
Canis, 1991[52]	76	30.3%		
Chong, 1991[53]	34	32.4%	18.2%	
Total	1903	34.0%		

*Ectopic rate represents the proportion of total pregnancies that are extrauterine.

TABLE 14-8. **Laparotomy Versus Laparoscopy for Tubal Disease**

	N	Pregnancies	Ectopic	Follow-up
Laparotomy				
Swolin, 1975[34]	33	63%	24%	> 8 y
Rock, 1978[18]	87	28%	6%	> 4 y
Gomel, 1977[54]	41	29%	12%	> 1 y
Jansen, 1980[55]	91	18.7%	?	> 10 y
DeCherney, 1981[32]	54	44%	17%	2 y
Kelly, 1983[56]	28	11%	4.5%	1 y
Mage, 1986[19]	68	37%	9%	1.5 y
Tulandi, 1984[43]	45	24.5%	2.2%	1 y
Tulandi, 1985[57]	67	26%	4.4%	2 y
Boer-Meisel, 1986[16]	108	46.3%	38%	
Schlaff, 1990[17]	95	27%	26%	
Audibert, 1991[51]	211	40.8%	24%	2 y
Canis, 1991[52]	76	30.3%		
Total	1011	33.7%		
Laparoscopy				
Gomel, 1977[54]	9	44.4%	0	1 y
Mettler, 1979[58]	38	26%	?	> 1 y
Fayez, 1983[59]	19	10%	10%	2 y
Daniell, 1984[60]	21	24%	5%	6–18 mo
Dubuisson, 1990[61]	65	33.8%	18.2%	
Audibert, 1991[51]	55	20%	15%	2 y
Canis, 1991[52]	87	33.3%	6.9%	
McComb, 1991[62]	22	22.7%	?	> 1 y
Nezhat, 1992[63]	42	35.7%	15.4%	
Total	370	30.3%		

deagglutination of the fimbria is obtained (Figure 14–7). Gentle manipulation decreases the chance of bleeding.[64]

Neosalpingostomy. Once the laparoscope is inserted and two to three suprapubic trocars are placed, the suction-irrigator and grasping forceps can be introduced. Adhesions surrounding the tubes and ovaries are lysed using the CO_2 laser (30 to 80 W). Once the adnexa are freely mobile, the distal portion of the tube is manipulated into position with the grasper or the uterine fundus as a shelf. Fluid distention of the tube using chromopertubation allows identification of the avascular central point, which is generally the thinnest portion of the tube (Figure 14–8). A cruciate incision using the CO_2 laser or scissors creates several flaps

TABLE 14-9. **Results of CO_2 Laser and Electrosurgery by Laparoscopy for Tuboplasty**

	N	Pregnancies	Ectopic	Follow-up
Laser				
Tulandi, 1985[57]	37	29.7%	18.2%	2 y
Mage, 1986[19]	38	42.1%	18.8%	18 mo
Electrosurgery				
Tulandi, 1985[57]	30	23.3%	14.3%	2 y
Mage, 1986[19]	30	30.0%	33.3%	18 mo

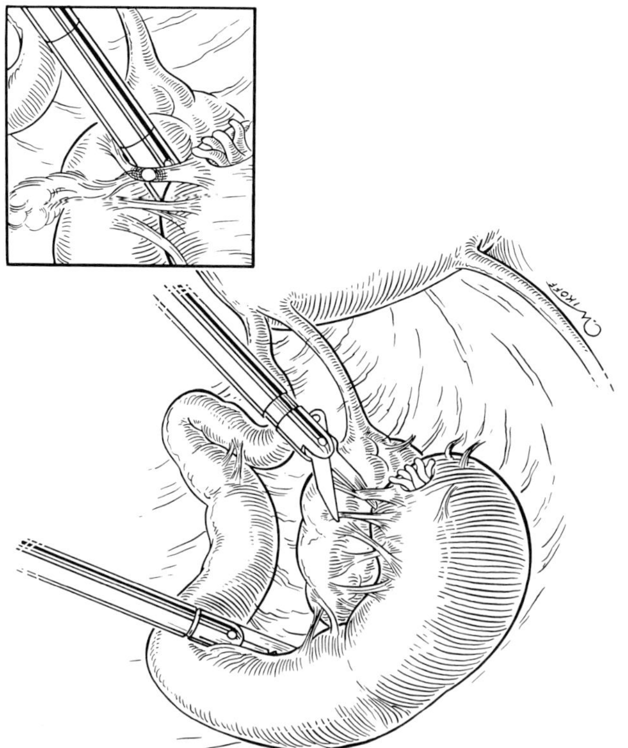

Figure 14-6 Sharp microscissors or ultrapulse CO_2 laser (*inset*) is used. The tube is under traction.

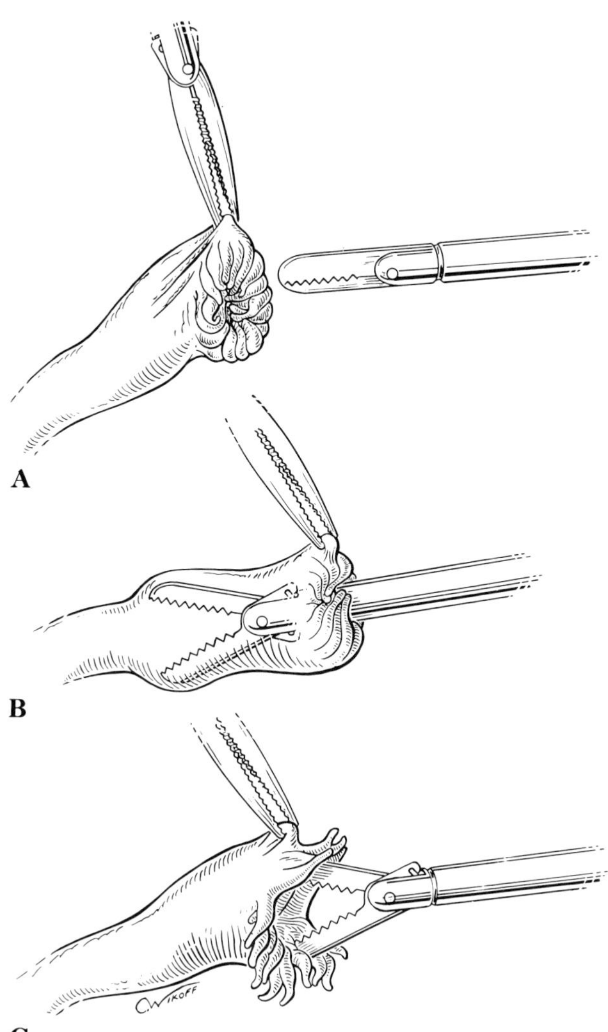

Figure 14-7 Steps in performing a fimbrioplasty. A, Introduction of grasping forceps. B, Opening forceps. C, Withdrawing forceps.

(Figure 14–9). The edges are flared back using the defocused laser (10 W; Figure 14–10). The defocused laser causes the serosa and superficial underlying tissue to shrink, thus everting the edges of the tube without suture.

Neosalpingostomy also can be performed by opening the distended end of the tube and then grasping the endosalpinx with an atraumatic grasping forceps, pulling it out and back over the tube like a sleeve.[64] The defocused laser is used to further evert the edges. If the tube is thick and does not flare back well with the laser, the edges are sutured to the tubal serosa using 4–0 PDS (Ethicon; Figure 14–11). Tubal patency is confirmed by injecting diluted indigo carmine through the cannula of the uterine manipulator. The presence of fimbrial adhesions may be assessed on close-up view of the fimbria as the dye is injected. The condition of the tubal mucosa can be evaluated by salpingoscopy.

Salpingoscopy

Until recently, it was not possible to examine the tubal mucosa endoscopically. As previously noted, the degree of tubal mucosa damage is probably the major factor in establishing a prognosis for tubal reconstructive surgery. It has been assumed that

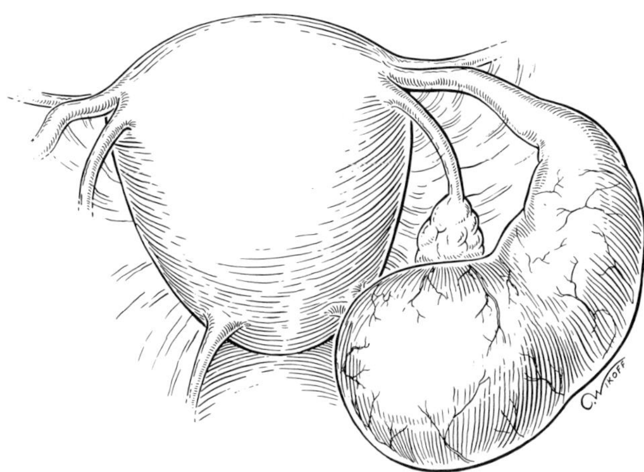

Figure 14-8 Chromopertubation is performed and an avascular central point of hydrosalpinx is identified.

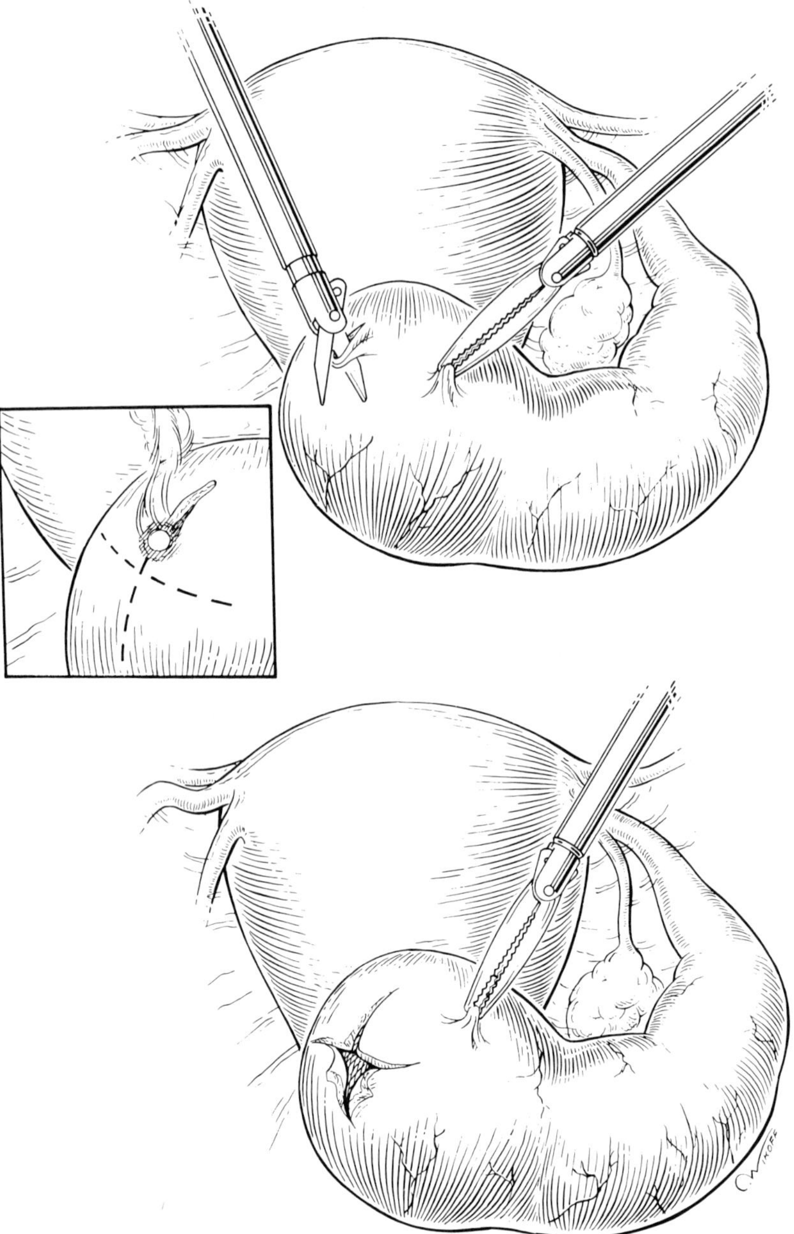

Figure 14-9 Production of cruciate incisions in distal end of tube. Sharp microscissors or ultrapulse CO_2 laser (*inset*) is used.

tubal patency on hysterosalpingogram (HSG) indicated tubal normality. Thus, the selection of patients who could benefit from tubal reconstructive surgery was based on preoperative HSG and laparoscopic appearance of the tubes. Although the mucosal folds can be outlined by HSG, the correlation between radiologic studies and endoscopy in assessing the tubal mucosa is poor.

The importance of salpingoscopy was demonstrated originally by Henry-Suchet and colleagues,[65] who examined 231 tubes during tubal microsurgery and found that lesions in the ampulla differed significantly from those predicted by HSG (Table 14–10). They found that if the tube had normal folds on HSG regardless of the presence of distal occlusion, there was agreement between the two diagnostic methods only 55% of the time. In other cases, salpingoscopy revealed various lesions such as synechiae and denuded areas that were unsuspected from HSG appearance, for a false negative rate of 45%. If the tubal mucosa seemed to have an abnormality on HSG, a normal mucosa was discovered at salpingoscopy 21% of the time. These data suggest that salpingoscopy more accurately indicates the condition of the tubal mucosa than HSG and that assessment of tubal status by salpingoscopy allows a better assessment of treatment options.

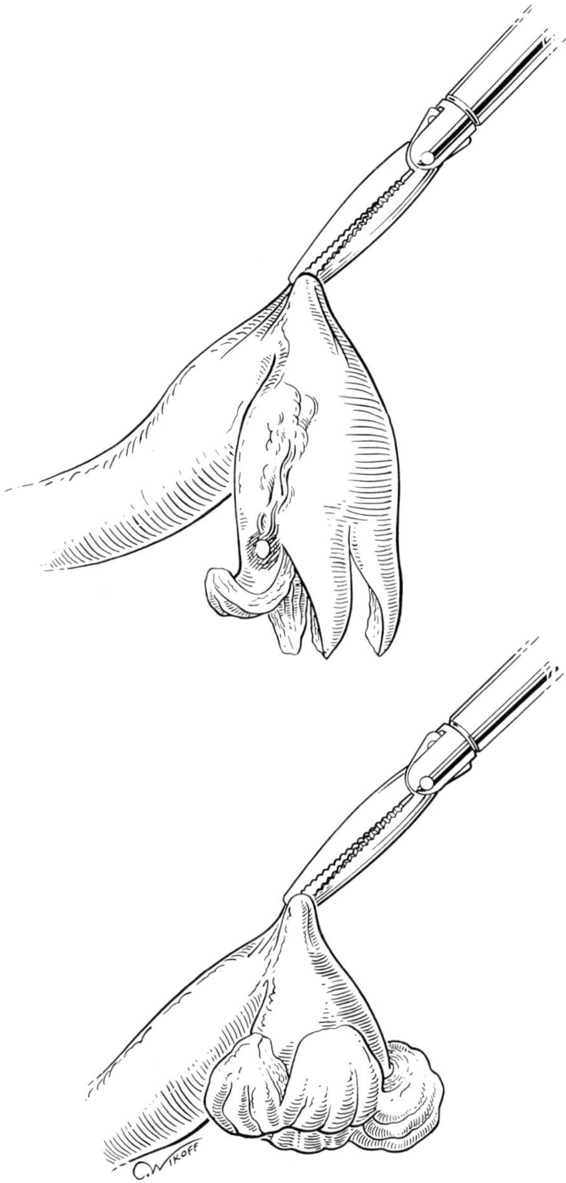

Figure 14-10 Ends of tube are everted using the defocused laser beam.

Figure 14-11 Eversion of tube with fine suture is shown.

TABLE 14-10. Salpingoscopy Compared to Hysterosalpingography

	Salpingoscopy Normal	Salpingoscopy Abnormal
HSG normal (n = 61)	58%	42%
HSG abnormal (n = 52)	39%	61%

Source: Henry-Suchet J, et al., 1985[65]

Currently, more infertility surgery is performed by laparoscopy than by laparotomy. Recently, endoscopic evaluation of the tubal mucosa during laparoscopy was described by Cornier,[66] who used a flexible bronchoscope and by Brosens and coworkers,[67] who used a specially designed rigid salpingoscope. Nezhat and colleagues[68] have successfully used a 3-mm 0-degree hysteroscope. Brosens[67] reported discrepancies between HSG diagnosis and salpingoscopic appearance of the tubal mucosa similar to those reported by Cornier.[66]

Indications. Laparoscopic salpingoscopy permits detailed examination of the ampullary portion of the tubal mucosa and is particularly useful to:

1. Detect unsuspected tubal lesions not previously identified on HSG.
2. Evaluate the extent of mucosal damage in a woman who has PID.
3. Evaluate the status of tubal mucosa in patients who have known tubal disease with or without a hydrosalpinx.
4. Decide on management of the contralateral tube in a woman with an ectopic pregnancy.
5. Examine tubes before the granulocyte immunofluorescence test.

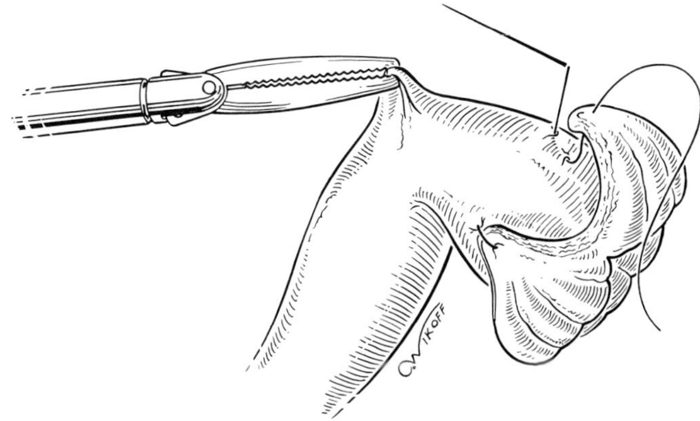

Technique. Laparoscopy is performed by introducing the laparoscope through the umbilicus and inserting the two suprapubic accessory trocars. The tube is manipulated gently with forceps applied to the antimesenteric serosal surface close to the fimbria (Figure 14–12). Then a 3-mm scope is inserted through the ipsilateral accessory trocar sleeve and gently placed in the tubal lumen. Saline is infused through the Cohen cannula (or similar device), which has been attached to the cervix. The saline infusion is an essential part of the procedure because it creates space and makes the anatomy of the mucosa fold more visible.

The distal end of the tube can be occluded with an atraumatic grasper if distention of the tube is inadequate. The scope is advanced slowly and gently under direct vision into the tubal infundibulum where the major and minor folds can be seen. In a normal tube, the folds are well formed, parallel to each other, and freely move in the distending fluid. The tubal lumen is followed into the ampulla by advancing the scope and carefully negotiating the bends. In the ampulla there are four to six major folds, each about 4 mm in height, with accessory folds arising from them. Between the major folds there are several minor folds approximately 1 mm in height. When the junction of ampulla and isthmus is reached, the major folds give way to three or four rounded folds 200 to 400 μm in height. With experience, it is usually possible to follow the lumen as far as the isthmic-ampullary junction.

Complications from this operation are rare; however, it is possible to damage the fimbriae with the forceps, causing minor bleeding or adhesion formation. The most serious complication, perforation of the tubal mucosa, may occur when the scope is advanced blindly or with unnecessary force. Occasionally, bleeding will occur at the level of the fimbria, but usually ceases spontaneously.

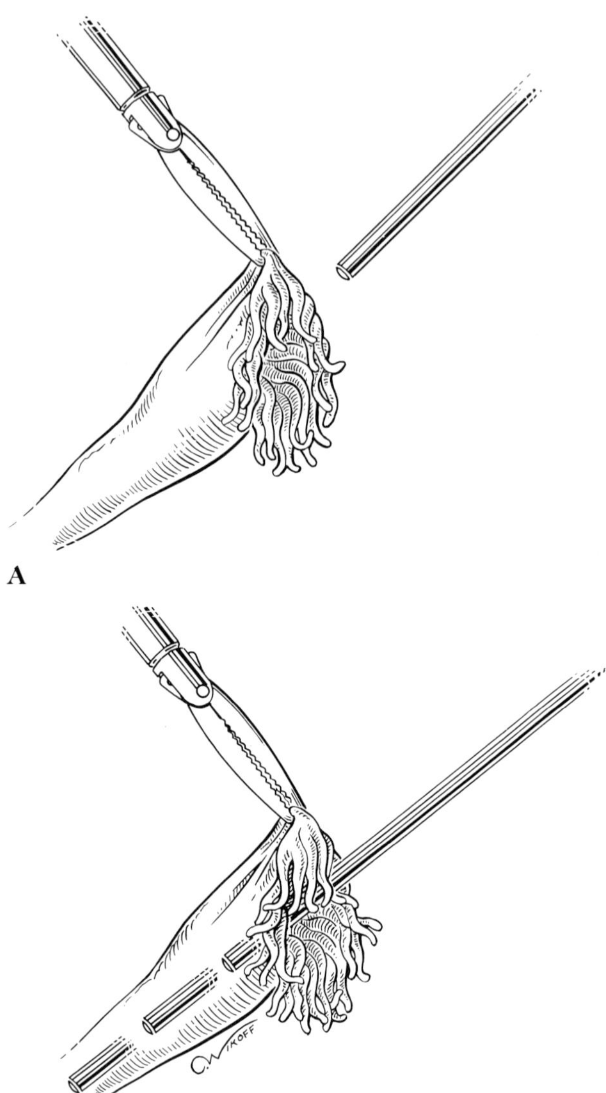

Figure 14-12 A, Salpingoscopy. Manipulation of the tube with grasping forceps and placement of salpingoscope. B, The salpingoscope is advanced under direct vision, and the tube extended with saline.

Salpingectomy

There are occasions when a fallopian tube is damaged to such an extent that its removal is indicated. Circumstances that frequently require salpingectomy include pathologic conditions such as ruptured ectopic pregnancy, more than two ectopic pregnancies in the same tube, severe tubal damage, particularly if the contralateral tube is normal, severe pelvic adhesions, pain caused by recurrent hydrosalpinx, and large hydrosalpinx or torsion with nonviability of the tube.

Salpingectomy is a relatively easy procedure, requiring those instruments commonly used to perform tubal electrocoagulation for sterilization.[69] The instruments necessary are bipolar electrocoagulator, grasping forceps, scissors, and laparoscope. A CO_2 laser can be used.

Once the patient is anesthetized, the laparoscope and 5-mm suprapubic trocars are placed, through which the graspers and bipolar electrocoagulator are inserted. Adhesions that limit mobility of the fallopian tube are lysed and it is grasped at the isthmic portion. The most proximal portion of the isthmus is coagulated and cut using either the scissors or laser (Figure 14–13). If scis-

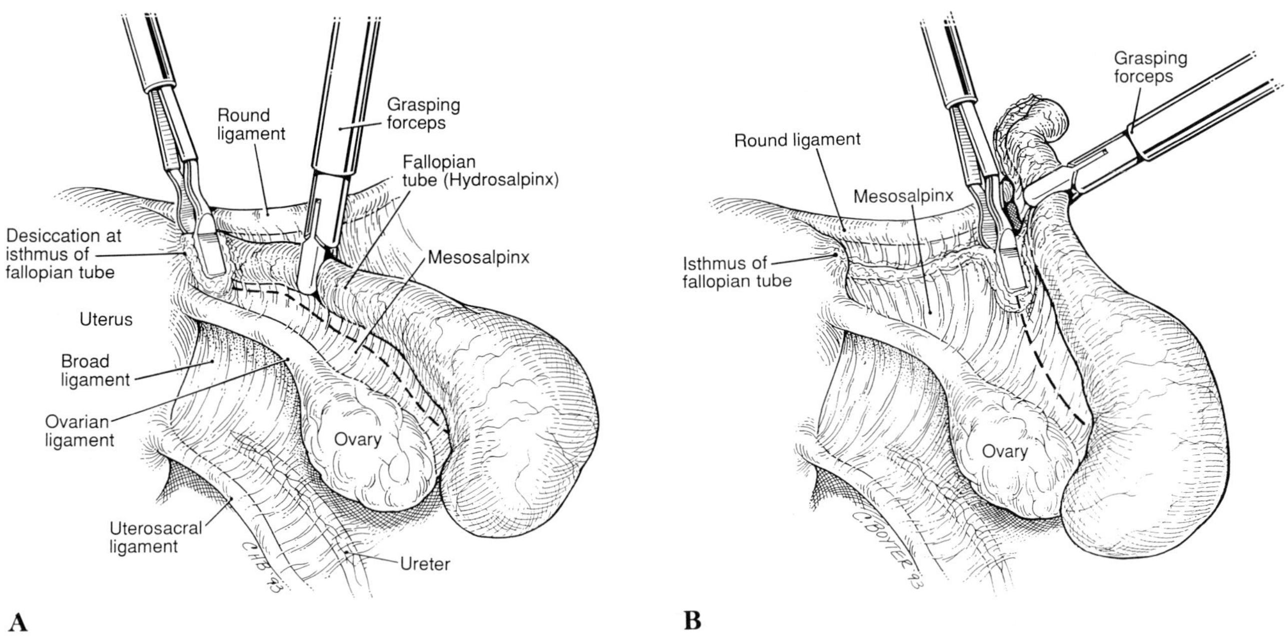

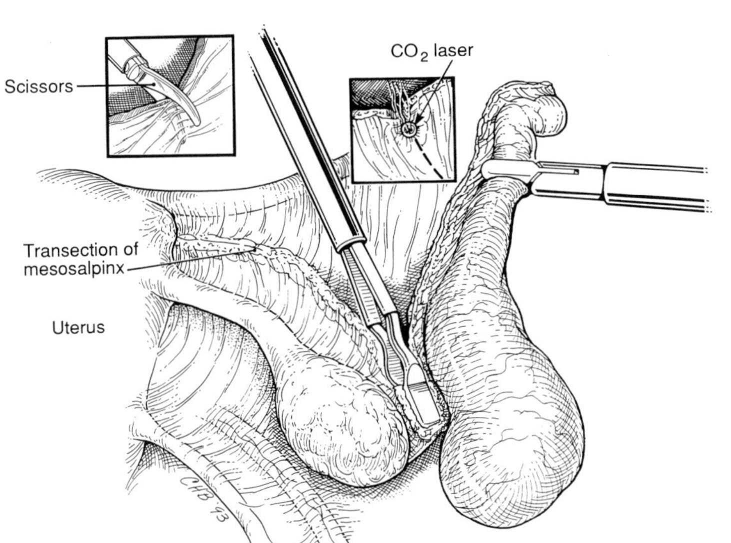

Figure 14-13 Salpingectomy using bipolar electrocoagulation for hemostasis. A, The isthmic portion of the tube is coagulated and cut close to the uterus. B, While the tube is under traction, the mesosalpinx is coagulated and cut. C, Sharp scissors (*inset*) or the ultrapulse CO_2 laser (*inset*) is used for cutting.

sors are used, the bipolar electrocoagulator must be removed and replaced with the scissors through the same secondary trocar, or a third accessory trocar is placed. The laser generally is faster and more precise than the scissors. Cutting is performed in layers so there is less chance to cut beyond the coagulated area. Once the isthmus of the tube is transected, the mesosalpinx is alternatively coagulated and cut at intervals of 1 to 2 cm in the direction of the tubo-ovarian ligament (see Figure 14–13C).[69]

Alternatives to bipolar electrocoagulation of the mesosalpinx are the automated stapling device (Endo-path ELC 35, Ethicon) and Endoloop suture (Ethicon). The stapling device is introduced through a 12-mm trocar incision. After lysing significant adhesions and mobilizing the tube, it is pulled up and put under traction. The stapler is used from the proximal to the distal end to staple and cut the tube. One to two applications are sufficient for the entire tube (Figure 14–14). Before using the Endoloop ligature, both the proximal portion of the tube and its distal attachment to the ovary (fimbria ovarica) are coagulated and cut (Figures 14–15A and B). The Endoloop is passed around the tube, and the mesosalpinx is ligated with one Endoloop and removed (Figure 14–15C). The mesosalpinx is cut above the ligature. An ade-

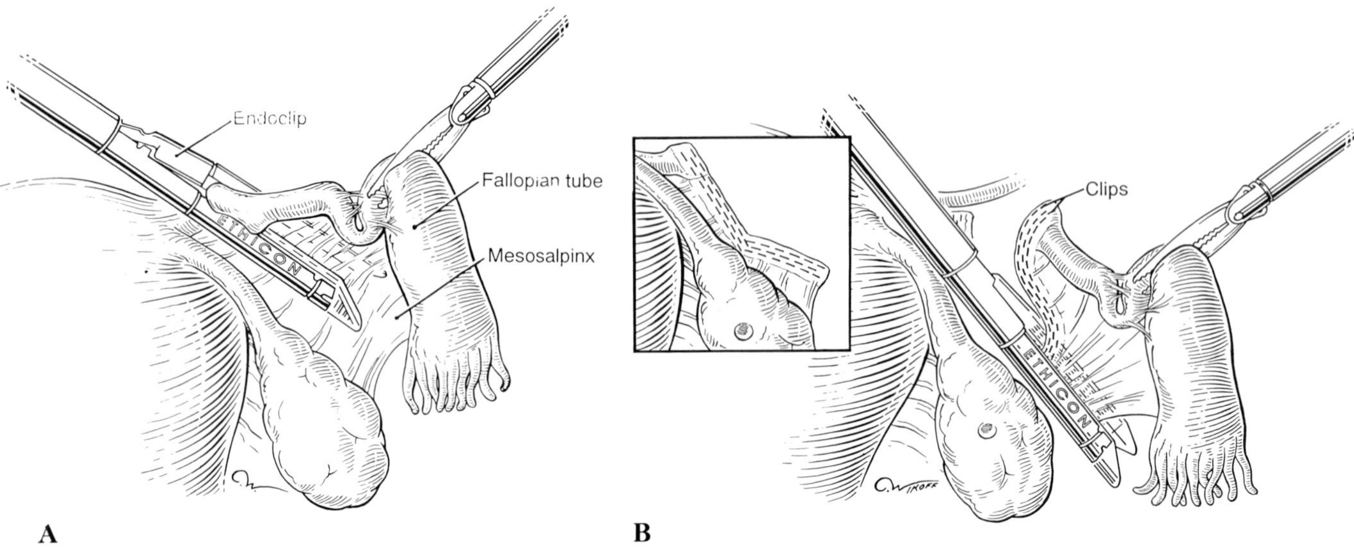

Figure 14-14 Salpingectomy using Endo-path ELC 35. A, The first application of the stapling device is to the proximal portion of the tube across the mesosalpinx. The tube is under traction. B, The second application completes the salpingectomy. *Inset*, A view of the mesosalpinx after the tube has been removed.

quate stump is left to prevent the ligature from slipping (Figure 14–15D).

Once detached, the fallopian tube is removed from the pelvis through one of the suprapubic trocar sleeves or the operating channel of the laparoscope. Removal of a larger tube (a ruptured tubal pregnancy or hydrosalpinx) may require an Endopouch (Ethicon) or another method of removal. Finally, the pelvic cavity is irrigated thoroughly. The intra-abdominal pressure is decreased to reveal any bleeding temporarily controlled by pneumoperitoneum, an important maneuver when using a stapling device.

Tubal Anastomosis

Cost containment pressures and a desire to perform less invasive surgery resulted in the continued performance of anastomosis by laparoscopy; however, the reproductive outcome after tubal anastomosis by laparoscopy has been poor. Sedbon and colleagues[70] reported five procedures performed with fibrin glue with no subsequent pregnancies. Successful tubal anastomosis depends on precise apposition of tissues to ensure and restore anatomic integrity. Fine suture material can minimize tissue reaction and excessive scar formation. Several obstacles have limited the performance of tubal anastomosis at laparoscopy. There were no laparoscopic needle-drivers available capable of manipulating 8–0 suture; it was difficult to tie suture laparoscopically and difficult to precisely align tissue.

Klink and coworkers[71] described a laser-welding technique to anastomose previously ligated rabbit uterine horns. This technique of laser welding rabbit uterine cornua and human fallopian tubes offered the theoretical advantages of reduced operating time, improved hemostasis, and precise microsurgery. More importantly, the technique presented options for performing anastomosis with the laparoscope without microsuturing. However, the results of laser welding have not been successful. Lyon and colleagues[72] compared patency in the uterine horns of 12 rats who were randomized to undergo anastomosis by argon photocoagulation or microsuture. All microsutured anastomoses were patent and contiguous with no apparent fibrosis. In contrast, four of six laser subjects had complete occlusion, and the other two had tubal stenosis. Although initially producing a satisfactory union, argon laser photocoagulation eventually proved traumatic and resulted in poor healing of the anastomosis. Other studies demonstrated that fallopian tube welding was accompanied by postoperative dehiscence.[73–75]

In Europe, the availability of fibrin glue has increased the options for joining tissues without suture. Tulandi[76] recently performed a randomized prospective study that compared microsurgical tubal anastomosis with anastomosis using fibrin glue. Postoperative adhesions and pregnancy rates did not differ between the two groups. Although this study was performed by laparotomy, it may encourage the study of fibrin glue for laparoscopic tubal anastomosis. Recently, with the development of the macro needle holder, we have

Figure 14-15 Salpingectomy by pretied Endoloop suture. After the proximal (A) and distal (B) portions of the tube are coagulated and cut, one Endoloop is placed around the mesosalpinx and tied (C). Using sharp scissors, the mesosalpinx is cut above the suture (D). An adequate stump is left so that the suture will not slip.

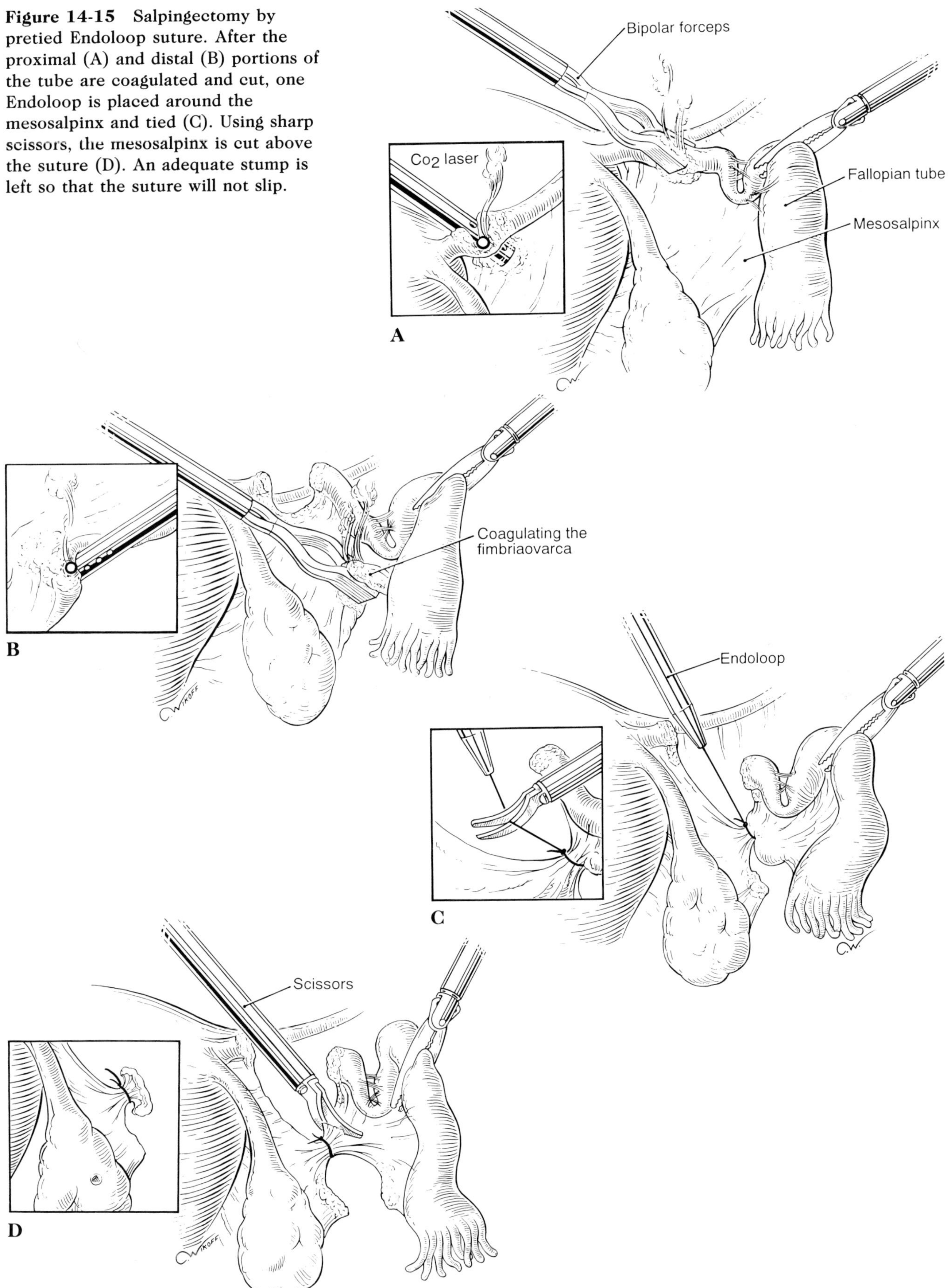

performed laparoscopic tubal anastomosis with good results.

Excising occluded portions of fallopian tubes (laser or cold knife) does not appear to alter the outcome when the tubal segments are approximated using microsurgical techniques[75,77] and some evidence indicates that the risk of adhesions may be less with laser preparation of the tubal segments prior to microsurgical anastomosis.[75,78] These authors noted improved hemostasis, precision, and enhanced preservation of normal tissue while using the laser as an adjunct to their microsurgical techniques. Scalpel preparation of the tubal ends may have a distinct advantage over CO_2 laser for interstitial-isthmic anastomoses because the CO_2 laser cannot slice the interstitial segment of tube like the scalpel.[77]

Silva and colleagues[79] described a combined laparoscopic/minilaparotomy outpatient reversal of tubal sterilization with a conception rate of 71%. Outpatient microsurgical reversal of tubal sterilization combining laparoscopy and minilaparotomy theoretically is safe. The non-microsurgical aspects are similar to tubal sterilization by minilaparotomy, which has an excellent safety record on an outpatient basis.[80–82] Importantly, the occluded portions of tube can be prepared laparoscopically by either sharp techniques or the CO_2 laser and the uterus or tubes can be delivered into the operative field so that the tubal lumen can be approximated by microsurgical procedures.

Candidates for tubal reversal by this method are less than 43 years old, are not more than 20% over ideal body weight, and have more than 2 cm of proximal fallopian tube. Original operative notes and pathology reports are reviewed to ascertain the type of sterilization procedure performed and the amount of tubal segment removed.

Patients are given one preoperative dose of prophylactic antibiotics. A single-toothed tenaculum with Cohen cannula or Humi cannula is attached to the cervix to aid in uterine manipulation and allow retrograde dye studies. Laparoscopy is performed to assess the length of distal tube present and to lyse adhesions. At this point, the procedure can be performed in one of two ways. The method described by Silva and coworkers[79] involves a minilaparotomy (5 to 6 cm) with uterine exteriorization with a Somers clamp. The adnexa can be exteriorized by traction on the utero-ovarian ligaments, if necessary. It is essential that significant adhesions are lysed laparoscopically to avoid blunt tearing of tissue. The uterus and adnexa are maintained in their exterior position by wedging gauze between the uterus and incision. During resection of the occluded tubal portions and microsurgical anastomosis, constant irrigation of the exposed organs is used to prevent desiccation. Etidocaine (1%) is injected into the peritoneal, fascial, and subcutaneous layers during closure of the abdominal wall to act as a long-acting anesthetic. Patients are monitored for 3 to 6 hours postoperatively before discharge or admitted overnight. Most patients returned to work within 1 to 2 weeks.

A similar procedure has been performed successfully in which the tubes are prepared laparoscopically using either sharp techniques, CO_2 laser, or microelectrocoagulation. Hemostasis is obtained using fine bipolar electrocoagulation. The ends of the tube are exteriorized through a minilaparotomy incision and the lumen are approximated with 8–0 or finer suture. Exteriorization is aided by using traction on the uterine manipulator (Cohen cannula or HUMI) to properly position the uterus. Patients are discharged the same day or the following morning.

The data from Silva's study[79] indicate that sterilization reversal by the laparoscopic/minilaparotomy approach compared to conventional laparotomy results in reduced cost, morbidity, and recuperation time. It can be used for 75% of sterilization reversals. Most importantly, the pregnancy rate of 71% is comparable to previously published rates using microsurgical techniques. With continuous progress in laparoscopic microinstruments, with refinement of video-cameras, and with further improvement of endoscopic surgical skills, it is possible that microsurgical tubal anastomosis will eventually be performed entirely by laparoscopy as it is now routinely performed at the Nezhat Institute for Special Pelvic Surgery. However, the success of the anastomosis should never be sacrificed for the sake of performing the procedure by laparoscopy.

References

1. Marana R, Muscatello P, Vanzetto M, et al. Laparoscopic salpingoscopy: Results. In: Marana R, Brosens A, Mancuso S, eds. *Diagnostic and Operative Gynecological Endoscopy.* Braun Druck; 1991:61.
2. Bateman BG, Nunley WC, Kitchin JD. Surgical management of distal tubal obstruction —are we making progress? *Fertil Steril.* 1987;48:523.
3. Tulandi T. Reconstructive tubal surgery by

laparoscopy. *Obstet Gynecol Surg.* 1987; 432:193.

4. Holst N, Maltau JM, Forsdahl F, Hansen LJ. Handling of tubal infertility after introduction of in vitro fertilization: changes and consequences. *Fertil Steril.* 1991;55:140.
5. Fayez JA, Suliman SO. Infertility surgery of the oviduct: comparison between macrosurgery and microsurgery. *Fertil Steril.* 1982;37:73.
6. Centers for Disease Control and Prevention. Pelvic inflammatory disease: guidelines for prevention and management. *MMWR.* 1991;40:1.
7. Walker CK, Landers DV. Pelvic abscesses: new trends in management. *Obstet Gynecol Surg.* 1991;46:615.
8. Allen LA, Schoon MG. Laparoscopic diagnosis of acute pelvic inflammatory disease. *Br J Obstet Gynecol.* 1983;90:966.
9. Jacobson L, Westrom L. Objective diagnosis of acute pelvic inflammatory disease. *Am J Obstet Gynecol.* 1969;105:1088.
10. Livengood CH, Hill BG, Addison WA. Pelvic inflammatory disease: finding during inpatient treatment of clinically severe, laparoscopy-documented disease. *Am J Obstet Gynecol.* 1992;166:519.
11. Henry-Suchet J, Soler A, Loffredo V. Laparoscopic treatment to tubo-ovarian abscesses. *J Reprod Med.* 1984;8:579.
12. Droegmueller W. Pelvic inflammatory disease: changing management concepts. *Drug Ther.* 1984; June:67.
13. Anducci JE. Laparoscopy in the diagnosis and treatment of pelvic inflammatory disease with abscess formation. *Int Surg.* 1981; 66:359.
14. Mecke H, Semm K, Freys I, et al. Pelvic abscesses: pelviscopy or laparotomy. *Gynecol Obstet Invest.* 1991;31:231.
15. Vasilev SA, Roy S, Essin DJ. Pelvic abscesses in postmenopausal women. *Surg Gynecol Obstet.* 1989;169:243.
16. Boer-Meisel ME, teVelde ER, Haffeman JDF, et al. Predicting the pregnancy outcome in patients treated for hydrosalpinx: a prospective study. *Fertil Steril.* 1986;45:23.
17. Schlaff WD, Hassiakos DK, Damewood MD, et al. Neosalpingostomy for distal tubal obstruction: prognostic factors and impact of surgical technique. *Fertil Steril.* 1990; 54:984.
18. Rock JA, Katayma KF, Martin EJ, et al. Factors influencing the success of salpingostomy techniques for distal fimbrial obstruction. *Obstet Gynecol.* 1978;52:591.
19. Mage G, Pouly JL, DeJolinieres JB, et al. A preoperative classification to predict the intrauterine and ectopic pregnancy rates after distal tubal microsurgery. *Fertil Steril.* 1986;46:807.
20. Palmer R. Salpingostomy: a critical study of 396 personal cases operated upon without polyethylene tubing. *Proc R Soc Med.* 1960;53:357.
21. Mulligan WJ. Results of salpingostomy. *Int J Fertil.* 1966;11:424.
22. Garcia CR. Surgical reconstruction of the oviduct in the infertile patient. In: Behrman SJ, Kistner RW, eds. *Progress in Infertility.* Boston: Little, Brown; 1968:255.
23. Crane M, Woodruff JD. Factors influencing the success of tuboplastic procedures. *Fertil Steril.* 1968;19:810.
24. O'Brien JR, Arenet GH, Eduljee SY. Operative treatment of fallopian tube pathology in human fertility. *Am J Obstet Gynecol.* 1969;103:520.
25. Young DE, Egan JE, Barlow JJ, et al. Reconstructive surgery for infertility at the Boston Hospital for Women. *Am J Obstet Gynecol.* 1970;108:1092.
26. Grant A. Infertility surgery of the oviduct. *Fertil Steril.* 1971;22:496.
27. Lamb EJ, Moscovitz W. Tuboplasty for infertility. *Int J Fertil.* 1972;17:53.
28. Umezaki C, Katayama KP, Jones HW. Pregnancy rates after reconstructive surgery on the fallopian tubes. *Obstet Gynecol.* 1974;43:418.
29. Comninos AC. Salpingostomy: results of two different methods of treatment. *Fertil Steril.* 1977;28:1211.
30. Siegler AM, Kontopoulos V. An analysis of macrosurgical and microsurgical techniques in the management of tuboperitoneal factor in infertility. *Fertil Steril.* 1979;32:377.
31. Spadoni LR. Tubal and peritubular surgery without magnification: an analysis. *Am J Obstet Gynecol* 1980;137:198.
32. DeCherney AH, Kase N. A comparison of treatment for bilateral fimbrial occlusion. *Fertil Steril.* 1981;35:162.
33. Wallach EE, Manara LR, Eisenberg E. Experience with 143 cases of tubal surgery. *Fertil Steril.* 1983;39:609.
34. Swolin K. Electromicrosurgery and salpingostomy: long-term results. *Am J Obstet Gynecol.* 1975;121:418.

35. Marik J. Microsurgical repair of hydrosalpinx. In: Phyllips JM, ed. *Microsurgery in Infertility.* St. Louis: St. Louis Board of Publication; 1977;19:147.
36. Salat-Baroux J, Cornier E, Rotman J: Analyse de 65 salpingostomies microchirugicales. *J Gynecol Obstet Biol Reprod.* 1979;8:647.
37. Betz G, Engel T, Penney LL. Tuboplasty comparison of the methodology. *Fertil Steril.* 1980;34:534.
38. Gomel V. Clinical results of infertility microsurgery. In: Crosignani PG, Rubin BL, eds. *Microsurgery in Female Infertility.* London: Academic Press; 1980:77.
39. Frantzen C, Schlosser HW. Microsurgery and postinfectious tubal infertility. *Fertil Steril.* 1982;38:397.
40. Hulka JF. Adnexal adhesions: a prognostic staging of fertility surgery results at Chapel Hill, North Carolina. *Am J Obstet Gynecol.* 1982;144:141.
41. Verhoeven HC, Berry H, Frantzen C, et al. Surgical treatment for distal tubal occlusion: a review of 167 cases. *J Reprod Med.* 1983;28:293.
42. Bellina JH. Microsurgery of the fallopian tube with the carbon dioxide laser: analysis of 230 cases with a two-year follow-up. *Laser Surg Med.* 1983;3:255.
43. Tulandi T, Farag R, McInnes RA, et al. Reconstructive surgery of hydrosalpinx with and without the carbon dioxide laser. *Fertil Steril.* 1984;42:839.
44. Russell JB, DeCherney AH, Laufer N, et al. Neosalpingostomy: comparison of 24 and 72 month follow-up time show increased pregnancy rate. *Fertil Steril.* 1986;45:296.
45. Donnez J, Casanas-Roux F. Prognostic factors of fimbrial microsurgery. *Fertil Steril.* 1986;46:200.
46. Kitchin JD, Nunley WC, Bateman BG. Surgical management of distal tubal occlusion. *Am J Obstet Gynecol.* 1986;155:524.
47. Daniell JF, Diamond MP, McLaughlin DS, et al. Clinical results of terminal salpingostomy with the use of the CO_2 laser: report of the intraabdominal laser study group. *Fertil Steril.* 1986;45:175.
48. Carey M, Brown S. Infertility surgery for pelvic inflammatory disease: success rates after salpingolysis and salpingostomy. *Am J Obstet Gynecol.* 1987;156:296.
49. Jacobs LA, Thie J, Patton PE, et al. Primary microsurgery for postinflammatory tubal infertility. *Fertil Steril.* 1988;50:855.
50. Williams KM, Griffin WT. Distal tuboplasty: is it appropriate? *South Med J.* 1988;81:872.
51. Audibert F, Hedon B, Arnal F, et al. Therapeutic strategies in tubal infertility with distal pathology. *Hum Reprod.* 1991;6:1439.
52. Canis M, Mage G. Pouly JL, et al. Laparoscopic distal tuboplasty: report of 87 cases and a 4 year experience. *Fertil Steril.* 1991; 46:616.
53. Chong AP. Pregnancy outcome in neosalpingostomy by the Cuff vs Bruhat technique using the carbon dioxide laser. *J Gynecol Surg.* 1991;7:207.
54. Gomel V. Salpingostomy by laparoscopy. *J Reprod Med.* 1977;18:265.
55. Jansen RPS. Surgery-pregnancy time interval after salpingolysis, unilateral salpingostomy, and bilateral salpingostomy. *Fertil Steril.* 1980;34:222.
56. Kelly RW, Roberts DK. Experience with the carbon dioxide laser in gynecologic microsurgery. *Am J Obstet Gynecol.* 1983; 145:585.
57. Tulandi T, Vilos GA. A comparison between laser surgery and electrosurgery for bilateral hydrosalpinx: a 2 year followup. *Fertil Steril.* 1985;44:846.
58. Mettler L, Giesel H, Semm K. Treatment of female infertility due to tubal obstruction by operative laparoscopy. *Fertil Steril.* 1979;32:384.
59. Fayez JA. An assessment of the role of operative laparoscopy in tuboplasty. *Fertil Steril.* 1983;39:476.
60. Daniell JF, Herbert CM. Laparoscopic salpingostomy utilizing the CO_2 laser. *Fertil Steril.* 1984;41:558.
61. Dubuisson JB, DeJolinieres JB, Aubriot FX, et al. Terminal tuboplasties by laparoscopy: 65 consecutive cases. *Fertil Steril.* 1990;54:401.
62. McComb PF, Paleologou A. The intussusception salpingostomy technique for the therapy of distal oviductal occlusion at laparoscopy. *Obstet Gynecol.* 1991;78:443.
63. Nezhat C, Nezhat F, Nezhat C. Operative laparoscopy (minimally invasive surgery): state of the art. *J Gynecol Surg.* 1992;8:111–141.
64. Gomel V. *Microsurgery in Female Infertility.* Boston: Little, Brown; 1983:141.
65. Henry-Suchet J, Loffredo V, Tesquier L, et al. Endoscopy of the tube (tuboscopy): its prognostic value for tuboplasties. *Acta Eur Fertil.* 1985;16:139.

66. Cornier E. L'amullosalpingoscopie per-coelioscopique. *J Gynecol Obstet Biol Reprod.* 1985;14:459.
67. Brosens IA, Broeck W, Delattin P, et al: Salpingoscopy: a new preoperative diagnostic tool in tubal infertility. *Br J Obstet Gynaecol.* 1987;94:760.
68. Nezhat F, Winer WK, Nezhat C. Fimbrioscopy and salpingoscopy in patients with minimal to moderate pelvic endometriosis. *Obstet Gynecol.* 1990;75:15.
69. Nezhat C, Nezhat F, Winer W. Salpingectomy via laparoscopy: a new surgical approach. *J Laparosc Surg.* 1991;1:91.
70. Sedbon E, Delajolinieres JB, Boudouris O, et al. Tubal desterilization through exclusive laparoscopy. *Hum Reprod.* 1989;4:158.
71. Klink F, Grosspietzsch R, von Klitzing L, et al. Animal in vivo studies and in vitro experiments with human tubes for end-to-end anastomotic operation by a CO_2 laser technique. *Fertil Steril.* 1978;30:100.
72. Lyon DR, Vontver LA, Patton DL, et al. A comparison between argon laser and microsuture anastomosis of the rat uterine horn. *Fertil Steril.* 1987;47:329.
73. Baggish MS, Chong AP. Carbon dioxide laser microsurgery of the uterine tube. *Obstet Gynecol.* 1981;58:111.
74. Fayez JA, McComb JS, Harper MA. Comparison of tubal surgery with the CO_2 laser and the unipolar microelectrode. *Fertil Steril.* 1983;40:476.
75. Choe JK, Dawood MY, Bardawil WA, et al. Clinical and histologic evaluation of laser reanastomosis of the uteri tube. *Fertil Steril.* 1984;41:755.
76. Tulandi T. Effects of fibrin sealant on tubal anastomosis and adhesion formation. *Fertil Steril.* 1991;56:136.
77. Chong AP, Pepi M, Lashgari M. Pregnancy outcome in microsurgical anastomosis using cold knife versus CO_2 laser. *J Gynecol Surg.* 1989;5:99.
78. Choe JK, Dawood MY, Andrews AH. Conventional versus laser reanastomosis of rabbit ligated uterine horns. *Obstet Gynecol.* 1983;61:689.
79. Silva PD, Schapes AM, Meisch JK, et al. Outpatient microsurgical reversal of tubal sterilization by a combined approach of laparoscopy and minilaparotomy. *Fertil Steril.* 1991;55:696.
80. Penfield AF. Minilaparotomy for female sterilization. *Obstet Gynecol.* 1979;54:184.
81. Uchida HL. Uchida tubal sterilization. *Am J Obstet Gynecol.* 1975;121:153.
82. Osathanondh V. Suprapubic minilaparotomy, uterine elevation technique: simple, inexpensive and outpatient procedure for interval female sterilization. *Contraception.* 1974;10:251.

15

Uterine Surgery

Benign diseases of the uterus are encountered commonly in gynecologic practice and account for a large proportion of laparotomies and hysterectomies. Most of these procedures can be performed laparoscopically, with results equivalent to laparotomy, shorter hospitalization, and financial savings. This chapter describes laparoscopic myomectomy, treatment of adenomyosis and the noncommunicating rudimentary uterine horn, uterine suspension, and hysterectomy.

Myomectomy

Fibroids are the most common uterine neoplasm, affecting approximately 20% to 25% of women of reproductive age.[1,2] Fibroids arise from the benign transformation and proliferation of a single smooth muscle cell. The growth and development of myomas are influenced by many factors, some of which are not well defined. Increased estrogen stimulation alone or acting synergistically with growth hormone or human placental lactogen appear to be the major growth regulators. In contrast, progesterone appears to inhibit the growth of fibroids,[1] although some evidence indicates that under certain circumstances it can promote their growth.[3]

The severity of symptoms associated with uterine leiomyomas depends on the number of tumors, their size, and location. They may cause abdominal pressure, urinary frequency, or constipation or alter blood flow to the uterus and endometrium, resulting in menorrhagia. Uterine leiomyomas are seldom the only cause of infertility, but data from several studies demonstrate a link between fibroids, fetal wastage, and premature delivery.[1] Indications for treatment are summarized (Table 15-1).

Preoperative Evaluation

In women with menorrhagia, the hematocrit is used to assess the degree of anemia. Patients with large broad ligament fibroids may require an intravenous pyelogram to search for ureteral obstruction. Periodic pelvic and ultrasound examinations help monitor the growth rate of asymptomatic leiomyomas.

Factors such as the size, number, and location of leiomyomas will influence the decision to perform a myomectomy by laparotomy, hysterectomy, or laparoscopy. Submucous fibroids can be detected by ultrasound, hysterosalpingography, or hysteroscopy. Small intramural myomas may be palpated during laparotomy and missed at laparoscopy. Therefore, a vaginal ultrasound should be performed preoperatively.[4,5]

Laparoscopically Assisted Myomectomy (LAM), Laparoscopic Myomectomy (LM), and Myomectomy by Laparotomy

Patients with uterine myoma who desire future fertility present a challenge to most physicians who attempt a laparoscopic approach. The risk of a future uterine rupture is a major concern following any operation involving the myometrium.[6] The difficulties of adequately closing all layers laparoscopically and using electrocoagulation for hemostasis may contribute to the risk of uterine rupture.[7,8]

TABLE 15-1 Indications for Myomectomy

Menometrorrhagia and anemia
Pelvic pain and pressure
Enlarging leiomyoma and possibility of neoplasia
Associated fetal wastage or infertility
Gestational size more than 12 wks and inability to evaluate the adnexae
Obstructed ureter

Uteroperitoneal fistulas may follow laparoscopic myomectomy because meticulous laparoscopic approximation of all layers is impossible. The use of electrocoagulation for hemostasis inside the uterine defect may also increase the risk of uteroperitoneal fistula formation.

Postoperative adhesions increase when sutures are placed in the serosal layer.[7,9] A single uterine incision for removal of multiple leiomyomas and subserosal approximation of the uterine defect is advised.

A combination of laparoscopy and minilaparotomy may reduce some of these problems. The simpler procedure and reduced operative time will enable more gynecologists to apply this technique. The uterine closure also is improved when a minilaparotomy is used for conventional suturing in two or three layers, thereby decreasing the possibility of uterine dehiscence, fistulas, and adhesions. Pelvic observation during the laparoscopic portion of the procedure allows the diagnosis and treatment of associated endometriosis or adhesions.

As a safe alternative to LM, LAM is a less technically difficult procedure and may require less time to complete. A decrease in operative time results from removing the myomas from the abdomen through a minilaparotomy incision. Further, the risk of uterine rupture is lowered by suturing the uterine defect in layers and avoiding excessive electrocoagulation. These considerations are summarized (Table 15-2).

The decision to proceed with LAM usually is made in the operating room after the diagnostic laparoscopy and treatment of associated pathology are completed. The criteria for LAM are myoma greater than 5 cm or numerous myomas requiring extensive morcellation, deep intramural myoma, and removal that requires uterine repair with sutures.

Charts from 143 patients who had either myomectomy by laparotomy (22; 15.3%), LM (64; 44.7%), or LAM (57; 39.8%) were evaluated.[5] The 22 myomectomies by laparotomy were performed before the development of the LAM technique. The data are summarized (Table 15-3). The leiomyoma weight was greater in the LAM than LM group ($P < .05$). LAM replaced myomectomy by laparotomy, patient selection criteria were comparable, and the myoma weights of these two groups were similar.

The mean estimated blood loss of the LAM and laparotomy groups was not different. In contrast, blood loss among the LM patients was significantly

TABLE 15-2 Results of Types of Myomectomy

Studied Parameter	LAM (57) mean ± SEM	LM (64) mean ± SEM	Lap (22) mean ± SEM	P(LM)* P(Lap)†
Leiomyoma weight (g)	247 ± 30.1	58 ± 7.16	337 ± 77.4	P(LM) < .00001 P(Lap) ± .27
Uterine size (wks)	12 ± 26	8 ± 14	10 ± 24	
Operative time (min)	127 ± 7.62	136 ± 9.6	134 ± 9.95	P(LM) = .36 P(Lap) = .59
Blood loss (mL)	267 ± 54.4	143 ± 35.6	245 ± 56.1	P(LM) = .0068 P(Lap) = .78
Postoperative hospital stay (days)	1.28	0.91	3.3 ± 0.39	P(LM) = .0141 P(Lap) = .00004
Days to resume normal activity	12.2	11.2	39.2	P(LM) = .43 P(Lap) < .0001
Days for complete "100%" recovery	23.1	20.9	70.0	P(LM) = .41 P(Lap) = .00002

*P(LM) compares LAM and LM.
†P (Lap) compares LAM and myomectomy by laparotomy.
LAM, laparoscopically assisted myomectomy; LM, laparoscopic myomectomy.

TABLE 15-3 Comparison of Hysterectomy, Abdominal Myomectomy, and Laparoscopic Myomectomy for the Management of Symptomatic Leiomyomas

	Hysterectomy	Abdominal Myomectomy	LM
Degree of difficulty	Low	Moderate	High
Patient age	>45 y	Childbearing	>45 y
Recurrence (%)	None	10–15	10–15
Blood loss	<500 mL	Occasionally > 500 mL	<500 mL
Postoperative adhesion formation	Minimal	>30%	>30%
Postoperative hospitalization (days)	3–4	3–4	1–2
Type of myoma	All types	Intramural, subserosal, pedunculated	Subserosal, pedunculated
Uterine rupture	None	1%	Risk of uteroperitoneal fistula

lower and may be attributed to the smaller leiomyomas (see Table 15-3). Previous studies[7,10] have underscored the need to decrease the operative time of LM. Although subserosal myomas less than 5 cm can be managed easily laparoscopically, larger and intramural lesions require prolonged morcellation and laparoscopic suturing of the uterine defect. The largest reported myomas removed by laparoscopy were 15 to 16 cm[7,10] and one group reported that 10 cm was their limit.[11] Both laparoscopic morcellation and myometrial suturing are difficult and prolong operations. LAM, with conventional morcellation and suturing through the minilaparotomy incision, reduces the duration of the operation and the need for extensive laparoscopic experience. Similar mean operating times for LM and LAM techniques were observed despite larger myomas and their intramural positions, adjunctive laparoscopy, and the smaller incisions of the LAM group (see Table 15-2).

Hospitalization was longer for the patients who underwent myomectomy by laparotomy ($P < .05$) compared to both LAM and LM groups. When comparing the hospitalization time of the LAM and LM patients, the LAM group was longer ($P(\text{LM}) = .014$). This may be explained by the initial reluctance of some physicians to discharge LAM patients on the day of surgery or on the first postoperative day. After the initial 10 to 15 cases, all women underwent LAM on an outpatient basis. In fact, by removing the initial 15 cases from the LAM group, the mean hospital stay drops to 1.06 days, a time period not statistically different from the LM group.

The comparison of postoperative recovery time is important between the LAM and LM groups. Here, despite the differences in size and location of myoma, the recovery time can be compared because of the different incisions. The time elapsed before patients resumed work or regular activity is similar ($P > .05$). Introducing a 4-cm incision in the LAM group only slightly prolonged ($P > .05$) the subjectively perceived time for the women to achieve 100% recovery.

Three major objectives of LAM are: minimizing blood loss, preventing postoperative adhesions, and maintaining uterine wall integrity.

Minimizing blood loss. Significant intraoperative blood loss can occur during the excision of subserosal and intramural leiomyomas. Depending on the tumor size and location, preoperative autologous blood donation is suggested. Patients are counseled regarding the consequences of intraoperative and postoperative bleeding and the possible need for a laparotomy. For anemic patients, preoperative treatment with gonadotropin-releasing hormone (GnRH) may enable restoration of a normal hematocrit, decrease the size of the myoma,[12] and reduce the need for transfusion.[13] Intraoperatively, the use of dilute vasopressin helps to minimize blood loss. Vertical uterine incisions bleed less than transverse incisions,[1] and pneumoperitoneum seems to decrease intraoperative bleeding.

Preventing postoperative adhesions. Although myomectomy is performed to preserve fertility, postoperative adhesion formation often jeopardizes this goal. Several procedures can minimize postoperative adhesions. Single, vertical, anterior, and midline uterine incisions are least likely to

TABLE 15-4 Incidence of Adhesion Formation after Laparoscopic Myomectomy with or without Use of Suture

	No Suture Used				Suture Used			
Leiomyoma Size	**0***	**1**	**2**	**3**	**0**	**1**	**2**	**3**
<3 cm	18/21	3/21	0/21	0/21	N/A	N/A	N/A	N/A
>3 cm	10/16	5/16	1/16	0/16	0/19	4/19	12/19	5/19

*Adhesion score: 0, no adhesions; grade 1, filmy and nonvascular; grade 2, thick and nonvascular; grade 3, thick, vascular, and bowel.
N/A, suture was not used for myomas < 3 cm in size.

cause adhesions.[14] Although sutures predispose patients to adhesions, they are often necessary to close the uterine defect (Table 15-4).[7] While there are several adhesion barriers available or currently under development, none have proven effective.[15,16]

Maintaining uterine wall integrity. Uterine rupture following myomectomy is rare, accounting for about 2% of all pregnancy-related uterine ruptures.[17] Inadequate approximation of the uterine wall and poor healing[8] predispose patients to uterine rupture.

Second-look laparoscopies performed on post-myomectomy patients who had pedunculated and superficial subserosal myomas show complete uterine healing. In contrast, intramural and deep subserosal myomas are associated with evidence of granulation tissue and indentation of the uterus proportional to the size of the leiomyoma removed, unless sutures have been used to approximate the edges. The use of sutures is associated with a higher rate of adhesions (see Table 15-4).[7] In patients with intramural fibroids and significant uterine wall defects, an unacceptably high rate of endometrial-serosal fistula formation occurs. At present, the meticulous suturing made possible during laparotomy is not possible at laparoscopy.

During an abdominal myomectomy, if the endometrial cavity is entered or a submucous myoma or large intramural myomas are removed, a patient who subsequently becomes pregnant should undergo a cesarean delivery.[7] Similar guidelines should be followed for laparoscopic myomectomies. Currently, women with large intramural fibroids should be managed laparoscopically only if they no longer wish to have children.

Preoperative Therapy with Gonadotropin-Releasing Hormone

Preoperative GnRH agonists have been used to decrease myomas and intraoperative blood loss,[4,18] simplify leiomyoma removal,[19] and treat severe anemia.[20] Some studies show a decrease in intraoperative blood loss following a course of GnRH therapy,[18] but others do not.[4] GnRH therapy is expensive, is associated with hypoestrogenic side effects,[12] and possibly causes an increased risk of fibroid recurrence.[4] Preoperatively, GnRH is indicated mainly to arrest menorrhagia and is given to women who can be managed with less invasive surgery such as hysteroscopic myomectomy.

Laparoscopic Myomectomy

Nezhat and colleagues have reported data on myomectomy in 137 women from whom 196 leiomyomas were removed.[7] The fibroids ranged in size from 2 to 14 cm. The operations lasted from 50 to 160 minutes (mean 116 minutes). Estimated blood loss was between 10 and 600 mL, and 2 women received transfusions because of intraoperative blood loss. The postoperative hospital stay ranged from 7 to 48 hours, with a mean of 19.6 hours.

Excision of myomas. Essential instruments include a CO_2 laser or other instrument for cutting, bipolar Kleppinger forceps, and clawed grasping forceps. In addition, dilute vasopressin (1 IU in 100 mL lactated Ringer's) helps control uterine bleeding.

Pedunculated leiomyomas are easiest to remove by coagulating and cutting the stalk. Dilute vasopressin (3 to 5 mL) is injected into the base of the stalk, at the junction of the uterine fundus. The pedicle is coagulated with bipolar forceps and cut, or cut and coagulated with the CO_2 laser (40 to 80 W, superpulse or ultrapulse mode). Bleeding points are coagulated with bipolar forceps.

Depending on the size and depth of penetration into the myometrium, removing subserosal and intramural fibroids may require more manipulation to control bleeding. Dilute vasopressin is injected in multiple sites between the myometrium and the fibroid capsule (Figure 15-1). An incision is made

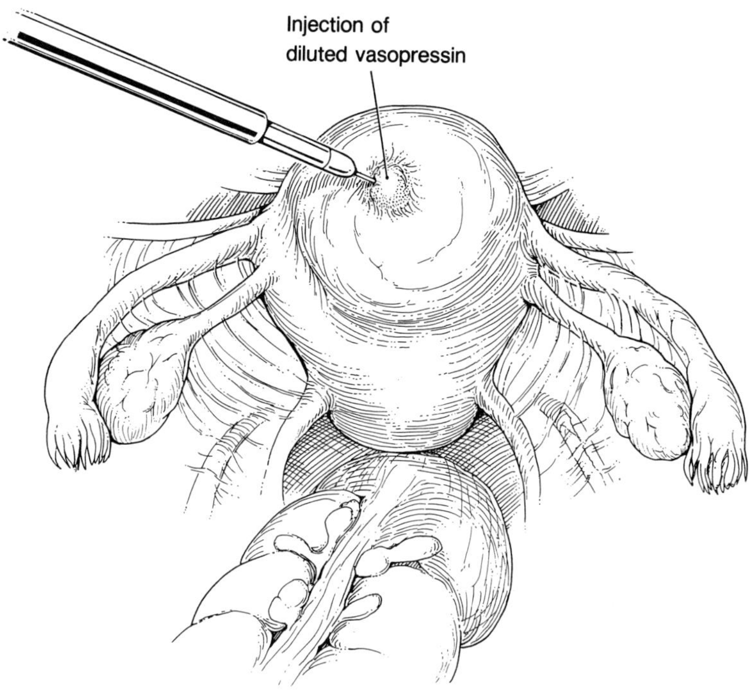

Figure 15-1 The base of the fibroid is injected with dilute vasopressin.

on the serosa overlying the leiomyoma using the CO_2 laser (superpulse or ultrapulse mode) (Figure 15-2), a monopolar electrode, or fiber laser. The incision is extended until it reaches the capsule. The myometrium retracts as the incision is made, exposing the tumor. Two grasping toothed forceps hold the edges of the myometrium and the suction-irrigator is used as a blunt probe, to shell the leiomyoma from its capsule. A myoma screw is inserted into the fibroid to apply traction while the suction-irrigator is used as a blunt dissector (Figures 15-3 and 15-4). The CO_2 laser is used to further dissect capsular attachments. Vessels are electrocoagulated before being cut. After complete myoma removal, the uterine defect is irrigated. Bleeding points are identified and con-

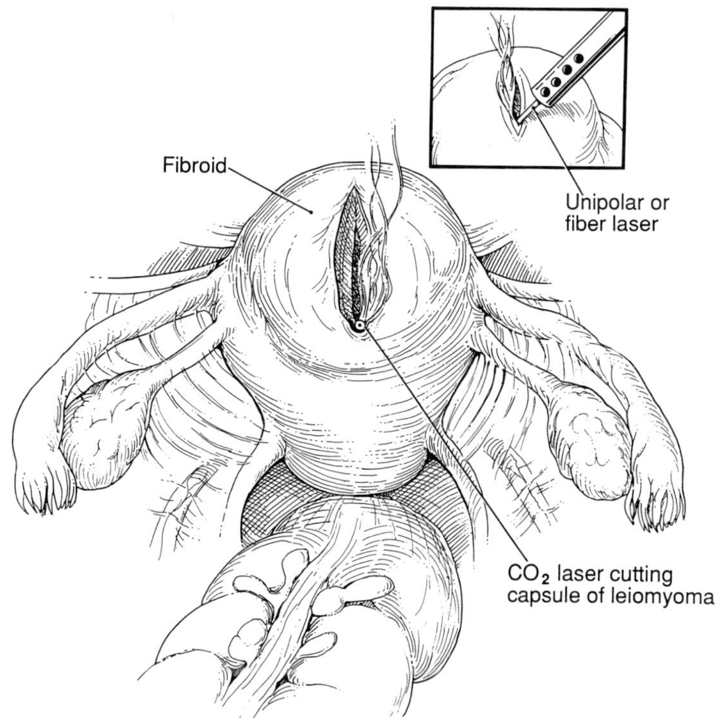

Figure 15-2 Incision of the myometrium to remove an intramural fibroid.

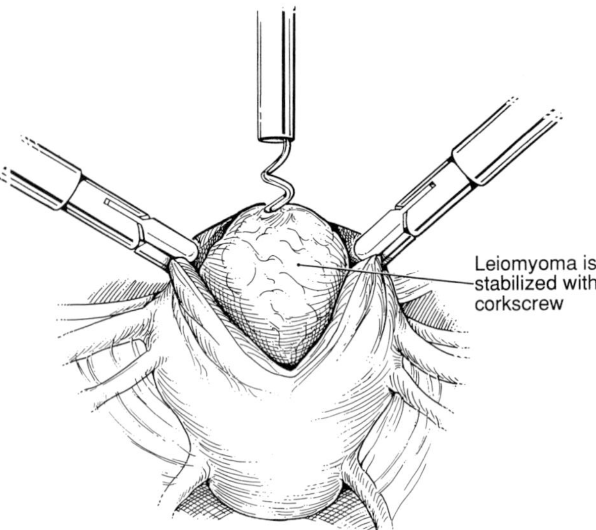

Figure 15-3 Use of a myoma screw to facilitate fibroid excision.

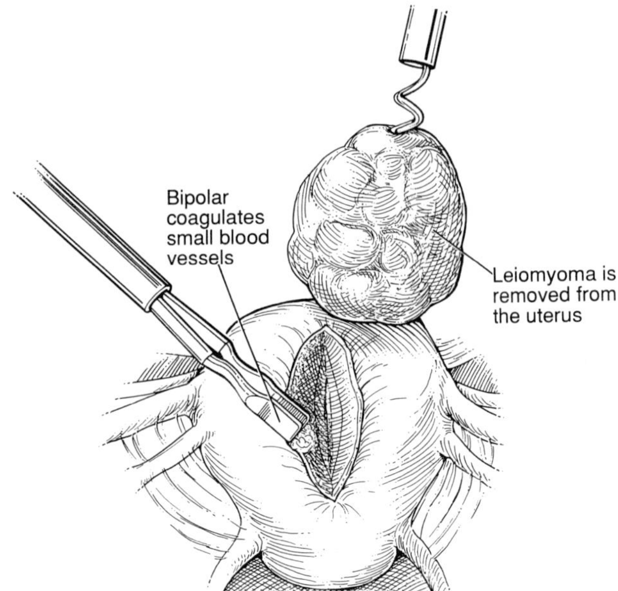

Figure 15-5 Obtaining hemostasis using bipolar forceps.

trolled with electrocoagulation (Figure 15-5). If the leiomyoma is small and the patient does not desire future fertility, the edges of the uterine defect are approximated by coagulating the myometrium without suturing (Figure 15-6).

If the defect is deep or large, the myometrium and serosa are approximated using 4–0 polydioxanone or 1–0 polyglactin suture on a straight or curved needle. The repair mainly involves the serosal and subserosal layers and can be accomplished in one layer. The sutures are applied in 1 cm increments using extracorporeal or intracorporeal knot tying (Figures 15-7 and 15-8). Following repair, the uterine surface is irrigated with warmed lactated Ringer's (Figure 15-9) and Interceed (Johnson & Johnson) is applied over the suture line. Spraying 10,000 IU of thrombin over the Interceed is used for further hemostasis. Suturing is limited because of the high incidence of postoperative adhesions (see Table 15-4). In contrast, the defect heals better and with less uterine muscle deformity when the edges are approximated.

Even under ideal circumstances, laparoscopic closure of the myometrial defect is difficult. Approximating the edges of the defect often requires a considerable amount of force. Through the laparoscope, this degree of tension is difficult to achieve without tearing the tissue. Often, the re-

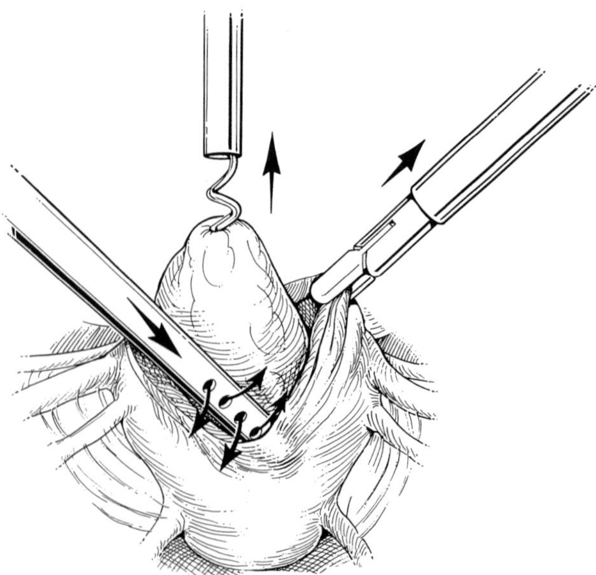

Figure 15-4 Fibroid removal using the suction-irrigator as a blunt probe and for hydrodissection.

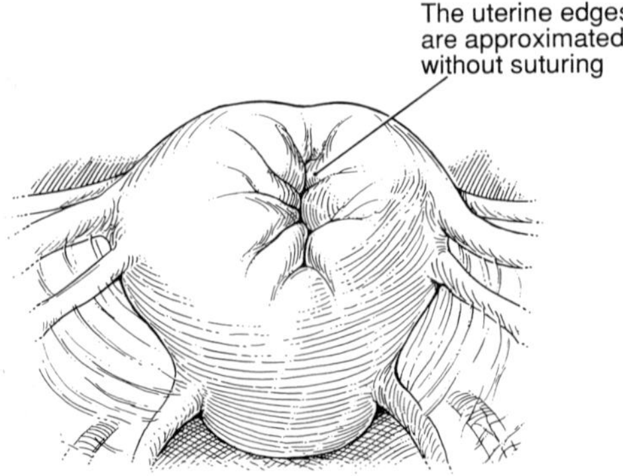

Figure 15-6 Uterine serosa is approximated without suturing.

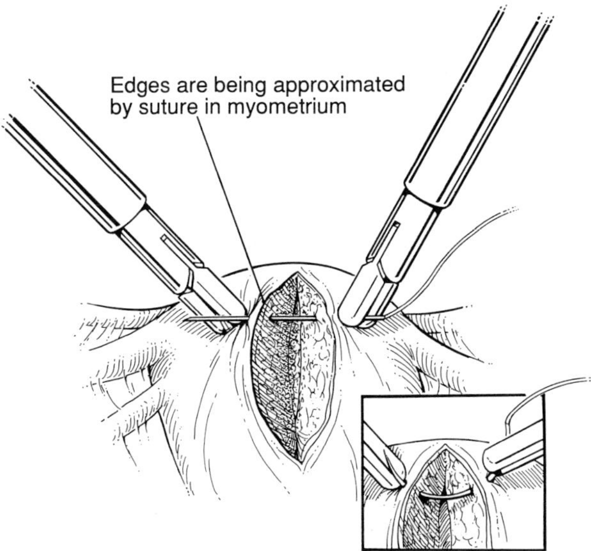

Figure 15-7 Repair of uterine defect using straight or curved needle.

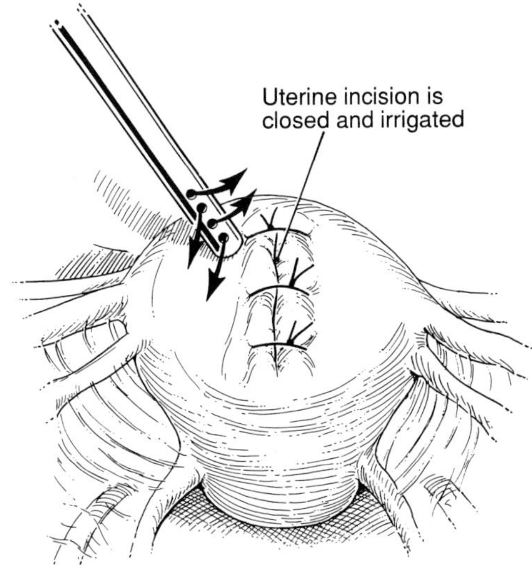

Figure 15-9 Uterine incision is closed and irrigated.

sult is increased bleeding or a defect with significant gaps. This aspect of the procedure is tedious and may lead to endometrial-serosal fistula formation. Precise suturing of several layers is almost impossible.

Intraligamentous and broad ligament fibroids are challenging to remove because of potential ureteral and vascular damage. Following a thorough laparoscopic delineation of the ureters and large blood vessels and depending on the location of the myoma, an incision is made on the anterior or posterior leaf of the broad ligament. The leiomyoma is shelled as described for subserosal and intramural fibroids. Throughout the procedure, the location of the ureter is monitored. Bleeding points are controlled by the laser or bipolar forceps. The broad ligament and peritoneum are not closed but allowed to heal spontaneously.

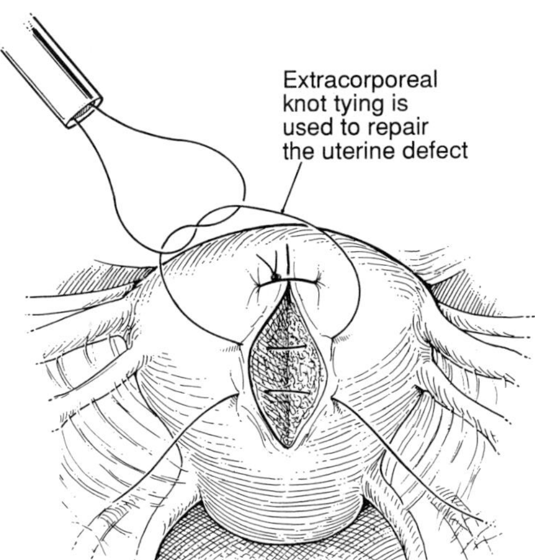

Figure 15-8 Uterine repair using extracorporeal knot tying.

None of the available lasers, regardless of the power setting or focus of the beam, adequately coagulate myometrial bleeding vessels because of their large caliber. The bipolar electrocoagulator is excellent for this purpose. The endocoagulator is an alternative for hemostasis but the effect is quite slow. If postoperative oozing is likely, a Jackson-Pratt drain is inserted through one of the suprapubic punctures and removed before the patient is discharged.

Removal of myoma from the abdomen. Removal of leiomyoma(s) from the abdominal cavity is one of the procedure's most time-consuming aspects and no methods or instruments ideally are suited to this purpose. Different methods of removal include the use of the claw-toothed forceps inserted through a 10-mm sleeve for myomas 5 cm or less in size. Alternatively, the trocar sleeve is removed and a long Kocher clamp inserted through one of the suprapubic incisions. The midline incision is preferred to avoid injury to the inferior epigastric artery and this technique is quick. However, the suprapubic incision often must be extended. Larger myomas are removed through a posterior colpotomy[21] (Figures 15-10 A and B and 15-11), which increases operative time, infectious morbidity, and risk of bowel and ureteral injury. In women with concurrent posterior cul-de-sac pathology, colpotomy is not safe. Medium and large myomas are morcellated using a

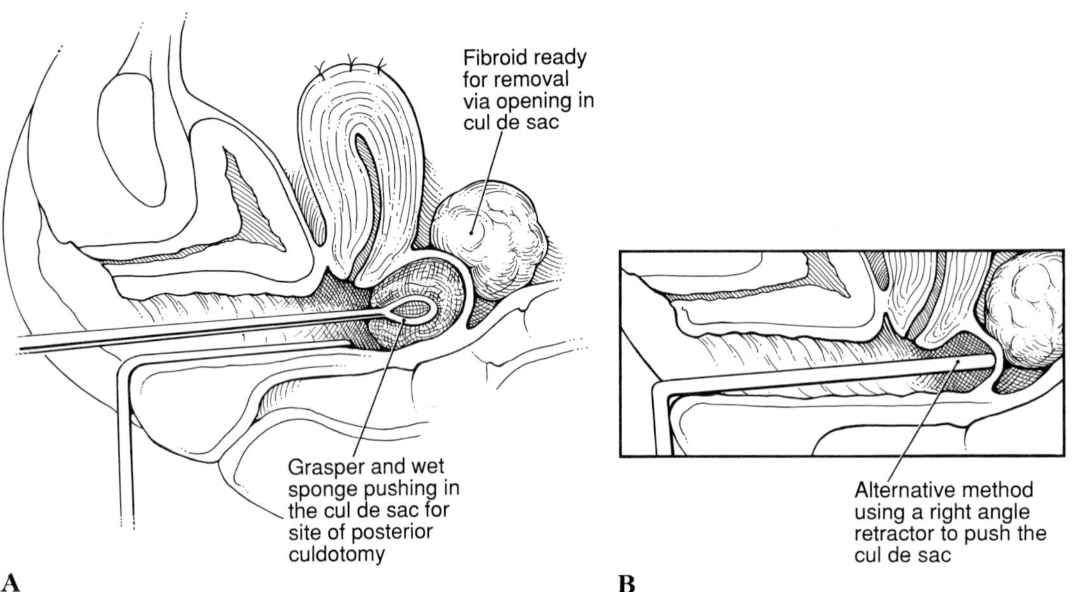

Figure 15-10 Folded gauze on sponge forceps (A) or Heaney right angle retractor (B) is used in performing posterior culdotomy.

morcellator, scalpel, or scissors (Figure 15-12). The process is ineffective for reducing calcified myomas.

Laparoscopically Assisted Myomectomy

The leiomyoma, or in cases of multiple myomas, the most prominent one, is injected at its base with 3 to 7 mL diluted vasopressin. A vertical incision is made with the CO_2 laser (or other modality) over the uterine serosa until the capsule of the leiomyoma is reached. A corkscrew manipulator is inserted into the leiomyoma and used to elevate the uterus toward the midline suprapubic puncture. With the trocar and manipulator attached to the myoma, this midline 5-mm puncture is enlarged to 4 to 5 cm transverse incision. Following the incision of the fascia transversely at 4 to 5 cm, the rectus muscles are separated at the midline.

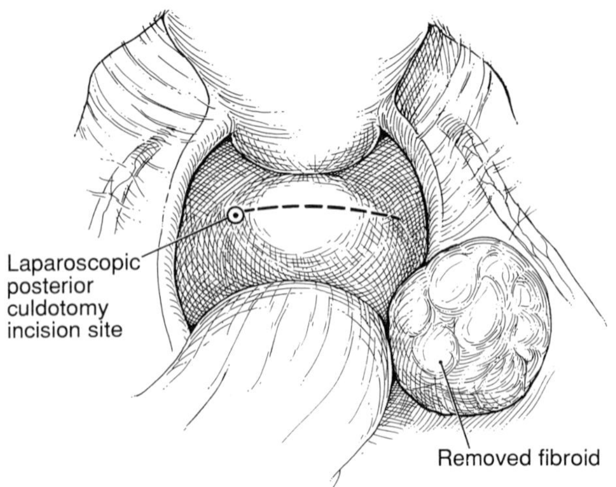

Figure 15-11 Location of posterior culdotomy.

The peritoneum is entered transversely, and the leiomyoma is located and brought to the resulting incision using the corkscrew manipulator. The uterine manipulator is used to raise the uterus. The corkscrew manipulator is replaced with two Lahey tenacula. The leiomyoma is shelled sequentially and morcellated, gradually exposing new areas. After complete removal of the leiomyoma, the uterine wall defect is seen through the incision. If uterine size allows, the uterus is brought to the skin through the minilaparotomy incision to complete the repair. When multiple leiomyomas are found, as many as possible are removed through a single uterine incision. When the leiomyomas are in distant locations and identification is impossible, the minilaparotomy incision is closed temporarily by one layer of running suture. The laparoscope is reintroduced, and the leiomyomas identified and brought to the incision. Posterior leiomyomas are difficult to reach with the minilaparotomy incision and are removed completely laparoscopically, allowing exteriorization of the uterus through the minilaparotomy incision.

The uterus is reconstructed in layers using 4–0 to 2–0 and 0 polydioxanone suture without sutur-

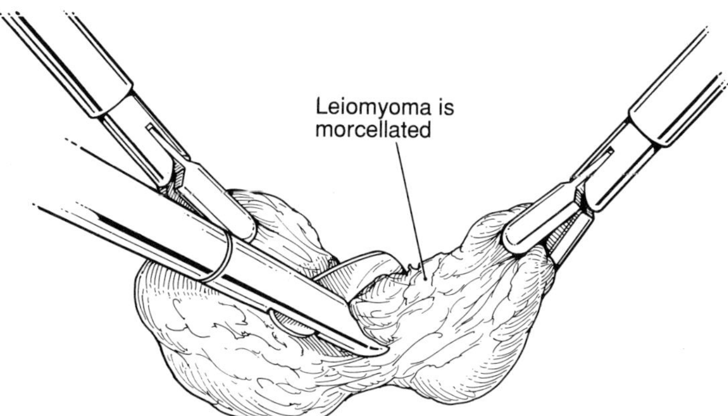

Figure 15-12 Leiomyoma morcellation using scissors.

ing the serosa, and the uterus is palpated to insure that there are no small intramural leiomyomas. The uterus is returned to the peritoneal cavity, and the fascia and skin are closed in layers. The fascia is closed with 1–0 polyglactin suture and the skin is closed in a subcuticular manner. The laparoscope is used to evaluate the uterus and ensure final hemostasis. At this time, the pelvis is evaluated to detect and treat endometriosis and adhesions that may have been obscured previously by leiomyomas. Copious irrigation is performed, blood clots are removed, and Interceed is applied over the uterus to help prevent adhesion formation.

Women are observed postoperatively for possible complications. A complete blood count is obtained the day of or following surgery. When the women awaken, an oral medication is prescribed for pain. In the developmental stages of this procedure, myomectomy patients were admitted to the hospital so that their postoperative course could be monitored closely. Currently, patients are observed in an outpatient unit and discharged the morning following surgery. Some women are allowed to leave the afternoon or evening of surgery provided their condition is stable.

Recommendations

Several concerns must be addressed before laparoscopic myomectomy will be accepted in place of laparotomy. Uterine healing and the extent of adhesion formation associated with laparotomy must be compared with the laparoscopic approach in which sutures are used. Women of childbearing age who require a myomectomy for an intramural fibroid should undergo either an abdominal myomectomy or a modified laparoscopic procedure to ensure proper closure of the myometrial defect. The laparoscopic approach is appropriate for pedunculated or subserosal fibroids when myometrial closure does not affect uterine healing.

Adenomyosis

Adenomyosis is a difficult diagnosis to make preoperatively and most often the effective treatment is a hysterectomy. Theoretically, if the misplaced endometrial tissue could be destroyed, the dysmenorrhea and menorrhagia caused by adenomyosis could be relieved. The neodymium: yttrium-aluminum-garnet (Nd:YAG) laser can penetrate deeply and coagulate large volumes of tissue,[22] which is useful in treating adenomyosis. A preliminary study was conducted in patients who presented with dysmenorrhea and menorrhagia and in whom other causes were excluded by hysteroscopy and laparoscopy. These women did not desire future fertility. Pain relief was achieved in 75% of the women using the following technique.[22]

A green-tinted filter and goggles are added to the operating room setup. A bare Nd:YAG fiber laser set at 50 W is inserted 1 to 1.5 cm into the myometrium repetitively, at 15 to 25 random sites, for 3 to 10 seconds each. The myometrium is approached from both the serosal and endometrial surfaces (Figures 15-13 and 15-14). The fiber is inserted through the hysteroscope for the endometrial approach. Constant laparoscopic surveillance helps prevent perforation or fiber contact with adjacent structures. The same procedure can be performed using a 14- to 18-gauge electrosurgical needle.

Noncommunicating Rudimentary Uterine Horn

Congenital uterine anomalies are caused by failure of müllerian fusion and absorption or development during the eighth week of intrauterine development.[23,24] It is estimated that 20% to 25% of patients with müllerian anomalies have reproductive

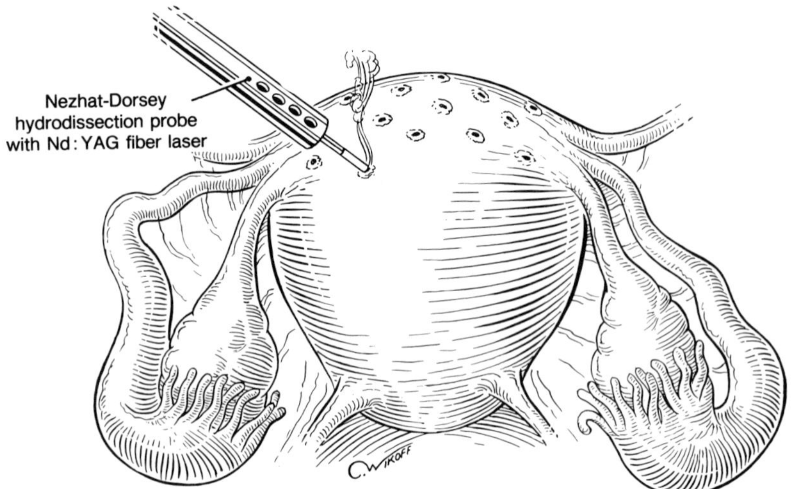

Figure 15-13 An Nd:YAG fiber laser is inserted into the myometrium repetitively.

irregularities, the most common being fetal wastage.[24] In patients with a unicornuate uterus, the incidence of spontaneous abortion may approach 50%.[23,24]

Abnormal mesonephric development can result in a uterus with a unilateral hypoplastic horn. Despite the rudimentary development, the horn may contain functional endometrial glands, and if it is noncommunicating, hematometra or hematosalpinx can result in severe dysmenorrhea. The high incidence of associated endometriosis has been documented in cases of obstructive müllerian anomalies.[23] It is possible that removing the obstructed cornu may reduce the incidence or severity of endometriosis.

The management of a rudimentary horn may involve amputation of the aplastic cornu to avoid associated endometriosis and possible cornual pregnancy.[25,26] Although laparotomy has been advocated,[26] Canis and colleagues[27] reported laparoscopic amputation of a rudimentary horn in a patient who presented with a 15-cm endometrioma. Intraoperatively, it was diagnosed as a nondistended, noncommunicating rudimentary uterine horn. The authors performed laparoscopic removal following diagnosis made by hysterosalpingography.

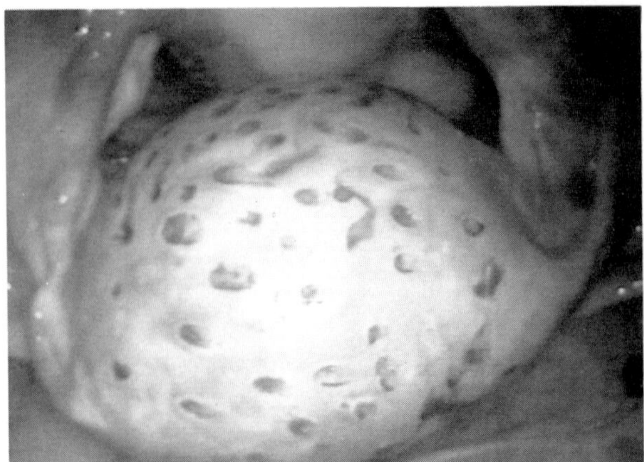

Figure 15-14 Adenomatous uterus after treatment with the Nd:YAG laser.

Management of an occluded rudimentary horn, severely dilated by hematometra and complicated by a long history of endometriosis was reported by Nezhat and colleagues.[28] A simultaneous laparoscopic and hysteroscopic evaluation revealed the presence of a rudimentary, noncommunicating horn previously diagnosed as a bicornuate uterus by hysterosalpinogram.

Removal of the rudimentary horn was performed by coagulating and cutting the right round ligament and developing the bladder flap, followed by coagulating and cutting the right utero-ovarian and broad ligaments and uterine artery on the right. While the cosurgeon was monitoring the procedure with the hysteroscope, an incision was made between the rudimentary and left horn. This incision was lengthened using sequential bipolar electrocoagulation and CO_2 laser to develop a distinct plane between the two horns. The dilated right horn was amputated at the level of internal cervical os. It was cut into several parts and removed from the abdomen through the infraumbilical incision. Five 4–0 polydioxanone sutures were used to close the muscularis and the serosa of the left uterine horn. Chromopertubation showed left tubal patency and no damage to the left uterine wall. The patient was discharged on postoperative day 1 following an uncomplicated hospital course. At 2-year follow-up, she was pain free with regular menses and was planning a pregnancy.

Uterine Suspension

Indications for uterine suspension are limited to dyspareunia secondary to severe uterine retroversion in the absence of other cul-de-sac disease and in selected cases of severe endometriosis involving the cul-de-sac and rectum. At laparoscopy, adhesions, endometriosis, and hydrosalpinx can be corrected and the uterine suspension accomplished during the same operation.

Women with dyspareunia secondary to the uterine position will have a retroverted, retroflexed uterus, and palpation of the uterine-cervical junction on vaginal examination will reproduce the pain. Although some authors have advocated placement of a pessary before attempting to surgically correct the retroversion,[29] others have noted that the dyspareunia was eliminated in the patient but the male partner was disturbed by the pessary during coitus.[30] Complete or partial relief of dyspareunia[30–32] from laparoscopic uterine suspension has been reported in approximately 90% of patients, but two reports showed no relief.[33,34] The three most effective methods are fallope rings, ventrosuspension of the round ligament, and modified Olshausen uterine suspension.

Fallope Rings

Fallope rings have been used for many years in laparoscopic tubal sterilization. A special instrument that fits through a 5-mm accessory trocar sleeve simultaneously grasps the tube, retracts it into the instrument, and places a small, tight silicone band around the knuckle of the tube. A similar procedure shortens the round ligaments (Figure 15-15).[35] It may be necessary to place multiple fallope rings to achieve the proper tension on the round ligaments. Placing the rings on the round ligaments can lacerate the broad ligament or the round ligament. Bipolar electrocoagulation is used for hemostasis.

Ventrosuspension of the Round Ligament

This procedure involves the placement of two 5-mm suprapubic trocars through which grasping forceps are introduced,[30,36–38] or long Kelly clamps are inserted through suprapubic stab incisions. Both round ligaments are grasped near their midpoint and the pneumoperitoneum is allowed to partially escape. The knuckle of the round ligament is pulled gently and firmly through the incision in the fascia (Figure 15-16). The round ligaments are sutured to the rectus fascia with 2–0 Ethibond nonabsorbable sutures. Uterine position is confirmed with the laparoscope, and one must avoid kinking the fallopian tubes.

Potential complications with this procedure include avulsion of the round ligament secondary to an inadequate fascial incision and undue tension or positioning of the round ligaments with a full pneumoperitoneum. The inferior epigastric arteries may be lacerated during placement of the suprapubic trocars. Transillumination of the abdomen often helps prevent this complication, but it is difficult in obese patients. Although nonabsorbable suture is recommended, one patient had chronic pain at an incision site, which abated on

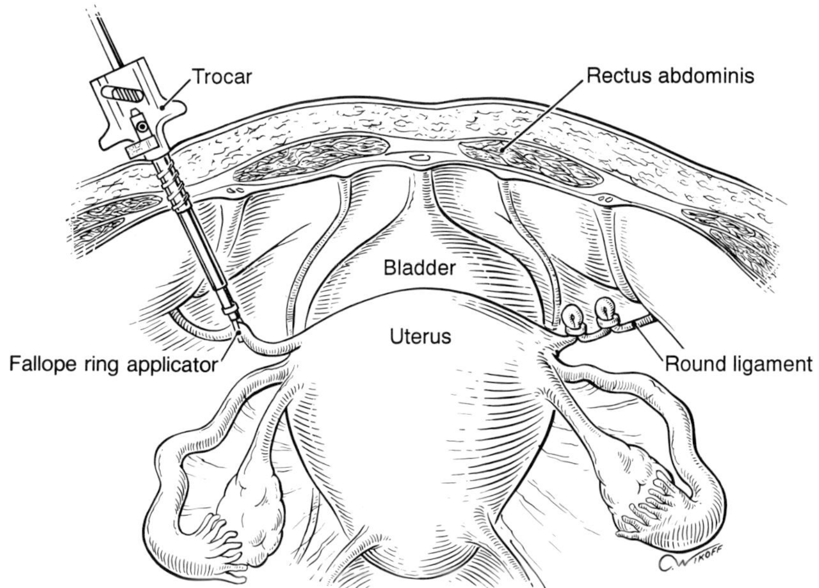

Figure 15-15 Shortening the round ligaments with fallope rings.

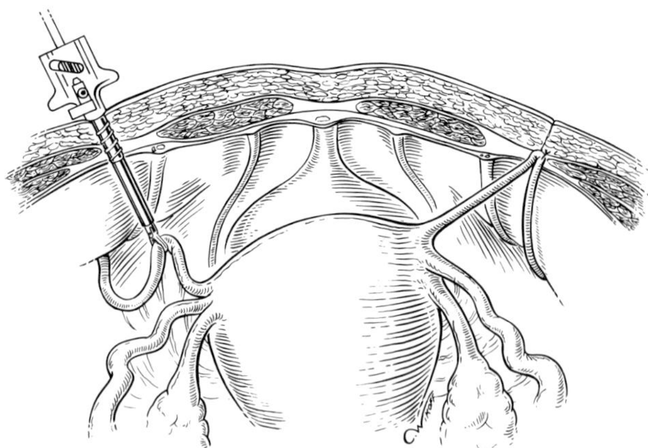

Figure 15-16 The round ligaments at midpoint are pulled through the suprapubic incision and tied to the rectus fascia.

suture removal. For most patients, incisional pain and discomfort are managed with mild analgesics and a heating pad. Occasionally, patients who experience more significant postoperative pain from secondary spasms of the recti muscles are relieved with heat, muscle relaxants, and analgesics. Women are advised to avoid strenuous exercise for 4 to 6 weeks postoperatively.

Lose and Lindholm[39] reported a case of intermittent urinary retention in a young woman with a retroverted, retroflexed uterus who had undergone a uterine suspension for dyspareunia. At the time of corrective surgery, it appeared that the rearranged uterus caused an obstruction that may have been exacerbated by the patient's low voiding pressures.

Modified Olshausen Uterine Suspension

Either delayed absorbable or permanent suture is passed transabdominally at the suprapubic trocar site using a swaged needle. While the surgeon places the round ligament on stretch, several areas are taken where the round ligament enters the inguinal canal moving toward the uterus. Approximately 2 cm from the uterus, the direction of the needle is reversed and a similar maneuver is performed along the length of the round ligament to the inguinal canal. The needle is passed transabdominally. Once both sides are completed, the pneumoperitoneum is decreased and the suture is tied above the fascia (Figure 15-17). The result is a plication of the round ligaments.

This procedure is an alternative to ventrosuspension of the uterus. It is associated with the same risk of complications, except that the risk of round ligament avulsion is lower. This procedure also requires more surgical skill than others because intracorporeal suturing techniques are used.

Hysterectomy

Hysterectomy is one of the most frequently performed major surgical procedures. The rate varies among different regions and cultures[40–43] reflecting differences in health care systems, education, and psychosocial attitudes toward the procedure.[44–46] The highest rates of hysterectomy are found in the United States and Australia (36% and 40%, respectively)[40,42,43] in contrast with European rates, which range from 5.8% (France) to 15.5% (Italy).[41]

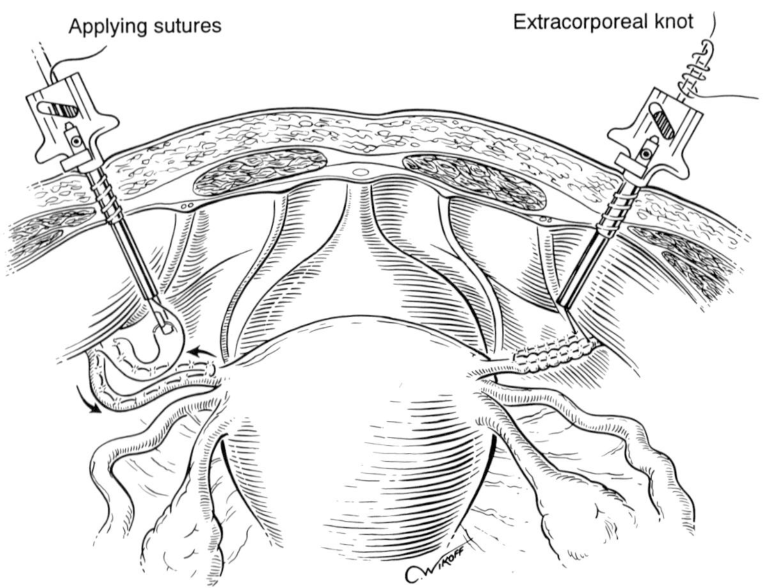

Figure 15-17 Modified Olshausen technique.

TABLE 15-5 Indications for Hysterectomy

	Abdominal Hysterectomy[57] (%)	Vaginal Hysterectomy[57] (%)
Leiomyomata	38	1
Uterine prolapse	1	76
Endometriosis	3	0
Abnormal bleeding	13	9
Adenomyosis	9	8
Pelvic pain/adhesions	5	0
Ovarian tumors	10	0
Uterine neoplasia	15	3

Indications

Most hysterectomies are performed for leiomyomas, uterine prolapse, endometriosis, gynecologic cancer, or adenomatous endometrial hyperplasia.[43] Other indications including abnormal uterine bleeding, diseases of the parametrium or pelvic peritoneum, pelvic infection and its sequelae, ovarian tumors, and complications of pregnancy account for 15% to 21% of hysterectomies.[42] The number of hysterectomies performed for endometriosis doubled between 1965 and 1984, exceeding the increase observed for any other indication and probably reflecting an increased recognition of endometriosis.[42]

Current Approach

About 75% of hysterectomies are accomplished abdominally and 25% vaginally,[43,44] the latter being performed mainly for uterine prolapse and other indications depending on uterine size, coexistent adnexal disease, and the surgeon's skill and preference. Abdominal hysterectomy usually is performed for women having significant pelvic disease that may make vaginal removal more difficult. These diseases include endometriosis, adhesions, or other pelvic abnormalities that cannot be treated during vaginal hysterectomy (Table 15-5).[47] Compared to vaginal hysterectomy, women having an abdominal hysterectomy have more febrile morbidity, receive more blood transfusions,[44,48] and have a longer postoperative hospitalization and convalescence. If more women underwent vaginal rather than abdominal hysterectomy, considerable therapeutic, economic, and social benefits would result.[49–53]

The decision to perform abdominal rather than vaginal hysterectomy is based on clinical assessment of the pelvic disorder from the medical history, pelvic examination, ultrasound studies, review of prior surgical notes, and the surgeon's experience in vaginal surgery.[54] Kovac and associates[49] performed diagnostic laparoscopy in 46 patients scheduled for abdominal hysterectomy who, based on clinical indicators, were thought to have serious pelvic abnormality that contraindicated vaginal hysterectomy. Based on the laparoscopic findings, 42 of the 46 (91%) women were candidates for vaginal hysterectomy, which was performed under the same anesthesia. Because clinical assessment of pelvic disease may not be accurate, laparoscopy may reveal that a vaginal approach is appropriate.

However, vaginal hysterectomy is sometimes contraindicated because of severe endometriosis, lack of uterine prolapse, prior abdominal surgery, previous cesarean, pelvic adhesions, or large leiomyomas. For these women, diagnostic or operative laparoscopy provides the benefits of both the vaginal and abdominal approaches without the disadvantages (Table 15-6).

There are many variations of a laparoscopically assisted hysterectomy and it is almost impossible to accurately compare published results. A review of the literature reveals many definitions. Several

TABLE 15-6 Advantages and Disadvantages of Abdominal, Vaginal, and Laparoscopically Assisted Vaginal Hysterectomy (LAVH)

	Abdominal	Vaginal	LAVH
Exposure	Excellent	Limited	Excellent
Associated pelvic disease	Easily treated	Reduced access	Easily treated
Incision	Abdominal	Vaginal	Abdominal/vaginal
Hospitalization (days)	3	2–3	1–2
Cost	Average	Average	More expensive
Morbidity (%)	30	10	10
Surgical expertise	Average gynecologist	Average gynecologist	Experienced endoscopist
Oophorectomy	Easy	<25%	Easy

authors have refined their nomenclature as their experience broadened. A set of definitions identifying various degrees of laparoscopic and vaginal dissection according to the seven basic steps of hysterectomy follows (Table 15-7).

1. *Total laparoscopic hysterectomy* (TLH)—All steps are performed laparoscopically, including vaginal cuff closure.
2. *Subtotal laparoscopic hysterectomy* (SLH)—Supracervical hysterectomy is performed laparoscopically.
3. *Vaginally assisted laparoscopic hysterectomy* (VALH)—Four or more steps are performed laparoscopically and the procedure is completed vaginally.
4. *Laparoscopically assisted vaginal hysterectomy* (LAVH)—The hysterectomy is begun by laparoscopy but four or more steps are performed vaginally.

Patients with suspected pelvic endometriosis undergo a diagnostic laparoscopy to inspect the pelvis. Significant pelvic disease is treated endoscopically, and if necessary, adnexectomy is performed and the hysterectomy is completed vaginally.[49] Usually, a combined laparoscopic and vaginal approach is used to dissect and remove uterine attachments.[50–53,55,56] The extent of laparoscopic and vaginal dissection should be based on the surgeon's preference and experience with laparoscopic and vaginal surgery.[57] TLH can be time consuming for the novice laparoscopist, especially if the uterus is more than 16 to 18 weeks gestational size. Laparoscopic hysterectomy is useful when the vagina is small and narrow, if there is significant, infiltrative pelvic endometriosis and vaginal surgery is difficult, and when the surgeon is very experienced in operative laparoscopy, including suturing. Almost all abdominal hysterectomies for endometriosis can be converted to LAVH, VALH or TLH.[52] Patients who have indications for traditional vaginal hysterectomy do not need LAVH, VALH or LH.[56]

TABLE 15-7 Seven Basic Steps of Hysterectomy

1. Severing the round ligaments and dissection of the upper portion of the broad ligament.
2. Severing the tubouterine junction and the utero-ovarian ligament if the adnexa are to be preserved, or severing the infundibulopelvic ligaments.
3. Severing the uterine vessels.
4. Preparation of the bladder flap and severing the bladder pillars.
5. Severing the cardinal-uterosacral ligament complex.
6. Performing anterior and posterior culdotomy and separation of the cervix from the vaginal membrane.
7. Closure of the vaginal cuff.

Preoperative Evaluation

Patients are evaluated as they would be for major abdominal surgery. Routine preoperative tests include a complete blood count with differential, serum electrolytes, bleeding time, and urinalysis. More comprehensive blood studies, thrombin time, partial thrombin time, electrocardiogram, chest X-ray, and endometrial biopsy are done as indicated. A mechanical and antibiotic bowel preparation is advised. Consultations with a urologist, bowel surgeon, and oncologist are sought as necessary. Appropriate informed consent is obtained from the patient following a thorough explanation of the planned operation, its potential risks and benefits, the possibility of laparotomy, and therapeutic alternatives. Following an overnight fast, patients are admitted to the ambulatory surgical unit the morning of surgery.

Positioning of the Patient

The patient's initial positioning is the same as for standard laparoscopy. The 10-mm trocar is inserted infraumbilically for placement of the operative laparoscope, and two to four accessory trocars are positioned suprapubically. For the vaginal portion, the patient's legs are readjusted to allow vaginal access (Allen universal stirrups). With an adjustment under the drapes, the legs can be flexed and abducted without redraping. Some surgeons prefer to place the patient in candy-cane stirrups for the vaginal portion.

Every operative laparoscopy begins with a thorough exploration of the abdominal and pelvic cavity to assess the extent of disease. Important anatomic landmarks, anomalies, distortions, and alterations are identified. The locations of the bladder, ureters, colon, rectum, and major blood vessels are noted. The omentum and small bowel are evaluated for disease and checked for Veress needle or trocar injury.

Operative Technique

Following the diagnostic laparoscopy, the surgeon uses the CO_2 laser and hydrodissection to resect, ablate, or coagulate any endometriosis implants. An electrocoagulator, clips, staplers, Endoloops (Ethicon), monopolar electrodes, or fiber lasers are used for coagulating or ligating large vessels. At CSPS, the CO_2 laser is used through the operative channel of the laparoscope as a long knife and bipolar forceps through the mid suprapubic port for hemostasis. We have used both with few complications.[58] Other instruments include suction-irrigator probe (left), and grasping forceps (right). The bowel is freed from the pelvic organs to expose the pelvis. The ovaries and tubes are dissected from the cul-de-sac or pelvic sidewall and endometriosis and other abnormalities are treated. Once the uterus and adnexae are separated from adhesions, hysterectomy is performed.

Ureteral Evaluation and Dissection

The direction and location of both ureters are identified from the pelvic brim to the cardinal ligaments where they are no longer visible. The course of the ureters is marked superiorly with laser or electrocoagulation so they can be identified while the broad ligament and adnexa are dissected (Figure 15-18). When the ureters cannot be identified clearly because of severe scarring or endometriosis, they are dissected retroperitoneally, using sharp or blunt dissection, or hydrodissection[59] (Figure 15-19 A, B, and C). For extensive endometriosis, very wide dissection as performed during radical hysterectomy is necessary.[51,53] To identify the ureters at the level of the cardinal ligaments, the peritoneum is opened above or below the ureter and hydrodissection performed. A peritoneal incision is made and the ureter is identified toward its course to the bladder. Small bleeders are controlled by laser or electrosurgery. If the uterosacral ligaments are dissected, the ureter is retracted laterally and the uterosacral ligaments are dissected at their connection to the back of the cervix. The uterine vessels, which run superiorly, are isolated and safely coagulated. When pelvic anatomy is distorted, it may be safer to perform a cystoscopy and place catheters in both ureters for better identification.

Upper Broad Ligament and Adnexa

If adnexectomy is indicated, following electrodesiccation and cutting of the round ligament 2 to 3 cm from the uterus, the infundibulopelvic ligament is electrodesiccated and cut, taking progressive bites of tissue starting at the pelvic brim and moving toward the round ligament. If the endoscopic linear stapler is used, the adnexa is grasped with forceps. It is retracted medially and caudally to stretch and outline the infundibulopelvic ligament, which is grasped and secured with the stapler. The stapler is not fired until the contained tissue is identified and the ureter's safety is confirmed. Once transected, the staple line should be examined closely for placement and hemostasis. Following infundibulopelvic ligament transection, the adnexa and uterine fundus are retracted in the opposite direction and the tissue of the upper broad ligament, including the round ligament, is

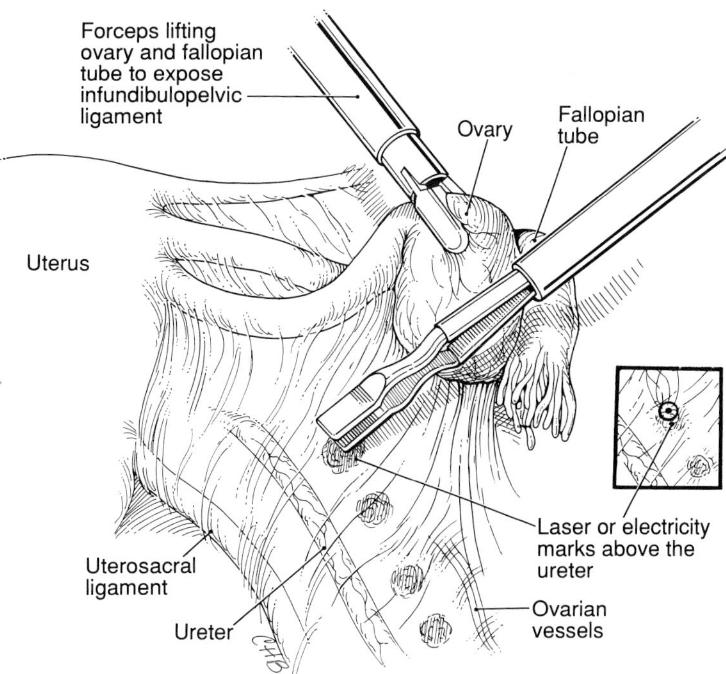

Figure 15-18 Marking the direction and location of the ureter by making a superficial peritoneal coagulation above it.

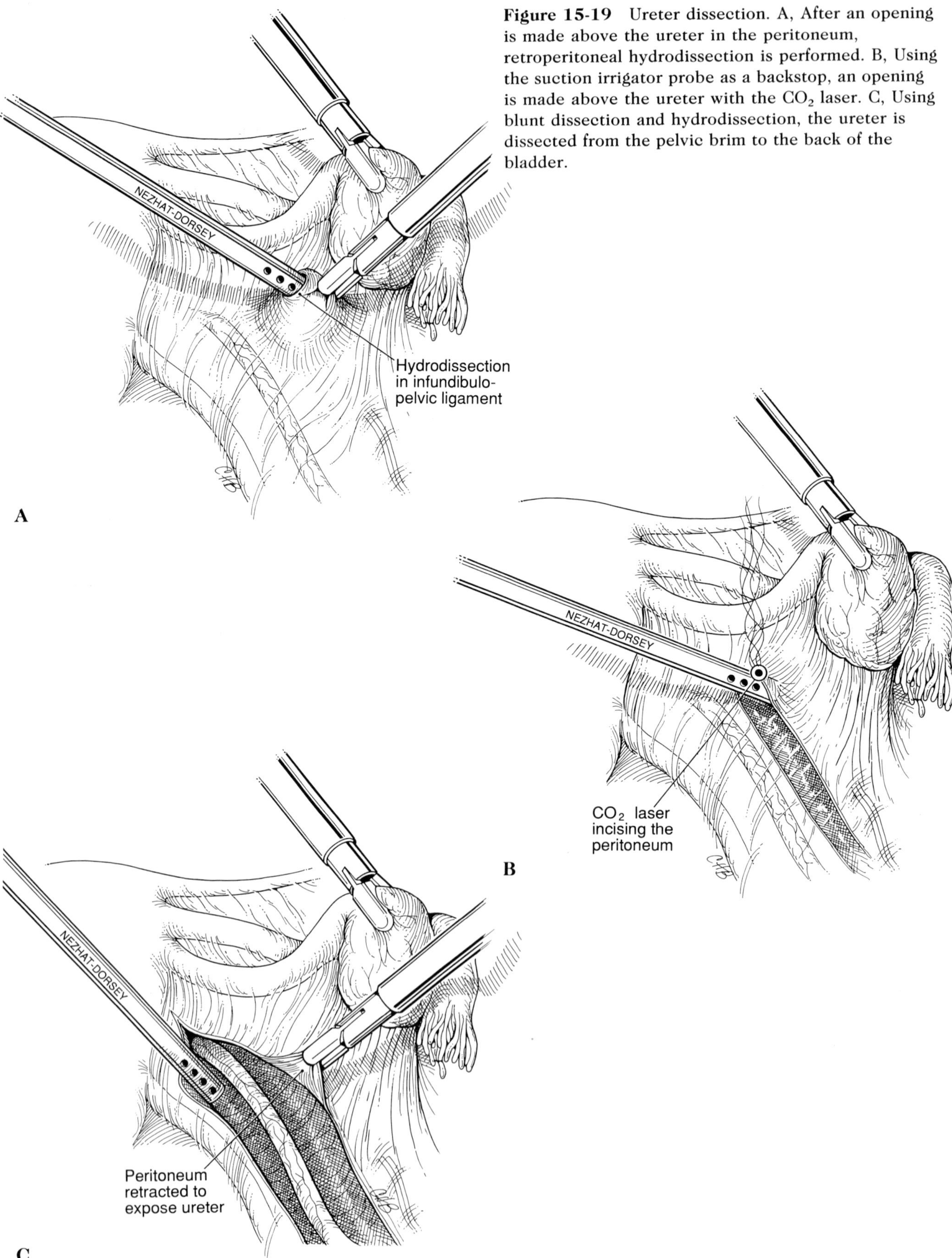

Figure 15-19 Ureter dissection. A, After an opening is made above the ureter in the peritoneum, retroperitoneal hydrodissection is performed. B, Using the suction irrigator probe as a backstop, an opening is made above the ureter with the CO_2 laser. C, Using blunt dissection and hydrodissection, the ureter is dissected from the pelvic brim to the back of the bladder.

grasped, secured, and cut after safe margins are established (Figure 15-20A). The infundibulopelvic and the round ligament occasionally are cut with a single staple application (Figure 15-20B).

Development of the Bladder Flap

If the adnexae are preserved, the round ligament is electrodesiccated and cut approximately 3 cm from the uterus (Figure 15-21). By the surgeon's use of hydrodissection, the anterior leaf of the broad ligament is opened toward the vesicouterine fold and the bladder flap is developed (Figure 15-22). The anterior leaf of the broad ligament is grasped with forceps, elevated, and dissected from the anterior lower uterine segment with hydrodissection and CO_2 laser (Figure 15-23). The utero-ovarian ligament, proximal tube, and mesosalpinx are progressively electrodesiccated and cut, and the posterior leaf of the broad ligament is opened (Figure 15-24). Similarly, the round ligament, fallopian tube, and utero-ovarian ligament are grasped close to their insertion into the uterus with the endoscopic linear stapler, then secured, stapled, and severed (Figure 15-25 A and B). The distal end of the stapler or bipolar forceps must be kept free of the bladder and ureter.

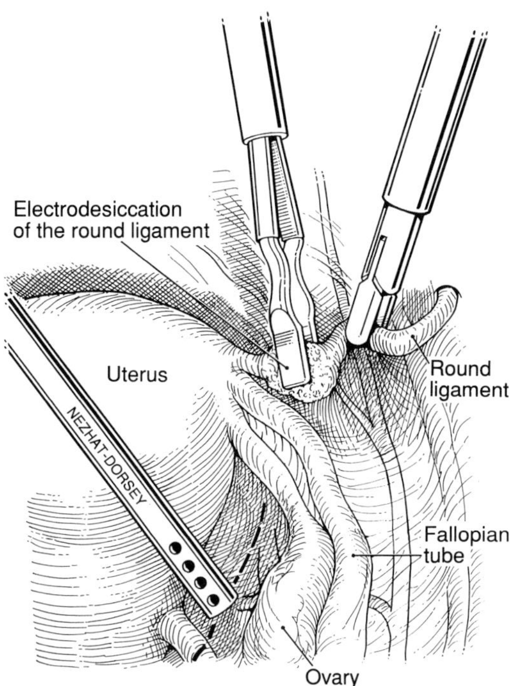

Figure 15-21 The round ligament is electrodesiccated and cut 2 to 3 cm lateral to the uterus.

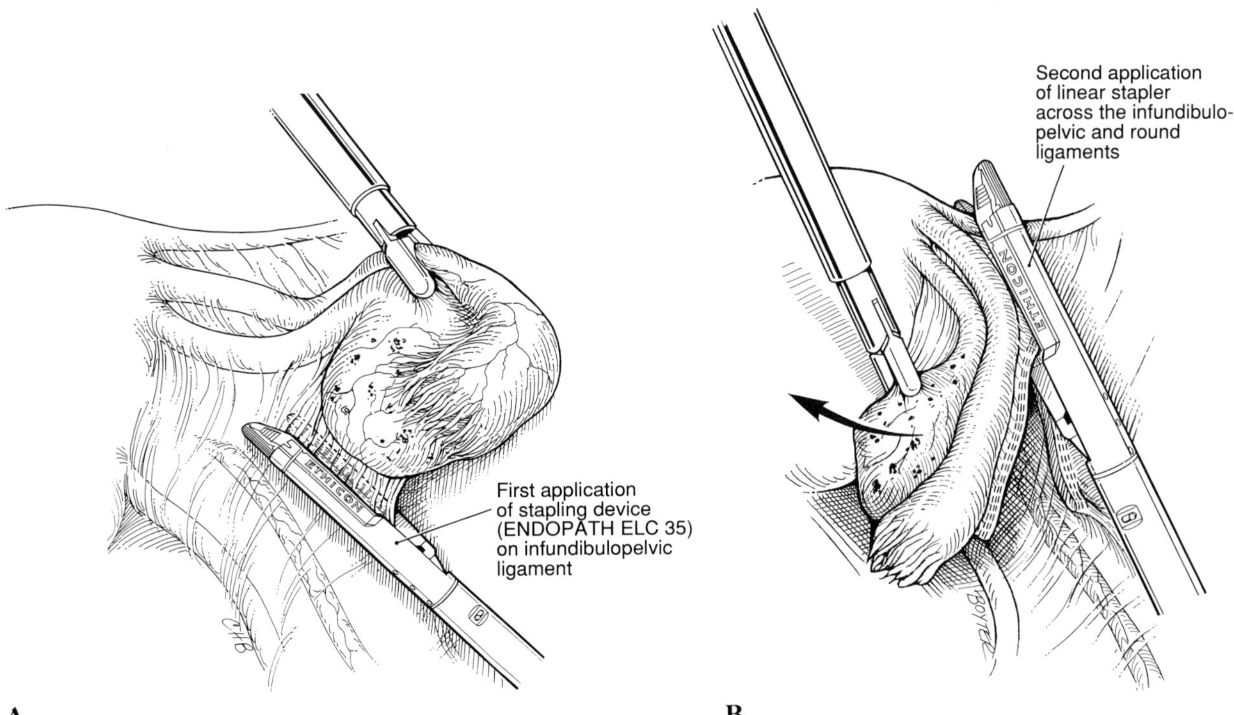

Figure 15-20 A, The linear stapler is applied across the infundibulopelvic ligament. Ureter evaluation before transection of the ligament is very important. B, Second application of the stapler across the infundibulopelvic ligament. The round ligament may be included.

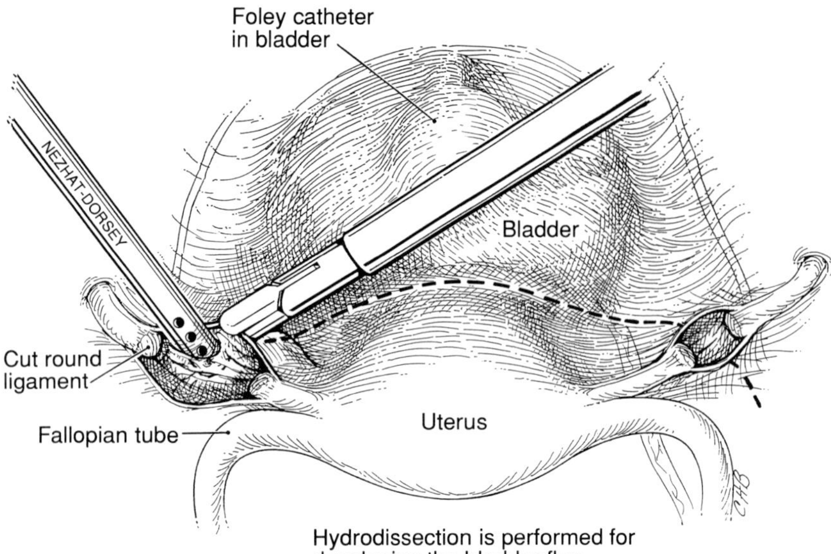

Figure 15-22 While the anterior leaf of the broad ligament is elevated using hydrodissection, it is opened toward the vesicouterine fold.

The uterovesical junction is identified, grasped, and elevated with forceps while being cut with scissors, laser, or electrode. The bladder pillars are identified, desiccated, and cut, completely freeing the bladder from the uterus by pushing downward with the tip of a blunt probe along the vesicocervical plane until the anterior cul-de-sac is exposed completely (Figure 15-26).

In patients with severe anterior cul-de-sac endometriosis, previous cesarean, or adhesions, sharp dissection of the vesicouterine fold is often necessary. Injecting 5 mL of indigo carmine in the patient's IV helps detect bladder trauma. Alternatively, sterile milk (infant formula) is instilled through the Foley catheter to detect bladder leaks.

Uterine Vessels

After dissecting the bladder from the anterior cervix, the uterine vessels, which vary in size and location, are identified, desiccated, and cut to free the lateral borders of the uterus (Figure 15-27). If sutures, single clips, or linear staplers are used, it is important to skeletonize the vessels. As the uterine vessels are grasped and cut, the safety and position of the ureters should be checked, which is done more easily if they are marked, exposed, or catheterized at the beginning of the procedure.

Cardinal Ligament

At the level of the cardinal ligaments, the ureter and the descending branches of the uterine artery

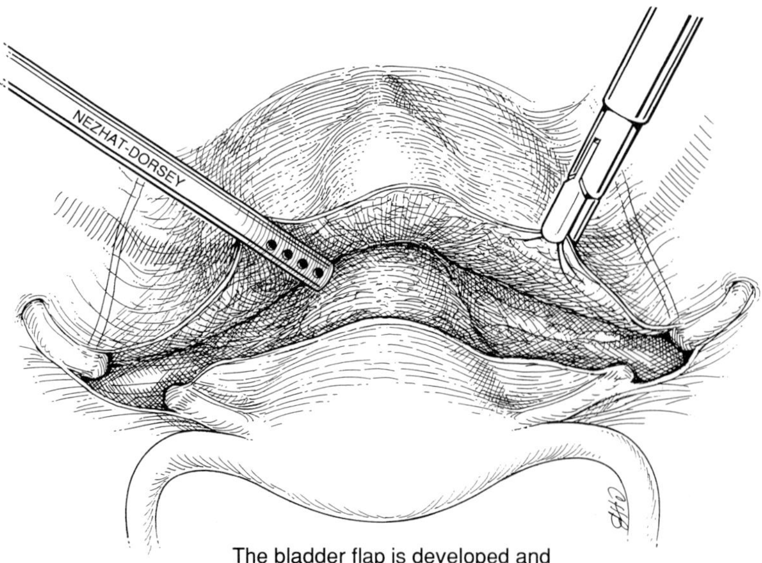

Figure 15-23 The bladder is elevated and further separated from the cervix, and pushed downward using sharp and blunt dissection and hydrodissection.

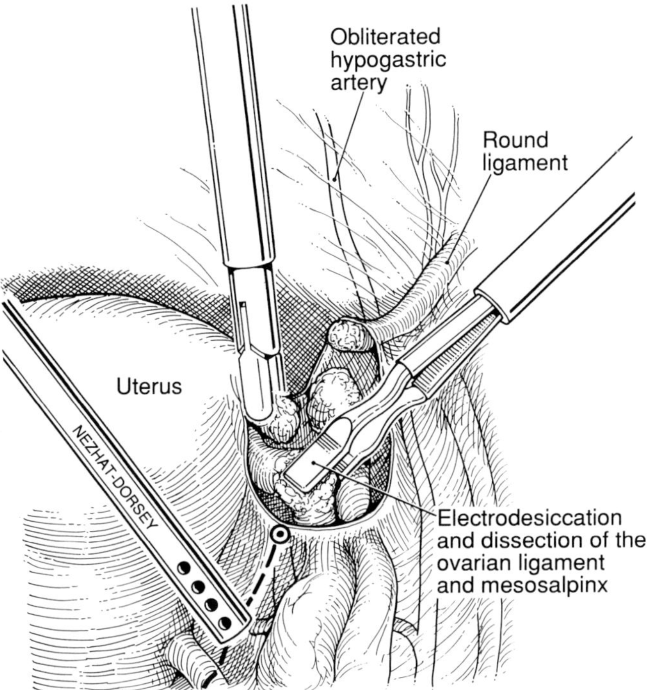

Figure 15-24 The proximal tube, mesosalpinx, and utero-ovarian ligament are electrodesiccated and cut.

are close to one another and the cervix. Therefore, cardinal ligament dissection must be precise to prevent bleeding and ureteral injury. The linear stapler is used only if the parametrium has been dissected with ample margins, as in cervical malignancy. The linear stapler is 12 mm wide which, considering the short distance between the cervix and ureter, increases the risk of ureteral injury by the stapler. Using contralateral retraction of the uterus, the cardinal ligament is dissected to identify tissue planes, vessels, and the ureter. Once the ureter is displaced laterally, the cardinal ligament

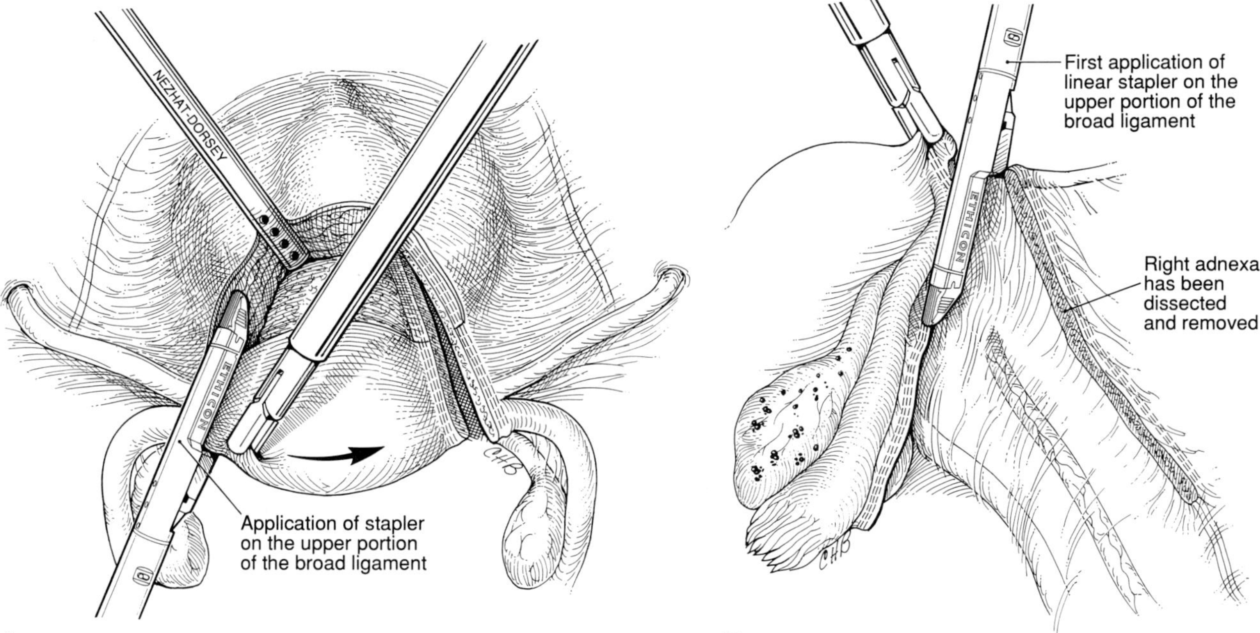

Figure 15-25 A, Application of the linear stapler on the upper portion of the broad ligament while preserving the adnexa. B, Application of the linear stapler on the upper broad ligament while removing the adnexa.

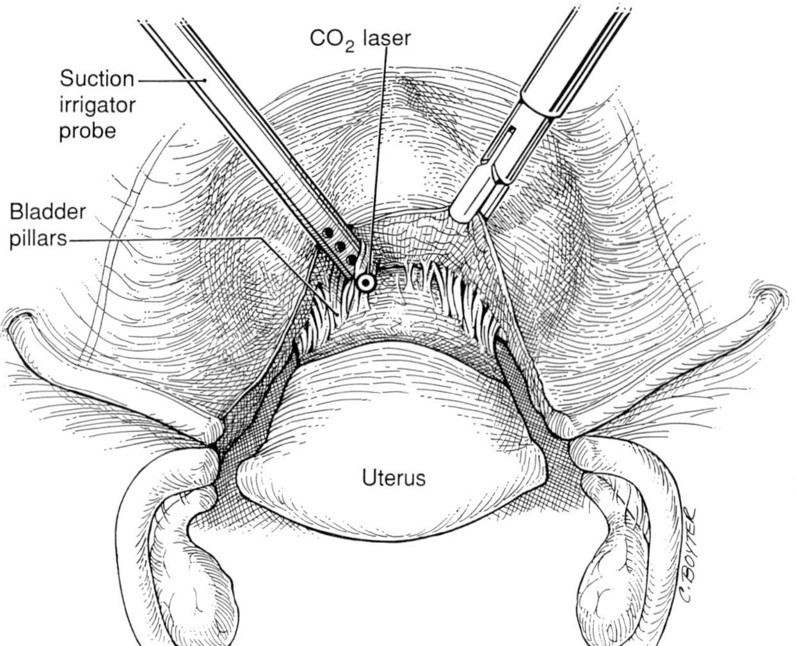

Figure 15-26 The bladder pillars are identified and cut close to the cervix using the CO_2 laser.

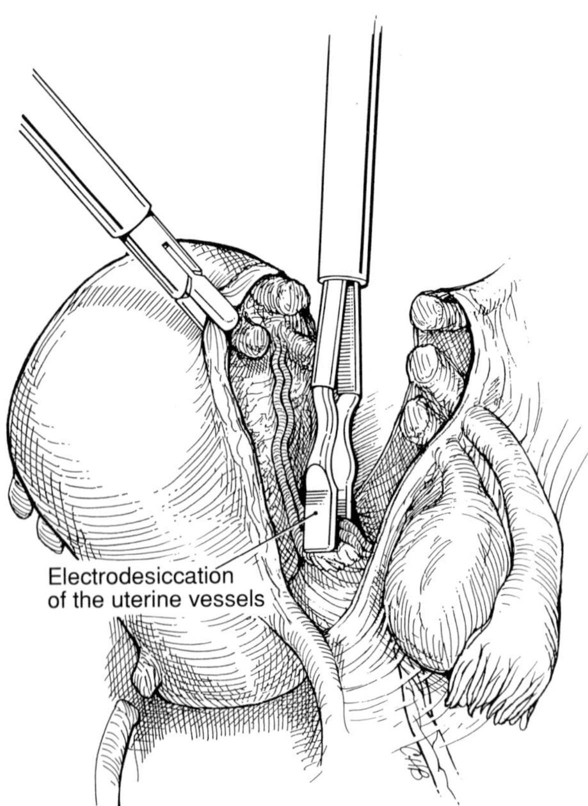

Figure 15-27 While observing the ureter, the uterine vessels are skeletonized, electrodesiccated, and cut.

tissue closest to the cervix is electrodessicated and transected (Figure 15-28). Alternatively, the linear stapler can be applied both on the uterine vessels and cardinal ligament (Figure 15-29).

Anterior and Posterior Culdotomy

A folded wet gauze in a sponge forceps, or the tip of a right angle Heaney retractor, is used to mark the anterior or posterior vaginal fornix. The vaginal wall is tented and transected horizontally with laser or knife electrode (Figures 15-30 and 15-31).

Vaginal Portion of the Hysterectomy

Once the dissection is extended to the lower uterine segment or to the level of the cardinal ligaments, the laparoscopic portion temporarily is terminated before or after performing the anterior or posterior culdotomy. Dissecting and resecting the uterus can be completed vaginally using standard techniques. Once the uterus is removed, the vaginal cuff is closed. To ensure support of the vaginal vault, the vaginal angles are attached to the uterosacral and cardinal ligaments with absorbable sutures. The vaginal cuff is closed transversely, and any coexisting cystocele or rectocele is repaired. Once vaginal surgery is completed and the cuff is closed, the laparoscopic procedure is resumed.

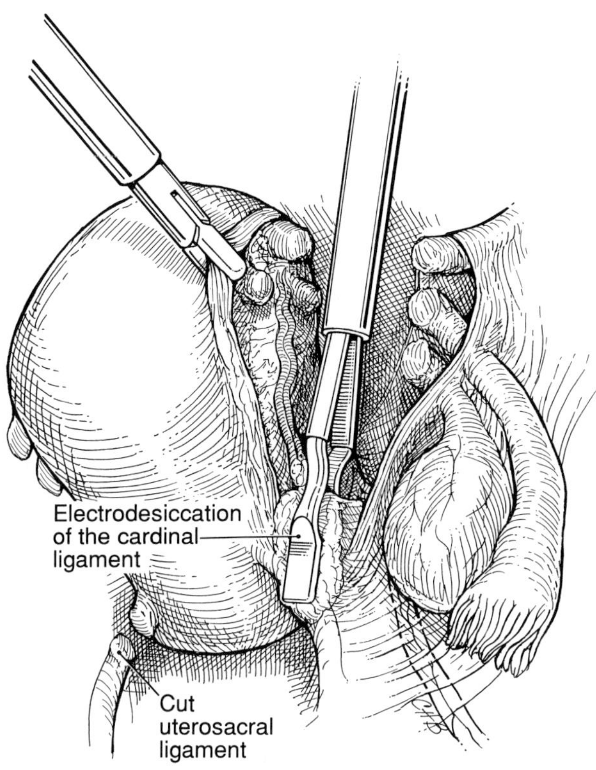

Figure 15-28 While pulling the uterus to the opposite side using a grasping forceps, and electrodesiccating and cutting the cardinal ligament, the ureter must be observed to ensure that it is not damaged by the bipolar forceps.

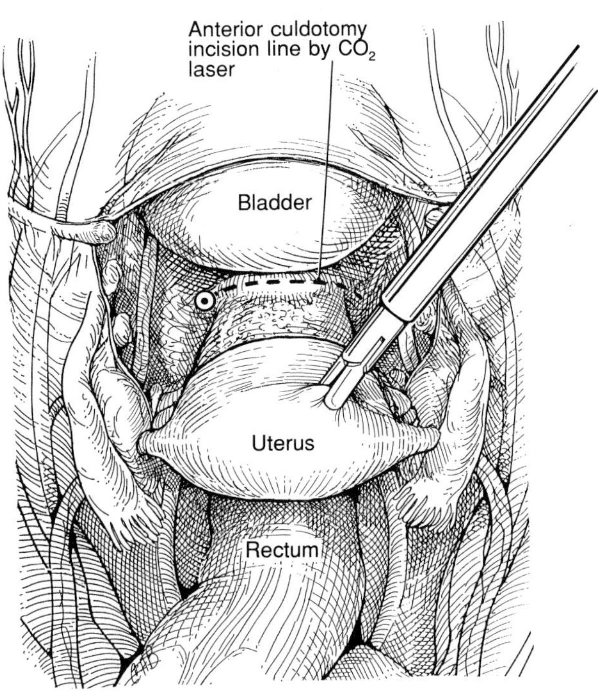

Figure 15-30 The uterus is completely mobilized, and as it is pushed down, a laparoscopic anterior culdotomy is performed using the CO_2 laser.

Figure 15-29 The linear stapler is applied across the uterine vessels and cardinal ligament. The ureter is dissected and held away from the stapler jaws.

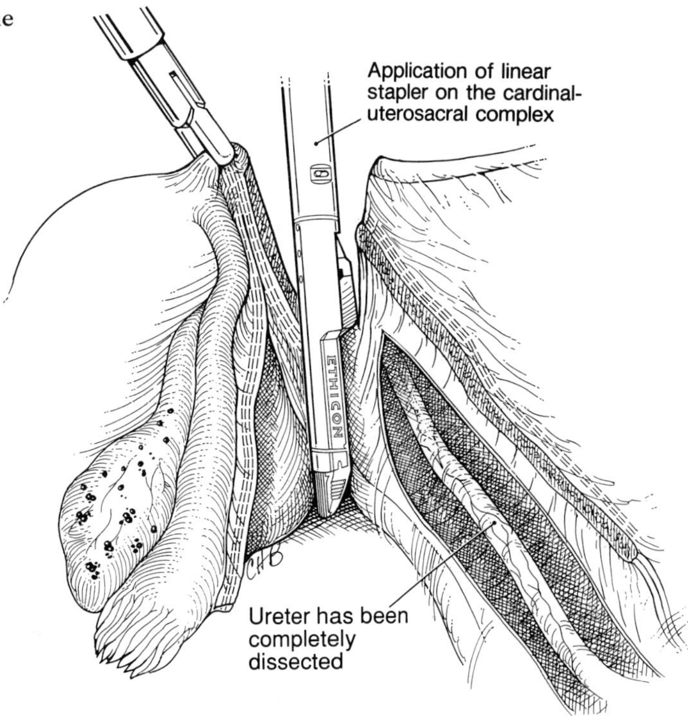

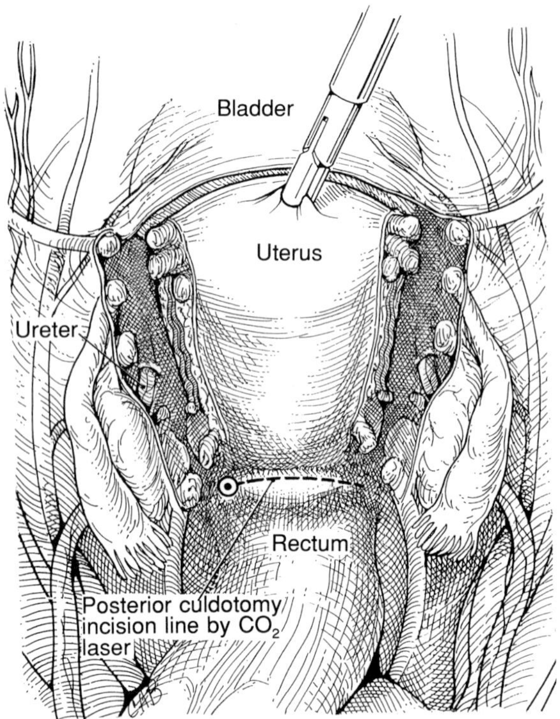

Figure 15-31 The uterus is elevated, and as the assistant identifies the posterior fornix, a laparoscopic posterior culdotomy is performed. The surgeon must ensure that the correct location is selected and that the rectum is not involved.

Hysterectomy for Extensive Pelvic Endometriosis and Adhesions

In women who have extensive endometriosis, the rectosigmoid colon often is densely adherent to the posterior aspect of the uterus (Figure 15-32). Similarly, if the ovaries are affected by endometriosis and endometriomas, they may attach to the pelvic side wall. To desiccate the uterine artery, it is necessary to develop the paravesical space and identify the uterine vessel at its origin from the hypogastric artery. Bipolar forceps, clips, or sutures are used. The rectosigmoid colon is separated from the posterior uterus incrementally, and the bowel endometriosis is resected or vaporized (Figures 15-32 and 15-33). The high-power ultrapulse CO_2 laser is precise, and with a penetration of only 100 μm, the possibility of delayed bowel necrosis is low. Any excess bleeding not controlled by the CO_2 laser is controlled with application of the bipolar electrocoagulator. Endometriosis of the rectum, rectovaginal septum, and uterosacral ligament is treated by vaporization, excision, or a combination, and the posterior cul-de-sac is freed

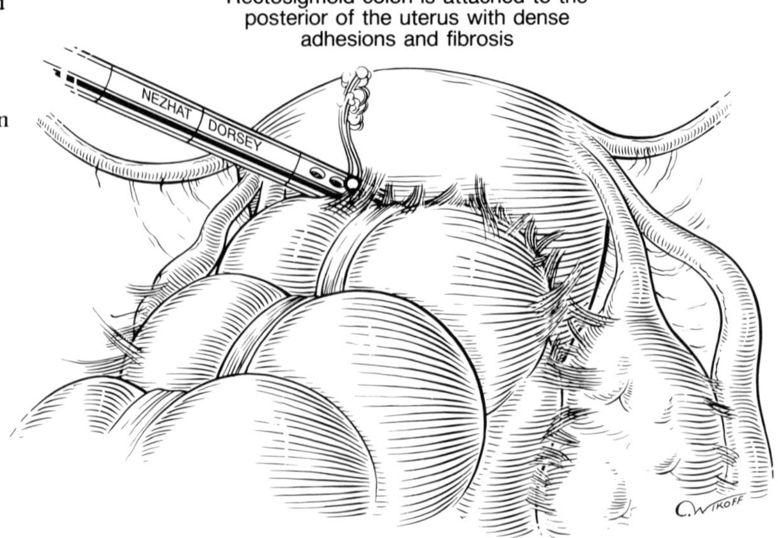

Figure 15-32 Rectosigmoid colon is attached to the posterior aspect of the uterus with dense adhesions and endometriosis. Using the hydrodissection probe and CO_2 laser, the adhesions are lysed and the rectosigmoid colon is separated from the uterus.

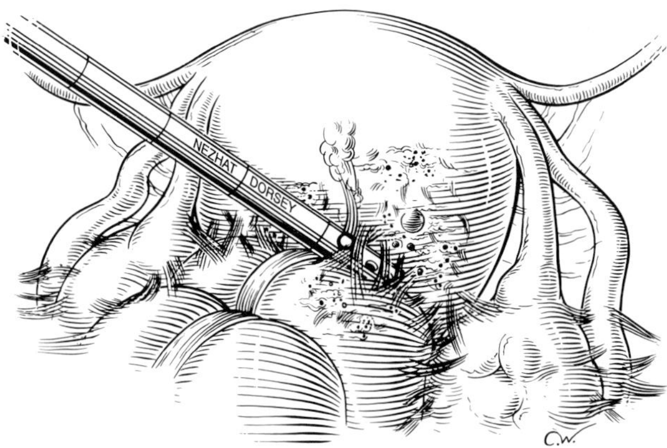

Figure 15-33 The dissection of the rectosigmoid colon is continued.

(Figures 15-34 and 15-35). Bipolar forceps are used for achieving hemostasis. If the endometriosis penetrates deeply to the bowel muscularis or mucosa and causes stricture requiring anterior or complete resection and repair, this procedure is performed after the hysterectomy.[60,61]

The hysterectomy starts with electrodesiccation and transection of the round ligament close to the pelvic sidewall (Figure 15-36). The peritoneum is opened, and the paravesical spaces are dissected by blunt dissection, hydrodissection, and CO_2 laser. This technique allows excellent skeletonization of the obliterated hypogastric artery (Figure 15-37).[51,53]

The bladder serosa is injected with lactated Ringer's.[59] The bladder flap is developed using the CO_2 laser or sharp scissors and countertraction. After division of scar tissue in the vesicouterine fold, the suction-irrigator probe is used for blunt dissection and mobilization of the bladder (Figure 15-38). The infundibulopelvic ligaments are electrodesiccated with bipolar electrocoagulation and transected with the laser (Figure 15-39).

The uterine vessels are retracted medially and removed from the ureter using the CO_2 laser. The anterior parametrium is transected using the laser, with the suction-irrigator probe as a backstop to protect the ureter. The ureters are freed from the peritoneum and skeletonized down to the bladder using the suction-irrigator probe and the laser. The uterine vessels are electrodesiccated close to the hypogastric artery (Figure 15-40).

Cardinal Ligaments

At the level of the cardinal ligaments, the ureter and the descending branches of the uterine artery are close to one another and the cervix. Therefore, cardinal ligament dissection must be precise to prevent bleeding and ureteral injury. The linear stapler is used only if the parametrium has been dissected with ample margins, as in cervical malignancy. The linear stapler is 12 mm wide, which

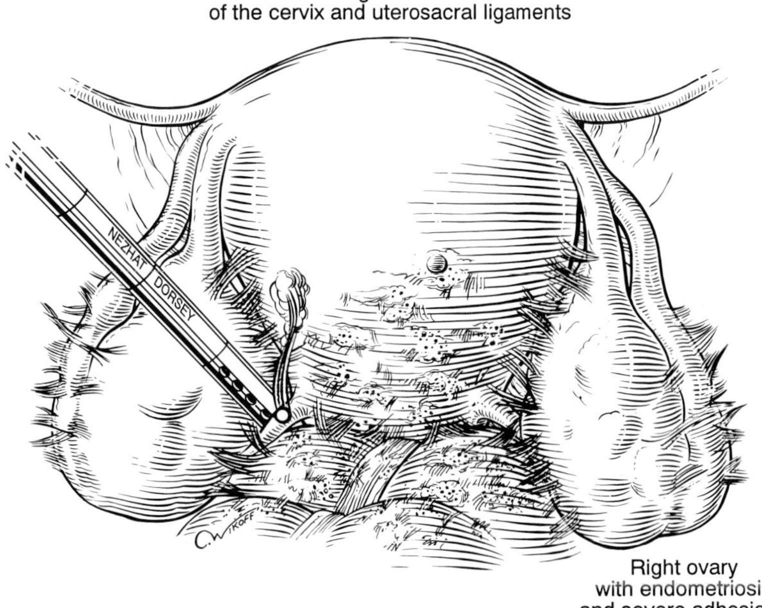

Figure 15-34 The rectum, which is severely attached to the back of the cervix and uterosacral ligaments, is dissected.

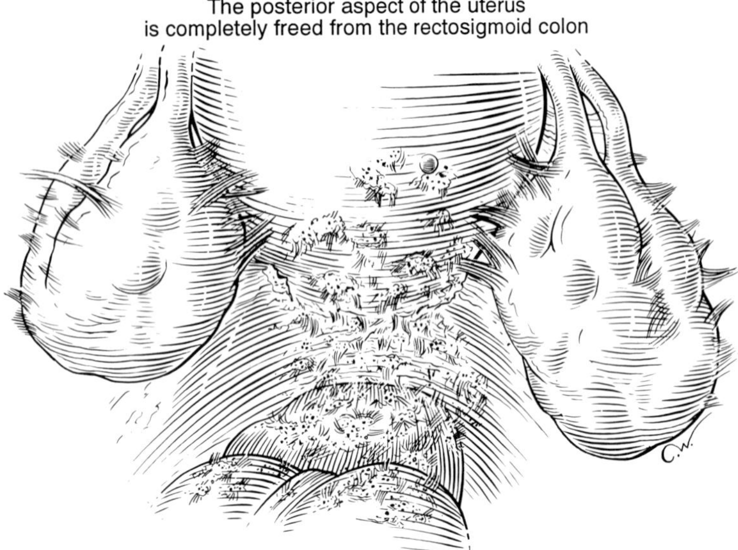

Figure 15-35 The rectosigmoid colon is freed from the posterior aspect of the uterus and cervix.

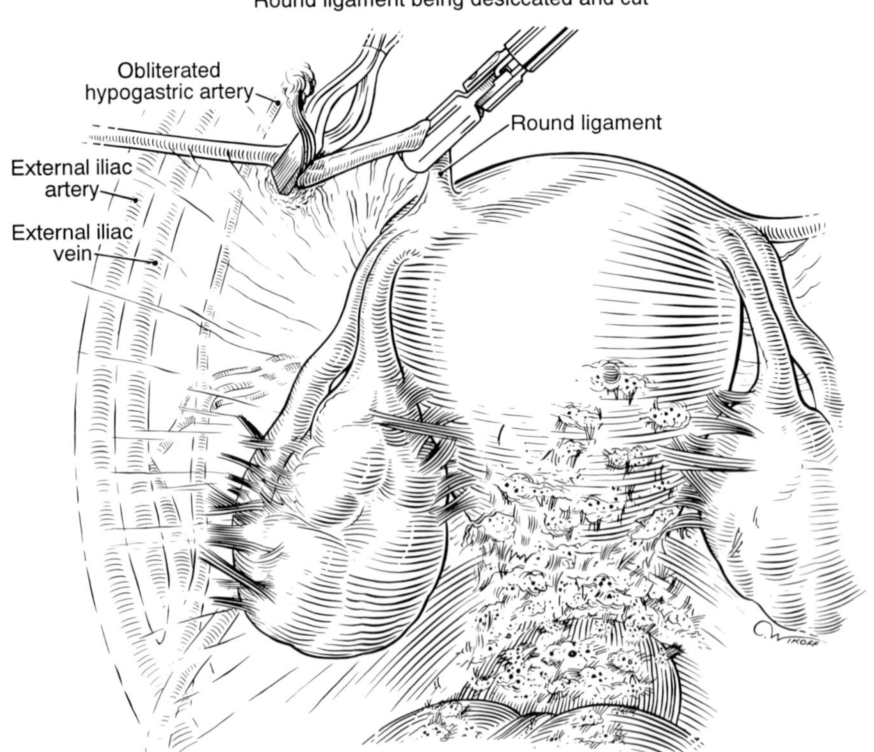

Figure 15-36 While the uterus is pulled to the right, the left round ligament is electrodesiccated close to the pelvic sidewall.

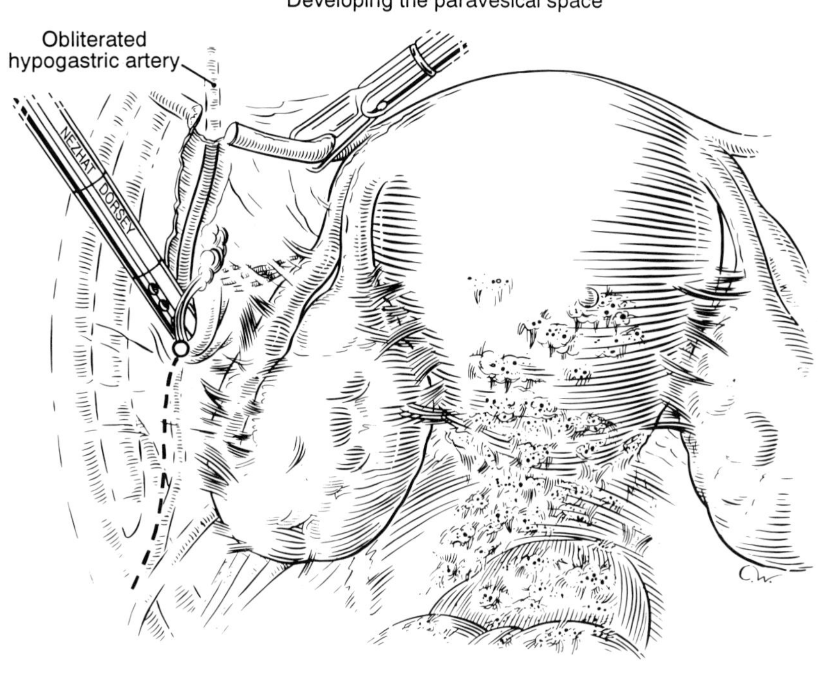

Figure 15-37 The hydrodissection probe is used as a backstop for the CO_2 laser to develop the paravesical space. The surgeon must be careful to avoid injury to the major pelvic sidewall vessels and the ureter.

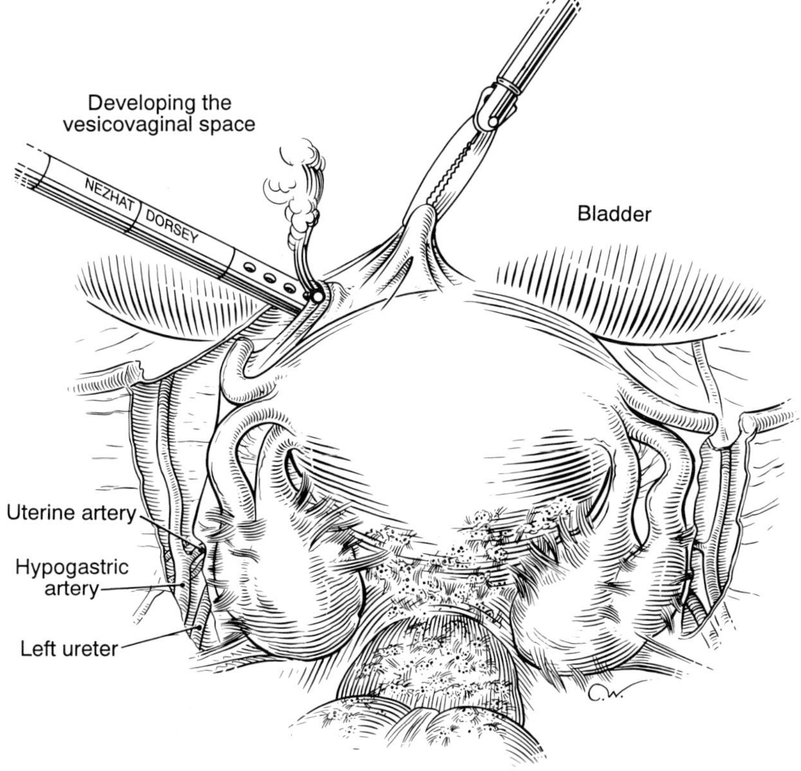

Figure 15-38 Preparation for developing the vesicovaginal space. The anterior leaf of the left broad ligament is dissected using hydrodissection and the CO_2 laser.

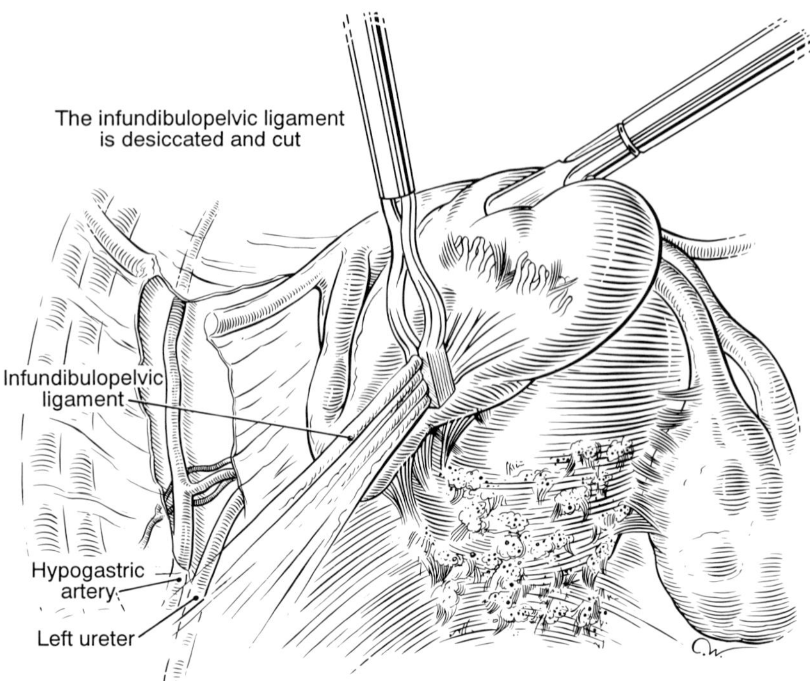

Figure 15-39 Desiccation of the infundibulopelvic ligament. The left infundibulopelvic ligament is electrodesiccated close to the ovary using bipolar forceps.

considering the short distance between the cervix and ureter, increases the risk of ureteral injury by stapler. Using contralateral retraction of the uterus, the cardinal ligament is dissected to identify tissue planes, vessels, and the ureter (Figure 15-41). Once the ureter is displaced laterally, the cardinal ligament tissue closest to the cervix is electrodesiccated and transected (Figure 15-42). The bladder pillars, which can be very thick and involved with endometriosis, are transected close to the cervix (Figure 15-43).

Culdotomy with Cuff Closure

After the uterosacral ligaments are dissected completely, and a folded wet gauze in a sponge forceps, or the tip of a right angle Heaney retractor, is used to mark the anterior or posterior vaginal fornix, the vaginal wall is tented and transected horizontally with laser or electrode (Figures 15-44 and 15-45). Bipolar electrocoagulation is used to control bleeding. The remainder of the procedure is performed vaginally if it is possible or if the operator prefers.

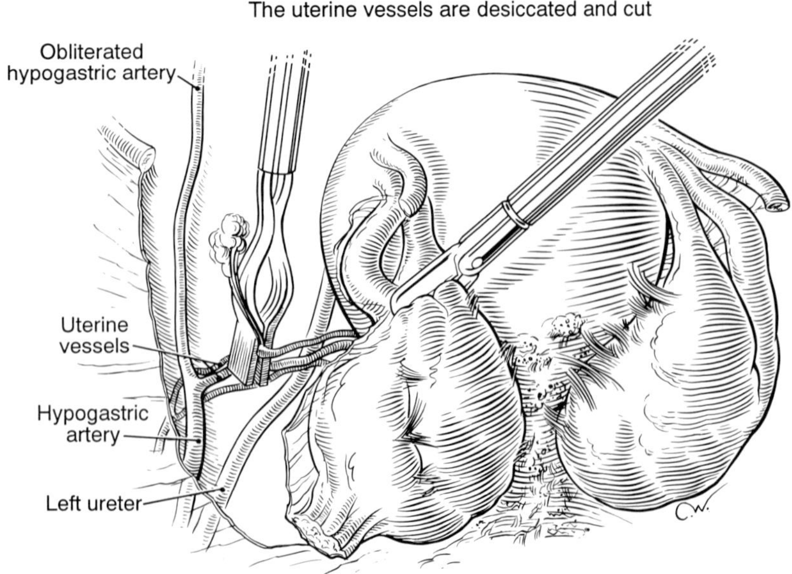

Figure 15-40 Desiccation of the uterine vessels. The paravesical space is developed and the uterine vessels identified. The uterine artery at its origin from the hypogastric artery is electrodesiccated using bipolar forceps. The ureter must be observed and excessive heat avoided to prevent ureteral injury.

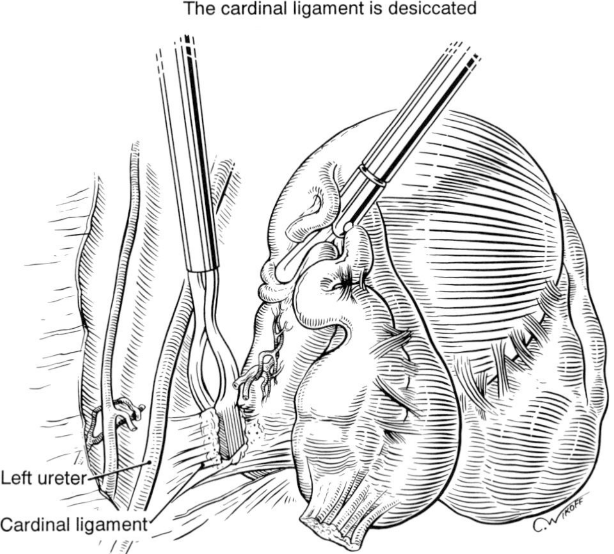

Figure 15-41 Electrodesiccation of cardinal ligament. While the uterus is pulled to the right, bipolar forceps are used to desiccate the cardinal ligaments close to the cervix. The ureter is distanced from the bipolar forceps.

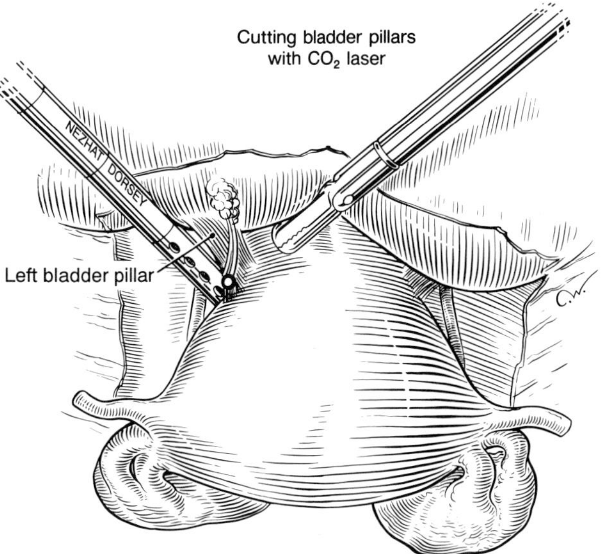

Figure 15-43 The vesicocervical fascia (bladder pillars) is dissected close to the cervix using the CO_2 laser.

Total Laparoscopic Hysterectomy

If TLH is performed, we place two 4 × 4 wet sponges in a glove and insert it into the vagina to prevent loss of pneumoperitoneum. By applying contralateral retraction to the uterus, the vaginal wall surrounding the cervix is outlined, coagulated with unipolar scissors or bipolar forceps, and cut circumferentially until the cervix is separated (Figure 15-46). The specimen is pulled to mid-vagina but not removed to preserve pneumoperitoneum. The vaginal cuff is irrigated and inspected for active bleeding. Once hemostasis is achieved, vaginal angles are sutured to the adjacent cardinal and uterosacral ligaments; care is taken to avoid the ureters. The rest of the vaginal cuff is closed with O Vicryl (Ethicon) suture on a straight or curved needle using extracorporeal knotting (Figures 15-47 and 15-48). Endoscopic suturing can

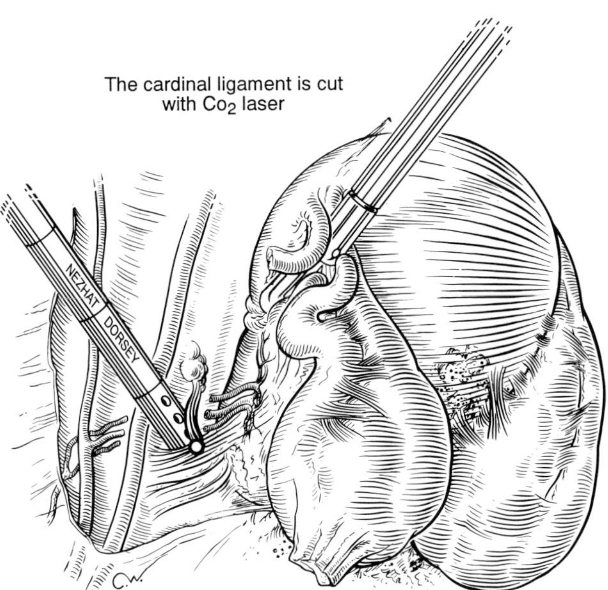

Figure 15-42 The cardinal ligament is dissected with the CO_2 laser.

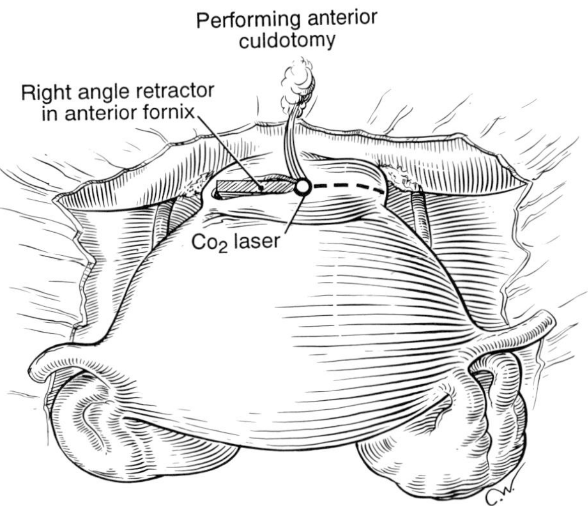

Figure 15-44 Laparscopic anterior culdotomy. An assistant places a right angle Heaney retractor in the anterior fornix and the CO_2 laser is used to perform an anterior culdotomy.

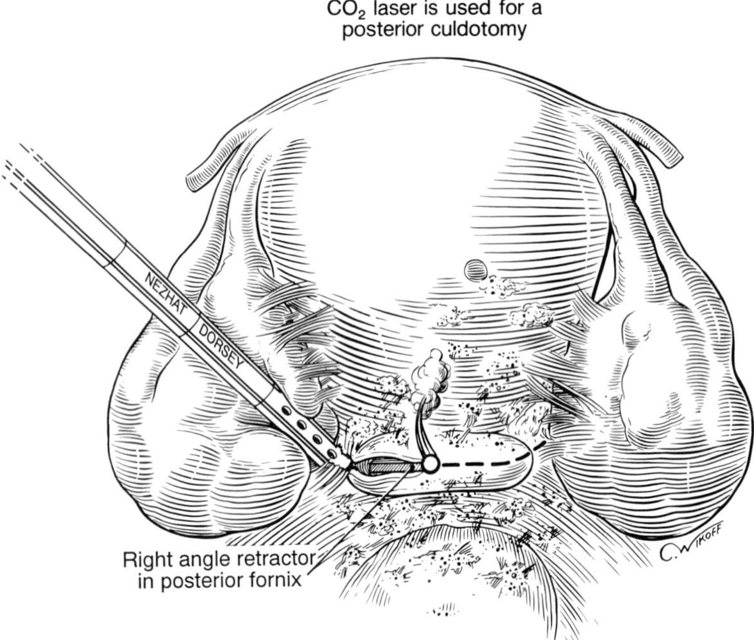

Figure 15-45 Posterior culdotomy. A right angle Heaney retractor is used to help identify the site for a posterior culdotomy. The CO_2 laser is used to cut the remainder of the uterosacral and cardinal ligament.

be difficult and time consuming and is performed in selected cases, such as in women with severe vaginal stenosis. Bipolar electrocoagulation is used cautiously at the vaginal cuff to prevent tissue necrosis and subsequent wound breakdown if sutures are placed in nonviable tissue.

Moschcowitz Procedure

By obliterating the posterior cul-de-sac, this procedure may prevent enterocele, especially in patients with a deep pelvis. A continuous nonabsorbable or delayed absorbable suture is placed through the various structures of the posterior cul-de-sac, preventing herniation into the rectovaginal space. The suture is started laterally over the periureteral area after the ureter is located. It is passed through the serosa of the rectosigmoid colon posteriorly, the contralateral side to include the opposite periureteral area, and the anterior vaginal wall. When tied, the posterior cul-de-sac is

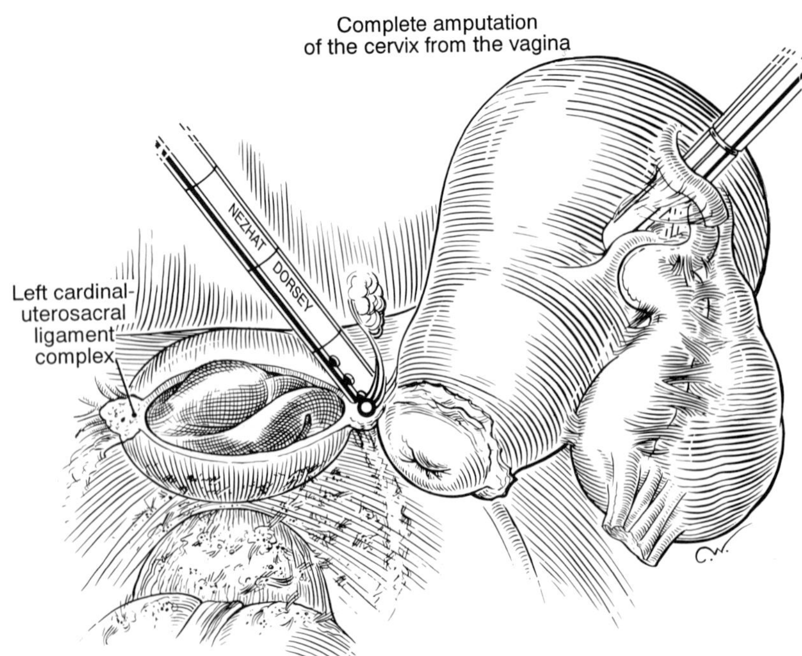

Figure 15-46 The cervix is amputated from the vagina. After anterior and posterior culdotomy are performed, the remainder of the cardinal and uterosacral ligaments on each side are dissected and the uterus is removed.

Figure 15-47 Laparoscopic vaginal cuff closure. After the uterus is removed, two sponges are placed in a surgical glove and left inside the vagina to prevent the loss of pneumoperitoneum. The vaginal angles are sutured to the uterosacral-cardinal ligament complex and the cuff is closed using 0 Vicryl laparoscopic sutures and intracorporeal or extracorporeal knot tying.

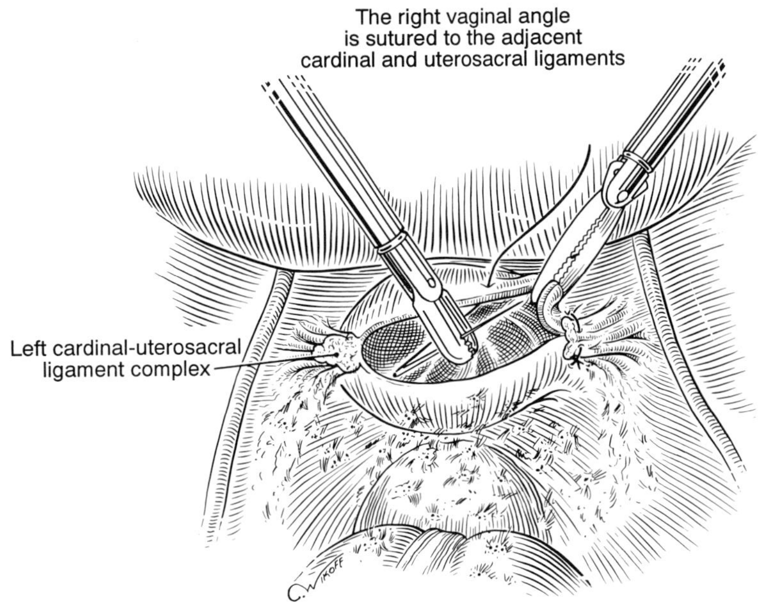

obliterated. Injury to the ureter, rectum, and bladder is avoided by meticulous suturing.

Final Laparoscopic Evaluation

The vaginal cuff is closed from below or above, and pneumoperitoneum is restored. The pelvic and abdominal cavities are evaluated laparoscopically, copiously irrigated, and cleared of blood clots and debris. Bleeding is controlled and the pelvis is filled with 300 to 500 mL lactated Ringer's before reevaluating and inspecting the pedicles and vaginal cuff under low pneumoperitoneal pressure.[52,62] The vaginal cuff is examined to ensure that no small bowel or omental tissue is included in its closure. At this point, the fluid in the pelvis should be clear and a final look at the ureters should confirm normal peristalsis and anatomic integrity. If the stapling device has been used, the stapler line is evaluated for hemostasis under low pneumoperitoneal pressure. To avoid incisional omental or bowel strangulation after the removal of any trocar(s) more than 5 mm in size, the fascia is repaired with delayed absorbable sutures.[63]

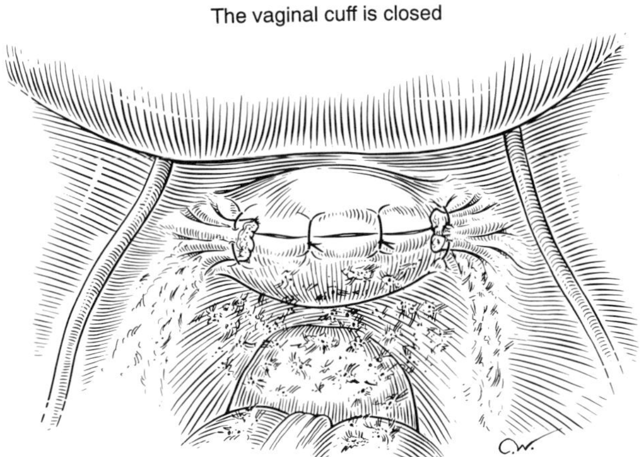

Figure 15-48 The vaginal cuff is repaired laparoscopically.

Subtotal Hysterectomy

Supracervical hysterectomy is requested by patients and performed by some gynecologists who believe that the cervix affects sexuality and orgasm and helps provide better vaginal support. The procedure is performed laparoscopically with the difficulty of removing the specimen through a small abdominal incision.

After desiccating and cutting the uterine vessels at the level of the cardinal ligaments above the uterosacral ligaments, the uterus is retracted and its lower segment amputated with scissors, unipolar endoscopic electrode, or laser. After transecting the uterus from the cervix, the uterine manipulator is removed vaginally, the cervical stump irrigated, and hemostasis is achieved. The endocervical epithelium lining the cervical canal is vaporized or coagulated with laser or electrosurgery. The rest of the endocervical canal is ablated vaginally to reduce the risk of intraepithelial cervical neoplasia. The cervical stump is closed with interrupted absorbable sutures and covered with peritoneum, which is sewn transversely with either continuous or interrupted sutures. The uterus is morcellated and removed through a 10-mm trocar, minilaparotomy, or posterior colpotomy. Copious peritoneal washing and thorough inspection of the pelvis and abdomen are performed at the end of the procedure. If the vagina is not entered, there are fewer sexual restrictions. These patients are advised of the continued risk of cervical neoplasia and the need for annual examinations and Papanicolaou smears.

Hysterectomy for Large Myomas

At CSPS, the largest uterus that has been treated by this method was 26 weeks gestational size (1530 g). The following factors are considered when selecting patients for this procedure:

1. The patient must have an adequate hemoglobin and hematocrit.
2. GnRH analogs can be used if the uterus is more than 18 weeks gestational size.
3. The primary trocar is inserted between the umbilicus and xyphoid when the uterus is more than 18 weeks gestational size. The secondary trocars are placed higher than usual.

A uterus of more than 16 weeks gestational size with multiple large leiomyomas is more difficult to manipulate laparoscopically. Three, and at times, four secondary trocars are introduced to provide adequate traction to the uterus. The anatomy can be distorted and ureteral dissection may be necessary, although the ureters usually can be seen more easily in patients with large myomas. Although it is possible to dissect the uterus laparoscopically, it may take longer than a combined laparoscopic and vaginal approach. If there is a large pedunculated leiomyoma that interferes with the exposure and laparoscopic manipulation, myomectomy is performed first. The laparoscopic approach is continued until the cardinal ligaments are reached and the remaining portion of the procedure is completed vaginally. After the uterosacral and cardinal ligaments are ligated and cut vaginally, the uterus is morcellated and removed vaginally.

Current Experience

The first publication of a randomized series comparing abdominal hysterectomy (10 patients) to LAVH (10 patients) in 1992 by Nezhat and coworkers,[52] established the validity of LAVH and suggested that it could replace most abdominal hysterectomies for benign lesions. The indications for laparoscopic hysterectomy in this series were similar to those listed for abdominal rather than vaginal hysterectomy. All hysterectomies in the LAVH group were completed endoscopically without significant complications. These patients had minimal morbidity, blood loss, postoperative discomfort, hospitalization, and recovery time. Following submission of this report, an additional 96 hysterectomies were completed laparoscopically without major complications.

A slightly less optimistic experience with laparoscopic hysterectomy was reported by Bruhat and colleagues[64] in a series of 36 patients of whom 27 (75%) were treated successfully by laparoscopy and 9 (25%) were converted to laparotomy. Surgeons had difficulty achieving hemostasis (6 cases) and locating anatomic landmarks (3 cases) because of a large uterus, myoma, or long cervix.[64] Nevertheless, the authors concluded that LAVH is a viable option to abdominal hysterectomy in properly selected patients.

Although laparoscopic hysterectomy compares favorably to abdominal hysterectomy, offering reduced morbidity, expenses, and discomfort, the opposite is true when LAVH is compared to standard vaginal hysterectomy, as reported by Summit and associates.[56] Of 56 women scheduled to undergo vaginal hysterectomy in an outpatient setting, 29 were randomized to LAVH and 27 to standard vaginal hysterectomy. In the latter group, all surgical procedures were completed and patients were discharged within 12 hours of admission. In the LAVH group one patient suffered a bladder laceration, which was repaired, and the hysterectomy was completed endoscopically. A second patient experienced bleeding from the inferior epigastric vessels. It could not be controlled endoscopically, and she underwent exploratory laparotomy with abdominal hysterectomy. When the two groups were compared, the LAVH group required more pain medication, experienced greater blood loss and more intraoperative complications, and incurred higher surgical expenses, a mean of $7905 versus $4891 for the standard vaginal group. These results strongly support the recommendation that LAVH should not replace vaginal hysterectomy.

At CSPS in Atlanta, 361 women fulfilled criteria for abdominal hysterectomy but underwent LAVH (24), VALH (148), TLH (176), or SLH (13) from July 1987 through July 1993 (Table 15-8). Bipolar forceps and CO_2 laser were used for hemostasis and cutting, respectively. Cases that required suturing, staples, or clips for hemostasis or had malignancy were excluded from the study. Preoperative indications for hysterectomy included chronic pelvic pain (116 women), chronic pelvic pain with abnormal uterine bleeding (148 women), abnor-

TABLE 15-8 Type of Laparoscopic Hysterectomy Performed

		BSO	RSO	LSO
LAVH	24	14	2	3
VALH	148	94	12	13
TLH	176	114	15	29
SLH	13	6	0	1
TOTALS	361	228	29	46

BSO, bilateral salpingo-oophorectomy; LAVH, laparoscopically assisted vaginal hysterectomy; LSO, left salpingo-oophorectomy; RSO, right salpingo-oophorectomy; SLH, subtotal laparoscopic hysterectomy; TLH, total laparoscopic hysterectomy; VALH, vaginally assisted laparoscopic hysterectomy.

mal uterine bleeding (40 women), and enlarging leiomyoma (28 women). Other indications were endometrial hyperplasia, cervical dysplasia, pelvic abscess, ectopic pregnancy, and pelvic relaxation (Table 15-9). There were no conversions to laparotomy, although one patient with bowel endometriosis and stricture underwent laparotomy for bowel resection and anastomosis. Intraoperative and pathologic findings are summarized in Table 15-10. Most patients underwent one or more additional procedures (Table 15-11) and the complication rate was 10% (Table 15-12).

Vaginal cuff dehiscence is a rare posthysterectomy complication that has been reported following both abdominal and vaginal hysterectomies, and may occur spontaneously or postcoitally. We recently noted vaginal cuff dehiscence following total laparoscopic hysterectomy in two women, who were not included in this study, at 2 and 4 months postoperatively. Both presented with vaginal bleeding and abdominal pain. One occurred following vaginal intercourse, and the other was apparently spontaneous. In one woman, a portion of the small bowel protruded into the vagina; the other woman only had opening of the vaginal cuff. In each case, repair was accomplished vaginally using 0 polydioxanone. Both women continue to do well.

TABLE 15-9 Summary of 361 Women Who Underwent LAVH, VALH, TLH, or SLH

Mean age	42.5 (25–72) y
Gravidity	1.6 (0–7)
Parity	1.3 (0–5)
Mean duration of procedure	2.3 h (55 min to 6.5 h)
Uterine size	4–26 wks gestational size
Mean uterine weight	178.38 g (36–1530 g)
Average blood loss	73 mL (50–800 mL)
Average hospital stay*	21 h (20 h to 5 days)
Postoperative full recovery†	3.3 wk (3 d to 13 wks)
Need for postoperative pain medication‡	3.3 d (0–21 days)

*From termination of procedure until discharge from hospital.
†This information was obtained during office visits, written questionnaires, and telephone interviews.
‡After the patient was discharged from the hospital.
Abbreviations are defined in text and in Table 15–8.

TABLE 15-10 Intraoperative and Pathologic Findings in 361 Women

Mild to extensive endometriosis	212
Mild to extensive adhesions	189
Uterine fibroids (uterine size 8–26 wks)	116
Uterine adenomyosis	119
Endometriomas (5–15 cm diameter)	22
Endometrial polyp	13
Endometrial hyperplasia	2
Cervical dysplasia	4
Large cornual pregnancy	1
Hydrosalpinx	7
Pelvic abscess	1
Asherman syndrome	2
Benign cystic teratoma	3
Serous cyst	2
Mucinous cyst	2
Paraovarian cyst	2

Concluding Remarks

An estimated one in five women will undergo hysterectomy, making hysterectomy the second most

TABLE 15-11 Additional Procedures Performed at the Time of Hysterectomy

Treatment of mild to extensive endometriosis	212
Lysis of mild to extensive abdominal and/or pelvic adhesions	189
Ureterolysis	129
Moschcowitz procedure	88
Appendectomy	47
Marshall-Marchetti-Krantz or Burch procedure	43
Rectocele repair	24
Cystocele repair	13
Bowel resection	11
Enterocele repair	6
Removal of ovarian remnant	4
Vaginal sacral colposuspension	2
Cholecystectomy	2
Removal of pelvic abscess	1
Removal of ectopic pregnancy	1

TABLE 15-12 Complications Following Hysterectomy in 361 Women

	Number	Incidence/ 100 Women
I. Mortality	0	0.00
II. Intraoperative		
A. Vascular		
1. Inferior epigastric vessel injury	3	0.83
2. Hemorrhage requiring transfusion	2	0.55
3. Major blood vessel injury	0	0.00
B. Gastrointestinal		
1. Small bowel injury	1	0.27
2. Large bowel injury	0	0.00
C. Urological		
1. Bladder	1	0.27
2. Ureter	0	0.00
III. Postoperative		
A. Vascular		
1. Vaginal cuff bleeding	3	0.83
2. Delayed incisional bleeding	1	0.27
3. Abdominal wall ecchymosis	4	1.12
B. Gastrointestinal		
1. Gastroenteritis	1	0.27
C. Urological		
1. Cystitis	6	1.66
2. Urinary retention	3	0.83
3. Fistula	0	0.00
D. Febrile Morbidity and Infection		
1. Vaginal cuff cellulitis and pelvic infection	0	0.00
2. Transient high fever (38 degrees Celsius) after 24 hours	5	1.39
E. Cardiopulmonary		
1. Transient tachycardia	1	0.27
2. Pneumonia, bronchitis	4	1.12
F. Others		
1. Ovarian remnant syndrome	2	0.55
Total	37	10.23

commonly performed surgical procedure in the United States. Currently, 25% of hysterectomies are performed vaginally, the least traumatic, safest, and most cost-effective way to remove the uterus. But 75% of hysterectomies continue to be performed abdominally. VALH or LH are excellent alternatives when the standard vaginal approach is contraindicated. However, the endoscopic approach may be more difficult in women with extensive abdominal and pelvic adhesions or in women with uteri of more than 22 weeks gestational size. Laparoscopic complications occur mostly during an endoscopic surgeon's early experience. Nevertheless, these operations offer many advantages and efforts should no longer be directed toward validating LAVH, but rather toward providing gynecologic surgeons with more opportunities for training.

References

1. Buttram VC, Reiter RC. Uterine leiomyomata: etiology symptomatology and management. *Fertil Steril.* 1981;36:433.
2. Vollenhoven BJ, Lawrence AS, Healy DL. Uterine fibroids: a clinical review. *Br J Obstet Gynaecol.* 1990;97:285.
3. Cramer SF, Robertson AL, Ziats NP, et al. Growth potential of human uterine leiomyomas: some in vitro observations and their implications. *Obstet Gynecol.* 1990; 97:393.
4. Fedele L, Vercellini P, Bianchi S, et al. Treatment with GnRH agonists before myomectomy and the risk of short-term myoma recurrence. *Br J Obstet Gynaecol.* 1990;97: 393.
5. Fedele L, Bianchi S, Dorta M. Transvaginal ultrasonography versus hysteroscopy in the diagnosis of uterine submucous myomas. *Obstet Gynecol.* 1991;77:745.
6. Nezhat CR, Nezhat F, Bess O, et al. Laparoscopically assisted myomectomy: a comparison of a new technique to myomectomy by laparotomy and laparoscopy. *Int J Fertil.* 1994;39:39.
7. Nezhat C, Nezhat F, Silfen SL, et al. Laparoscopic myomectomy. *Int J Fertil.* 1991; 36:275–280.
8. Harris WJ. Uterine dehiscence following laparoscopic myomectomy. *Obstet Gynecol.* 1992;80:545–546.
9. Nezhat CR, Nezhat F. Laparoscopic myomectomy complications. *Int J Fertil.* 1991;37:64. (Letter).
10. Hasson HM, Rotman C, Rana N, et al. Laparoscopic myomectomy. *Obstet Gynecol.* 1992;80:884–888.
11. Dubuisson JB, Lecuru F, Herve F, et al. Myomectomy by laparoscopy. *Fertil Steril.* 1991;56:827–830.

12. Friedman AJ, Rein NS, Harrison-Atlas D, et al. A randomized, placebo-controlled, double blind study evaluating leuprolide acetate depot treatment before myomectomy. *Fertil Steril.* 1989;52:728.
13. Shaw RW. Mechanism of LHRH analogue action in uterine fibroids. *Horm Res.* 1989; 32:150.
14. Operative laparoscopy study group. Postoperative adhesion development after operative laparoscopy: evaluation at early second-look procedures. *Fertil Steril.* 1991;55: 700–704.
15. Linsky CB, Diamond MP, DiZerega GS. Effect of blood on the efficacy of barrier adhesion reduction in the rabbit uterine horn model. *Infertility.* 1988;11:273.
16. Bayers SP, Jansen D. Gore-Tex surgical membrane. In: DeCherney A, Diamond MP, eds. *Treatment of Post-Surgical Adhesions.* New York: Wiley Liss; 1990:93.
17. Georgakopoulous PA, Bersis G. Sigmoido-uterine rupture in pregnancy after multiple myomectomy. *Int Surg.* 1981;66:367–368.
18. Lumsden MA, West CP, Baird DT. Goserelin therapy before surgery for uterine fibroids. *Lancet.* 1987;1:36.
19. Rock JA. Gonadotropin-releasing hormone agonist analogs in the treatment of uterine leiomyomas. *J Gynecol Surg.* 1991;7:147.
20. George M, Lhomme C, Lefort J, et al. Long-term use of an LH-RH agonist in the management of uterine leiomyomas: a study of 17 cases. *Int J Fertil.* 1989;34:19.
21. Davis, GD, Hruby PH. Transabdominal laser colpotomy. *J Reprod Med.* 1989;34:438.
22. Nezhat C, Nezhat F. Videolaseroscopy for the treatment of adenomyosis. Abstract presented at the 19th annual meeting of the American Association of Gynecologic Laparoscopists, Orlando, FL, 1990.
23. Ansbacher R. Uterine anomalies and future pregnancies. *Clin Perinatol.* 1983;10: 295–304.
24. Rock JA, Schlaff WD. The obstetric consequences of uterovaginal anomalies. *Fertil Steril.* 1985;43:681–691.
25. Buttram VC, Gibbons WE. Müllerian anomalies: a proposed classification. *Fertil Steril.* 1979;32:40–46.
26. Mattingly RF, Thompson JD, eds. Surgery for anomalies of the müllerian ducts. In: *Te-Linde's Operative Gynecology*, 6th ed. Philadelphia: JB Lippincott; 1985.
27. Canis M, Wattiez A, Pouly JL, et al. Laparoscopic management of unicornuate uterus with rudimentary horn and unilateral extensive endometriosis: case report. *Hum Reprod.* 1990;5:819–820.
28. Nezhat F, Nezhat C, Bess O. Laparoscopic amputation of a noncommunicating rudimentary horn after a hysteroscopic diagnosis. A case study. *Surg Laparosc Endosc.* 1994; 4:155–156.
29. Donaldson JK, Sanderlin JH, Harrell WB. A method of suspending the uterus without open abdominal incision. *Am J Surg.* 1942; 15:537.
30. Smith DB, Kelsey JF, Sherman RL, et al. Laparoscopic uterine suspension. *J Reprod Med.* 1977;18:98.
31. Paterson MEL, Jordan JA, Logan-Edwards R. A survey of 100 patients who had laparoscopic ventrosuspension. *Br J Obstet Gynaecol.* 1978;85:468.
32. Servy EJ, Aksu MF, Tzingounis VA. Laparoscopic hysteropexy and the position of the fallopian tubes. In: Phillips JM, ed. *Endoscopy in Gynecology.* Sante Fe Springs, CA: American Association of Gynecologic Laparoscopists Department of Publications; 1978:87.
33. Gleeson NC, Gaffney GMN. Ventrosuspension—five years of practice at the Rotunda Hospital reviewed. *J Obstet Gynecol.* 1990;10:415.
34. Yoong AFE. Laparoscopic ventrosuspension: a review of 72 cases. *Am J Obstet Gynecol.* 1990;163:1151.
35. Massouda D, Ling FW, Muram D, et al. Laparoscopic uterine suspension with fallope rings. *J Reprod Med.* 1987;32:859.
36. Steptoe PC. *Laparoscopy in Gynecology.* London: Livingstone; 1967:78.
37. Candy JW. Modified Gilliam uterine suspension using laparoscopic visualization. *Obstet Gynecol.* 1976;47:242.
38. Mann WJ, Stenger VG. Uterine suspension through the laparoscope. *Obstet Gynecol.* 1978;51:563.
39. Lose G, Lindholm P. Impaired voiding efficiency and urinary retention after laparoscopic ventrosuspension ad modum Steptoe. *Acta Obstet Gynecol Scand.* 1984;63:371.
40. Selwood T, Wood C. Incidence of hysterectomy in Australia. *Med J Aust.* 1978;2:201.
41. van Keep PA, Wildemeersch D, Lehert P. Hysterectomy in six European countries. *Maturitas.* 1983;5:69.
42. Porkas R, Hufnagel VG. Hysterectomy in the

United States, 1964–84. *Am J Public Health.* 1988;78:852.

43. Bachmann GA. Hysterectomy: a critical review. *J Reprod Med.* 1990;35:839.
44. Dicker RC, Scally MJ, Greenspan JR, et al. Hysterectomy among women of reproductive age. *JAMA.* 1982;248:323.
45. Palmer RH, Kane G, Churchill H, et al. Cost and quality in the use of blood bank services for normal deliveries, cesarean sections, and hysterectomies. *JAMA.* 1986;256:219.
46. Dranov P. Change of life: for some women hysterectomy has profound consequences. *New York Magazine*, October 1987.
47. White SC, Wartel LJ, Wade ME. Comparison of abdominal and vaginal hysterectomy—a review of 600 operations. *Obstet Gynecol.* 1971;37:530.
48. Wingo PA, Huezo CM, Rubin GL, et al. The mortality risk associated with hysterectomy. *Am J Obstet Gynecol.* 1985;152:803.
49. Kovac RS, Cruikshank SH, Retto FH. Laparoscopy-assisted vaginal hysterectomy. *J Gynecol Surg.* 1990;6:185.
50. Nezhat C, Nezhat F, Silfen SL. Laparoscopic hysterectomy and bilateral salpingo-oophorectomy using multifire GIA surgical stapler. *J Gynecol Surg.* 1990;6:287.
51. Nezhat C, Burrell MO, Nezhat FR, et al. Laparoscopic radical hysterectomy with paraaortic and pelvic node dissection. *Am J Obstet Gynecol.* 1992;166:864–865.
52. Nezhat C, Nezhat F, Gordon S, et al. Laparoscopic versus abdominal hysterectomy. *J Reprod Med.* 1992;37:247–250.
53. Nezhat CR, Nezhat FR, Ramirez CE, Burrell M, Carrodeguas J, Nezhat CH. Laparoscopic radical hysterectomy and laparoscopic assisted vaginal radical hysterectomy with pelvic and paraaortic node dissection. *J Gynecol Surg.* 1993;9:105–120.
54. Lee NC, Dicker RC, Rubin GL, et al. Confirmation of the preoperative diagnoses for hysterectomy. *Am J Obstet Gynecol.* 1984; 150:283.
55. Nezhat C, Nezhat F, Burrell M. Laparoscopically assisted hysterectomy for the management of a borderline ovarian tumor: a case report. *J Laparoendosc Surg.* 1992;2: 167–169.
56. Summit RL, Stovall TG, Lipscomb GH, et al. Randomized comparison of laparoscopy-assisted vaginal hysterectomy with standard vaginal hysterectomy in an outpatient setting. *Obstet Gynecol.* 1992;80:895.
57. Nezhat C, Nezhat F, Nezhat C. Operative laparoscopy (minimally invasive surgery): state of the art. *J Gynecol Surg.* 1992; 8:111–141.
58. Nezhat F, Nezhat C, Levy JS. A report of laparoscopic injuries and complications over a 10-year period. Presented at 41st annual clinical meeting of American College of Obstetricians and Gynecologists, Washington, DC, May 3–6, 1993.
59. Nezhat C, Nezhat F. Safe laser excision or vaporization of peritoneal endometriosis. *Fertil Steril.* 1989;52:149–151.
60. Nezhat F, Nezhat C, Pennington E, et al. Laparoscopic segmental resection for infiltrating endometriosis of the rectosigmoid colon: a preliminary report. *Surg Laparosc Endosc.* 1992;2:212–216.
61. Nezhat C, Nezhat F, Pennington E, et al. Laparoscopic disk excision and primary repair of the anterior rectal wall for the treatment of full thickness bowel endometriosis. *Surg Endosc.* 1994;8:682.
62. Nezhat C, Nezhat F, Winer W. Salpingectomy via laparoscopy: a new surgical approach. *J Laparosc Surg.* 1991;1:91–95.
63. Nezhat C, Nezhat F, Bess O, et al. Injuries associated with the use of a linear stapler during operative laparoscopy: review of diagnosis, management, and prevention. *J Gynecol Surg.* 1993;3:145–150.
64. Bruhat MA, Mage G, Pouly JL, et al. Duvivier R, Vancaillie TG, trans. *Laparoscopic Hysterectomy in Operative Laparoscopy.* New York: McGraw-Hill; 1992:217–221.

16

Appendectomy

There are few areas in which the indications for and management by endoscopy are changing as rapidly as suspected appendicitis. As gynecologic and general surgeons perform more endoscopic procedures, the benefits and risks of laparoscopic appendectomy should be considered. This chapter describes the value of laparoscopy for diagnosis, discusses the indications for laparoscopic appendectomy, and illustrates the techniques.

Why Laparoscopy

Acute appendicitis is difficult to diagnose in women because many gynecologic disorders cause symptoms and signs indistinguishable from those of appendicitis.[1] In the general population, 15% to 20% of appendices removed by laparotomy for suspected appendicitis show no abnormality compared to 30% to 45% in young women.[2] The type and location of pain or discomfort associated with ovulation, ovarian cysts, endometriosis, salpingitis, and urinary tract disorders are not always easily differentiated from acute appendicitis. Accurate diagnosis and prompt management help prevent complications from perforation, including significant postoperative morbidity and an increased risk of tubal infertility.[3–5]

The sequelae from removing a normal appendix usually are not serious, although a 1% to 17% morbidity rate from such operations has been reported.[6,7] These observations and concern about postoperative adhesions have increased the use of laparoscopy for the diagnosis of the cause of pelvic and abdominal pain prior to definitive therapy.[8–10]

In a suspected appendicitis, laparoscopy can reduce the need for laparotomy because the surgeon inspects the peritoneal cavity and pelvis with the laparoscope and avoids even a McBurney or small laparotomy incision.[11,12] However, observation of the entire appendix is only possible in 90% to 95% of patients.[13] In addition, some visually normal appendices have been removed in which histologic examination revealed acute or chronic inflammation.[10,14]

In a series of 100 incidental appendectomies, 52 appendices were normal, 28 had adhesions, 14 showed foci of endometriosis, 4 showed focal chronic inflammation, and 1 contained a benign mucocele, and another a carcinoid.[7] These findings demonstrate the potential yield of appendiceal disease associated with the grossly normal appendix. A similar abnormality rate was reported by Krone[15] in his series of 1718 incidental appendectomies: 21.4% were normal, but 65.1% showed evidence of chronic disease and 5.6% had a carcinoid, a mucocele, or endometriosis.

Therefore, without an obvious appendiceal abnormality or other explanation for an acute abdomen, prophylactic laparoscopic appendectomy should be considered. It eliminates the chance of missing an early appendicitis and can remove the source of chronic right lower quadrant pain.

Prophylactic Appendectomy

Laparoscopic appendectomy is relatively simple and safe and could set a precedent for modern ambulatory surgery. Because disease is found in grossly normal appendices, excision removes both a potential site of disease and confusion in future diagnoses of right lower quadrant pain. With the expansion of procedures made possible by operative laparoscopy, the transition from laparoscopic diagnosis to laparoscopic appendectomy is logical.

Women with chronic right lower quadrant pain also have a high rate of gross or microscopic appendiceal abnormalities. In a series of 62 laparoscopic appendectomies performed for acute and chronic pain,[16] 38 were associated with entrapping adhesions, 12 showed evidence of chronic inflammation, and 5 were involved with endometriosis. Only 7 were normal. Of the 55 patients with predominantly right lower quadrant or flank pain, 53 had either complete or significant pain relief on long-term follow-up (1 to 6 years). These results indicate that when there are no other pelvic abnormalities, appendectomy should be considered. Prolonging laparoscopy for 4 to 21 minutes to perform an appendectomy adds minimal stress to the patient.[7]

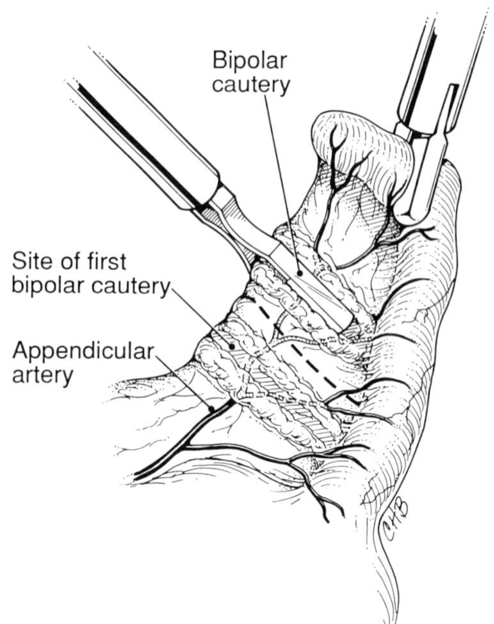

Figure 16-1. The mesoappendix is coagulated with bipolar forceps.

Technique

Prophylactic laparoscopic appendectomy is similar in principle to appendectomy by laparotomy. Prophylactic antibiotics are administered preoperatively to patients who complain of right lower quadrant pain. The operation is performed under general anesthesia. Appendectomy is advisable after other laparoscopic procedures and copious irrigation to minimize bacterial contamination.

After the pelvis is inspected, the appendix is identified, mobilized, and examined. Periappendiceal or pericecal adhesions are lysed using either the laser or scissors. Mobilization and exposure are essential, particularly if the appendix is attached to the pelvic sidewall or if it is retrocecal. The mesoappendix is coagulated with bipolar forceps or clipped and cut with laparoscopic scissors or laser to skeletonize the appendix (Figures 16-1 and 16-2). Fecal contents are milked out using a grasper over an area of 2 cm from the cecum. Two Endoloop sutures (Ethicon) are passed sequentially through one of the 5-mm suprapubic trocar sleeves and looped around the base of the appendix on top of each other (Figure 16-3). A third Endoloop suture is applied 5 mm distal to the first two sutures. Hulka tubal clips (used for tubal sterilization) also can be used to secure the proximal and distal portions of the appendix.[8,17] The appendix is cut between the two sets of sutures, using the laser or laparoscopic scissors (Figure 16-4). The luminal portion of the appendiceal stump is seared with the CO_2 laser, Betadine is applied, and the tissues copiously irrigated with lactated Ringer's solution (Figure 16-5).

A purse-string or Z-suture can be placed in the cecum to bury the appendiceal stump[18] although there appears to be no advantage to its invagination.[19] Countersinking the stump does not guarantee that adhesions or complications will be avoided. If the stump is to be buried, polydioxanone Endosuture (Ethicon) is used with two needleholders or graspers inserted through the suprapubic trocar sleeves. The stump is invaginated with a grasper, and the purse-string suture tied using an instrument tying method or extracorporeal suturing. A significant difference was found in the incidence of postoperative small bowel obstruction when invagination was compared to stump ligation. The invagination group had six cases (1.6%), and the stump ligation group had only one (0.3%). This difference in complications may be related to the high incidence of adhesions found in over 70% of patients with purse-string or Z-suture placement.[14]

Simple ligation simplifies the technical procedure and shortens the operating time. It produces no deformation of the cecal wall that might, in later contrast radiography, arouse suspicion of a neoplasm.

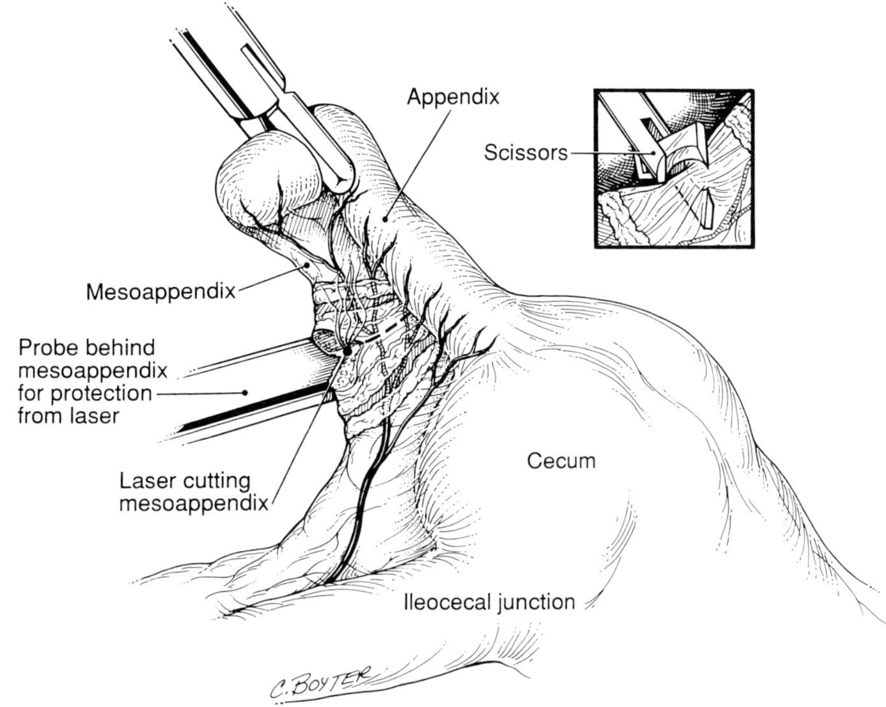

Figure 16-2. The mesoappendix is cut with CO_2 laser or laparoscopic scissors.

Stapling devices make laparoscopic appendectomy simpler and faster. The multifire stapler is introduced through a 12-mm suprapubic midline incision and applied directly across the entire mesoappendix and appendix (Figure 16-6). In a single motion, the entire appendix and its mesoappendix are clipped and cut (Figure 16-6, *inset*). It is important to ensure that the stapler's operation will not be hindered by contact with surrounding tissue and the cecum is free from attachments. Appendiceal contents do not leak intraperitoneally and the larger trocar sleeve allows easier removal of the separated appendix. Two disadvantages to the stapling device are its cost and the need to use a 12-mm trocar.

The appendix can be removed from the abdo-

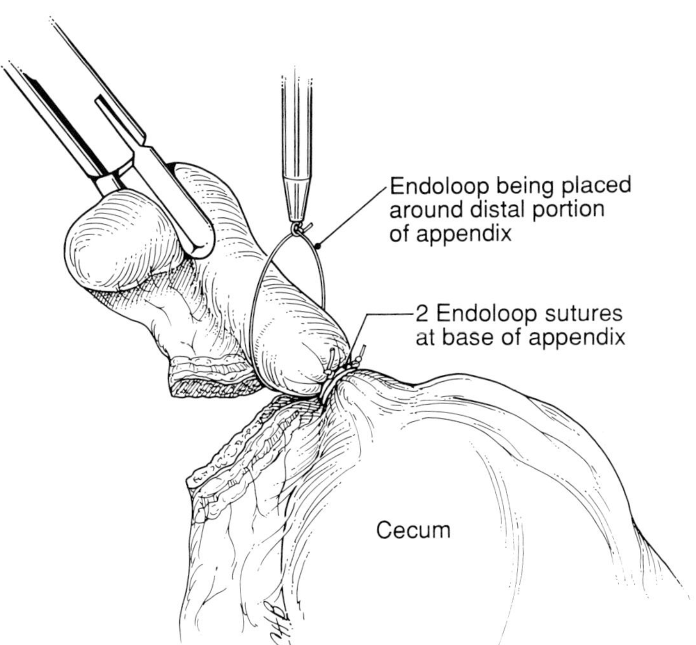

Figure 16-3. Endoloop sutures are placed around the base of appendix.

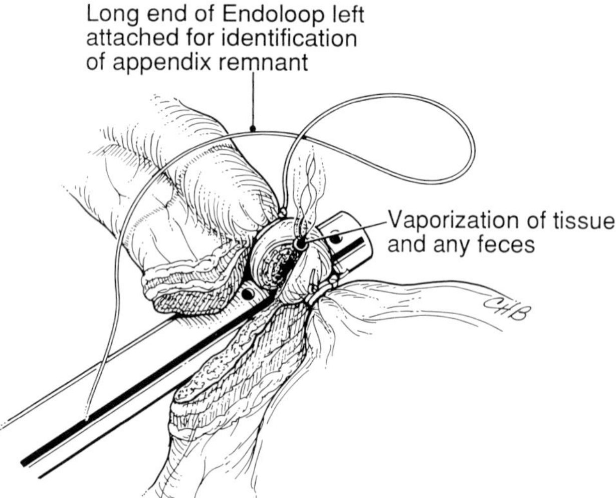

Figure 16-4. The appendix is excised with a CO_2 laser or scissors.

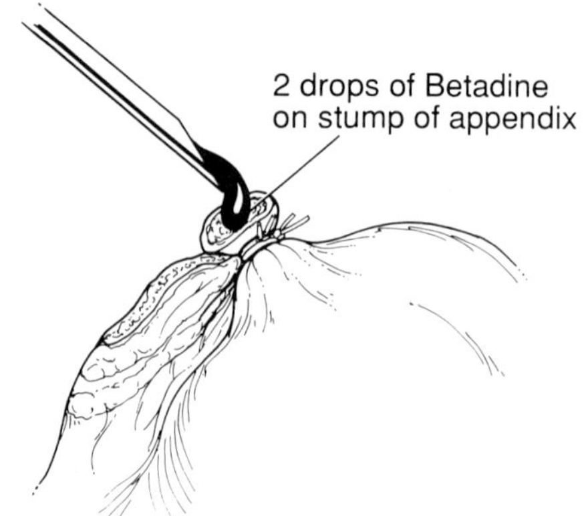

Figure 16-5. The appendiceal stump is seared with CO_2 laser or rinsed with Betadine.

men with long grasping forceps placed through the operating channel of the laparoscope. However, this method contaminates both the graspers and the operating channel. Alternately, an Endoloop suture can be placed around the distal tip of the appendix as a substitute for a grasping instrument during initial mobilization and excision of the appendix. Once the appendix is free, the suture is used to pull the appendix into a 5- or 10-mm accessory trocar sleeve. The trocar sleeve is removed from the suprapubic incision with the appendix contained within. Endobags (Ethicon) that minimize contact between contaminated tissue and the pelvis are available. Traction on the purse-string of the bag will allow it to be drawn

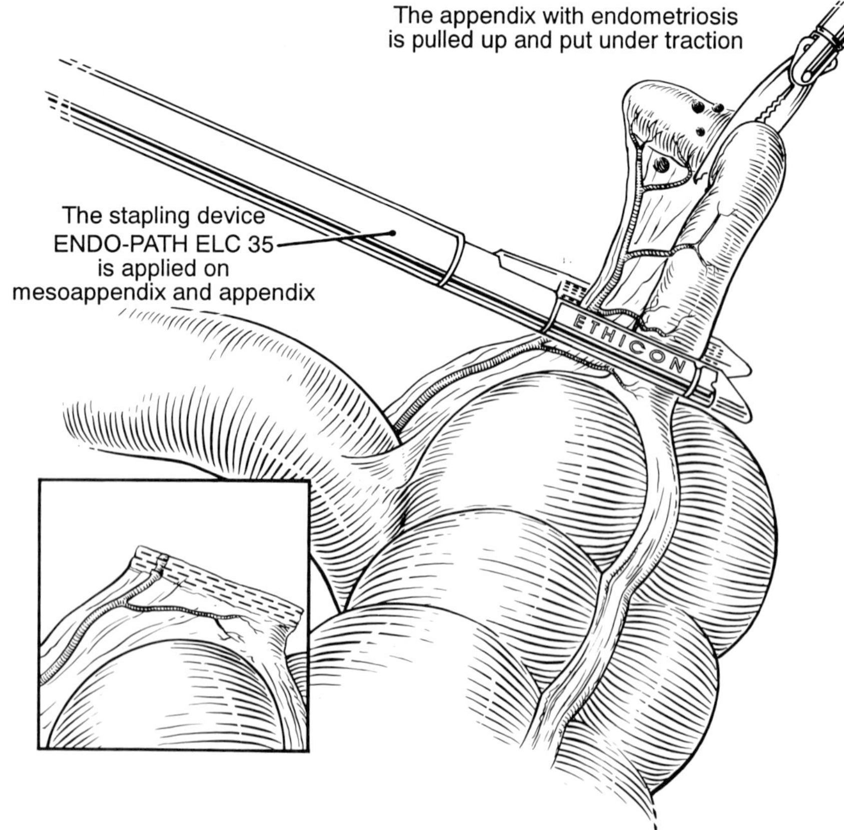

Figure 16-6. The stapling device is applied directly across the mesoappendix and appendix. *Inset,* The appendix and mesosalpinx are clipped and cut.

TABLE 16-1. **Outcome of Laparoscopic Appendectomy**

Author	No. of Patients	Complications
Bryson[16]	62	2 vulvovaginitis, 1 cystitis
Fleming[22]	15*	0
Gotz et al.[23]	388*	3 intraoperative bleeding, 1 intraoperative stump failure
Leahy[8]	4*	0
Nezhat, Nezhat[7]	100	1 postoperative febrile morbidity, 1 periumbilical ecchymosis
Nowzaradan[13]	43*	6 postoperative febrile morbidity
Schreiber[14]	70	1 electrosurgical thermal injury to cecum, 3 laparotomies
TOTAL	692	.027%

*Series with acute appendicitis

through small skin incisions without contaminating the incision.

The patient is discharged either the day of surgery or after an overnight stay and should avoid solid food for 24 hours. In a series of 100 patients (CSPS), all were discharged within 24 hours, although 7 remained overnight because of their own preference or late surgery.[7]

Although the procedure has a favorable cost-benefit ratio, complications including stump blowout, wound infection, hemorrhage, and postoperative ileus have been described (Table 16-1).[20,21]

Appendectomy for Appendicitis

Laparoscopy for appendicitis is similar to an incidental appendectomy, except that the appendix is edematous and possibly more fragile. The presence of gross inflammation, ease of excision, and absence of abscess formation influence the decision to perform laparoscopic appendectomy. Two or three accessory trocars are required, with the laparoscope in the umbilicus. Adhesions are lysed with the laser or scissors so that the appendix is mobile. In removing the appendix at its base, a sufficient stump is left to prevent spillage of luminal contents from the pedicle.

An alternative procedure[17] is to place clips on the base of the inflamed appendix, and then control the blood supply in the mesoappendix with electrocoagulation, hemoclips, or a multifire stapling device. If an inflamed appendix is removed laparoscopically, and 18- to 20-mm trocar (Ethicon) is inserted to ease its removal[22] and the operative site is irrigated.

A retrocecal appendicitis makes laparoscopic appendectomy more difficult. Gotz and colleagues[23] noted that complications requiring laparotomy (including bleeding, adhesions, abnormal position of the appendix) occurred early in their series of 388 patients with appendicitis. These findings prompted them to emphasize the significant learning curve and the long period needed to become proficient in laparoscopic appendectomy for a ruptured appendix, in the presence of extensive adhesions, or if the appendix is relatively inaccessible.

Laparoscopically assisted appendectomy has been described for cases in which the proper endoscopic instruments and sutures are unavailable.[22] The laparoscope facilitates the definitive diagnosis of appendicitis and a grasper is passed through an accessory trocar located over McBurney's point. The tip of the appendix is grasped and then pulled from the trocar insertion along with the trocar sleeve and grasper. Routine appendectomy can be performed through a small abdominal incision. The procedure usually takes 5 to 20 minutes or longer if the appendix is ruptured or an abscess is present.

References

1. Bongard F, Landers DV, Lewis F. Differential diagnosis of appendicitis and pelvic inflammatory disease: a prospective analysis. *Am J Surg.* 1985;150:90.
2. Condon RE. Appendicitis. In: Sabiston DG, ed. *Textbook of Surgery*, 13th ed. Philadelphia: WB Saunders; 1986:967.
3. Mueller BA, Daling JR, Moore DE, et al. Appendectomy and the risk of tubal infertility. *N Engl J Med.* 1986;315:1506.

4. Geerdsen J, Hansen JB. Incidence of sterility in women operated on in childhood for perforated appendicitis. *Acta Obstet Gynecol Scand.* 1977;56:523.
5. Powley PH. Infertility due to pelvic abscess and pelvic peritonitis in appendicitis. *Lancet.* 1965;1:27.
6. Chang FC, Hogle HH, Welling DR. The fate of the negative appendix. *Am J Surg.* 1973;126:752.
7. Nezhat C, Nezhat F. Incidental appendectomy during videolaseroscopy. *Am J Obstet Gynecol,* 1991;165:559.
8. Leahy PF. Technique of laparoscopic appendectomy. *Br J Surg.* 1989;76:616.
9. Paterson-Brown S, Thompson JN, Eckersley JRT, et al. Which patients with suspected appendicitis should undergo laparoscopy? *Br Med J.* 1988;296:1363.
10. Whitworth CM, Whitworth PW, Sanfilippo J, et al. Value of diagnostic laparoscopy in young women with possible appendicitis. *Surg Gynecol Obstet.* 1988;167:187.
11. Deutsch AA, Zelikovsky A, Reiss R. Laparoscopy in the prevention of unnecessary appendectomies: a prospective study. *Br J Surg.* 1982;69:336.
12. Leape LL, Ramenofsky MD. Laparoscopy for questionable appendicitis—can it reduce the negative appendectomy rate? *Ann Surg* 1980;191:410.
13. Nowzaradan Y. Laparoscopic appendectomy for acute appendicitis: indications and current use. *J Laparoendosc Surg.* 1991;7:247.
14. Schreiber JH. Early experience with laparoscopic appendectomy in women. *Surg Endosc.* 1987;1:211.
15. Krone HA. Preventive appendectomy in gynecologic surgery report of 1718 cases. *Geburtshilfe Frauenheilkd.* 1989;49:1035.
16. Bryson K. Laparoscopic appendectomy. *J Gynecol Surg.* 1991;7:93.
17. Schultz LS, Pietrafitta JJ, Graber JN, et al. Retrograde laparoscopic appendectomy: report of a case. *J Laparoendosc Surg.* 1991;1:111.
18. Semm K. Endoscopic appendectomy. *Endoscopy.* 1983;15:59–64.
19. Engstrom L, Fenyo G. Appendectomy: assessment of stump invagination versus simple ligation: a prospective, randomized trial. *Br J Surg.* 1985;72:971.
20. Fisher KS, Ross DS. Guidelines for therapeutic decision in incidental appendectomy. *Surg Gynecol Obstet.* 1990;171:95.
21. Nezhat C, Nezhat F, Nezhat CH. Operative gynecology (minimally invasive surgery): state of the art. *J Gynecol Surg.* 1992;8:111.
22. Fleming JS. Laparoscopically directed appendectomy. *Aust N Z Obstet Gynecol.* 1985;25:238.
23. Gotz F, Pier A, Bacher C. Modified laparoscopic appendectomy in surgery: a report on 388 operations. *Surg Endosc.* 1990;4:6.

17

Presacral Neurectomy and Uterosacral Transection and Ablation

Presacral Neurectomy

Dysmenorrhea, severe enough to limit social activities, affects more than 18 million women in the United States.[1] Surgical management of dysmenorrhea was reviewed by Fontaine and Herrmann.[2] In 1899, Jaboulay[3] described severance of sacral sympathetic afferent fibers using a posterior extraperitoneal approach, and in the same year Ruggi[4] described resection of the utero-ovarian plexus to relieve dysmenorrhea. Leriche[5] advocated periarterial sympathectomy of the internal iliac (hypogastric) arteries, and Cotte[6] reported that results following transection of the superior hypogastric plexus were highly effective in relieving severe dysmenorrhea. Cotte claimed that his technique was simpler and as effective as the Leriche operation. Other surgical procedures were reported,[7,8] but interest in pelvic neurectomy for relieving primary and secondary dysmenorrhea waned because of the introduction of nonsteroidal anti-inflammatory medications, oral contraceptives, danazol, and gonadotropin-releasing hormone (GnRH) analogs. Although highly effective in most patients, medical therapy fails to relieve dysmenorrhea in 25% to 30% of women. As a consequence of the advances in minimally invasive surgery, there is a reviving interest for including neurectomy in the treatment of disabling pelvic pain.

Cotte did the first "presacral neurectomy" in 1924. In the absence of precise physiologic data concerning the presacral nerve (superior hypogastric plexus of Hovelacque), it is difficult to explain the successful results obtained by presacral neurectomy.[9] Cotte emphasized that only nerve tissue within the interiliac triangle should be removed, and resection of all nerve elements within the triangle was essential. Both measures tend to maximize effectiveness and minimize complications.

Davis[10] claimed that it was not necessary to extend a presacral neurectomy beyond the interiliac triangle. In his early cases, he reported a cure rate of 50%, but in subsequent operations, the results improved to 75%.

Anatomy

Pain impulses from the cervix, body of the uterus, and the proximal fallopian tube are transmitted through afferent fibers that accompany sympathetic nerves into the spinal cord at the thoracic and lumbar levels. The sympathetic nerves emerging from the uterus pass through the uterosacral ligaments along the cardinal ligament to join the pelvic plexus. Parasympathetic fibers from S-1 through S-4 travel with the phrenic nerve through the pelvic plexuses (Frankenhauser's ganglia) lateral to the cervix to reach the bladder, rectum, and uterus.[11]

The presacral nerve is not a single nerve, but rather a plexus of nerve fibers called the superior hypogastric plexus. Elaut,[12] Davis,[13] Labate[14] and Curtis and coworkers,[15] among others, reported results based on cadaver dissections. The variable anatomic findings emphasized differences surgeons might encounter. Sometimes fibers of the superior hypogastric plexus were not found on the right, but 75% were located on the left and 50% were seen in the midline. In some dissections, one third to two thirds of the fibers were in left or central locations. In 8% to 15% of cases, the mesocolon was over the triangle making neurectomy difficult or impossible. Findings of a single nerve were reported in 8% to 13%.[14] Labate performed 75 dissections and described a plexus in 84%, parallel nerve trunks in 8%, and single nerves in 8%. In 27 presacral neurectomies, Black[16] found 3 (11.1%) single nerves and 23 (85.2%) plexiform elements. Davis[7] reported an accessory ureter lying in the midline in one instance during 20 presacral neurectomies.

Within the interiliac trigone, the common iliac artery and ureter are on the right and the common iliac vein is on the left. The inferior mesenteric, superior hemorrhoidal, and mid-sacral arteries are in the center of the prelumbar space. This trigone is defined caudally by the sacral promontory and laterally by the common iliac arteries meeting at the aortic bifurcation above.[12] Centrally and to the left, multiple nerve fibers, sometimes in bundles, run caudally from the aortic plexus above, through the interiliac trigone to form the superior hypogastric plexus. They continue anteriorly to comprise the inferior hypogastric plexus. These fibers, representing the presacral nerve, are buried in loose areolar tissue. They display no particular patterns and vary among individuals. To the left and right of the trigone, both ureters are identified before transecting the nerve bundle. The left ureter is more difficult to see because it is under the rectosigmoid and mesocolon.

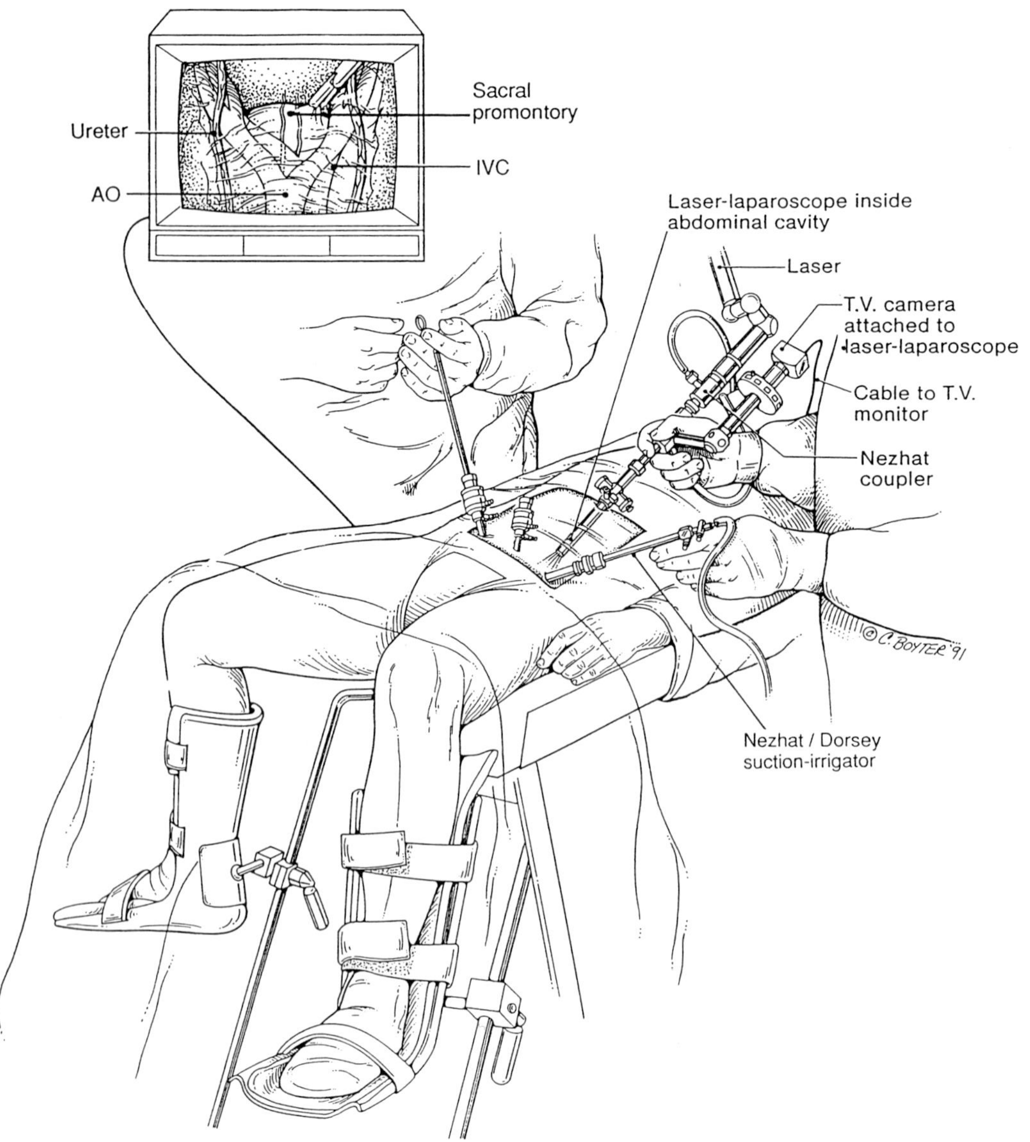

Figure 17-1. Instrument placement.

Indications

Presacral neurectomy is indicated for patients who have disabling midline dysmenorrhea and pelvic pain, and who have not responded to appropriate and adequate medical therapy. The success rate is difficult to predict even though the operation is likely to be very effective in 50% to 75% of patients.

Primary dysmenorrhea or dysmenorrhea related to endometriosis may be an indication for endoscopic corrective surgery, followed by presacral neurectomy. In most patients, dyspareunia is decreased and chronic pain is alleviated.

Assuming that laparoscopic presacral neurectomy is as effective as laparotomy, the convenience of outpatient surgery and shortened convalescence with minimal morbidity may alter the risk-benefit value.

Technique

The instruments are placed as shown in Figure 17-1. After treating associated pelvic abnormalities, steep Trendelenburg position is used and the patient is tilted slightly to the left. The aortic bifurcation, the common iliac arteries and veins, the ureters, and the sacral promontory are identified; the peritoneum overlying the promontory is elevated with grasping forceps and a small opening is made with the CO_2 laser (Figure 17-2), a knife electrode, or scissors. Through this, the suction irrigator is inserted and the peritoneum elevated by hydrodissection.[17] The peritoneum is incised horizontally and vertically, and the opening extended cephalad to the aortic bifurcation (Figure 17-3). Bleeding from peritoneal vessels is controlled with the CO_2 laser or a bipolar electrocoagulator. Retroperitoneal fatty tissue is removed before the hypogastric plexus is reached. Hemostasis is obtained with bipolar electrocoagulation.

The nerve plexus is grasped with atraumatic forceps. Using blunt dissection and the CO_2 laser, the nerve fibers are skeletonized, coagulated, and excised with either the CO_2 laser (Figure 17-4), knife electrode, or scissors. All the nerves that lie within the boundaries of the interiliac triangle are removed, including fibers entering the area from under the common iliac arteries (Figure 17-5). The retroperitoneal space is irrigated and bleeding points are coagulated. Sutures are not required. Excised tissue is sent for histologic confirmation of nerve removal. At second look laparoscopy, the presacral area is healed with usually no small bowel attached to this area. If mesocolon detachment is required at the initial procedure, the mesocolon usually reattaches itself to the presacral area.

In most patients, the mesocolon does not cover the sacral promontory. In a recent laparoscopic evaluation of 50 consecutive laparoscopic presacral neurectomies by Nezhat et al., the mesocolon was located completely in the left side of the sacral promontory in 31 (62%). In the remaining 19 (38%) patients, the sacral promontory was covered by the mesocolon to some degree: completely

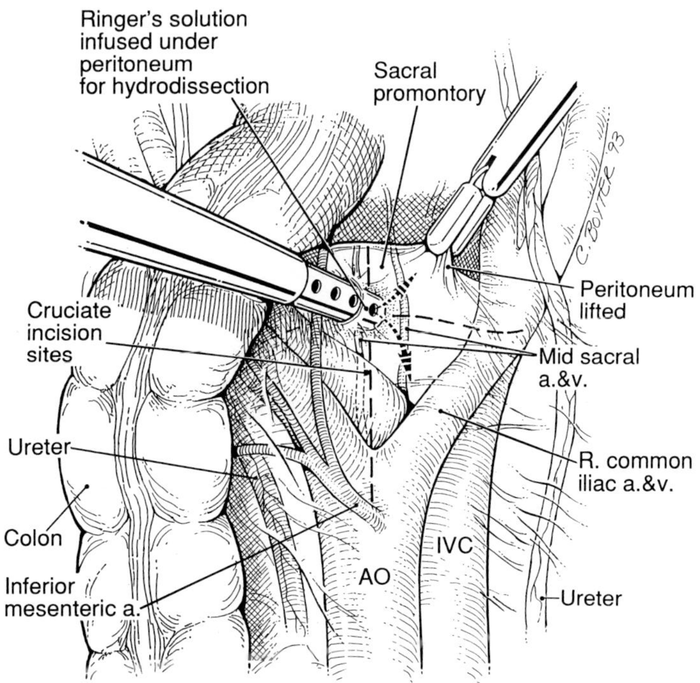

Figure 17-2. The peritoneum overlying the promontory is elevated with grasping forceps and opened with the CO_2 laser.

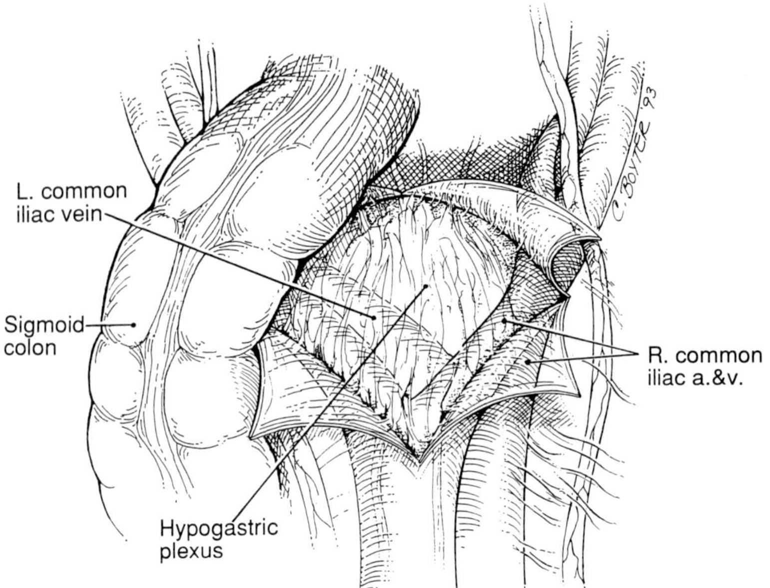

Figure 17-3. Location of the superior hypogastric nerve.

covering it in three patients (6%), less than half covering it in eight (16%), and covering 50% to 75% of the sacral promontory in the remaining eight women. Whenever the mesocolon covers the sacral promontory, the procedure is more difficult and the surgeon must avoid injuring the inferior mesenteric artery and its branches.

Results

Fifty-two women had excision of visible endometriosis and a presacral neurectomy. Thirty-one patients had minimal disease, 13 had mild endometriosis, 5 had moderate, and 3 had severe endometriosis (Table 17-1).[18] Forty-eight of 52 women (92.3%) reported relief of dysmenorrhea. Of these 52, 27 (51.9%) noted 100% pain relief of dysmenorrhea in one follow-up. Sixteen (66.7%), 6 (25%), and 3 (12.5%) had minimal, mild, and moderate endometriosis, respectively. These results indicate there may be a 50-50 chance for long-term, complete pain alleviation in selected patients with endometriosis undergoing a presacral neurectomy.

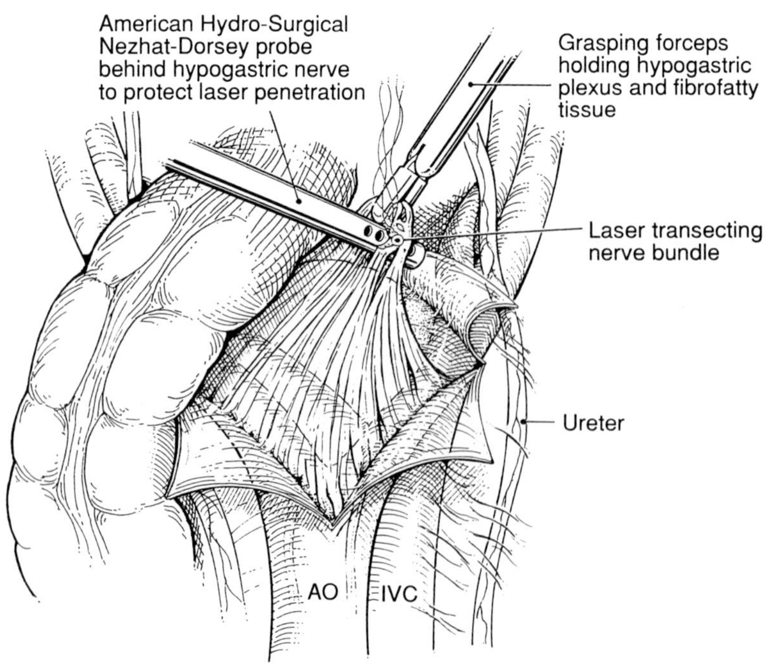

Figure 17-4. Excision of the superior hypogastric nerve.

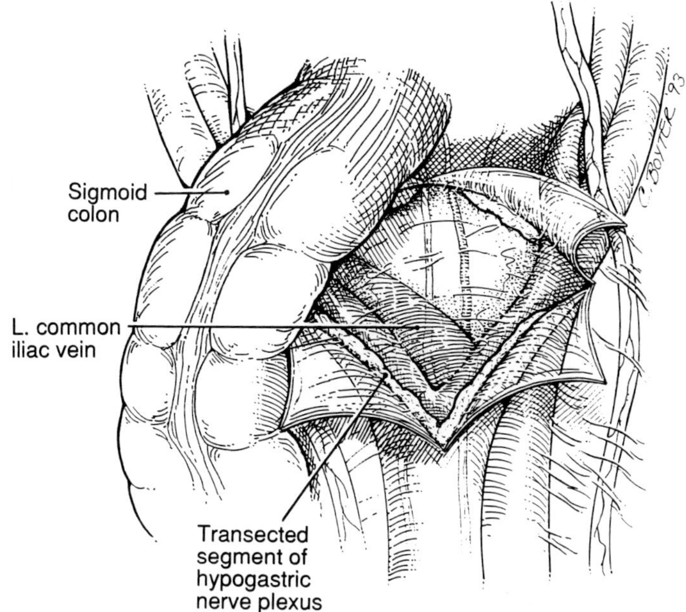

Figure 17-5. All nerves between the two ureters that lie within the interiliac triangle have been removed.

A number of studies describe the potential of presacral neurectomy for severe pelvic pain. Cotte[19] reported only 2% failure in 1500 patients using presacral neurectomy. Black[20] collected 2516 cases from the world literature (1936–1963) in which treatment of primary and secondary dysmenorrhea included presacral neurectomy. Positive results were noted in 70% of cases; 19% were improved and 11% had no relief. Lee and coworkers[8] tabulated pelvic denervation data from 11 studies (1939–1985) covering 576 cases, including 40 patients of their own. The combined figures reveal a success rate of 74%. Partial success was 14% and failures were seen in 12%.

Perez[21] described a laparoscopic approach for doing a presacral neurectomy. Results in 25 endo-

TABLE 17-1. Patient Estimated Relief of Menstrual/Overall Pelvic Pain at a Minimum of One Year After Surgery

Stage of Endometriosis*	Patients, n (%)†	Age (Years) Mean (Range)	Estimated Relief (%)	Dysmenorrhoea Relief, n (%)	Overall Pelvic Pain Relief, n (%)
Minimal	31 (60)	27.4 (18–38)	100	16 (52)	17 (55)
			50–80	10 (32)	7 (22)
			>50	3 (10)	5 (16)
			0	2 (6)	2 (6)
Mild	13 (25)	33.6 (33–39)	100	6 (46)	6 (46)
			50–80	6 (46)	4 (31)
			>50	0	2 (15)
			0	1 (8)	1 (8)
Moderate	5 (10)	30.5 (22–34)	100	3 (60)	2 (40)
			50–80	2 (40)	0
			>50	0	3 (60)
			0	0	0
Severe	3 (9)	35.3 (31–45)	100	2 (67)	2 (67)
			50–80	0	0
			>50	0	1 (33)
			0	1 (33)	0

*Revised American Fertility Society Staging (American Fertility Society, 1985).
†Percentages may not total 100 due to rounding.

metriosis patients with dysmenorrhea in which adnexal pain was minimal and medical treatment unsatisfactory were assessed using a 0 to 10 pain scale. The mean preoperative score was 8.4 (7 to 10) compared with a postsurgical figure of 2.2 (0 to 8), that is, all patients initially had incapacitating pain that kept them from school or work, and with one exception (4.0%), each patient resumed and maintained near-normal activity over a follow-up of 3 to 12 months. A retroperitoneal hemorrhage in one patient required a laparotomy.

Meigs[22] studied 20 women who had primary dysmenorrhea in whom therapy was limited to presacral neurectomy and noted 17 patients (85%) experienced relief and 3 (15%) had no relief. Black[20] reported positive results in 20 of 24 cases with a failure in 14%. Patients were observed for 10 years and Black attributed relief solely to the sympathectomy because the procedure was used alone or with a prophylactic appendectomy. Tjaden and colleagues[23] initiated a prospective study to ascertain the efficacy of presacral neurectomy in patients with stage III or IV endometriosis and midline dysmenorrhea. Although the intention was to include 60 to 80 patients in each randomized group, the study was terminated by the monitoring committee at the first 6 weeks' review because it was deemed unethical to deny patients with midline dysmenorrhea pain relief provided by presacral neurectomy. Among 26 patients, 17 received only presacral neurectomy; 15 (88%) noted relief and 2 (12%) had no improvement. Nine patients did not undergo presacral neurectomy and reported no pain relief. Meigs[22] also reported seven cases of dysmenorrhea in which other operative procedures were combined with presacral neurectomy. Six women (86%) noted complete relief but one patient (14%) had no relief. The author concluded "it is obvious that the correction of all pelvic pathology is better than presacral neurectomy alone."

Pain relief in patients with dysmenorrhea, endometriosis, and other disorders has been documented by Polan and DeCherney.[24] They reported that 14 (70%) of 20 patients who underwent corrective surgery plus presacral neurectomy were relieved of pain. Comparative control groups experienced pain relief in only 14 (26%) of 54 patients having infertility surgery without presacral neurectomy. The authors emphasized that presacral neurectomy plus reconstructive pelvic surgery was more effective than infertility laparotomy alone in the treatment of pelvic pain, but that presacral neurectomy did not increase the chance for pregnancy.

Lichten and Bombard[25] assessed the presacral neurectomy results of Black[20] and the uterosacral results noted by Doyle.[26] The authors thought a 30% failure to achieve pain relief was caused by individual anatomic variations including the role played by nociceptive afferents associated with the major pelvic arteries.

Complications

The most common intraoperative complication is excessive bleeding. The middle sacral vessels are located in the midline between the "presacral nerve" and the periosteum of the sacral promontory. Usually, the nerve is dissected anterior to the vessels and ligation is not necessary. Should bleeding occur, hemostasis is obtained by ligation or coagulation. However, an injury to the common iliac vein or vena cava may require an immediate laparotomy. Ureteral injury is also possible.

Meigs[22] noted urinary urgency in some women that persisted for 7 years after surgery and persistent postoperative constipation in 32% of cases. Black[16,20] reported catheterization in 13 of 26 cases postoperatively: 4 for 1 day, 6 for 2 days, and 1 each for 3, 5, and 6 days. In a discussion published at the end of Black's 1964 paper, Ranney noted three complications: one transient "poor bladder emptying" and permanent constipation and painless labor in two patients who, unwarned by labor pains, delivered at home. In the same discussion, Pratt remarked that he had cared for one case of intermittent ileal obstruction because of adhesions involving the fifth lumbar vertebra just above the sacral promontory following a presacral neurectomy. Lee and associates[8] noted similar complications in 4% of 50 patients. Eight (18%) of 45 patients who benefited from presacral neurectomy developed a return of pain laterally within 19 months for a mean follow-up time of 31 months. Cotte's recurrence rate was 2%.[19] Jones and Rock[27] cited vaginal dryness usually resolving within 6 months as a complication in 10% to 15% of presacral neurectomy cases.

Lee and colleagues[8] noted one acute operative complication involving an estimated 1500 mL blood loss from a damaged presacral vein. Davis[7] noted a vascular injury to the left common iliac vein that was repaired successfully. Cotte[19] reported one instance of damage to the left ureter among 1500 operations. He noted postoperative bleeding in four other patients. Two required a second operation and repair of the posterior peritoneum. The other two, involving subperitoneal blood infiltrating the posterior rectal areas, resolved spontaneously.

Wetherell[28] noted he had been "unable to find a mortality in the American literature" following removal of the superior hypogastric plexus. Bonica[29] tabulated 165 cases from six authors and found no mortality among four of them. However, Fontaine and Herrmann[2] reported a fatality in one patient, which occurred on the second postoperative day. At autopsy, cerebral edema was found. In over 300 patients, Cotte[9] described data on two patients who died from acute pulmonary complications.

Summary

Although the data and preceding discussions touch on past and present controversies regarding pelvic sympathectomy, presacral neurectomy competently performed is an effective option for selected patients with refractory, incapacitating central dysmenorrhea. For a given case, the procedure remains empirical in that success rates and short- and long-term complications are not predictable. Fortunately, complication and mortality rates have been minimal.

Inappropriate patients and incomplete neurectomy, either because of neurologic variability or failure to remove all nerve tissue within the Cotte triangle, are the most frequent reasons for poor result. Presacral neurectomy is a safe operative procedure with an enhanced laparoscopic visibility. Minimal patient stress and morbidity and a short recovery time make presacral neurectomy a viable alternative to laparotomy.

Uterosacral Transection/Ablation

Uterosacral transection was developed and popularized as an alternative to presacral neurectomy with Doyle's vaginal approach that involved transecting the uterosacral ligaments.[26] His results were as good as those obtained with presacral neurectomy. Lichten and Bombard[25] reported relief of incapacitating primary dysmenorrhea in 9 of 11 (81%) patients who underwent uterosacral nerve transection, but no dysmenorrhea relief in the control group who had only a diagnostic laparoscopy. However, one year later fewer than half the patients who originally experienced improvement were pain free.[25] Gurgan and colleagues[30] reported that 17 of 23 women reported relief of dysmenorrhea. The subjects quantified their pain preoperatively and postoperatively; the mean preoperative score was reduced by 33%. In a similar study, Sutton[31] reported a 63% reduction in the initial average score. Uterosacral transection should be performed as a secondary procedure that may provide partial or temporary relief of central dysmenorrhea and used in conjunction with nonsteroidal anti-inflammatory analgesics.

Technique

A standard three-puncture technique is used. The procedure is performed by placing the uterosacral ligaments on stretch by anteverting the uterus with the uterine manipulator. The CO_2 laser (40 to 60 W) or another cutting instrument transects the ligaments at their insertion into the cervix, using a vertical motion from medial to lateral (Figure 17-6). Transection at this location maximizes the number of nerve fibers transected because the fibers disperse as they pass along the uterosacral ligaments. Unfortunately, this segment of the uterosacral ligament is closest to the uterine vessels and ureter. The suction-irrigator is used as a backstop to make the uterosacral ligament more prominent and to protect the ureter. The depth of incision should be examined frequently because the goal is to completely transect the uterosacral ligament (Figure 17-7). Blood vessels run along the medial aspect of the uterosacral ligament, and, bleeding in this area must be controlled very carefully because of the proximity of the ureter and rectum. Some gynecologists also vaporize a path across the base of the cervix between the uterosacral ligaments. If the uterosacral ligaments are difficult to identify, uterosacral transection is not recommended. When the uterosacral ligament is cut, a blood vessel inside it tends to bleed. To determine if this has occurred, uterine traction should be released and pneumoperitoneum decreased.

Because ureteral injury is a serious complication associated with this procedure,[32] the direction of the ureter should be identified from the pelvic brim to the bladder. There is usually a distance of 2 to 3 cm between the ureter and the uterosacral ligaments. However, this proximity varies significantly. If the ureter is close to the uterosacral ligament, a "relaxing" incision is made along the outer side of the uterosacral ligament (Figure 17-8). The ureter is retracted laterally before the ligament is transected. Occasionally, the rectum may appear similar to the uterosacral ligament.

If uterosacral transection is unsuccessful, it is presumed that either interruption of the nerve fibers was incomplete or that the nerves regenerated. Lichten[33] reported that repeating the procedure did not relieve dysmenorrhea, implying that the course of the nerve fibers in these individuals

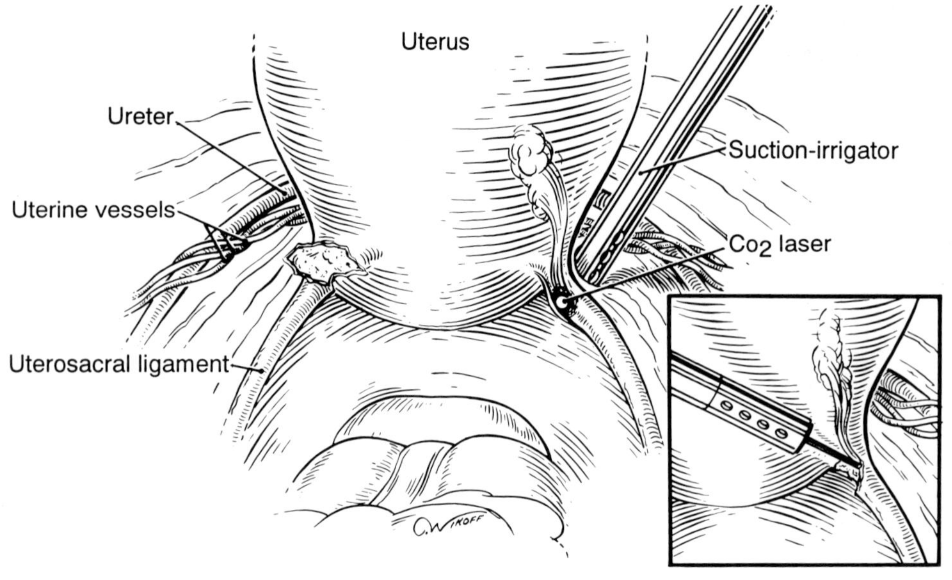

Figure 17-6. The CO_2 laser is being used to transect the uterosacral ligament. *Inset*, Fiber laser.

Figure 17-7. The uterosacral ligaments have been transected.

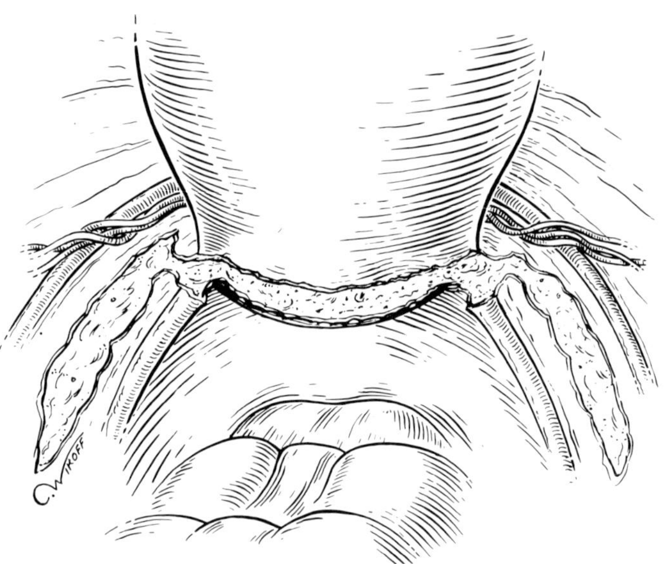

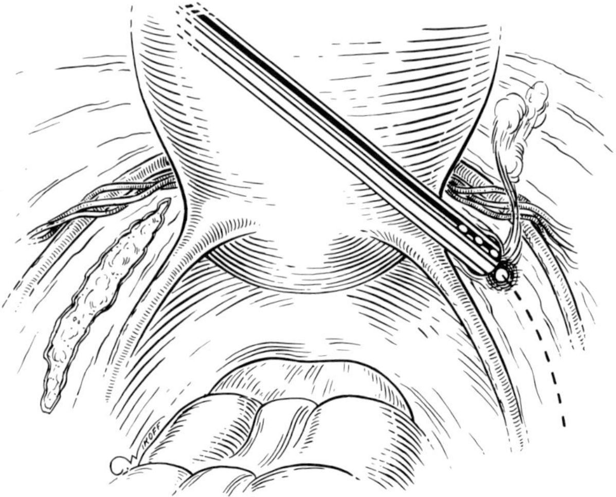

Figure 17-8. A relaxing incision is made along the outer side of the uterosacral ligament.

may not be normal. Several patients with failed uterosacral transection did obtain relief from a subsequent presacral neurectomy.[21] Complications may include loss of uterine support, adhesion formation, and ureteral transection.

Summary

These procedures benefit only women with midline pain because adnexa are innervated mostly by nerve fibers traversing the infundibulopelvic ligaments. The difference in innervation accounts for the anatomic and physiologic differences between lateral and midline pain.

References

1. Henzl MR. Dysmenorrhea: achievements and challenge. *Sex Med Today*. 1985;9:8.
2. Fontaine R, Herrmann LG. Clinical and experimental basis for surgery of pelvic sympathetic nerves in gynecology. *Surg Gynecol Obstet*. 1932;54:133.
3. Jaboulay M. Le traitement de la nevralgie pelvienne par la paralysie du sympathetique sacre. *Lyon Med*. 1899;90:102.
4. Ruggi G. Della sympatectamia al collo ed ale adome. *Policlinico* 1899;1:193.
5. Leriche R. Resultant eloigne cinq ans et demi d'une sympathectomie des deux arteres hypogastriques pour dysmnenorrhee douloureuse. *Lyon chirurgie*. 1927;XXIV:360.
6. Cotte MG. Sur le traitement des dysmenorrhees rebelles par la sympathectomie hypogastrique periarterielle ou la section du nerf presacre. *Lyon Med*. 1925;135:153.
7. Davis AA. The technique of resection of the presacral nerve (Cotte's operation). *Br J Surg*. 1933;20:516.
8. Lee RB, Stone K, Magelssen D, et al. Presacral neurectomy for chronic pelvic pain. *Obstet Gynecol*. 1986;68:517.
9. Cotte MG. Resection of the presacral nerve in the treatment of obstinate dysmenorrhea. *Am J Obstet Gynecol*. 1937;33:1030.
10. Davis AA. *Dysmenorrhea: Its Aetiology, Pathology and Treatment*. London: Oxford University Press, 1938.
11. Bonica JJ. Neurologic and pathologic aspects of chronic pelvic pain. *Arch Surg*. 1977; 112:750.
12. Elaut L. Surgical anatomy of the so-called presacral nerve. *Surg Gynecol Obstet*. 1933;57:581.
13. Davis AA. Discussion on sympathectomy for dysmenorrhea. *Proc Reg Soc Med*. 1934; 27:258.
14. Labate JS. The surgical anatomy of the superior hypogastric plexus—"presacral nerve." *Surg Gynecol Obstet*. 1938;67:199.
15. Curtis AH, Anson BJ, Ashley FL, et al. The anatomy of the pelvic autonomic nerves in relation to gynecology. *Surg Gynecol Obstet*. 1942;75:743.
16. Black WT. Presacral sympathectomy for dysmenorrhea and pelvic pain. *Am Surg*. 1936;103:903.
17. Nezhat C, Nezhat F. Safe laser excision or vaporization of peritoneal endometriosis. *Fertil Steril*. 1989;52:149.
18. Nezhat C, Nezhat F. A simplified method of laparoscopic presacral neurectomy for the treatment of central pelvic pain due to endometriosis. *Br J Obstet Gynaecol*. 1992; 99:659–663.
19. Cotte MG. Technique of presacral neurectomy. *Am J Surg*. 1949;78:50.
20. Black WT. Use of presacral sympathectomy in the treatment of dysmenorrhea—a second look after 25 years. *Am J Obstet Gynecol*. 1964;89:16.
21. Perez JJ. Laparoscopic presacral neurectomy: results of the first 25 cases. *J Reprod Med*. 1990;5:625.
22. Meigs JV. Excision of the superior hypogastric plexus (presacral nerve) for primary dysmenorrhea. *Surg Gynecol Obstet*. 1939; 68:723.
23. Tjaden B, Schlaff WD, Kimball A, et al. The efficacy of presacral neurectomy for the relief of midline dysmenorrhea. *Obstet Gynecol*. 1990;76:89.
24. Polan ML, DeCherney A. Presacral neurectomy for pelvic pain in infertility. *Fertil Steril*. 1980;34:557.
25. Lichten EM, Bombard J. Surgical treatment of primary dysmenorrhea with laparoscopic uterine nerve ablation. *J Reprod Med*. 1987;32:37.
26. Doyle EB. Paracervical uterine denervation by transection of the cervical plexus for the relief of dysmenorrhea. *Am J Obstet Gynecol*. 1955;70:11.
27. Jones HW, Rock JA. *Reparative and Constructive Surgery of the Female Generative Tract*. Baltimore and London: Williams & Wilkins; 1983:136.
28. Wetherell FS. Relief of pelvic pain by sympathetic neurectomy. *JAMA*. 1933;101:1255.

29. Bonica JJ. The management of pain, 2d ed; vol II. Malvern: Lea & Febiger; 1990:1327.
30. Gurgan T, Urman B, Aksu T, et al. Laparoscopic CO_2 laser uterine nerve ablation for treatment of drug resistant primary dysmenorrhea. *Fertil Steril.* 1992;58:422.
31. Sutton C. Laser uterine nerve ablation. In: Donnez J, ed. *Laser Operative Laparoscopy and Hysteroscopy*. Leuven: Nauwelaerts Printing; 1989:43.
32. Nezhat C, Nezhat F. Laparoscopic repair of resected ureter during operative laparoscopy to treat endometriosis. A case report. *Obstet Gynecol.* 1992;80:543.
33. Lichten E. Three years experience with L.U.N.A. *Am J Gynecol Health.* 1989;3:9.

18

Reconstructive Pelvic Surgery

Retropubic Urethral Suspension

Urinary incontinence is becoming more prevalent as the population ages.[1,2] Up to 20% to 40% of women have reported urine loss.[1–4] A significant improvement in the psychological status of these patients after the successful surgical cure of stress incontinence has been demonstrated.[5] With more than 160 operations available to correct stress urinary incontinence, an optimal approach has not been developed.[6] Retropubic urethropexy (Marshall-Marchetti-Krantz[7] or Burch,[8,9]) has the best outcome and relatively few complications. Needle urethropexy[10–14] is a shorter operation and is less invasive; recovery is rapid. However, needle urethropexy is less effective than the abdominal approach and is associated with more complications.[15–18] Tanagho's modification of the Burch procedure[19] reported the best outcome in patients with urinary stress incontinence with intact urethral sphincteric mechanism, poor urethral support, and a displaced urethrovesical junction.[19–23]

Recently, Nezhat and Vancaillie[24,25] described a procedure in which retropubic urethral suspension was performed laparoscopically. This development combines an outpatient procedure that has the potential to be a long-term solution to stress urinary incontinence. Moreover, when performed laparoscopically, the retropubic exposure is excellent, and videolaparoscopic magnification enhances the surgeon's ability to precisely place the sutures. The improved exposure enables support restoration with limited mobility and avoids urethral obstruction and compression. Patients receive the advantage of a quick recovery. At CSPS, laparoscopic modifications of the Marshall-Marchetti-Krantz and Burch procedures have been developed.[26]

Preoperative Evaluation and Procedure

Postmenopausal women receive at least 3 months of estrogen replacement therapy. Preoperative evaluation includes history, physical, gynecologic, and neurologic examinations. We emphasize evaluating and correcting (if possible) any factor contributing to urinary incontinence (medication, respiratory disease, etc). Office tests include stress test, Q-tip test, urinalysis, urine culture and sensitivity, and SMA22.[27] All women undergo a urodynamic evaluation[28–30] with emphasis on voiding time, voiding volume, and postvoid residual urine volume. Stress incontinence is diagnosed by a positive stress test in the absence of simultaneous detrusor contractions or pressure equalization on the stress urethral closure pressure profile. Symptom diaries for the previous 48 hours are obtained and placed in each woman's chart. The patients are instructed in self-catheterization and complete a questionnaire regarding their incontinence and its severity.

Operative Technique

Following the induction of general endotracheal anesthesia, the patient is placed in Allen stirrups to permit the assistant to perform a vaginal examination (Figure 18-1). A Foley catheter is placed in the bladder. A 10-mm operative videolaparoscope is inserted infraumbilically and three 5-mm accessory trocars are inserted suprapubically (Figure 18-2). The middle trocar is placed 5 to 6 cm above the symphysis pubis, and the other two 7 to 8 cm

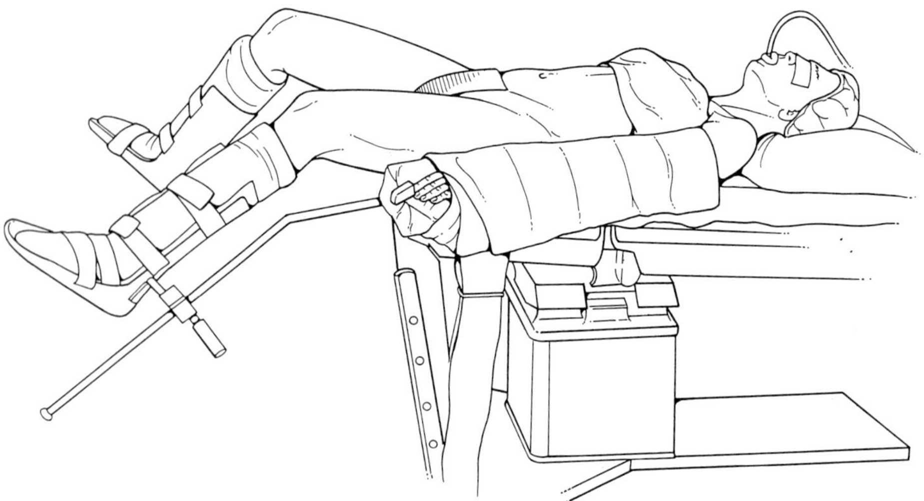

Figure 18-1. The patient is in a modified dorsal lithotomy position in Allen universal stirrups.

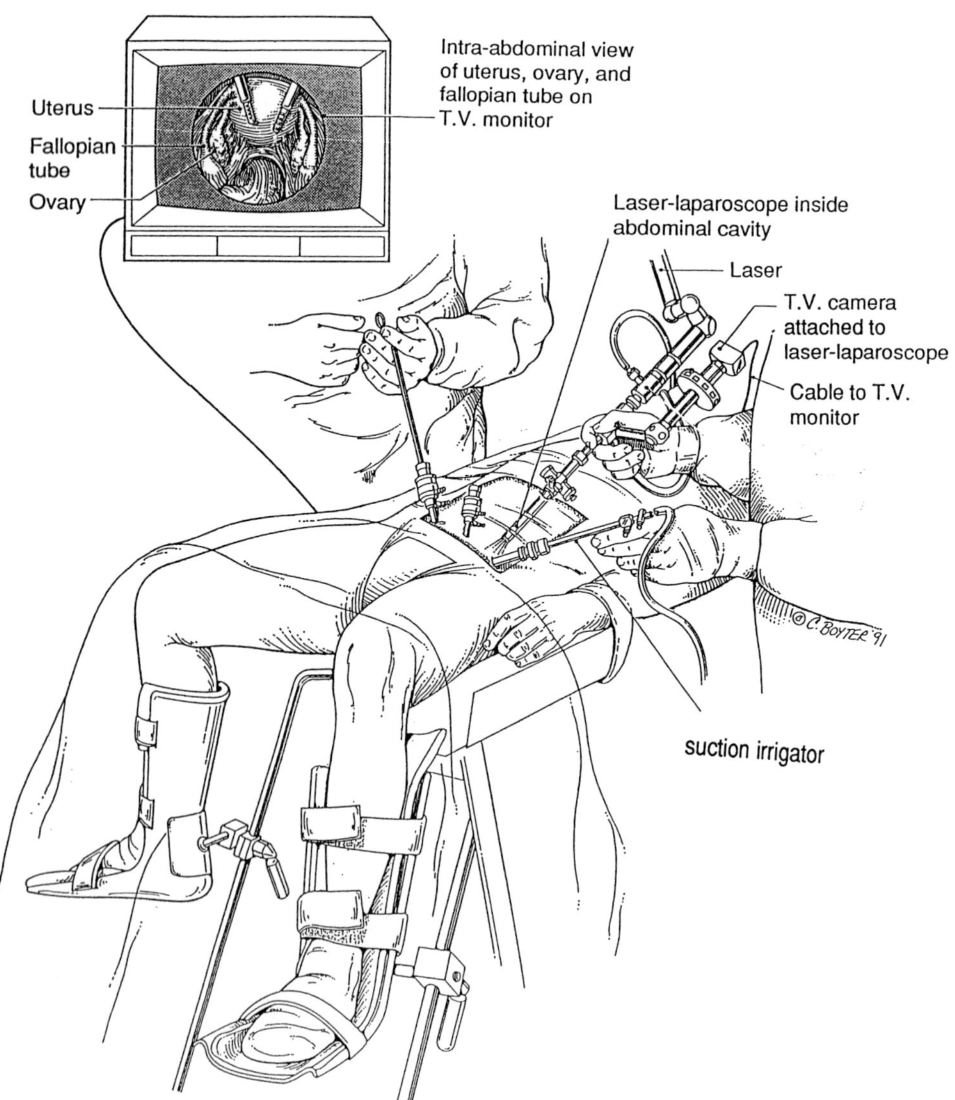

Figure 18-2. Room setup and location of the suprapubic incisions.

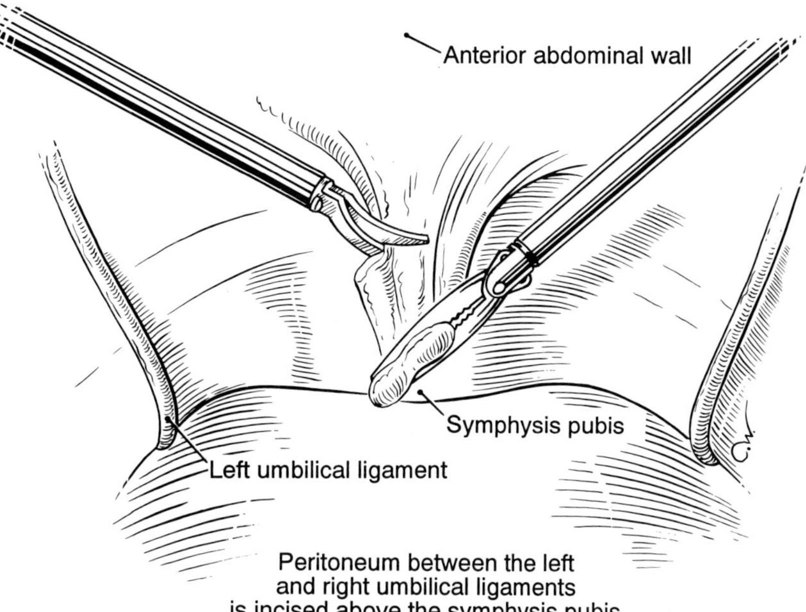

Figure 18-3. An incision is made in the peritoneum 3 to 5 cm above the symphysis pubis.

above the symphysis pubis lateral to the umbilical ligaments, avoiding injury to the inferior epigastric vessels. The CO_2 laser is placed through the operative channel of the 10-mm laparoscope. Through the accessory trocars, the suction irrigator, grasping forceps, needle holder, and bipolar electrocoagulator are introduced.[31] A Moschcowitz procedure is performed first.

To enter the space of Retzius intra-abdominally, the umbilical ligaments are identified laterally. The anterior abdominal wall peritoneum 3 to 5 cm above the symphysis pubis is pulled down with grasping forceps placed through a lateral accessory trocar (Figure 18-3). A transverse incision is made with the CO_2 laser or scissors caudal to the midsuprapubic trocar above the symphysis pubis on the peritoneum between the two umbilical ligaments. The midline trocar entry and anatomic landmarks, including the round ligament from the internal ring, are used to avoid bladder entry. Blunt dissection, hydrodissection, and the CO_2 laser for sharp dissection are used to expose the retropubic space (Figure 18-4). Stay close to the back of the pubic bone, dropping the anterior

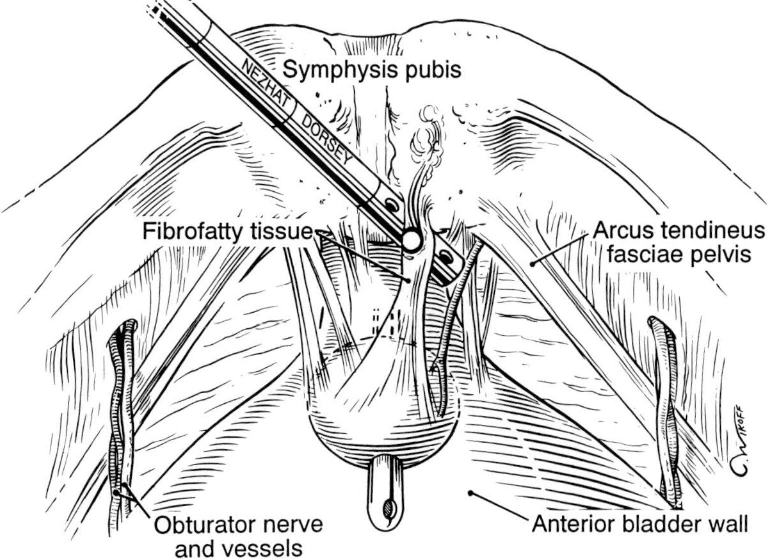

Figure 18-4. The space of Retzius is developed using blunt and CO_2 dissection of fibrofatty tissue. Care is taken to avoid obturator nerve and vessel injury.

bladder wall, vaginal wall, and urethra downward. Dissection is limited over the urethra in the midline, to approximately 2 cm lateral to the urethra to protect its delicate musculature. An assistant performs a vaginal examination with one finger on each side of the catheterized urethra, elevating the lateral vaginal fornix. The overlying fibrofatty tissue is cleared from the anterior vaginal wall under videolaparoscopic magnification. Beginning laterally, the bladder is dissected medially from the paravaginal fascia. The thin-walled venous plexus in this vascular area is identified and protected from surgical trauma. Pneumoperitoneal pressure and the CO_2 laser help control bleeding from small vessels. Hydrodissection, blunt dissection (suction-irrigator probe) and sharp dissection (CO_2 laser) are continued until the urethrovesical junction becomes apparent and the white glistening tissue of the paravaginal fascia appears. Every effort is made to protect the muscle fibers of the urethrovesical junction from surgical dissection. Bleeding in this area is controlled with bipolar electrocoagulation. After mobilizing the vesical urethral segment so that it can be lifted to a normal position, retropubic dissection is continued until Cooper's ligament is exposed. Dissection in the space of Retzius may be more difficult in patients who have undergone previous laparotomy, especially those who are obese. Pneumoperitoneal pressure provides exposure of the space and its contents out to the obturator nerve. This nerve and occasionally the aberrant obturator vein are identified and protected from surgical trauma. The space of Retzius also can be entered with a preperitoneal approach.

Alternatively, dissection in the space of Retzius may be achieved using the recently developed balloon dissector (General Surgical Innovations, Inc., Portola Valley, CA). The balloon dissector consists of a trocar, guide rod, and a balloon system. The dissector is inserted through a 1-cm infraumbilical incision. It is advanced between the rectus muscle and the anterior surface of the posterior rectus sheath to the symphysis pubis. The dissector's external sheath is removed, and the balloon is inflated with approximately 750 mL of saline solution. During inflation, the balloon unrolls sideways and exerts a perpendicular force that separates tissue layers. A blunt dissection of the connective tissues is propagated as the balloon expands. Full dissection takes about one minute. When maximal volume is reached, the balloon is deflated and removed through the incision. The dissected space is insufflated with CO_2 at a pressure of 8–10 mm Hg. The predefined shape of the balloon, its nonelastomeric material, and the incompressible character of the saline assure a large, relatively bloodless working space of predictable size and shape. The space is adequate for identification of pertinent landmarks and unencumbered manipulation of endoscopic surgical instruments.

After complete dissection, the paravaginal fascia is identified. Using an atraumatic grasping forceps, a bite of the paravaginal fascia is elevated and a suture placed at the level of the urethrovesical junction, approximately 1 to 1.5 cm from the urethra (Figure 18-5). This is facilitated by the Foley bulb with the catheter under gentle traction. This suture is placed perpendicular to the vaginal axis to include approximately 0.5 to 1 cm of tissue

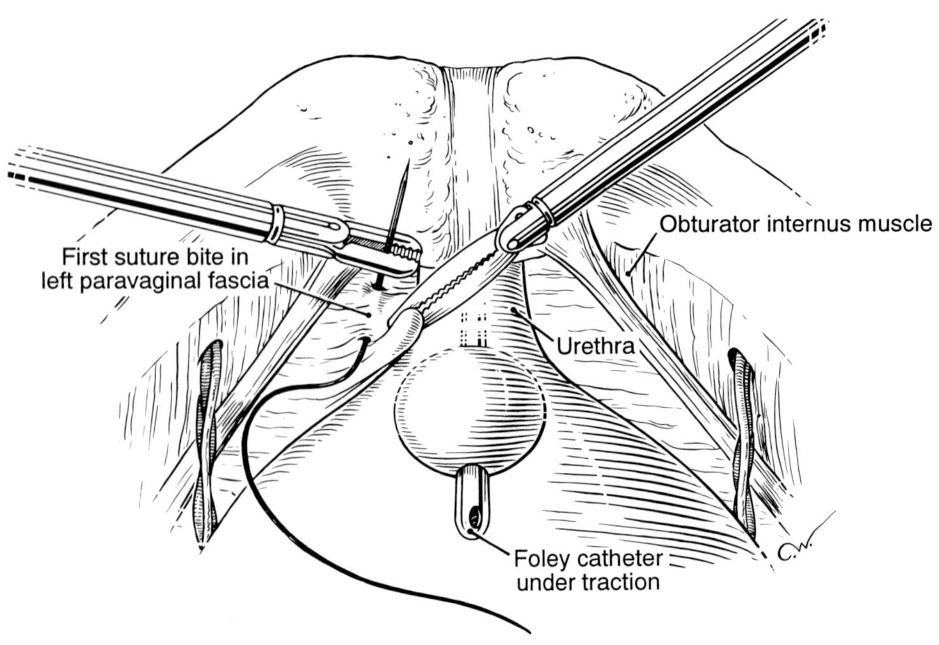

Figure 18-5. No. 0 Ethibond (Ethicon) suture is placed 1 to 1.5 cm from the urethra. The assistant's finger is used to elevate the paravaginal fascia and guide the surgeon.

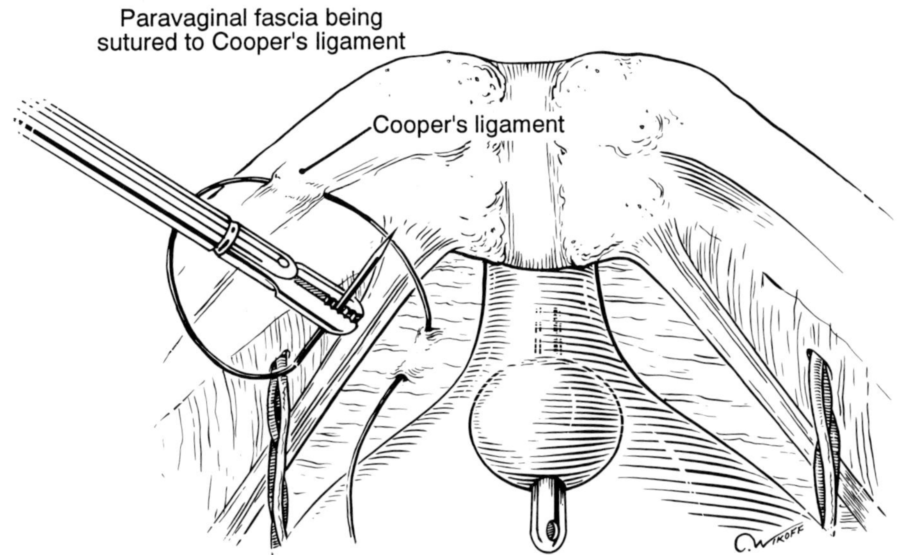

Figure 18-6. The suture is passed through Cooper's ligament in the Burch procedure.

(the complete vaginal fascia), but not to penetrate the vaginal mucosa. The patient is placed in steep Trendelenburg and rotated left to facilitate left-handed suture placement. The assistant's finger is used as a guide. The suture is fixed to Cooper's ligament (Figures 18-6 and 18-7) or the midline of the symphysis pubis fibrocartilage (Figure 18-8), depending on the surgeon's preference and whether a cystocele is present. If there is a low cystocele, a modified Burch technique is used. The sutures are tied either intracorporeally or extracorporeally with help from an assistant who lifts the vagina upward and forward. Direct observation assists the surgeon in avoiding excess tension in the vaginal wall while tying the suture. The urethra is observed to prevent it from being compressed against the pubic bone. This suturing is repeated on the opposite side, the goal being to create a platform on which the bladder neck can rest, while avoiding overcorrection. If the suspension is judged inadequate, a second and rarely, a third set of sutures is placed cephalad along the base of the bladder. Flexible cystoscopy is performed to ensure that there is no suture material in the bladder, to assess the urethrovesical junction angle, and to check ureteral patency. Pneumoperitoneal pressure is decreased and the retropubic space is evaluated. Bleeding is controlled with bipolar electrocoagulation. The peritoneal defect may be left open to heal spontaneously, or, if it is large, it may be closed laparoscopically with three to four interrupted 4-0 polydioxanone (Ethicon) sutures. The laparoscope is withdrawn from the abdomen and the procedure concluded. The Foley catheter remains in place for 2 to 3 days, except in women who have a cystotomy; then it is left in for 7 days.

Intercourse is contraindicated for 6 to 8 weeks postoperatively and the patients are advised to avoid heavy lifting or strenuous exercise for at least 2 months. Before their 2- and 6-week postop-

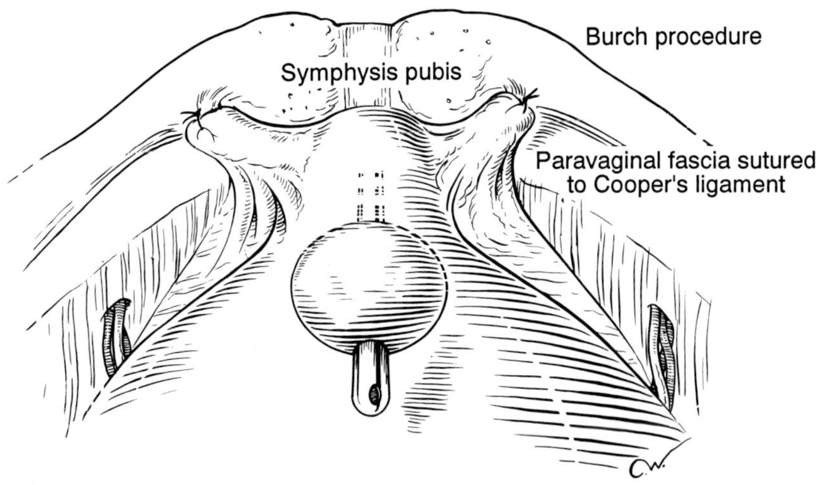

Figure 18-7. Suture is tied, extracorporeally or intracorporeally, elevating the ureterovesical angle.

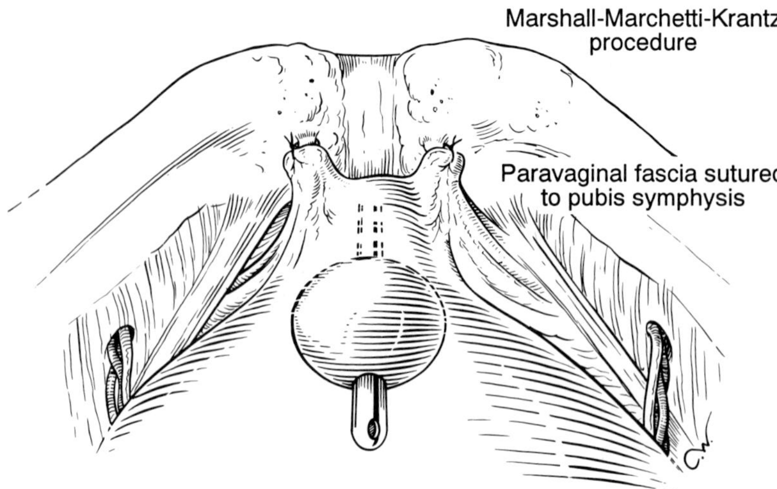

Figure 18-8. Marshall-Marchetti-Krantz procedure. Paravaginal fascia is sutured to the symphysis pubis.

erative visits, they are asked to keep a 24-hour symptom diary, in which they record their intake and urine output, urge to void, and leakage. It is similar to the one they kept preoperatively.

Prophylactic intravenous antibiotics are followed by a course of oral antibiotics for 5 days or until self-catheterization is discontinued.

Results

Sixty-two women, aged 34 to 69 years, gravidity 0 to 8 and parity 0 to 7, with gynecologic abnormalities requiring operative laparoscopy and stress incontinence were included in this study. Forty-eight (77.5%) were premenopausal and 14 (22.5%) were postmenopausal. They had distressing urinary stress incontinence with a positive stress test and normal detrusor function on cystometrogram.

A modified Moschcowitz procedure using 0 Vicryl Endoknot (Ethicon) or Ethibond (Ethicon) was used to obliterate the cul-de-sac.

The operative times for retropubic urethropexy procedure ranged from 30 to 45 minutes. The variation depended on the time necessary to dissect adipose tissue and the number of sutures placed. Blood loss ranged from 10 to 60 mL. All procedures were completed laparoscopically.

Intraoperative complications included one bladder perforation during bladder dissection (Table 18-1), which was repaired laparoscopically in one layer using 0 polyglactin interrupted sutures.[32] One patient developed an incisional hernia (see Table 18-1) at the site of the midline suprapubic trocar although the fascia had been repaired with one interrupted absorbable suture. The 5-mm trocar was exchanged for a 10-mm one to remove the adnexa, which had been placed in a bag. The hernia was repaired on an outpatient basis, and 8 months later, she is asymptomatic. Postoperatively, one 68-year-old woman was unable to void. She underwent bilateral salpingo-oophorectomy for a persistent ovarian cyst, a Moschcowitz procedure, and Burch retropubic urethropexy. She required self-catheterization for 10 days. Nine women had dysuria without infection which resolved with Pyridium treatment. Fifty-eight women voided following removal of the Foley catheter on the second or third postoperative day. Other than the woman noted above,

TABLE 18-1. Major Postoperative Complications

Pt. Age	G/P	Complication	Medical History	Concomitant Surgery	Type of Suspension
44	4/3	Cystotomy	TAH Hiatal hernia repair Endometriosis	BSO adhesiolysis	Marshall-Marchetti-Krantz
64	5/4	Hernia	TAH Arthritis Myocardial infarction	BSO adhesiolysis rectocele repair	Modified Burch

G/P, gravidity/parity; BSO, bilateral salpingo-oophorectomy; TAH, total abdominal hysterectomy

TABLE 18-2. Length of Hospital Stay in 62 Women Following Laparoscopic Retropubic Cystourethropexy

	No. of Patients	Length of Hospital Stay* (h/patient)	Total Hours/Group	Cumulative Average (h)
	17	19	323	19.0
	39	43	1677	35.7
	4	62	248	37.46
	1	77	77	38.1
	1	93	93	38.1
Total	62		2418	39

*Calculated from termination of operation to discharge.

three required self-catheterization (one 3 times, and two once) for inability to void and each kept a record of voided and residual urine volumes at home. They discontinued self-catheterization when postvoid residual urine was less than 100 mL. The average hospital stay, calculated from the end of the procedure until the patient was discharged from the hospital, was 39 hours (Table 18-2). No postoperative febrile morbidity was noted, and no patients required retropubic drainage. All women who were discharged with Foley catheter in situ were taught to remove it.

Five patients had symptomatic leakage with some or no relief postoperatively. Repeat urodynamic testing in four women confirmed suspected detrusor instability, which responded to Ditropan and bladder retraining. One patient reported no change in her preoperative and postoperative incontinence. Complete work-up including video urodynamic studies did not reveal any abnormality. She was placed on flavoxate (Urispas 100 mg, 2 tablets 3 to 4 times per day), which resolved her symptoms. Eleven months later she was continent.

Eighteen patients had symptoms of urgency and dysuria; these were relieved with Pyridium.

Postoperative evaluations were calculated as percentages and the total percentage of improvement subjectively and objectively (Table 18-3). In an 8- to 30-month follow-up, all women have reported satisfactory relief of symptoms and subjective and objective improvement. None noted urinary leakage during activities similar to those preoperatively associated with this condition. Subjective success was ascertained by a questionnaire about urine leakage and the absence of a need to wear pads. The perineal pad test was not used as its variability and high false positive rate renders its usefulness controversial.[33–35] Objective success was assessed using several criteria: comparison of preoperative and postoperative symptom diaries, urine characteristics by straight catheter (office dipstick for nitrate, leukocyte estrace, bacteria, white cell blood count, urine culture and sensitivity), postvoid residual volume (less than 100 mL was considered complete), urethrovesical junction angle as measured by catheter placement

TABLE 18-3. Percentage of Improvement

Percentage of Improvement	Activity	Leakage	Pad Required	No. of Times Changed/Day	No. of Patients
81-100	Sneezing, coughing, laughing	None to rare	No	N/A	57
61-80	Sneezing, coughing, laughing	Occasional	Rarely	N/A	1*
41-60	Sneezing, coughing, laughing	Predictable with activity	On occasion	1-3	0
21-40	Minimal activity (walking)	> 3 times/d	Yes	< 4	1*
0-20	At rest	Frequently	Yes	> 4	2*/1†

*All had detrusor instability with 90% to 100% relief by medical management.

†This patient had a normal intravenous pyelogram and videourodynamics; her symptoms resolved with Urispas.

(upward, downward, or straight); bladder support, and negative standing stress test. Emphasis was placed on the presence or absence of urine leakage and the need to wear a pad at rest, at different activity levels, and different urine volumes in the bladder (see Table 18-3).

Of the 11 patients reported by Vancaillie and Schuessler who underwent Marshall-Marchetti-Krantz procedure, a laparotomy was necessary for the first two of four patients to complete the surgery.[25]

Summary

Our study was undertaken to evaluate the efficacy of a laparoscopic retropubic cystourethropexy. We found it useful for selected women undergoing operative laparoscopy for concomitant pelvic abnormalities associated with stress incontinence and was better than abdominal retropubic urethropexy and needle urethropexy. Although the principles of an abdominal approach are followed, the disadvantages of a laparotomy incision are avoided. Because the sutures are deep in the pelvis, the problems with supports and sutures seen with needle procedures are unusual in laparoscopy. Elevation of the bladder neck depends on the adherence of the paravesical tissue to the symphysis pubis or pelvic sidewall, not on the two paraurethral sutures as in the needle procedure. Observation is better than that with laparotomy. The endoscopic approach appears less traumatic and invasive with decreased operative time and morbidity, and a more rapid recovery. The venous plexus can be identified with videolaparoscopic magnification and coagulated, which contributes to an almost bloodless operative field, eliminating the need for drainage or the formation of a postoperative hematoma. Other anatomic structures, such as the obturator nerve and venous plexus, are identified and protected from trauma. Although it has been reported that up to 5% of Marshall-Marchetti-Krantz procedures are associated with osteitis,[7] none of our patients experienced such a problem. The reported incidence of enterocele following the Burch procedure ranges from 3% to 17%.[8,9,36,37] In a recent study, up to 26.7% of women experienced genital prolapse after Burch colposuspension.[38] Concomitant assessment of the posterior cul-de-sac and performance of a Moschcowitz procedure can reduce the incidence of prolapse. Cordozo and colleagues[39] reported 18% postoperative detrusor instability after this procedure by laparotomy, but only 8% of our patients had this problem.

Preliminary results are promising with subjective and objective success rates averaging over 90% (see Table 18-3). Long-term follow-up studies are essential to decide if laparoscopic urethral suspension is equivalent to the same procedure performed by laparotomy. This procedure requires considerable experience in laparoscopic suturing techniques.

Vaginal Vault Suspension (Sacral Colpopexy)

Vaginal vault prolapse occurs when the apex of the vagina descends below the introitus. It is a rare sequela of hysterectomy and occurs in 900 to 1200 women in the United States annually because of disruption of the ligaments that maintain vaginal support.[40] Numerous surgical techniques have been proposed to prevent and correct this condition,[41–49] including abdominal sacral colpopexy with interposition of a synthetic suspensory hammock between the prolapsed vaginal vault and anterior surface of the sacrum.[40,41,50] However, this technique usually requires a midline abdominal incision, abdominal packing, and extensive bowel manipulation with morbidity, wound separation or dehiscence, and ileus or bowel obstruction.[40]

The advantages of a laparoscopic approach include a better view of the pelvis, precise hemostasis. a smaller incision, elimination of abdominal packing, and less manipulation of the viscera.[51] Sacral colpopexy involves placing a hammock of polypropylene mesh between the prolapsed vaginal vault and the anterior surface of the sacrum. Multiple permanent sutures attach one end of the mesh to the apex of the vaginal vault and the opposite end to either the hollow of the sacrum or the sacral promontory.

Patient Profile

Twelve women with symptomatic posthysterectomy vaginal vault prolapse underwent laparoscopic sacral colpopexy. Eight also had unilateral or bilateral adnexectomy.[51] One patient had cholecystectomy performed by a general surgeon at the same anesthesia. One woman had failed transvaginal sacrospinous colpopexy. The two women with complete genital procidentia who underwent laparoscopic hysterectomy also had removal of one or both adnexa and anterior and posterior repair.

Bothersome protrusion and pelvic pressure that worsened with ambulation and daily activity were the main presenting symptoms. Five women had difficulty walking, three had urinary incontinence, two had difficulty voiding, none had fecal incontinence, and two had difficulty defecating. All had recurrent mucosal irritation. Five women reported ulceration; one was frequent, three were occasional, and one rare. One of the women who had uterovaginal prolapse also had cervical ulceration and recurrent infection. The other wore a pessary, which she found inconvenient. Six noted coital difficulty, and two had problems with hygiene. Other symptoms included constipation and dyschezia. Physical examination focused on the degree of prolapse and associated rectocele, cystourethrocele, and incontinence (urinary or fecal).

Technique

Instructions for a preoperative mechanical and antibiotic bowel preparation are given.[24] The patient is placed in a supine position in Allen universal stirrups. The vagina is cleansed with an antiseptic before the procedure. The laparoscope is placed through an umbilical trocar, and other instruments through three suprapubic 5-mm accessory trocars.[24] The patient is placed in a steep Trendelenburg position and tilted to the left to move the bowel away from the operating field.

A diagnostic laparoscopy is performed. The vagina is pushed up by a sponge on a ring forceps in the vaginal vault and adhesiolysis is performed as necessary.[52] Peritoneum and connective tissue are removed from the vaginal apex until the vaginal fascia and scar are identified. While holding the vaginal apex with grasping forceps, the vesical peritoneum over the vaginal apex is incised using the CO_2 laser, hydrodissection, or scissors (Figure 18-9). The bladder is dissected from the anterior vaginal wall and the rectum from the posterior vaginal wall to expose approximately 4 cm of the vaginal vault. If an opening is made in the vagina, an inflated surgical glove is placed in the vagina to help maintain pneumoperitoneum.

If a coexisting enterocele is found, the repair is performed laparoscopically by excising the sac followed by a modified Moschcowitz[53] posterior cul-de-sac obliteration using Ethibond (Ethicon). After identifying the ureters, the lateral peritoneum is elevated, and the suture placed through the peritoneum, passed through the cul-de-sac base, the opposite side of the peritoneum, and the anterior rectosigmoid colon serosa. A continuous purse-string suture of 0 polybutilate-coated polyester is placed (Figure 18-10).

The posterior parietal peritoneum is lifted with grasping forceps and the anterior sacral fascia exposed. Care is taken to avoid injuring the presacral vessels. Bleeding is controlled with bipolar electrodesiccation suture or clips. The peritoneal incision is extended downward to the vagina through the presacral space (Figure 18-11). The presacral space is entered through a vertical peritoneal incision at the right pararectal area using hydrodissection combined with the CO_2 laser set at 40 to 80 W (this can be replaced by any cutting modality that the surgeon chooses). The following anatomic landmarks are identified to avoid bowel, ureter, and vessel injury: the right ureter, internal iliac artery and vein, descending colon, and presacral vessels. The sigmoid colon is reflected later-

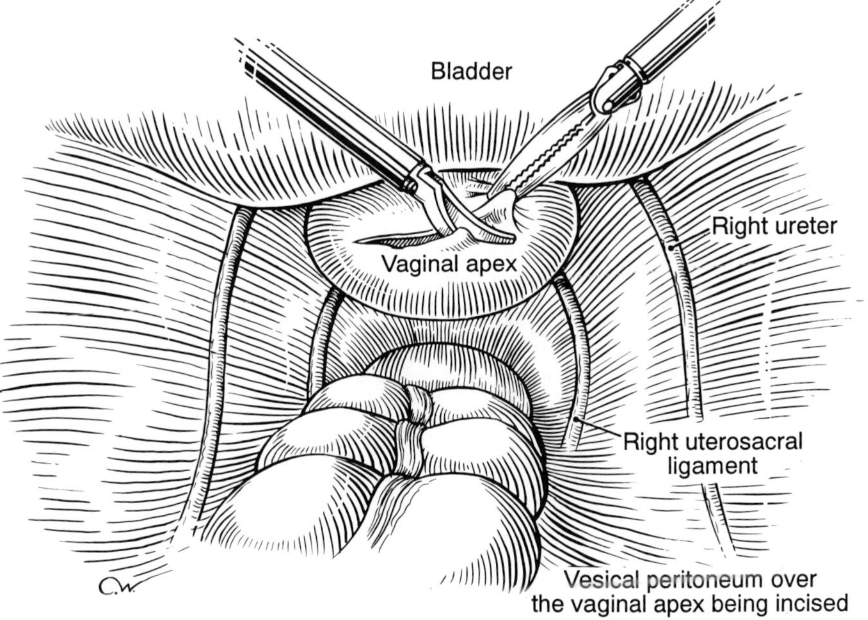

Figure 18-9. Vesical peritoneum over the vaginal apex is incised and vaginal apex is cleaned.

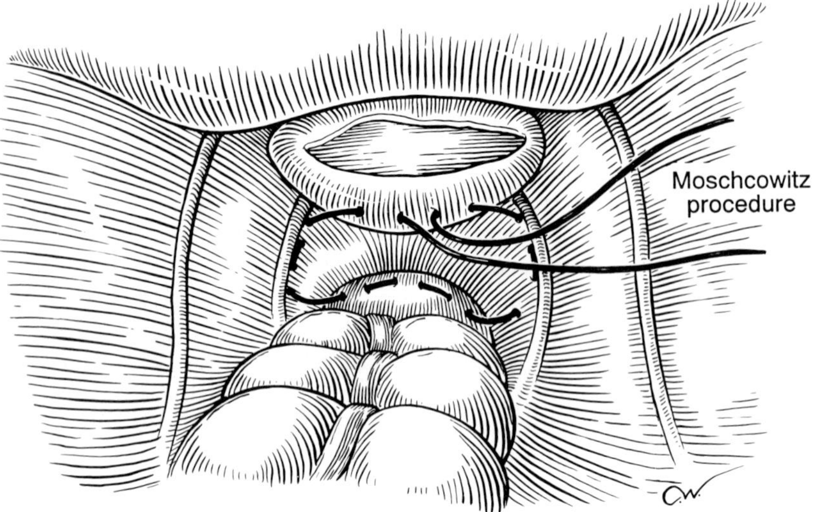

Figure 18-10. Posterior cul-de-sac is obliterated by Moschcowitz procedure using nonabsorbable suture.

ally to avoid injury to vessels in the sigmoid mesentery (see Figure 18-11).

The central 5-mm trocar above the symphysis pubis is replaced with a 10-mm trocar. The polypropylene mesh (Mersilene, Ethicon) is rolled and introduced into the abdomen through the 10-mm suprapubic port. Three to five 1–0 nonabsorbable polybutilate-coated polyester (Ethibond) sutures are placed in a single row in the vaginal wall apex (not including the vaginal mucosa) from one lateral fornix to the other (Figure 18–12). Each suture is placed through one end of the polypropylene mesh and tied loosely using extracorporeal or intracorporeal knot-tying techniques.

In most cases, other supportive measures in the lower vagina were necessary such as anterior and posterior colporrhaphy for the lower and middle third of the vagina. Partial vaginectomy was necessary in two patients, and this was done vaginally, with the mesh sutured to the posterior vaginal wall and placed intraperitoneally before closing the vaginal cuff.

Two permanent sutures or staples (Laptak, Surgin Surgical) are placed in the periosteum of the sacrum approximately 1 cm apart in the midline over S-3 and S-4 (Figure 18-13). Care is taken to avoid vascular injury to paravertebral and perforating blood vessels in this area. Hemostasis is dif-

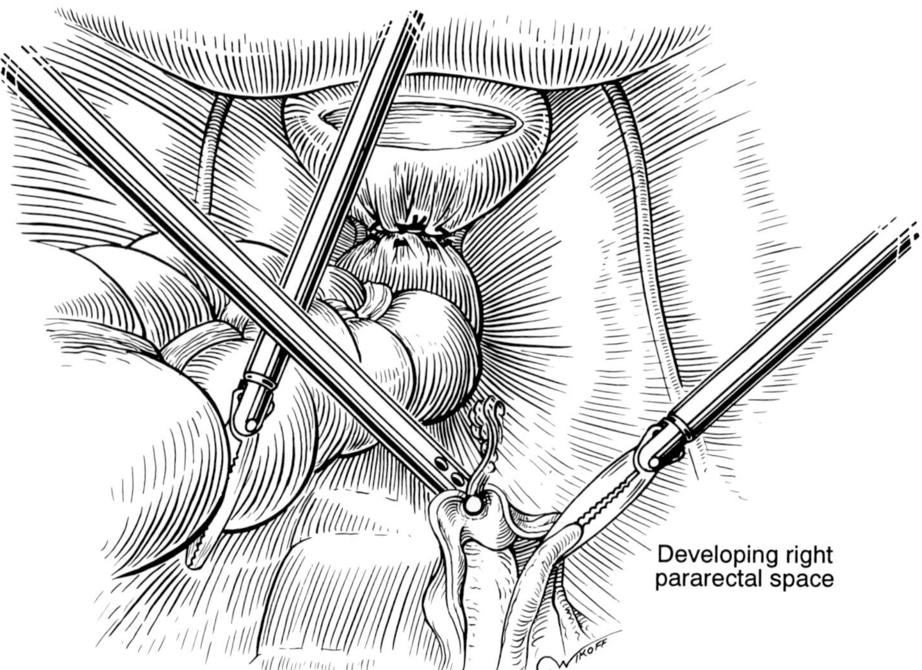

Figure 18-11. Using hydrodissection and the CO_2 laser, the right pararectal and presacral spaces are developed.

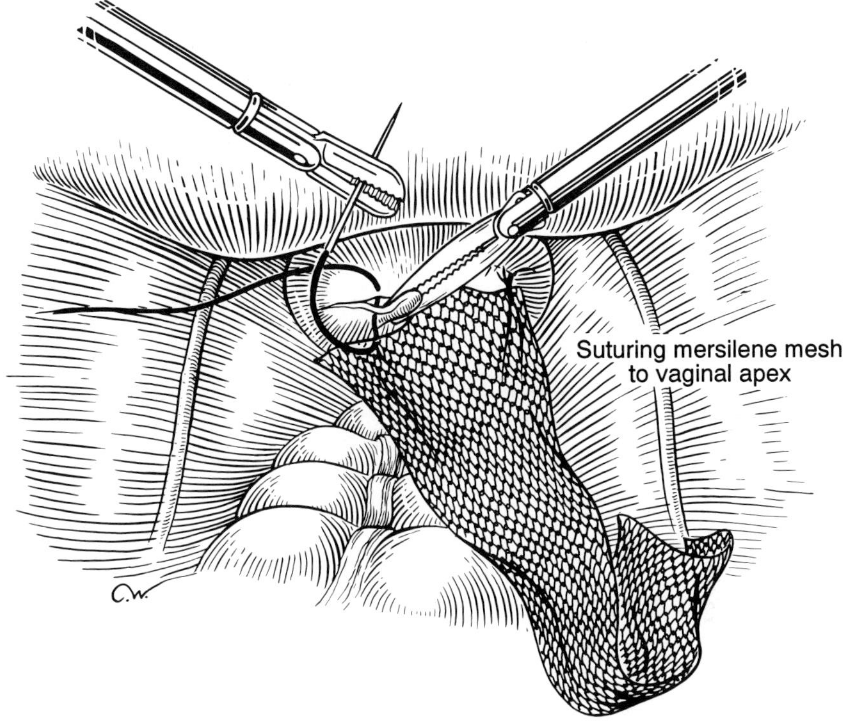

Figure 18-12. The polypropylene mesh is tied very loosely to the vaginal apex.

ficult even by laparotomy because of retraction of the severed vessels. The mesh is adjusted to hold the vaginal apex in the correct anatomic position without being tight. The excess mesh is trimmed from the strap. The peritoneum is closed over the strap using multiple interrupted sutures or clips.

Postoperatively, patients remain in bed for 24 hours. They are advised to avoid intercourse for 6

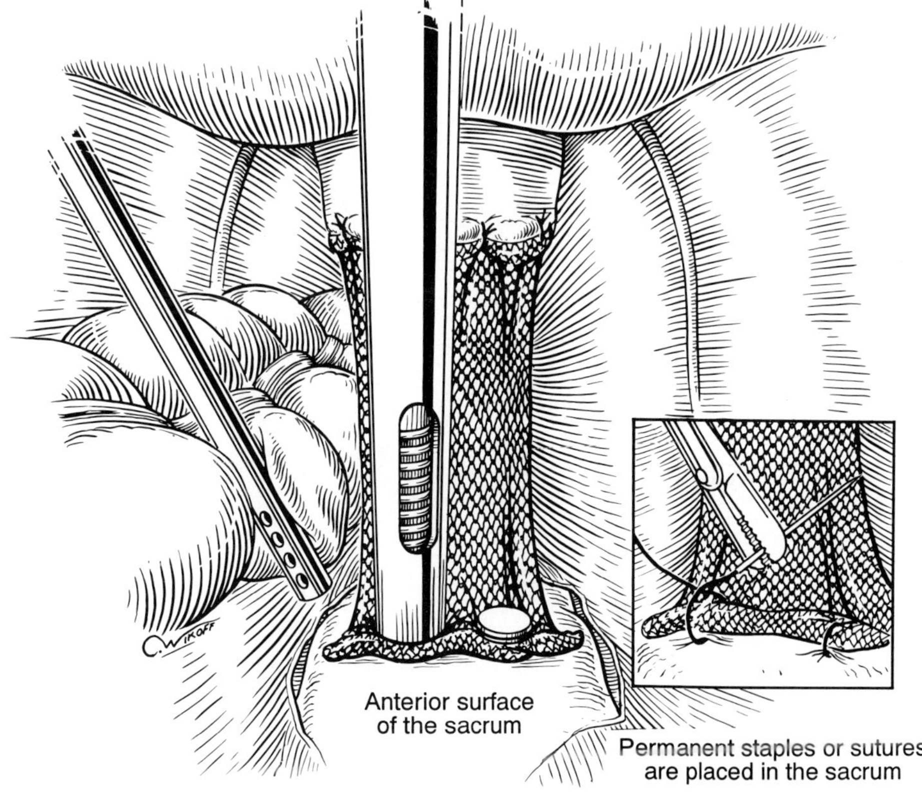

Figure 18-13. Two permanent sutures (inset) or staples are placed in the periosteum of the sacrum approximately 1 cm apart in the midline over S-3 and S-4.

TABLE 18-4. Summary of Patient History

Pt. No.	Age	G/P	Medical History	Medications	Previous Pelvic Surgery in Chronological Order
1	56	3/3	Arthritis, MVP, asthma	conjugated estrogen, antiasthmatic, ibuprofen	1. Laparotomy, left ovarian cystectomy, RSO 2. TAH, Burch retropubic, urethropexy. 3. APR
2	50	5/4	Hypertension, hypercholesterolemia	estradiol injections, diuretics	1. TVH 2. APR
3	77	3/3	Hypertension, polymyalgia, rheumatoid arthritis, osteoporosis, NIDDM, hypothyroidism	Prednisone, Synthroid, Zantac, Dyazide, Ativan, Hydergine, Citrucel, Flexeril, Didronel, Ocuvite, Premarin	1. TAH/BSO 2. Hernia repair 3. Cystocele repair, with Kelly-Kennedy plications
4	64	5/4	History of myocardial infarction, osteoporosis	ibuprofen, Premarin, Cardizem	1. Tubal ligation 2. TVH
5	48	1/1	None	none	1. Difficult forceps delivery 2. TVH 3. APR, with sacrospinous colpopexy
6	75	1/1	Arthritis, chronic bronchitis, HTN, recurrent cystitis, failed pessary	Lopressor, K-Dur, Synthroid, Premarin	1. Laparotomy/LSO
7	49	11/9	Recurrent cystitis, pelvic infection, chronic cervicitis, tuberculosis	none	None
8	61	6/4	Pneumonia, NIDDM	tetracycline, glyburide, ibuprofen, Premarin	1. TVH/APR 2. Rectocele, enterocele repair
9	66	4/4	Osteoporosis, HTN, hyperlipidemia	Premarin, Cardizem, cholestyramine	1. Transvaginal tubal ligation 2. TVH/APR 3. Cystocele, urethrocele repair
10	71	7/5	HTN, NIDDM, osteoporosis	Moduretic, Inderal, 1/2 estradiol tablet	1. TVH 2. APR
11	59	2/2	IDDM, HTN, interstitial cystitis	insulin, diuretic, Inderal, Urised, antibiotic	1. TVH 2. Laparoscopy, BSO, Burch
12	56	3/3	Arthritis, osteoporosis, irritable bowel, HTN, hypothyroid	estradiol, ibuprofen, Synthroid, Tenoretic	1. TAH/BSO 2. APR, Kelly-Kennedy

APR, anterior-posterior repair; G/P, gravidity/parity; HTN, hypertension; IDDM, insulin-dependent diabetes mellitus; LSO, left salpingo-oophorectomy; MVP, mitral valve prolapse; NIDDM, non–insulin-dependent diabetes mellitus; RSO, right salpingo-oophorectomy; TAH, total abdominal hysterectomy; TVH, total vaginal hysterectomy.

2 months. Their diet is advanced as tolerated and a mild laxative is prescribed to prevent constipation.

Results

To date, we have performed 12 sacral colpopexy procedures. Four patients also had anterior and posterior repair, and three had bladder neck suspension. The patients' medical and surgical histories are summarized in Table 18-4. With the exception of one case, all procedures were completed laparoscopically (Table 18-5). During application of the staples, patient number three had significant bleeding and eventually underwent laparotomy. She was 77 years old, obese, and had a complicated medical history (see Table 18-4). The intra-abdominal manipulation required to achieve hemostasis was difficult. Laparotomy was performed and, after bleeding was controlled, the procedure was completed. Patients received follow-up for 6 to 36 months and all had complete relief of their symptoms with excellent vaginal vault support. One patient had mild, temporary constipation for a few weeks, which gradually resolved. The 6- to 36-month follow-up was conducted by periodic examination, formal report by referring physician, and telephone interview.

Conclusion

Vaginal vault prolapse results from poor support of ligaments that normally maintain vaginal position.[40] Several operative techniques are available to correct this problem. Abdominal colpopexy by suspending a mesh hammock between the prolapsed vault and sacrum has been reported with good results.[53] The laparoscopic modification of this operation combines the advantages of several procedures. Proper anatomic relationships are restored by correcting enterocele, reconstructing paracolpium fibers, and directing the vaginal axis toward S-3 or S-4 by evenly distributing tension over vaginal vault, and the posterior cul-de-sac is obliterated using a Moschcowitz technique.

A laparoscopic approach has achieved favorable results[24] with minimal blood loss, reduced hospitalization, and rapid recovery. An overall decrease in complications such as wound infection and dehiscence, deep vein thrombophlebitis, and small bowel ileus was noted compared to laparotomy. Important patient selection factors include

Table 18-5. Results of Sacral Colpopexy Procedures

Pt. No.	Associated Operation	Operating Time (Minutes)	Complications		Hospital Stay (d)
			Intraoperative	Postoperative	
1	LSO, lysis of adhesions	115	None	None	2
2	BSO, enterolysis, ureterolysis	165	None	None	2
3	Extensive enterolysis, partial vaginectomy, exploratory laparotomy	240	Bleeding	Wound separation	7
4	BSO, APR, MMK, lysis of adhesions	200	None	Urinary retention, str. cath.	3
5	BSO, lysis of adhesions	105	None	None	2
6	TLH, RSO, APR	230	None	None	2
7	TLH, BSO, APR, perineorrhaphy		None	Atelectasis	3
8	BSO, Burch	150	None	None	2
9	BSO, ureterolysis, lysis of adhesions, posterior colporrhaphy	180	None	Constipation	3
10	BSO, enterolysis, ureterolysis, partial vaginectomy	180	None	None	2
11	Enterolysis, laparoscopy, cholecystectomy, APR	320	None	None	2
12	Enterolysis, partial vaginectomy, posterior colporrhaphy, Burch procedure	160	None	None	1.5

APR, anterior-posterior repair; BSO, bilateral salpingo-oophorectomy; LSO, left salpingo-oophorectomy; MMK, Marshall-Marchetti-Krantz; TLH, total laparoscopic hysterectomy.

an ability to tolerate prolonged general anesthesia and pneumoperitoneum.

Vesicovaginal Fistula Repair

Vesicovaginal fistulas are treated by different surgical techniques depending on their cause and location.[54] Small vesicovaginal fistulas unresponsive to nonsurgical management usually are repaired easily.[55] The edges of the fistula are removed and the defect is closed. Latzko's technique is the most commonly used vaginal approach[56] in which some fistulas are surrounded by severe fibrosis and are close to the bladder neck or urethral meatus. Lee and coworkers[57] recommended an abdominal approach for fistulas in the upper part of a narrow vagina, multiple fistulas, those associated with other pelvic abnormalities, and fistulas close to the ureter. A combined abdominal and vaginal approach has been recommended in some instances.[58]

Technique

The basic principles for fistula repair include suitable equipment and lighting, adequate exposure, excision of fibrous tissue from the edges of the fistula, approximation of the edges without tension, the use of suitable suture material, and efficient postoperative bladder drainage.[59]

A 10-mm infraumbilical incision is made for the insertion of the operative laparoscope coupled with the CO_2 laser. Three 5-mm trocars are inserted in the lower abdomen for the suction-irrigator probe, grasping forceps, and the bipolar forceps.[24] A simultaneous cystoscopy is performed and both ureters are catheterized to aid in their identification and protection during excision and closure of the fistula. A ureteral catheter is pulled through the fistula into the vagina to facilitate identification during excision.

A digital rectovaginal examination is performed to exclude rectal involvement. Using the CO_2 laser, an opening is made in the vagina, avoiding the bladder and rectum. An inflated glove in the vagina helps maintain pneumoperitoneum.

The anterior vaginal wall is elevated with a grasping forceps, and the fistula is identified with the help of the previously inserted catheter. It also delineates the posterior bladder wall. The bladder is filled with water, and a cystotomy is performed above the fistula using the CO_2 laser. The water is evacuated as the bladder is distended by the pneumoperitoneum from the cystotomy. The fistula tract, vesicovaginal space, and ureters are observed laparoscopically (Figures 18-14 and 18-15). The vesicovaginal space is developed laparoscopically using the CO_2 laser and hydrodissection. The bladder is freed posteriorly from the vaginal wall (Figure 18-16). The bladder fistula is identified, held with a grasping forceps, and excised using the CO_2 laser (Figure 18-17). Adequate bladder dissection and mobilization are performed to eliminate tension upon suturing.

Initially, the vaginal wall opening of approximately 1.5 cm is closed with one layer of interrupted polyglactin suture. Then, the vesical defect

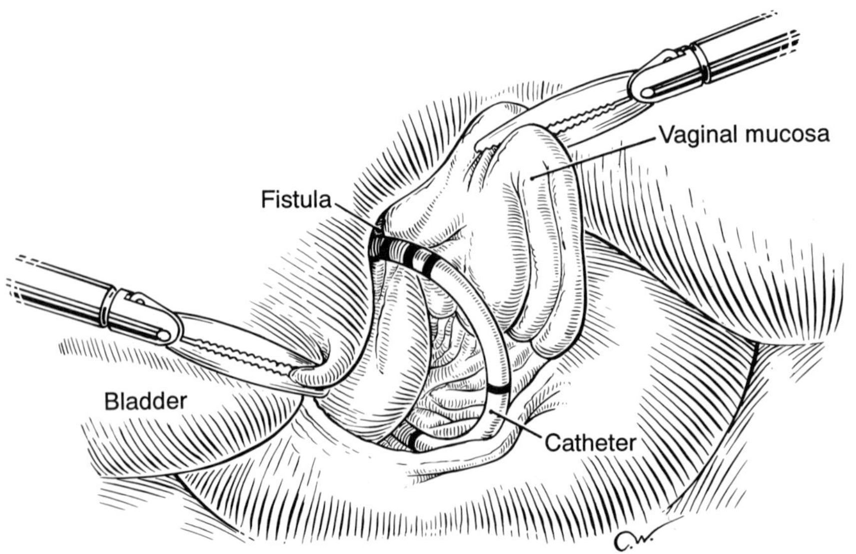

Figure 18-14. The fistula tract, vesicovaginal space, and ureters are observed laparoscopically.

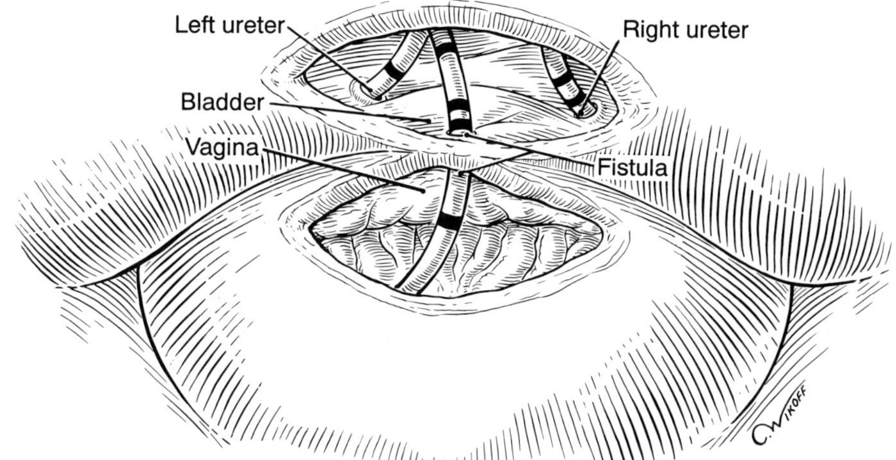

Figure 18-15. The bladder is freed posteriorly from the vaginal wall.

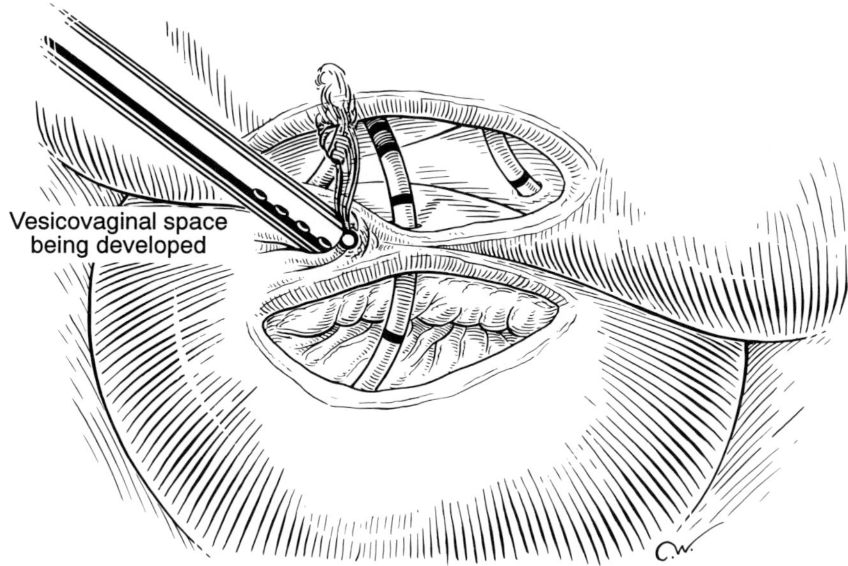

Figure 18-16. The bladder fistula is identified, held with a grasping forceps, and excised using the CO_2 laser.

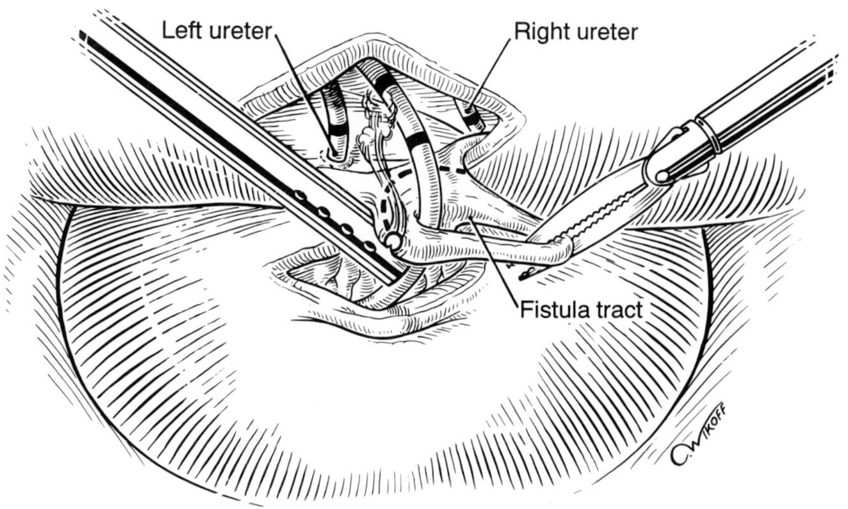

Figure 18-17. The vaginal wall repair is complete and the bladder opening repair is in progress.

is repaired in one layer with four interrupted 1–0 Endoknot polyglactin sutures (Ethicon) using extracorporeal knotting. It is important to close the defects in the vagina and bladder separately. Hemostasis of the vesicovaginal space and fistula area is essential. A peritoneal flap is obtained superior and lateral to the bladder dome close to the round ligament and diverted toward the bladder base. The flap is used to separate the vesicovaginal space, and it is secured with two interrupted polyglactin sutures. The dissected peritoneal area heals secondarily. No intraperitoneal drainage is used. Following the procedure, a suprapubic catheter is inserted and ureteral catheters are removed.

To date, we have performed laparoscopic repair of vesicovaginal fistula in two patients. Following a laparoscopic excision of an ovarian remnant, a 45-year-old patient developed a posterior vesicovaginal fistula in the upper third of the vagina, which failed to resolve with prolonged bladder drainage.[60] A vaginal approach was not appropriate because of the defects' complexity, location and condition. The morning after the repair of the fistula, the patient was discharged. Prophylactic antibiotics and estrogen were prescribed and on postoperative day 10, the Foley catheter was removed. A cystogram was performed and no evidence of fistula was seen. The patient was continent except for a short interval of urinary frequency.

The second patient was a 48-year-old woman who had a history of multiple previous abdominal operations. Following a total abdominal hysterectomy with bilateral salpingo-oophorectomy and cystotomy secondary to adhesions, she developed a high vesicovaginal fistula similar to the first patient. The repair was the same as in the first patient. Postoperatively, she did very well and has been asymptomatic for nine months.

Conclusion

Laparoscopy can be an alternative to laparotomy in managing several disorders.[24] The exposure and magnification afforded by videolaparoscopy provide direct access to the fistula. The videocystoscope enhances the access, eliminating the need for bladder dome incision for exposure. The fistula is resected under direct observation without ureteral trauma. An edge-to-edge approximation of the resected fistula is performed without difficulty. The magnification and exposure allow meticulous and atraumatic bladder dissection and fistula resection. The bladder capacity is not reduced significantly. There is no tension in the repair and it is vascularized.

References

1. Thomas TM, Plymat DR, Blannin J, et al. Prevalence of urinary incontinence. *Br Med J.* 1980;281:1243.
2. Diokno AC, Brock BM, Brown MD, et al. Prevalence of urinary incontinence and other urological symptoms in the noninstitutionalized elderly. *J Urol.* 1986;136:1022.
3. Yarnell JW, St. Leger AS. The prevalence, severity and factors associated with urinary incontinence in a random sample of the elderly. *Age Aging.* 1979;8:81.
4. Holst K, WIlson PD. The prevalence of female urinary incontinence and reasons for not seeking treatment. *N Z Med J.* 1988; 101:756.
5. Rosenzweig BA, Hischke MD, Thomas S, et al. Stress incontinence in women: Psychological status before and after treatment. *J Reprod Med.* 1991;36:835.
6. Horbach NS. Genuine SUI: best surgical approach. *Contemp Obstet Gynecol.* 1992; 37:53.
7. Marshall VF, Marchetti AA, Krantz KE. The correction of stress incontinence by simple vesicourethral suspension. *Surg Gynecol Obstet.* 1941;88:509–518.
8. Burch JC. Cooper's ligament urethrovesical suspension for stress incontinence. *Am J Obstet Gynecol.* 1968;100:764–772.
9. Stanton SL. Colposuspension. In: *Surgery of Female Incontinence.* New York: Springer-Verlag; 1986:95–103.
10. McGuire EJ, Lyton B. Pubovaginal sling procedure for stress incontinence. *Surg Gynecol Obstet.* 1973;136:547.
11. Pereyra AJ, Lebherz TB. Combined urethrovesical suspension and vaginourethroplasty for correction or urinary stress incontinence. *Obstet Gynecol.* 1976;30:537.
12. Raz S. Modified bladder neck suspension for female stress incontinence. *Urology.* 1981; 17:82.
13. Hohnfellner R, Petrie E. Sling procedures in surgery. In: Stanton SL, Tanagho E, eds. *Surgery of Female Incontinence,* 2d ed. Berlin: Springer-Verlag, 1986:105–113.
14. Gittes RF, Loughlin KR. No incision pubovaginal suspension for stress incontinence. *J Urol.* 1987;138:568.
15. Bhatia NN, Bergman A. A modified Burch versus Pereyra retropubic urethropexy for stress urinary incontinence. *Obstet Gynecol.* 1980;66:255.

16. Mundy AR. A trial comparing the Stamey bladder neck suspension procedure with colposuspension for the treatment of stress incontinence. *Br J Urol.* 1983;33:687–690.
17. Green DF, McGuire EJ, Lytton B. A comparison of endoscopic suspension of the vesical neck versus anterior urethropexy for the treatment of stress urinary incontinence. *J Urol.* 1986;136:1205–1207.
18. Karram MM, Bhatia NN. Transvaginal needle bladder neck suspension procedures for stress urinary incontinence: a comprehensive review. *Obstet Gynecol.* 1989;73: 906–914.
19. Tanagho EA. Colpocystourethropexy: the way we do it. *J Urol.* 1976;116:751–753.
20. Bergman A, Ballard C, Koonings P. Primary stress urinary incontinence and pelvic relaxation: prospective randomized comparison of three different operations. *Am J Obstet Gynecol.* 1989;161:97–101.
21. Bergman A, Ballard C, Koonings P. Comparison of three different surgical procedures for genuine stress incontinence: prospective randomized study. *Am J Obstet Gynecol.* 1989;1102–1106.
22. Penttinen J, Lindholm EL, Kaar K, Kauppila A. Successful colposuspension in stress urinary incontinence reduces bladder neck mobility and increases pressure transmission to the urethra. *Acta Gynecol Obstet.* 1989; 244:233–238.
23. Van Geelen JM, Theeuwes AGM, Eskes TKAB, Martin CB. The clinical and urodynamic effects of anterior vaginal repair and Burch colposuspension. *Am J Obstet Gynecol.* 1989;159:137–144.
24. Nezhat C, Nezhat F, Nezhat C. Operative laparoscopy (minimally invasive surgery): state of the art. *J Gynecol Surg.* 1992; 8:111–141.
25. Vancaillie TG, Schuessler W. Laparoscopic bladder neck suspension. *J Laparoendosc Surg.* 1991;1:169.
26. Nezhat CH, Nezhat F, Nezhat C, Rottenberg H. Laparoscopic retropubic cystourethropexy. *Journal of the American Association of Gynecologic Laparoscopists.* 1994. Accepted for publication.
27. Walters M, Shields L. The diagnostic value of history, physical examination and the Q-Tip cotton swab test in women with urinary incontinence. *Am J Obstet Gynecol.* 1988; 159:145–149.
28. Hilton P, Stanton SL. A clinical and urodynamic assessment of the Burch colposuspension for genuine stress incontinence. *Br J Obstet Gynaecol.* 1983;90:934–939.
29. Bergman A, Bhatia NN. Uroflowmetry for predicting postoperative voiding difficulties in women with SUI. *Br J Obstet Gynaecol.* 1985;92:835.
30. Bhatia NN, Bergman A. Use of preoperative uroflowmetry and simultaneous urethrocystometry for predicting risk of prolonged postoperative bladder drainage. *Urology.* 1986; 28:440.
31. Nezhat C, Nezhat F. Operative laparoscopy for the management of ovarian remnant syndrome. *Fertil Steril.* 1992;57:1003–1007.
32. Nezhat F, Nezhat C. Laparoscopic segmental bladder resection for endometriosis: a report of two cases. *Obstet Gynecol.* 1993;81: 882–884.
33. Wall LL, Wank K, Robson I, Stanton SL. The Pyridium pad test for diagnosing urinary incontinence. A comparative study of asymptomatic and incontinent women. *J Reprod Med.* 1990;35:682–684.
34. Walters MD, Dombroski RA, Prihoda TJ. Perineal pad testing in the quantitation of urinary incontinence. *Int Urogynecol J.* 1990:1:3–6.
35. Griffiths DJ, McCracken PN, Harrison GM. Incontinence in the elderly: objective demonstration and quantitative assessment. *Br J Urol.* 1991;67:467–471.
36. Burch JC. Urethrovaginal fixation to Cooper's ligament for correction of stress incontinence, cystocele, and prolapse. *Am J Obstet Gynecol.* 1961;81:281–290.
37. Stanton SL. The Burch colposuspension procedure. *Acta Urol Belg.* 1984;52:280–282.
38. Wiskind AK, Creighton SM, Stanton SL. The incidence of genital prolapse after the Burch colposuspension. *Am J Obstet Gynecol.* 1992;176:399–405.
39. Cordozo LD, Stanton SL, William JE. Detrusor instability following surgery for genuine stress urinary incontinence. *Br J Urol.* 1979;51:204.
40. Timmons MC, Addison WA, Addison SB, et al. Abdominal sacral colpopexy in 163 women with post-hysterectomy vaginal vault prolapse and enterocele. *J Reprod Med.* 1992;37:323.
41. Arthure HGE, Savage D. Uterine prolapse and prolapse of vaginal vault treated by sacral hysteropexy. *J Obstet Gynaecol Br Emp.* 1957;64:335.

42. Lane FE. Repair of posthysterectomy vaginal vault prolapse. *Obstet Gynecol.* 1962;22:72.
43. Langmade CF. Cooper ligament repair of vaginal vault prolapse. *Am J Obstet Gynecol.* 1965;92:601.
44. Richardson AC, Williams GA. Treatment of prolapse of the vagina following hysterectomy. *Am J Obstet Gynecol.* 1969; 105:90–93.
45. Birnbaum SJ. Rational therapy for the prolapsed vagina. *Am J Obstet Gynecol.* 1973; 115:411–419.
46. Randall CL, Nichols DH. Surgical treatment of vaginal inversion. *Obstet Gynecol.* 1971; 38:327–332.
47. Beecham CT, Beecham JB. Correction of prolapsed vagina or enterocele with fascia lata. *Obstet Gynecol.* 1973;42:542–546.
48. Ridley JH. A composite vaginal vault suspension using fascia lata. *Am J Obstet Gynecol.* 1976;126:590–596.
49. Symmonds RE, Williams TJ, Lee RA, et al. Post hysterectomy enterocele and vaginal vault prolapse. *Am J Obstet Gynecol.* 1981; 140:852–859.
50. Feldman GB, Birnbaum SJ. Sacral colpopexy for vaginal vault prolapse. *Obstet Gynecol.* 1979;53:399–401.
51. Nezhat F, Nezhat C, Silfen SL. Videolaseroscopy for oophorectomy. *Am J Obstet Gynecol.* 1991;165:1323–1330.
52. Nezhat C, Nezhat F, Gordon S, Wilkins E. Laparoscopic versus abdominal hysterectomy. *J Reprod Med.* 1992;37:247–250.
53. Nichols DH. Enterocele and massive eversion of the vagina. In: Thompson JD, Rock JA, eds. *Te Linde's Operative Gynecology.* 7th ed. Philadelphia: JB Lippincott; 1992: 855–885.
54. Drutz, HP. Urinary fistulas. *Obstet Gynecol Clin North Am.* 1989;16:911–921.
55. Falk HC, Orkin LA. Nonsurgical closure of vesicovaginal fistulas. *Obstet Gynecol.* 1957; 9:538–541.
56. Latzko W. Behandlund Hochsitzender Blasen und Mastdarmscheidenfisteln nach Uterusseztipation mit hohom Schedienverschluss. *Zentralbl Gynak.* 1914;38:904–911.
57. Lee RA, Symmonds RE, William TJ. Current status of genitourinary fistula. *Obstet Gynecol.* 1988;72:313–319.
58. Taylor JS, Hewson AD, Rachow P. Synchronous combined transvaginal repair of vesicovaginal fistulas. *Aust N Z J Surg.* 1980; 50:23–25.
59. Moir JC. Principles and methods of treatment of vesico-vaginal fistulae. In: *The Vesico-Vaginal Fistula.* London: Bailliere, Tindall and Cassell; 1967:52.
60. Nezhat CH, Nezhat F, Nezhat LC, Rottenberg H. Laparoscopic repair of a vesicovaginal fistula. A case report. *Obstet Gynecol.* 1994; 83:899.

19

The Role of Laparoscopy in the Management of Gynecologic Malignancy

Most gynecologic oncologists have been reluctant to use operative laparoscopy in the management of pelvic malignancy. Nevertheless, advanced laparoscopic operative techniques have been developed, and proper application in selected instances of pelvic malignancies is feasible and safe. The use of operative laparoscopy for gynecologic malignancies is new and this endoscopic approach should be performed only at centers whose surgeons have adequate experience and under certain research protocols.

Pelvic and abdominal anatomy are magnified with the videocamera and laparoscope. The upper abdomen, surfaces of the liver and the diaphragm, posterior cul-de-sac, and posterior aspect of the broad ligaments can be inspected for metastatic lesions. Laparoscopic access to the rectovaginal space is as good as at laparotomy. The vesicovaginal, paravesical, and pararectal spaces are developed laparoscopically because of the magnification afforded by the videolaparoscope. The pneumoperitoneal pressure decreases bleeding from small vessels and provides a dry operating field. Technological advances, such as the development of the CO_2 laser, enable disease to be treated precisely and with a great margin of safety. Eliminating the large abdominal incision avoids wound infection and dehiscence, which are increased in these patients. Early ambulation reduces cardiovascular and pulmonary complications.

Historical Perspectives

The first radical hysterectomy with para-aortic and pelvic lymph node dissection was performed in June 1989, and since 1991, we have been performing most hysterectomies totally laparoscopically, including radical hysterectomies.[1,2] Laparoscopic pelvic lymphadenectomy was described by Dargent and Salvat in 1989[3] and Querleu and colleagues[4] published their experiences in 1991. The laparoscopic treatment of adnexal masses suspected or proven to be malignant[5–8] and other applications of videolaparoscopy in gynecologic oncology have been reported.[4,9–13]

Following experience with pelvic and para-aortic lymphadenectomy for cervical cancer,[1,10] operative laparoscopy has been performed for the treatment of endometrial malignancy, staging of ovarian cancer, and second-look laparoscopy following a course of chemotherapy for ovarian malignancy.

The consent for surgery states that laparoscopic treatment is not yet the standard of care in gynecologic oncology. If malignancy is found, intraoperative cancer cell spillage is possible and can influence prognosis. A repeat surgical procedure, a laparotomy, may be required. A 1- to 3-day bowel preparation is administered preoperatively. A laparotomy, in addition to a laparoscopy, is always a possibility.

Cervical Cancer

Operative laparoscopy can be used in the surgical staging of cervical cancer. Para-aortic nodal metastasis has been reported in 5% of women with stage IB, 16% with stage II, and 25% with stage III. Berman and coworkers[14] found that 40 of 47 women with involved para-aortic nodes also had pelvic node metastases. If a work-up in search of metastasis such as chest x-ray or computed tomography-guided needle aspiration fails to reveal metastatic disease, laparoscopic staging is an option. Pelvic and para-aortic lymphadenectomy is feasible and radiotherapy initiated, or in early stages, radical hysterectomy is performed. Access to the rectovaginal space is excellent with laparoscopy, and the vesicovaginal, paravesical, and pararectal spaces are developed laparoscopically because of excellent magnification afforded by videolaparoscopy. These features facilitate removal of a large portion of vagina.

Radical hysterectomy and laparoscopically assisted radical vaginal hysterectomy are feasible alternatives to laparotomy in treating certain stages of cervical carcinoma.[1,9,13] Further, stage IA2 cervical cancer with lymphatic channel involvement, stage IB, and stage IIA (especially when the lesion extends into the vagina) can be managed by operative videolaparoscopy. For stages IIB and higher, laparoscopy is useful for node dissection and to change the FIGO staging to clinical staging, avoiding unnecessary extended field irradiation. In addition, operative laparoscopy can assist pelvic exenteration.

Radical Hysterectomy

The mortality rate for radical hysterectomy is higher than that for abdominal or vaginal hysterectomy. Morbidity is common postoperatively and serious complications such as ureteral injury (1% to 2%) and vesicovaginal fistulas occur (less than 1%).[15] The major postoperative complication is bladder dysfunction. The incidence increases with the extent of surgery,[16] and approximately 3% of patients develop chronic bladder hypotonia.[15]

Patients who undergo radical hysterectomy are relatively young with low-grade disease. The 5-year survival rate for stage IB is between 85% and 90%, and for stage IIA between 70% and 75%.[17] Although patients can achieve a comparable survival rate following primary radiation therapy, the subsequent complications make surgery preferable. Radical hysterectomy enables premenopausal women to preserve their ovaries, postpone hormonal replacement therapy, and the option of motherhood remains after their recovery from disease because of in vitro fertilization and surrogates.

Ovarian Cancer

The staging procedure plays an important role in the prognosis and planned treatment, particularly if the disease appears to be limited to one ovary. Inadequate surgical exploration leads to suboptimal treatment. The incidence of positive lymph nodes may be as high as 24% in stage I disease.[11] The standard preoperative work-up includes history and physical, pelvic examination, Papanicolaou smear, complete blood count, SMA 12, chest x-ray, intravenous pyelogram, barium enema, and gastrointestinal series if indicated. Pelvic examination under anesthesia and peritoneal, pelvic, and upper abdominal washings are essential. Total hysterectomy and bilateral salpingo-oophorectomy, multiple peritoneal biopsies, appendectomy, omentectomy, and pelvic and para-aortic lymphadenectomy are performed. If necessary, tumor debulking is undertaken using CO_2 laser excision or vaporization and CUSA (Cavitational Ultrasonic Surgical Aspirator, Valley Lab, Boulder, CO) aspiration.

For peritoneal cytology, a long suction-irrigator probe is used to obtain washings from the pelvic, para-aortic, and subdiaphragmatic area. Lactated Ringer's with heparin solution is used. Peritoneal biopsies are obtained by using the CO_2 laser and hydrodissection in the pelvis and mid-abdomen. A diaphragmatic biopsy is taken with biopsy forceps, or with hydrodissection and the CO_2 laser. Although observation of the diaphragm is excellent at videolaparoscopy, an additional 5-mm trocar occasionally is necessary for direct access. During the omentectomy, the patient is placed in a straight supine position. A subcolonic omentectomy is performed using sutures, bipolar forceps, or a linear stapling device (Ethicon). All specimens are removed without contaminating the abdominal wall. A laparoscopic Endobag (Ethicon) adequately confines excised tissue. Our preliminary results include laparoscopic surgical staging of 10 women with different stages and types of ovarian malignancy. This series includes stage IA serous cystadenoma of low malignant potential (one patient), stage IA, grade 1 mucinous cystadenocarcinoma (two patients), stage IA, grade 1 serous cystadenocarcinoma (one patient), stage IC clear cell adenocarcinoma (one patient), stage III papillary serous cystadenoma of low malignant potential (one patient), and stage IIIC epithelial adenocarcinoma (three patients). Laparoscopic hysterectomy and unilateral or bilateral salpingo-oophorectomy was performed in four patients. Peritoneal washings, multiple peritoneal biopsies, omentectomy, appendectomy, para-aortic and pelvic lymphadenectomy, or evaluation was performed in all cases. All procedures were completed laparoscopically without complication and the women were discharged within 24 hours with no short- or long-term complications to date (follow-up of 1 to 36 months). Six women did not have a hysterectomy. Three patients wanted to preserve their child-bearing capacity; two had a well-differentiated stage IA carcinoma and the other woman had borderline stage III serous papillary cystadenoma. Three women had previously undergone a total abdominal hysterectomy and bilateral salpingo-oophorectomy for a presumed benign adnexal mass. Although these preliminary results are promising, a longer follow-up period is needed.

All procedures were completed laparoscopically. Three patients underwent laparoscopically assisted placement of peritoneal infusion ports. Two patients underwent chemotherapy within 48 hours of their procedure; one began chemotherapy on the day of her surgery and the other on postoperative day 2. Because these patients were receiving chemotherapy, they were not discharged home until postoperative days 3 and 4, respectively. A third patient who had undergone sigmoidoscopy and anal fistulotomy at the time of her surgery was discharged home on postoperative day 2. The remaining 7 patients were discharged home on postoperative day 1. Complications occurred in only two patients. One patient with stage IIIC adenocarcinoma had an estimated blood loss of 800 mL and required a transfusion of 2 units of paced red blood cells intraoperatively and an additional 2 units postoperatively. A second patient with a stage IC clear cell adenocarcinoma had a mild corneal abrasion of her left eye, which required only overnight patching.

Second-Look Laparoscopy

Although the indication for second-look laparoscopy in patients with ovarian cancer after chemotherapy is debatable, it can be used safely in most cases. After the abdominal cavity is entered, the pelvic and abdominal cavity is evaluated for any gross disease, and peritoneal washings from the pelvis and upper abdomen are obtained. A biopsy is taken of any suspicious lesions. If no persistent disease is noted, multiple peritoneal biopsies are taken from the pelvis and upper abdomen, including any adhesions. Any remaining portion of the omentum is removed. If pelvic or para-aortic lymphadenectomy was not performed previously, it is, if possible, performed at this procedure. Tumor debulking can be performed using the CO_2 laser or CUSA, as long as the tumor is not too bulky.

Nineteen second-look laparoscopies following a laparotomy for ovarian cancer were performed. Peritoneal washings, multiple peritoneal biopsies from the upper abdomen, and pelvic and para-aortic node sampling were performed as indicated. In two patients, CUSA was used for debulking. One bowel perforation occurred that was repaired laparoscopically, and this patient was discharged home without sequelae. All patients were discharged from the hospital within 48 hours.

Endometrial Cancer

The standard treatment for endometrial carcinoma is peritoneal washings, total abdominal hysterectomy, bilateral salpingo-oophorectomy, and pelvic and para-aortic lymph node dissection. Endometrial carcinoma can be staged and treated laparoscopically. Clinical staging may be incorrect in many patients with stage I endometrial adenocarcinoma[19] so that surgical staging often is necessary. The use of the laparoscope enables conversion of abdominal hysterectomies to laparoscopic procedures, or at least, to laparoscopically assisted vaginal procedures. Usually, the laparoscopic approach to rectovaginal, vesicovaginal, paravesical, and pararectal spaces is adequate and exposure is improved. Almost all stages of endometrial carcinoma can be staged and managed laparoscopically.[20,21]

Fifteen women with stage I endometrial cancer, ranging in age from 51 to 76 years, were managed by laparoscopy. In nine women, peritoneal washing, total laparoscopic or vaginally assisted laparoscopy hysterectomy, and bilateral salpingo-oophorectomy were performed. Lymphadenectomy was not required in these women, but para-aortic and pelvic lymphadenectomy were necessary in the other six. No intraoperative or postoperative complications occurred. One woman with multiple medical conditions, including early heart failure, was observed in the coronary care unit overnight and discharged on the third postoperative day. In all women, the nodes were negative.

An additional patient was diagnosed with clinical stage IIIB, grade 1 adenocarcinoma of the endometrium. She underwent 5005 cGy of external beam radiation therapy followed by laparoscopic hysterectomy and bilateral salpingo-oophorectomy, with placement of perineal and suburethral interstitial needle implants delivering an additional radiation dose of 3000 cGy. Because of her marked obesity, the patient was observed overnight in the ICU. She had an uneventful recovery and was discharged home on postoperative day 5 after completing her interstitial brachytherapy and removal of the needle implants. One woman had undergone surgical staging at laparotomy revealing stage IVB poorly differentiated endometrial adenocarcinoma. At her initial presentation to us 3 months later, she was found to have persistent tumor. For symptomatic relief, it was decided to proceed with laparoscopic tumor debulking and peritoneal infusion port placement for future dose-intensive chemotherapy. At laparoscopy, however, the abdominopelvic organs were densely adherent and agglutinated leading to an enterotomy and a cystotomy. Given the extensive nature of the pathology, a laparotomy was performed allowing for completion of the debulking procedure, adhesiolysis, and peritoneal infusion port placement. The patient was discharged home in stable condition on postoperative day 7 after an uncomplicated recovery. This case illustrates that although laparoscopy can be of value in the treatment of endometrial cancer, there are still limits to its application. Large prospective controlled studies with long-term follow-up are necessary to further define the role and limitations of laparoscopy in the treatment of pelvic malignancies.

Para-aortic Lymphadenectomy

The room setup, patient position, and equipment require minor variations. These include an additional 5-mm trocar and placing the primary trocar 3 to 4 cm supraumbilically to improve access to the para-aortic area for node dissection. The surgeon stands on the right or left side of the patient, and two assistants are used. In some cases, the mid-suprapubic incision is used to insert the videolaparoscope and the surgeon stands at the foot of the patient. Accordingly, accessory trocars require minor adjustment.

After inserting the trocars, the upper abdomen and pelvis are inspected. For cervical and endometrial cancer, the nodes on both sides of the abdominal aorta up to the origin of the inferior mesenteric artery from right to left lumbar region and ureter should be removed. To expose the para-aortic region, the patient is tilted to the left and placed in a steep Trendelenburg position (35 to 40 degrees). The bowel is directed toward the diaphragm and held in place using an atraumatic grasping forceps. The ureters are identified through the peritoneum (Figure 19-1). An opening is made in the peritoneum just above the sacral promontory. Lactated Ringer's solution is injected into the retroperitoneal space[22]; the peritoneum above this opening is grasped and incised with the CO_2 laser or scissors toward the duodenal bulb (Figure 19-2).[1] The remaining retroperitoneum is opened. The aortic adventitial plane, from the origin of the inferior mesenteric artery to the common iliac arteries, is developed. The retroperitoneal fatty tissue below the bifurcation, which involves the hypogastric plexus nerve and lymph nodes, is removed. On the right side, the ureter must be identified and dissected from the underlying tissue and retracted laterally. It may be necessary to mobilize the small bowel and appendix and elevate them with an atraumatic grasping forceps to prevent them from falling into the operative field. The precaval node chain from the surface of the common iliac artery and vena cava are removed using blunt and sharp dissection and hydrodissection. The dissection is continued up to the origin of the mesenteric artery and para-aortic nodes in this area are removed (Figure 19-3). The aorta is retracted medially and nodes between this vessel and the vena cava are removed primarily by blunt dissection and hydrodissection. The perforating vessels are identified and desiccated using bipolar forceps, or clips can be used. The removed nodes are extracted through a 5- or 10-mm trocar sleeve without contaminating the abdominal wall. The left para-aortic and common iliac nodes are removed (Figure 19-4), from the inferior mesenteric artery to the left mid-common iliac artery. The removal of the left para-aortic nodes is difficult because of the location of the sigmoid colon, especially in obese patients. Caution must be exercised to avoid injuring the inferior mesenteric artery. The ureter and ovarian vessels are identified and separated from the psoas muscle. All nodes from the surface of the aorta and common iliac artery and vein are removed. Manipulation should be gentle to avoid injuring underlying major vessels, particularly the left common iliac vein, which is visible as a blue surface, "Big Blue." The small bowel is held up by an atraumatic grasp-

Figure 19-1 Anatomy of the pelvis and lower abdomen.

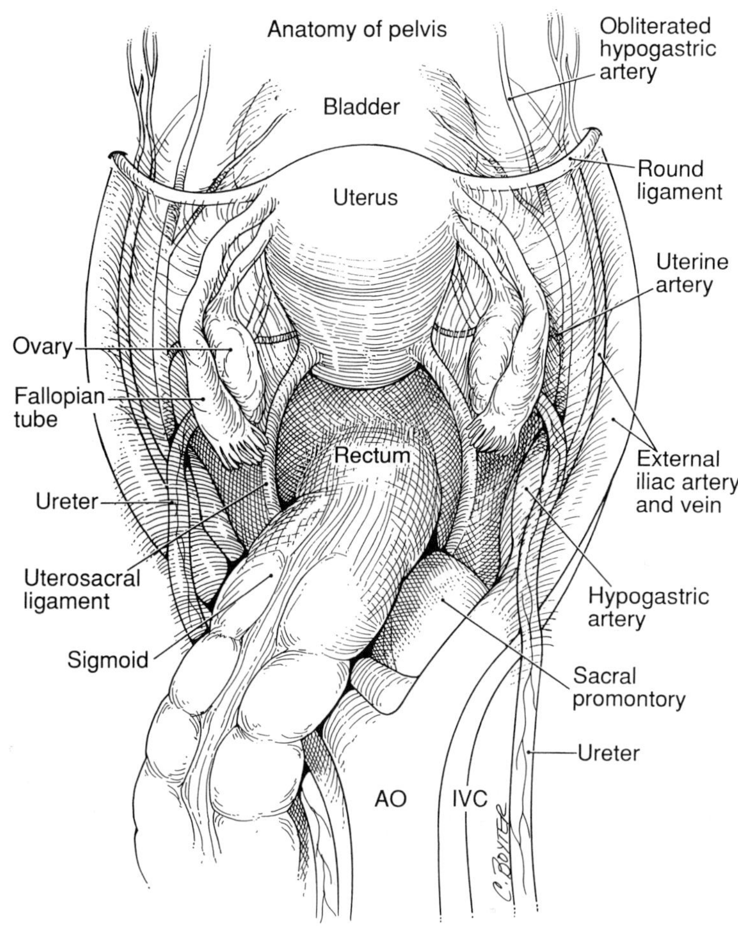

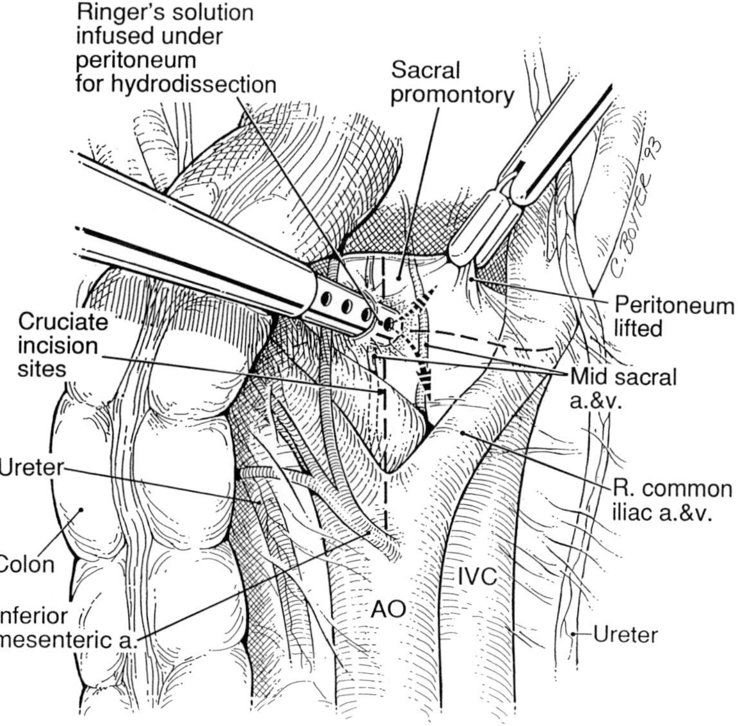

Figure 19-2 Para-aortic node dissection. After identifying the right ureter, the peritoneum above the sacral promontory is elevated using a grasping forceps and an opening is made. Hydrodissection is performed and the peritoneum is opened toward the duodenal bulb.

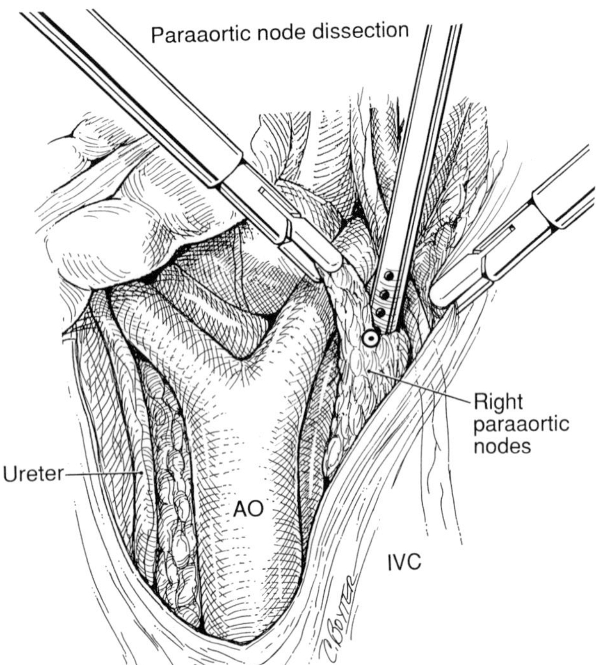

Figure 19-3 After removing the retroperitoneal fatty tissue and exposing the blood vessels, the right common iliac and para-aortic nodes between the aorta and vena cava are removed using gentle blunt and sharp dissection, and hydrodissection. The dissection can be extended to the renal vessels.

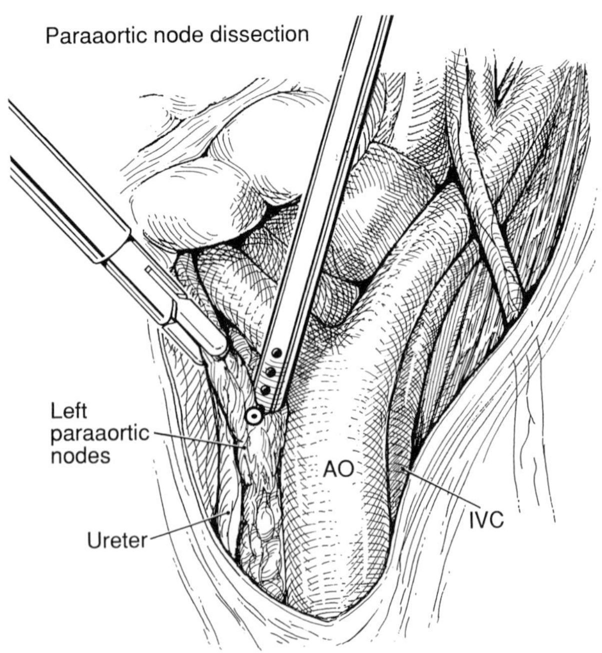

Figure 19-4 After the rectosigmoid colon is pushed laterally, the lymph nodes between the left ureter and aorta are removed.

ing forceps for better observation of this area. Pneumoperitoneal pressure decreases bleeding and hemostasis can be achieved with bipolar forceps or single vascular clips. For ovarian cancer staging, the para-aortic lymphadenectomy is extended above the origin of the mesenteric artery to the level of the left renal vein and right ovarian vein (Figure 19-5). Dissection is more difficult in this area, especially in obese patients, and care should be taken to avoid vascular injury. The vena cava and aorta must be separated from the transverse duodenum by blunt and sharp dissection. The assistant elevates the bowel with an atraumatic grasping forceps. On the right side, the dissection continues to the origin of the ovarian vein to the vena cava. On the left side, the dissection continues from the origin of the inferior mesenteric artery to the connection of the renal vein to the vena cava. Sometimes, it is necessary to clip or desiccate the left ovarian vein to be able to remove the nodes from this area safely. After lymphadenectomy, an evaluation under low pneumoperitoneal pressure is performed to search for bleeding. The peritoneum is not closed because it heals spontaneously. At second-look laparoscopy following a presacral neurectomy, these areas heal well with no significant bowel adhesions.

Pelvic Lymphadenectomy

In cases requiring hysterectomy, pelvic node dissection is performed after hysterectomy with or without oophorectomy. If hysterectomy is not necessary, lymphadenectomy is performed after developing the paravesical and pararectal spaces. The external iliac nodes between the external iliac vein and artery and obliterated hypogastric artery are excised to the deep circumflex veins. The obturator nerve behind the obliterated hypogastric artery is exposed bluntly and the hypogastric and obturator nodes removed (Figure 19-6).[1,3] The obturator nerve is dissected and cleaned caudally until its exit from the pelvis. The nodal and fatty tissue between the obturator nerve and external iliac vein is identified and completely dissected. The inferior aspect of the external iliac vein is separated using blunt dissection, CO_2 laser or scissors, and hydrodissection until the internal obturator muscle and pelvic bone are seen. Venous anastomosis between the obturator and external iliac veins is observed and saved from trauma. Bipolar electrodesiccation is used to facilitate the occlusion of larger vessels. Lymph nodes posterior to the obturator nerve also are excised. The lymph nodes are removed en bloc, labeled with an Endoloop, and placed laterally. They are removed after

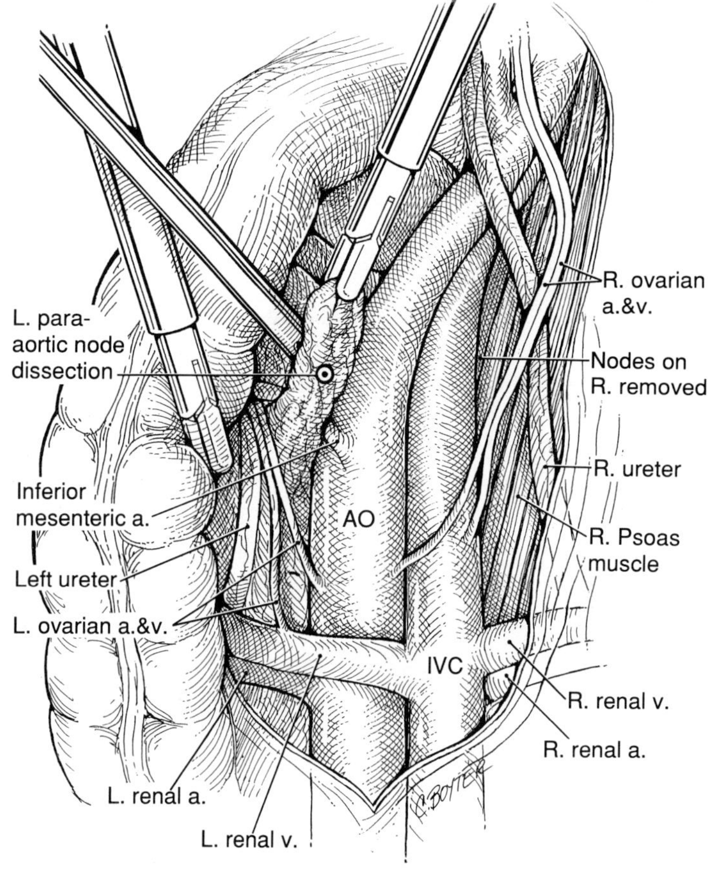

Figure 19-5 For ovarian cancer staging, the lymph nodes around the left renal vein and right ovarian vein should be removed.

the vagina is opened and the hysterectomy is completed.

Radical Hysterectomy

Technique. After inserting the trocars, the upper abdomen and pelvis are inspected, steep Trendelenburg (30 degrees) is obtained, and the bowel is displaced to the upper abdomen. Para-aortic node dissection (if indicated) is performed and specimens sent for frozen section. If they are negative, the operator proceeds with radical hysterectomy and pelvic node dissection. The rectovaginal, paravesical, and pararectal spaces are dissected. An assistant performs simultaneous rectal and vaginal examination, delineating the rectum and vagina.[23] The cul-de-sac is incised; the rectum is pushed from the posterior vaginal wall using CO_2 laser, blunt dissection, and hydrodissection to a level of 4 to 5 cm below the cervix (Figures 19-7 and 19-8).[23] For the paravesical space, the line of dissection is between the round ligament anteriorly, infundibulopelvic ligament medially and pelvic sidewall laterally (Figure 19-9). The round ligaments (Figure 19-10) are desiccated close to the pelvic side walls and transected. The peritoneum is opened and the paravesical and pararectal spaces dissected by blunt dissection, hydrodissection, and the CO_2 laser (Figures 19-10 and 19-11). This technique allows skeletonization of the obliterated hypogastric artery, which is grasped and traced until the uterine artery is reached. The uterine vessels are identified, skeletonized and electrodesiccated just medial to their origin and transected (Figure 19-12). They are grasped with the forceps and rotated anterior to the ureters (Figure 19-13). This separation from the ureters must be gentle. Small blood vessels from the uterine artery to ureter are desiccated with bipolar forceps.

To develop the vesicovaginal space, the bladder serosa is injected with lactated Ringer's.[22] The anterior leaf of the broad ligament is opened and the bladder flap is developed, using the CO_2 laser, blunt dissection, and hydrodissection.[22,24] After dividing scar tissue and the vesicouterine fold, the suction-irrigator probe pushes the bladder completely from the cervix and upper vagina (Figures 19-14 through 19-16).

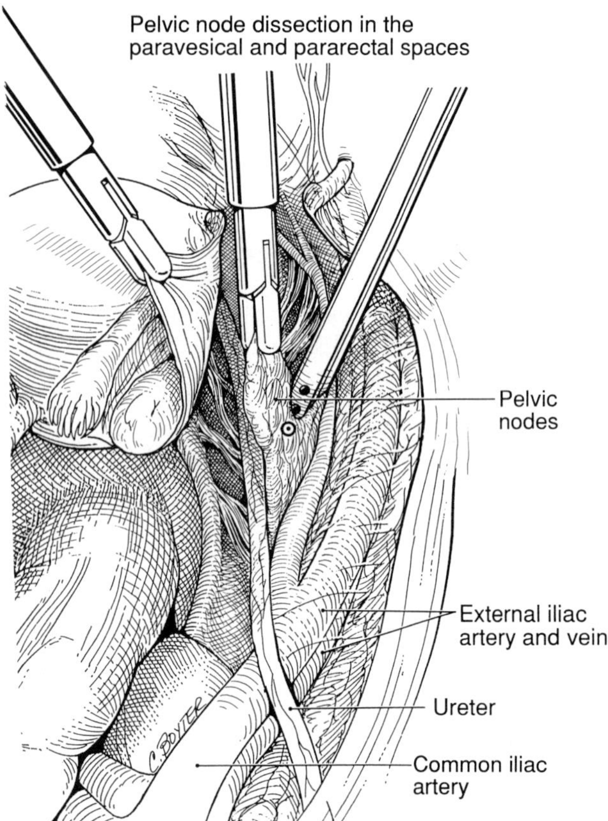

Figure 19-6 The lymph nodes anterior to the uterine artery between the bifurcation of the common iliac artery and nodes between and under the external iliac artery and vein, are removed.

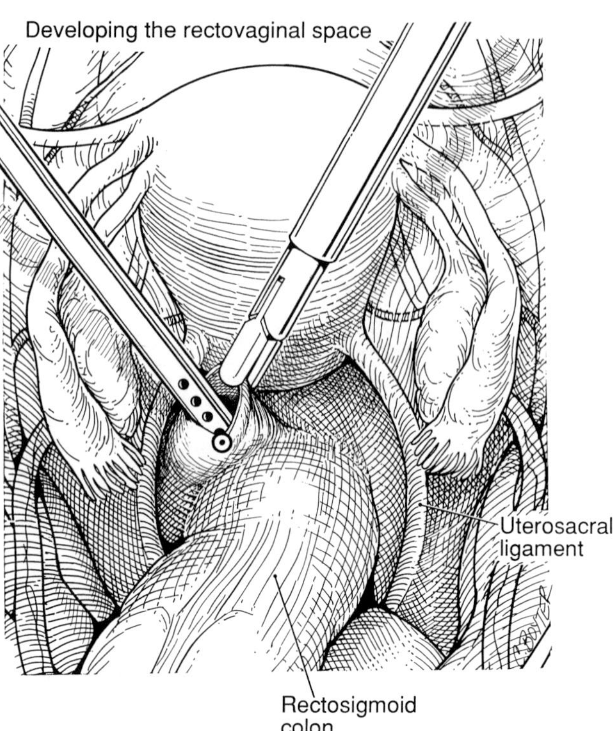

Figure 19-7 Development of the rectovaginal space. While an assistant performs the rectovaginal examination, an incision is made, hydrodissection is performed, and the rectovaginal space is developed.

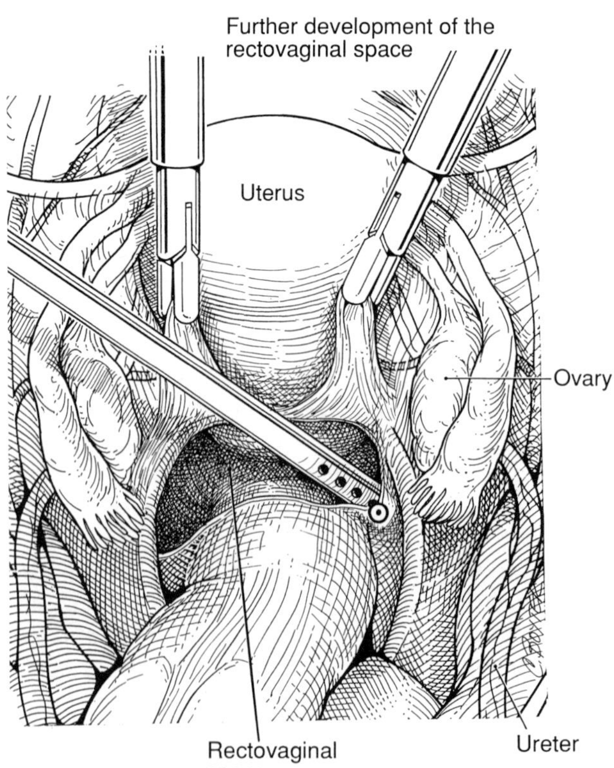

Figure 19-8 Complete development of the rectovaginal space. Sharp dissection with the CO_2 laser, blunt dissection, and hydrodissection are used.

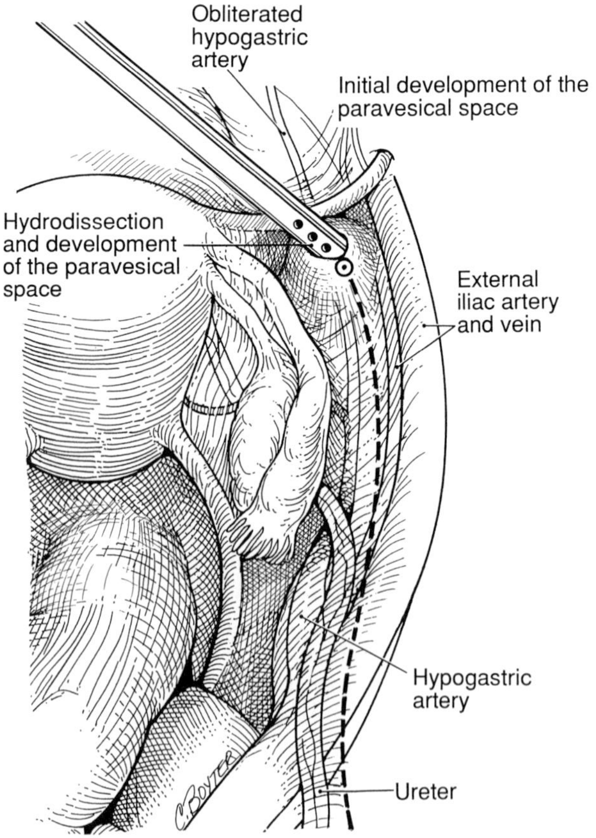

Figure 19-9 The right paravesical space is developed by opening the peritoneum and performing hydrodissection. The line is between the round ligament anteriorly, infundibulopelvic ligament medially, and pelvic side wall laterally.

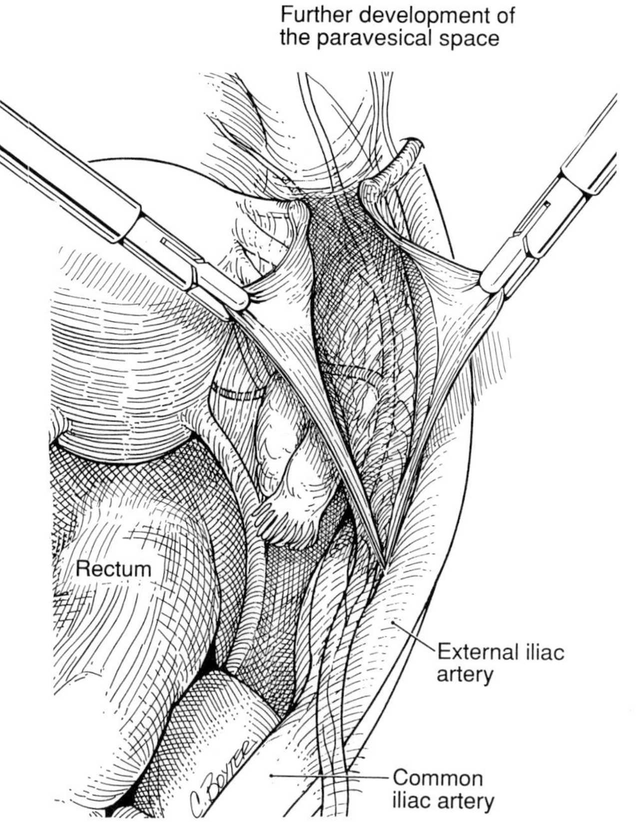

Figure 19-10 After electrodesiccation and cutting the right round ligament, the peritoneum is grasped laterally and the paravesical space is exposed.

Figure 19-11 The paravesical and pararectal spaces are developed. The retroperitoneal major blood vessels and ureter are identified.

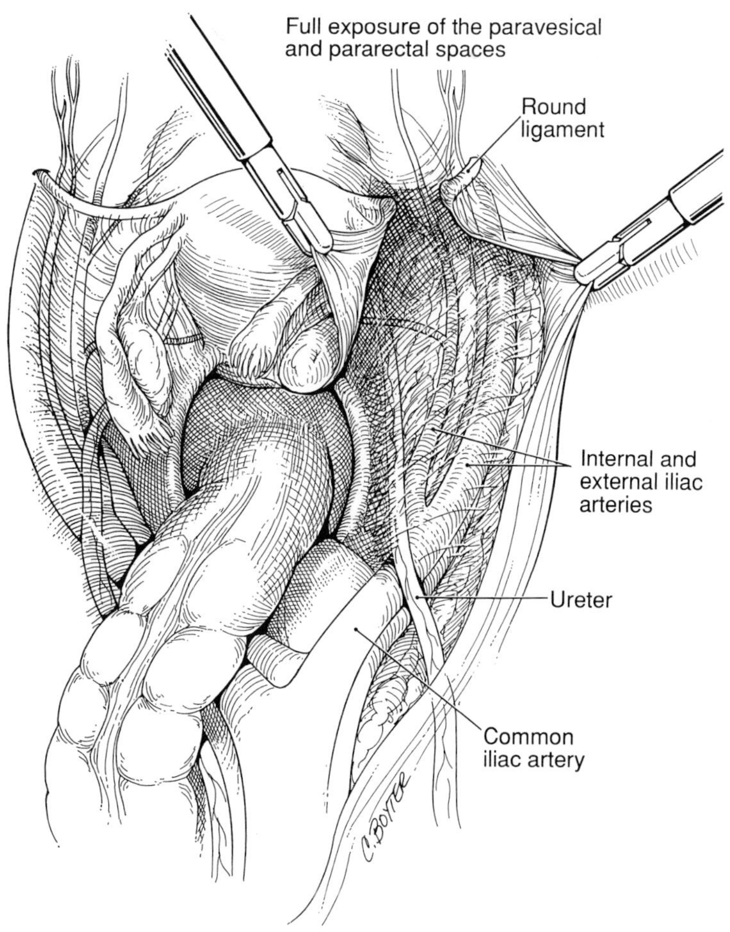

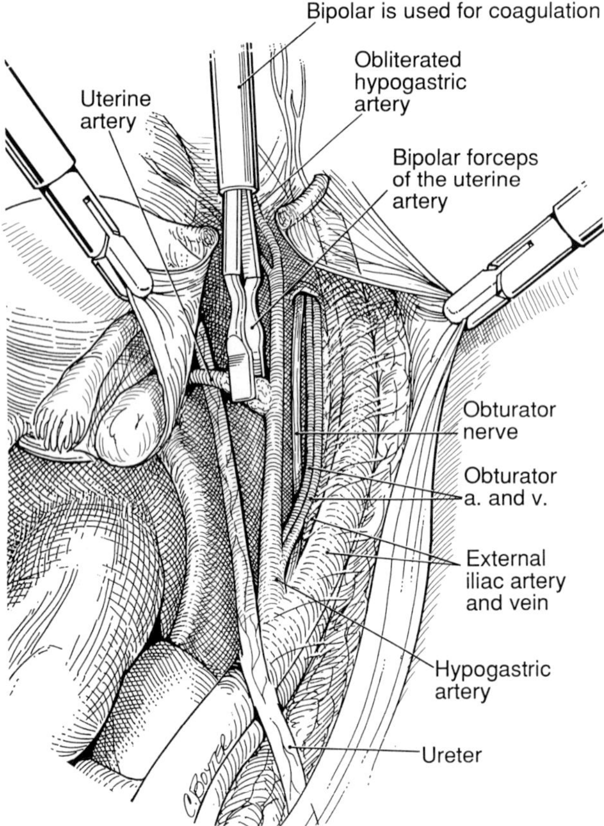

Figure 19-12 The uterine artery is electrodesiccated at its origin from the hypogastric artery using bipolar forceps.

The uterine vessels are retracted medially and removed from the ureter with the CO_2 laser. The anterior parametrium is transected with the laser and the suction-irrigator probe is used as a backstop. The ureters are freed from the peritoneum and skeletonized to the bladder with the suction-irrigator probe and the laser. The utero-ovarian or infundibulopelvic pedicles are electrodesiccated with bipolar forceps and transected with the laser.[20] Alternatively, a laparoscopic stapling device can achieve hemostasis and cut large pedicles.[25]

The uterosacral ligaments and lateral parametria are desiccated with bipolar forceps and sequentially transected approximately 1.5 to 2 cm lateral to the cervix. The dissection is taken to 2 to 3 cm below the cervix. The vagina is entered anteriorly and posteriorly with the CO_2 laser. A ring forceps or right angle retractor is placed into the vagina to push its walls anteriorly and posteriorly,[25] allowing it to be incised from above. Two wet sponges are placed in a surgical glove and inserted into the vagina to preserve the pneumoperitoneum.

The radical hysterectomy is completed vaginally by incising the vagina 3 cm distal to the cervix. The residual cardinal ligaments are mobilized anteriorly and posteriorly, then divided approximately 1.5 to 2 cm lateral to the cervix and suture ligated. The procedure is completed laparoscopically by incising the vagina laparoscopically while the assistant identifies the vagina by placing a sponge forceps in it. Manipulation can be difficult, particularly if the uterus is enlarged, and it may be easier to complete the procedure vaginally. After the uterus is removed, the vaginal cuff is left open until the lymph nodes are removed from the abdomen. Then, it is closed vaginally or laparoscopically with 0 Vicryl laparoscopic sutures. To preserve pneumoperitoneum, two wet sponges are

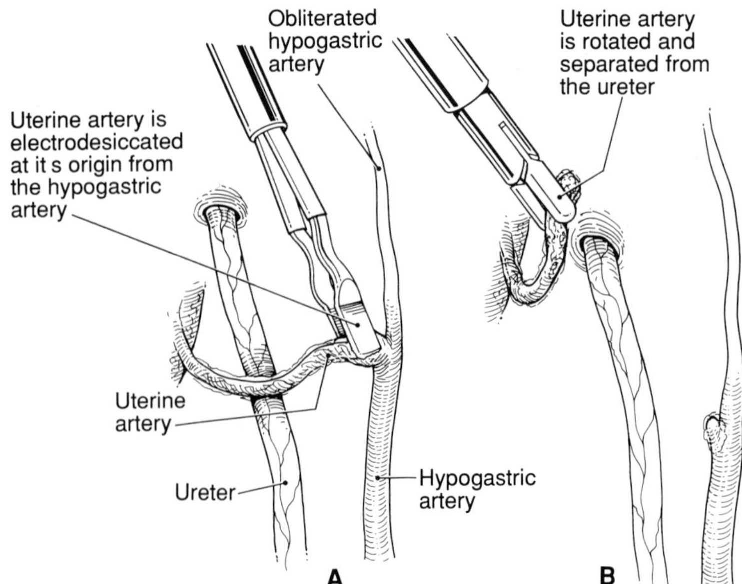

Figure 19-13 After the uterine artery is desiccated and transected, it is grasped with a forceps and rotated anterior to the ureter.

Figure 19-14 Developing vesicovaginal space. Anterior leaf of the broad ligament is elevated with grasping forceps and hydrodissection is performed. An incision is made toward the bladder using the CO_2 laser.

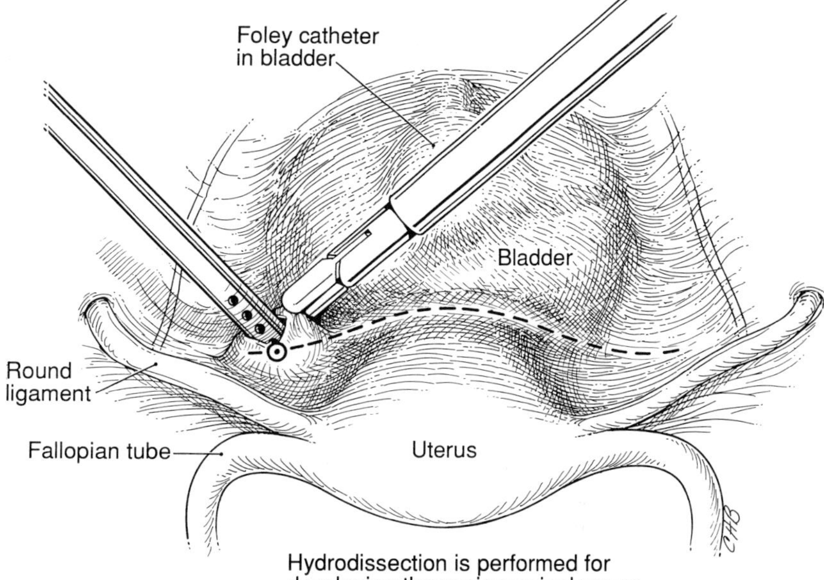

Figure 19-15 The peritoneum is elevated with the grasping forceps; using blunt and hydrodissection, the vesicovaginal space is developed.

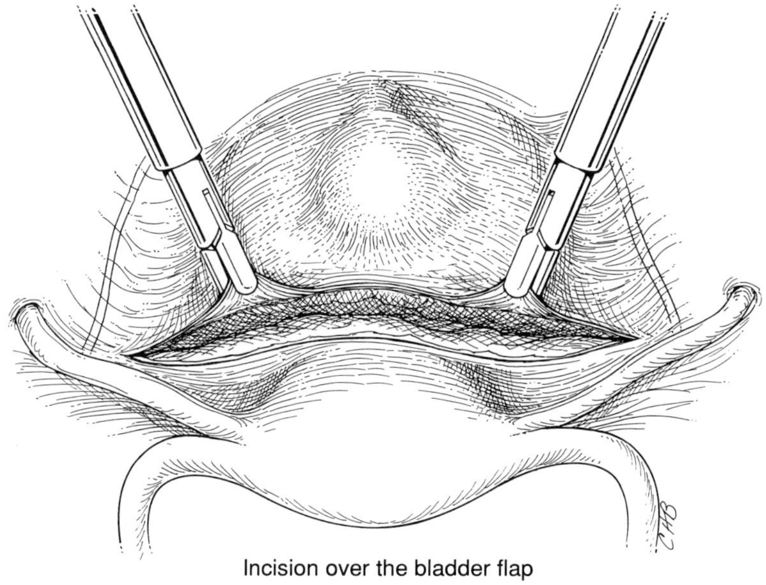

Incision over the bladder flap

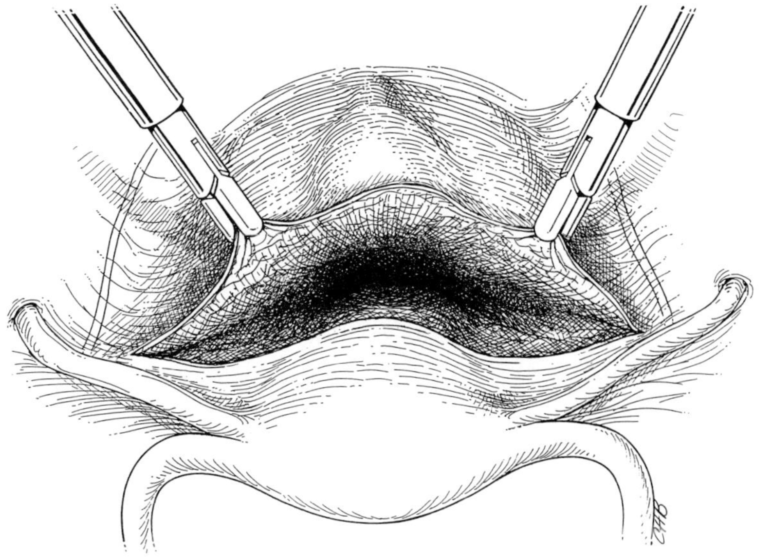

Figure 19-16 Further development of the vesicovaginal space.

placed in a surgical glove and placed in the vagina (Ceana's glove). Pelvic lymphadenectomy is performed at this stage.

Alternatively, the procedure is begun laparoscopically and completed vaginally. The laparoscopic portion includes uterine dissection to the cardinal ligament, separation and ligation of the uterine vessels at their origin, medial displacement of the ureters, and pelvic lymphadenectomy. The remainder of the operation is completed vaginally using a Schauta procedure,[26] including dissection of the vagina, uterosacral ligaments, and parametrium. After the vaginal portion is completed, laparoscopic evaluation is performed again. All pedicles and both ureters are evaluated and hemostasis ensured under low pneumoperitoneal pressure.[27] No drains are inserted, and the peritoneum is left open to allow lymph drainage into the peritoneal cavity and prevent lymphocyst formation. Suprapubic catheters are removed after 2 weeks and routine bladder training is performed.

Nezhat and coworkers reported 7 laparoscopic radical hysterectomies and 11 laparoscopically assisted vaginal radical hysterectomies. Laparoscopic pelvic-lymphadenectomy was performed in each case.[10] One patient with stage IIA disease, 7 with stage IB disease, and 3 with stage IA2 disease with lymphatic channel involvement underwent para-aortic node dissection (Table 19-1).[10]

Results. The average operative time for laparoscopic radical hysterectomy, including para-aortic and pelvic node dissection was approximately 5 hours (range, 4 to 8); the laparoscopic-assisted vaginal radical hysterectomy operations averaged 163 minutes (range, 125 to 214). The average specimen weight was 135 g (range, 120 to 155). Blood loss ranged from 30 to 250 mL. On average, 3 cm of vaginal tissue and 2 cm of paracervical and paravaginal tissue were removed on each side of the specimen. Between 3 and 9 para-aortic nodes were removed (average, 6); the number of pelvic nodes ranged from 11 to 33 (average, 22). The postoperative hospital stay averaged 2.1 days (range, 1 to 6). No major intraoperative or postoperative complications occurred.

Minor postoperative complications included bleeding from the umbilical incision on the first postoperative day, controlled by one suture applied using a local anesthetic. One patient remained hospitalized for 6 days because of febrile morbidity resulting from a urinary tract infection, which responded to medical therapy. The follow-up for all patients has included clinical examination and vaginal smear. There have been no signs of recurrence with the longest follow-up being 4.5

TABLE 19-1 Operative Laparoscopy for Cervical Cancer

	Age	Stage	Number of Nodes		Follow-up
			Pelvic	Para-aortic	(Mo)
1	24	IA2	17	NI*	4
2	33	IA2	15	NI	3
3	37	IA2	18	NI	3
4	40	IA2	22	NI	6
5	41	IA2	23	NI	4
6	34	IA2	33	NI	3
7	31	IA2	25	9	42
8	30	IA2	14	5	30
9	37	IA2	18	4	20
10	40	IA2	21	NI	11
11	26	IB	21	3	5
12	35	IB	27	4	5
13	41	IB	19	6	2
14	43	IB	25	4	2
15	47	IB	29	5	3
16	29	IB	27	8	18
17	34	IB	26	7	15
18	55	IIA	11	5	9

*Not indicated

years. Patients undergoing laparoscopic radical hysterectomy were told to expect neurogenic bladder dysfunctions, but these problems gradually resolved. The incidence of complications was lower than that reported at laparotomy.[28]

Conclusion. Operative mortality from radical hysterectomy has decreased from 8 in 473 cases reported in 1955 to zero in some recent studies.[29] Morbidity, as reflected by urinary fistula incidence, has decreased from more than 20% to less than 1%.[29] The goal of gynecologic oncologists has been to reduce surgical morbidity without compromising end results. For radical hysterectomy and lymphadenectomy performed laparoscopically to be effective, the extent of surgery must not be compromised by the new technology. The specimen removed must be as adequate as that achieved by laparotomy. The morbidity from the laparoscopic procedure must be no greater than with conventional techniques.

Details of pelvic anatomy are clearly visible with laparoscopy, and the number of lymph nodes removed, the size of parametrial tissue margins, and the width of the vaginal cuff are equal to those achieved by laparotomy. Therefore, the end results of a laparoscopic approach should be comparable. The possibility of postoperative adhesion formation with the technique is lower than with laparotomy.[30,31] Advantages of laparoscopy are decreased hospitalization, pain,[21] and morbidity.[9]

The only drawback to laparoscopy is the increased operative time, but as long as the tissue margins are adequate, the decrease in complications and morbidity support the laparoscopic approach. Although the skills to perform these procedures take time to acquire, encouraging preliminary results indicate that operative laparoscopy may benefit patients who require surgery for treating early stages of cervical carcinoma.

References

1. Nezhat C, Burrell MO, Nezhat FR, et al. Laparoscopic radical hysterectomy with paraaortic and pelvic node dissection. *Am J Obstet Gynecol.* 1992;166:864–865.
2. Nezhat C, Nezhat F, Silfen SL. Videolaseroscopy: the CO_2 laser for advanced operative laparoscopy. *Obstet Gynecol Clin North Am.* 1991;18:585–604.
3. Dargent D, Salvat J. *L'envahissement ganglionnaire pelvien.* Paris: MEDSI, 1989.
4. Querleu D, Leblanc E, Castelain B. Laparoscopic pelvic lymphadenectomy. *Am J Obstet Gynecol.* 1991;164:579–581.
5. Maiman M, Seltzer, V, Boyce J. Laparoscopic excision of ovarian neoplasms subsequently found to be malignant. *Obstet Gynecol.* 1991; 77:563–565.
6. Nezhat F, Nezhat C, Silfen SL. Videolaseroscopy for oophorectomy. *Am J Obstet Gynecol.* 1991;165:1323–1330.
7. Nezhat C, Nezhat F, Burrell M. Laparoscopically assisted hysterectomy for the management of a borderline ovarian tumor: a case report. *J Laparoendosc Surg.* 1992;2: 167–169.
8. Nezhat C, Nezhat F, Welander CE, et al. Four ovarian cancers diagnosed during laparoscopic management of 1,209 adnexal masses. *Am J Obstet Gynecol.* 1992;167:790–796.
9. Nezhat C, Nezhat F, Nezhat C. Operative laparoscopy (minimally invasive surgery): state of the art. *J Gynecol Surg.* 1992; 8:111–141.
10. Nezhat CR, Nezhat FR, Ramirez CE, et al. Laparoscopic radical hysterectomy and laparoscopic assisted vaginal radical hysterectomy with pelvic and paraaortic node dissection. *J Gynecol Surg.* 1993;9:105–120.
11. Querleu D. Laparoscopic paraaortic node sampling in gynecologic oncology: a preliminary experience. *Gynecol Oncol.* 1993; 49:24–29.
12. Childers JM, Hatch K, Tran A, et al. Laparoscopic para-aortic lymphadenectomy in gynecologic malignancies. *Obstet Gynecol.* 1993;83:741.
13. Canis M, Mage G, Wattiez A, et al. La chirurgie endoscopique a-t-elle une place dans la chirurgie radicale du cancer du col utérin? *J Gynecol Obstet Biol Reprod.* 1990;19:921.
14. Berman M, Keys H, Creasman W, et al. Survival and patterns of recurrence in cervical cancer metastatic to perioaortic lymph nodes: A Gynecologic Oncology Group study. *Gynecol Oncol.* 1984;19:8.
15. Hatch K, Hems CW. Cancer of the cervix—surgical treatment. In: Blackledge GRP, Jordan JA, Shingleton HM, eds. *Textbook of Gynecologic Oncology* London: WB Saunders; 1991:323.
16. DiSaia PJ, Creasman WT. In: *Clinical Gynecologic Oncology.* 2d ed. St. Louis: CV Mosby; 1984:82.
17. Thompson JD. Cancer of the cervix. In: Thompson JD, Rock JA, eds. *Te Linde's Op-*

erative Gynecology. 7th ed. Philadelphia; JB Lippincott; 1992:1247.
18. Nagano T, Nakai Y, Taniguchi F, et al. Diagnosis of paraortic and pelvic lymph node metastasis of gynecologic malignant tumors by ultrasound-guided percutaneous fine-needle aspiration biopsy. *Cancer.* 1991;18:2571.
19. Creasman WT, Super JT, Clarke-Pearson D. Radical hysterectomy as therapy for early carcinoma of the cervix. *Am J Obstet Gynecol.* 1986;155:964.
20. Nezhat C, Nezhat F, Gordon S, et al. Laparoscopic versus abdominal hysterectomy. *J Reprod Med.* 1992;37:247–250.
21. Childers JM, Brzechffa PR, Hatch KD, et al. Laparoscopically assisted surgical staging (LASS) of endometrial cancer. *Gynecol Oncol.* 1993;51:33–38.
22. Nezhat C, Nezhat F. Safe laser excision or vaporization of peritoneal endometriosis. *Fertil Steril.* 1989;52:149–151.
23. Nezhat C, Nezhat F, Pennington E. Laparoscopic treatment of lower colorectal and infiltrative rectovaginal septum endometriosis by the technique of videolaseroscopy. *Br J Obstet Gynaecol.* 1992;99:664–667.
24. Childers JM, Hatch K, Surwit EA. The role of laparoscopic lymphadenectomy in the management of cervical carcinoma. *Gynecol Oncol.* 1992;47:38–43.
25. Nezhat C, Nezhat F, Silfen SL. Laparoscopic hysterectomy and bilateral salpingo-oophorectomy using multifire GIA surgical stapler. *J Gynecol Surg.* 1990;6:287–288.
26. Schauta F. Die Operation des Gebarmutterkrebes mittels des Schuchardt'schen Paravaginalschnittes. *Montasschr Z Geburtschif Gynakol.* 1902;15:133.
27. Nezhat C, Nezhat F, Winer W. Salpingectomy via laparoscopy: a new surgical approach. *J Laparosc Surg.* 1991;1:92–95.
28. Mattingly RF, Thompson JD, eds. *Te Linde's Operative Gynecology.* 6th ed. Philadelphia: JB Lippincott; 1985:814.
29. Knapp RC, Berkowitz RS, eds. *Gynecologic Oncology.* New York: Macmillan, 1986;245.
30. Nezhat CR, Nezhat FR, Metzger DA, et al. Adhesion reformation after reproductive surgery by videolaseroscopy. *Fertil Steril.* 1990; 53:1008–1011.
31. Operative Laparoscopy Study Group. Postoperative adhesion development after operative laparoscopy: evaluation at early second-look procedures. *Fertil Steril.* 1991;55: 700–704.

20

Complications

Regardless of the degree of care and caution exercised, complications can occur. Timely recognition of a complication is essential to proper management. As laparoscopic surgery becomes more complex, the ability to handle an increasing number of complications endoscopically is essential.

Although it is generally agreed that diagnostic laparoscopy and laparoscopic tubal sterilization involve little risk, the potential for complication increases with the complexity of the procedures, the relative inexperience of some surgeons, and deviation from standard technique. The known rate of intraoperative and postoperative complications is less than 1% (Table 20-1), but the risk of complications for the average gynecologic surgeon probably is not reflected. Most reports are from large practices with experienced gynecologists,[1] surveys of members of the American Association of Gynecologic Laparoscopists (AAGL),[2,3] and reports from tertiary referral clinics.[4]

From July 1982 to December 1993 at CSPS in Atlanta and Stanford University in Palo Alto,[1] 6949 advanced operative laparoscopies were performed with a complication rate of 3.08%, significantly lower than that expected from laparotomy (Table 20-2). The most common complication was abdominal wall vascular injury (inferior epigastric vessels); none required laparotomy. Intestinal and urinary tract injuries were the second most common complication. Severe adhesions and endometriosis were the main contributing factors for these injuries; most injuries were intentional during the excision and treatment of urinary tract and rectosigmoid colon endometriosis. The incidence of laparotomy to manage the complications was only 0.23%; most occurred early in experiences with operative laparoscopy. For example, in the last 5000 operations performed, only one laparotomy was necessary to control bleeding. To date, no fatalities have occurred.

Complications associated with operative laparoscopy appear to be low when procedures are performed by an experienced laparoscopist. The incidence of complications is related directly to the severity of pelvic and abdominal pathology. Adhesions and endometriosis are contributing factors to urinary tract and intestinal injury. Certain complications are unavoidable, and surgeons must be prepared to manage them by laparotomy or laparoscopy. The incidence of conversion to laparotomy to manage complications or complete a procedure tends to be higher early in one's experience.[5]

In a study encompassing 17,521 diagnostic and operative procedures performed at seven centers, an overall complication rate of 3.2/1000 was found (Table 20-3).[6] The rate for diagnostic and minor procedures was 1.1/1000 and 5.2/1000 for major and advanced operations. Laparotomies were performed for hemorrhage (17) or visceral complications (40), and injury was most common following extensive adhesiolysis and advanced laparoscopic surgery; one fatality was reported.

In this chapter, situations are described in which the risk of complications is high. Techniques to avoid, minimize, recognize, and manage these possible complications are described.

Prevention

The best way to prevent complications is to avoid them. They may occur during simple procedures, and the surgeon must be prepared to deal with

TABLE 20-1 Major Complications per 1000 Operative Laparoscopies

By instrument	
Veress needle	2.7
Large trocar	2.4–2.7
Accessory trocar	2.5–6.0
Electrosurgery	0.5–2.8
Laser	1.2
Pneumoperitoneum	7.4
By site of injury	
Vessels/bleeding	2.6–11.0
Bowel	0.6–2.0
Genitourinary	0.6–1.6
Nerve	6.1
Uterine perforation	3.7
Other indicators	
Death	0.05–0.3
Hospitalization >72 h	4.2–27.0
Hospital readmission	3.1–5.0
Persistent β-human gonadotropin titers	63.2–144.0
Infection	1.4–6.5
Febrile	2.0

Sources: Goodman MP, Johns DA, Levine RL. Report of the study group: advanced operative laparoscopy (pelviscopy). *J Gynecol Surg.* 1989;5:353; Lehmann-Willenbrock et al, 1992[4]; Peterson et al, 1990[3]; CO_2 laser laparoscopy study group, 1989.

them. Thorough preoperative evaluation, consultation, and proper patient selection help minimize injury and possible subsequent litigation.

Success depends on the surgeon's familiarity with normal and abnormal anatomy, thorough evaluation of disease, meticulous dissection and vaporization, familiarity with instruments and energy sources, training under the supervision of a qualified surgeon, and a properly trained operating room staff and assistant.

Although most surgeons learn to perform operations under the supervision of residency programs, advanced laparoscopic procedures are learned in a clinical practice. The learning curve for laparoscopic surgery is long. The risk of complications is greatest early in a surgeon's experience and increases when new techniques or equipment are used.

Complications are reduced by becoming thoroughly familiar with all equipment, observing and scrubbing with a preceptor and performing initial complex procedures under supervision. Soderstrom and Butler[7] reported that the complication rate for laparoscopic sterilization was highest among physicians who had performed fewer than 100 procedures. It has been estimated that it takes 4 to 7 years to acquire sufficient laparoscopic surgical skills; several procedures should be performed each week with gradually increasing levels of complexity.[8]

Contraindications

In some cases, laparoscopy is not appropriate (Table 20-4). In patients who have generalized peritonitis, the bowel frequently is matted and adherent to the abdominal wall. Hemoperitoneum in an unstable patient is a contraindication because the bleeding source will be difficult to find and

TABLE 20-2 Summary of Complications and Method of Treatment

Complication	Vascular		Gastrointestinal		Genitourinary		
	Abdominal Wall	Intra-abdominal	Small Bowel	Large Bowel	Bladder	Ureter	Other*
Intraoperative	117	6	22	9	8	3	3
Laparoscopy	116	2	15	8	5	2	0
Minilaparotomy	1	0	3	1	0	0	0
Laparotomy	0	4	4	0	2	0	0
Medical Rx	0	0	0	0	1	1	3
Postoperative	12	5	6	5†	3	1	17‡
Laparoscopy	6	2	1	1	1	1	3
Laparotomy	1	2	1	3	0	0	3
Medical Rx	5	1	4	1	2	0	12

*Other includes pelvic infection, subcutaneous emphysema, pulmonary edema, incisional hernia, deep vein thrombosis, pleural effusion, vaginal cuff dehiscence, and severe dehydration.

†Some patients had a combination of laparoscopy and laparotomy or laparoscopy and medical treatment.

‡Three women had more than one complication.

TABLE 20-3 Complications of Gynecologic Laparoscopic Surgery

Laparoscopic Procedures	No. of Procedures	Laparotomies for Complications	Rate/1000
Diagnostic	4130	7	1.7
Minor	4213	2	0.5
Major extensive adhesiolysis	1910	16	8.4
Other	6370	24	3.8
Advanced	898	8	8.9

treat laparoscopically. It is, however, appropriate to diagnose and treat suspected intra-abdominal bleeding caused by ectopic pregnancies or a bleeding hemorrhagic corpus luteum. Intestinal obstruction and bowel distention are associated with an increased risk of perforation. Although laparoscopic surgery is less invasive than laparotomy and often the better of the two approaches, bowel obstruction not relieved by conservative decompression techniques may require laparotomy. Patients with class IV cardiac disease have a high risk of cardiac arrhythmias and failure as a result of Trendelenburg positioning, even for relatively short procedures. Class III patients can undergo procedures lasting less than 30 minutes. Acute pelvic inflammatory disease is not a contraindication and can be diagnosed appropriately and treated laparoscopically.

Patients who have relative contraindications (see Table 20-4) require extraordinary surgical care. Although benefits are derived from laparoscopic management, the risks for these individuals may be high. Some surgeons may view the relative contraindications as absolute.

TABLE 20-4 Absolute and Relative Contraindications to Laparoscopic Surgery

Absolute
- Generalized peritonitis
- Hypovolemic shock
- Intestinal obstruction
- Class IV cardiac disease

Relative
- Large pelvic or abdominal mass
- Intrauterine pregnancy >16 wks
- Pelvic abscess
- Multiple prior abdominal surgical procedures
- Diaphragmatic hernia
- Chronic pulmonary disease
- Extremes of body weight

Procedural Failure Leading to Complications

It is better to complete a procedure by laparotomy than to risk injury to the patient or be forced to proceed with emergency laparotomy because of a complication. However, this deviation from the surgical plan raises concerns about the adequacy of the presurgical evaluation, patient consent, and the surgeon's skill.

The most critical point of laparoscopy is abdominal cavity entry of the Veress needle and primary and secondary trocars. The possibility of complications is increased in patients with multiple previous laparotomies, a body mass index greater than 30, and those who are very thin. Bowel preparation is recommended if there is a risk of bowel injury. Veress needle and trocar insertion are modified in the presence of a large pelvic mass.

Veress Needle

Intra-abdominal placement of the Veress needle is required to establish a pneumoperitoneum. Because the Veress needle is inserted "blindly," the needle may enter other spaces or puncture organs. Further, instillation of CO_2 under pressure through the Veress needle can produce serious complications.

Prevention. To minimize the probability of Veress needle injury, the steps for placement of the Veress needle outlined in Chapter 8 should be followed. Factors that increase the risk of perforation or laceration with the Veress needle include bowel adhesions, lateral displacement of the Veress needle during insertion, too steep an insertion angle, or uncontrolled, sudden entry. The patient must be horizontal so that the sacral promontory and sacral curve are identified easily. Premature Trendelenburg positioning should be avoided (Figure 20-1).

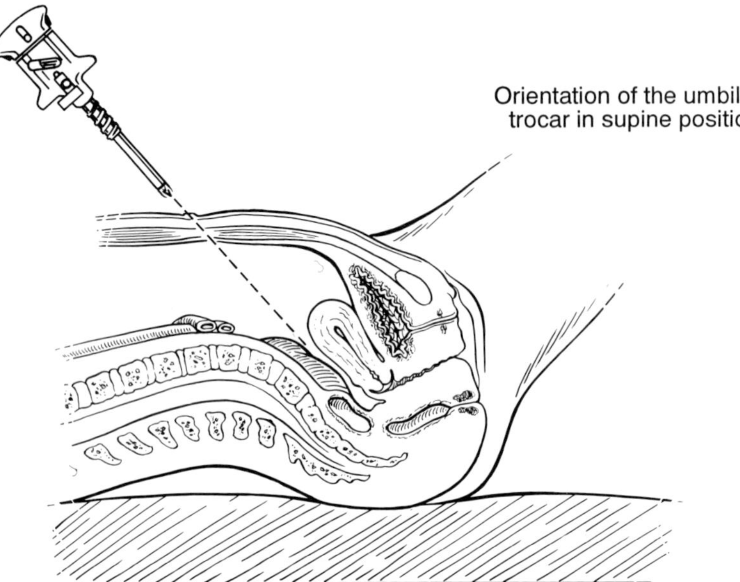

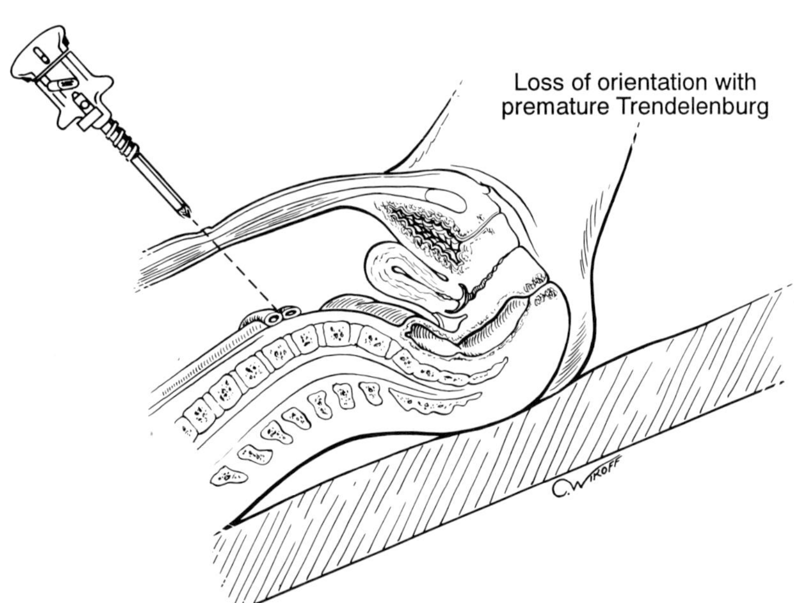

Figure 20-1 Patient must be horizontal so that the sacral promontory and sacral curve are clearly identified and the operator is not disoriented by premature Trendelenburg positioning.

When an upper abdominal site is used in establishing a pneumoperitoneum, the Veress needle may puncture the pleural cavity, stomach, liver, or spleen. The stomach becomes distended following prolonged manual ventilation with a mask or when endotracheal intubation is difficult. Puncture of the stomach may occur even with umbilical placement of the Veress needle. A distended stomach displaces the transverse colon toward the lower abdomen, increasing the probability of intestinal puncture (Figure 20-2). A nasogastric tube minimizes the risk of gastric distention. An overdistended bladder also is at risk for injury. Routine placement of a Foley catheter before the procedure should substantially eliminate the risk of inadvertent bladder injury.

Recognition. Veress needle punctures generally are not apparent until CO_2 insufflation or laparoscope insertion. Abnormally high insufflation pressures are encountered when the Veress needle is misplaced. During the initial examination of the pelvis, it is important to survey the mid and upper abdomen for signs of needle-induced trauma, such as hematomas, needle punctures, and collections of gas.

Management. Puncture of a hollow viscus with the Veress needle generally does not require anything more than examination of the puncture site

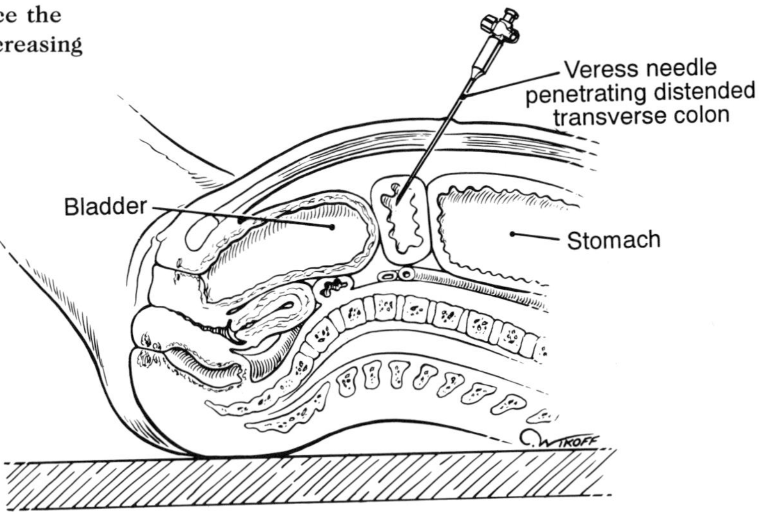

Figure 20-2 A distended stomach may displace the transverse colon toward the lower abdomen, increasing the probability of colon puncture.

to check for a bleeding vessel or leakage from the viscus. The patient can be discharged with instructions to call the physician in case of increasing abdominal pain or fever. If puncture with the Veress needle results in laceration of a viscus, repair is indicated, and the route of repair is based on the organ involved (small or large bowel, bladder, stomach, or major blood vessels), the nature of the fluid that is leaking, and operator experience. Many injuries may require immediate laparotomy for repair and adequate irrigation of the abdomen. Some surgeons may be able to repair injuries laparoscopically.

Establishing a Pneumoperitoneum

The complications that develop as a result of insufflating a space other than the abdominal cavity vary depending on the structure that has been punctured and the amount of CO_2 instilled.

Prevention. Intra-abdominal structures such as the bladder, stomach, or bowel may be punctured by the Veress needle. Placement of a Foley catheter before surgery practically eliminates bladder puncture. Aspiration generally facilitates early recognition of stomach or bowel penetration. However, this method is not infallible and stomach or bowel insufflation should be suspected when there is asymmetric abdominal distention, belching, or passing of flatus. If these signs develop, the gas should be allowed to escape, and once a proper pneumoperitoneum has been established, the laparoscope should be inserted and the suspected perforation site should be examined.

Recognition. Signs of potential complications generally are first apparent with instillation of CO_2. These signs include elevated CO_2 filling pressures, continued liver dullness after instillation of 1 L CO_2, subcutaneous crepitation, belching, passing flatus, asymmetric abdominal distention, hematuria or air bubbles in the Foley catheter line, sudden drop in blood pressure, tachycardia, cardiac arrest, or difficulty in ventilating the patient. However, the absence of these signs does not guarantee proper placement. Preperitoneal placement of the Veress needle with sufficient insufflation of CO_2 leads to the disappearance of liver dullness. If the Veress needle enters the bowel, this may not be recognized immediately because the large capacity of the bowel allows low filling pressures.

Even though the Veress needle may be placed correctly, the increased abdominal pressure and peritoneal irritation associated with instillation of CO_2 may result in bradycardia and hypotension. These signs respond readily to supportive measures.

Management. If the initial flow rate or intra-abdominal pressure is high (indicating improper Veress needle position), raising the abdominal wall may correct the placement of the Veress needle, particularly if it initially was placed within the omentum. If the pressure does not immediately fall to normal levels, the Veress needle should be withdrawn and examined to ensure that the spring-action of the device is working properly and that there is no tissue in the port or the tip. If a second placement attempt fails, consideration should be given to inserting the Veress needle at another site, open laparoscopy, or direct trocar entry.

The most common extraperitoneal site to be insufflated is the preperitoneal space. If recognized early, the CO_2 line should be disconnected and the gas allowed to escape. The Veress needle is removed and reinserted with particular attention paid to the "pop" that occurs when the needle has pierced the peritoneum. If not recognized early and if sufficient gas is instilled, the preperitoneal gas collection will be discovered following trocar placement and introduction of the laparoscope. The spider-web appearance of the tissue will be apparent, and as much gas as possible should be allowed to escape before attempting to reinsert the Veress needle. Preperitoneal insufflation can extend to the mediastinum and compromise cardiac function. If this occurs, the laparoscopy is abandoned and the gas allowed to escape.

Pneumo-omentum is a relatively common and benign occurrence unless a vessel is lacerated. Puncture of the omentum with the Veress needle may be associated with higher than normal filling pressures. Slight withdrawal of the needle or traction on the abdominal wall may release the omentum. Because this occurs frequently, the omentum and other structures in the path of the Veress needle and the trocar should be examined at initial exploration of the pelvis to rule out omental vessel laceration.

If a large vessel entry is not noticed on insertion of the Veress needle, intravascular insufflation with CO_2 may lead to gas embolism and even death. Transuterine insufflation is associated with a risk of gas embolism.[9] Gas embolism initially presents as cardiorespiratory distress associated with a classic "mill wheel" murmur. Once recognized, the patient needs to be placed in the left lateral decubitus position for possible immediate cardiac puncture to release the gas.

Laparoscopic Trocar

Punctures or lacerations of pelvic structures are potentially serious because of the large diameter of subumbilical trocars.

Prevention. Although an adequate pneumoperitoneum provides a safe distance between the anterior abdominal wall and the pelvic viscera, trocar injuries are caused generally by technical failure or adherent bowel (Figure 20-3).[10] The need for excessive force when inserting the trocar can result from an inadequate umbilical incision, scar tissue, or a dull trocar. Factors such as uncontrolled sudden entry of the trocar, lateral displacement of the trocar during insertion, or too steep an angle of placement increase the risk of injury. Even with meticulous technique, abdominal wall bleeding, hollow viscus perforation, blood vessel laceration, or liver and spleen injury can occur.

The trocar should be pyramidal tipped and sharp to penetrate muscle and fascia. Establishing a large pneumoperitoneum before trocar insertion and elevating the abdominal wall to increase the distance between the abdominal wall and viscera decrease the chance of bowel and vessel injury. The syringe test may indicate the presence of adhesions before trocar insertion. However, Nezhat and colleagues demonstrated that direct insertion of the umbilical trocar without prior pneumoperitoneum may be as safe as preliminary Veress needle insertion.[11]

Attention has been given to the disposable trocar because of its sharp tip and spring-loaded safety shield. Theoretically, a permanently sharp trocar that provides controlled entry should decrease the risk of injury to intra-abdominal structures.[12] However, no large-scale clinical trial has established its advantage over multiple-use trocars and the unexpected ease of insertion could result in inadvertent damage.

The first trocar should be inserted with the patient in a horizontal position because premature Trendelenburg can alter the relationship of the sacral promontory and sacral hollow. The abdominal wall is elevated on both sides of the umbilicus; the trocar is inserted and advanced toward the sacral hollow to provide the greatest distance between the trocar tip and solid tissue. Using this technique, the bowel slides away from the advancing trocar.

In the obese patient, the trocar is angled close to the vertical so that the distance between the sacral promontory, blood vessels, and trocar is relatively large (Figure 20-4). In thin patients, the distance between the anterior abdominal wall and sacral promontory is small and the force required to introduce the trocar is often less than anticipated so that controlled, angled entry is essential.[9]

A distended bowel is at increased risk for trocar injury. This condition may be iatrogenic, resulting from intraluminal placement of the Veress needle. The filling pressure of the small bowel may be the same as that of the abdominal cavity, because of the former's large capacity. Therefore, the surgeon may be unaware of this complication.

Recognition. When removing the trocar, signs of complications requiring immediate evaluation are bleeding from the trocar sleeve or a fecal odor. Insertion of the laparoscope allows assessment of the injury. If the laparoscope enters the bowel lumen, the instrument should be left in place to prevent the escape of bowel contents and to help identify the injury. In the presence of excessive bleeding, immediate laparotomy is indicated.

Figure 20-3 A trocar injury due to small bowel adhesions to anterior abdominal wall (A) directly beneath the umbilicus, or (B) caudal to the umbilicus.

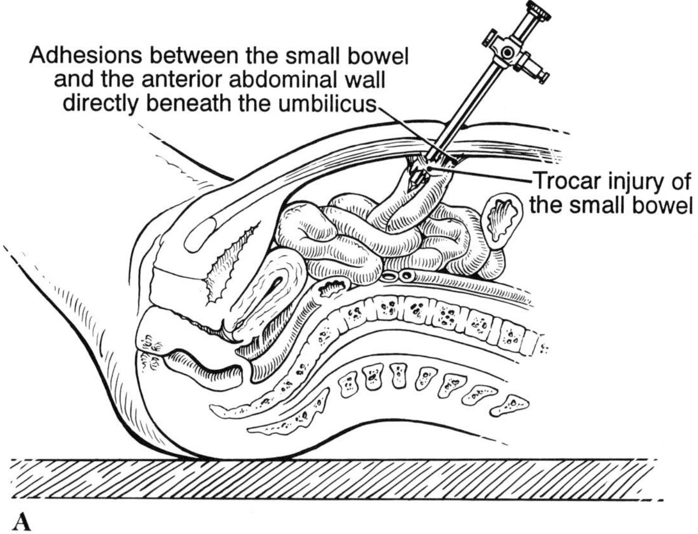

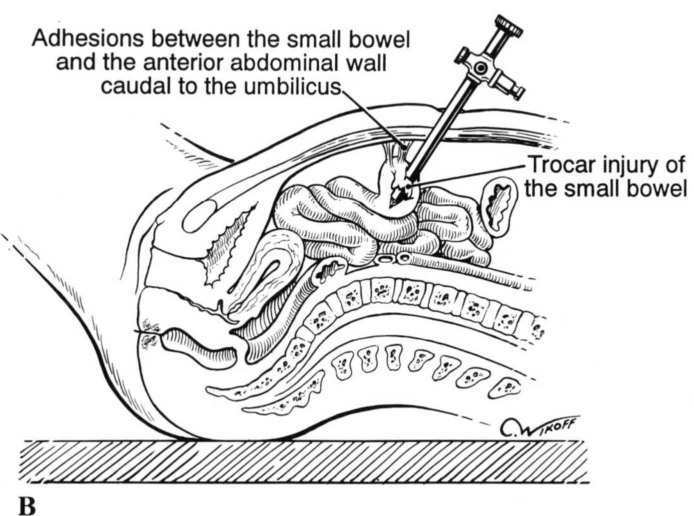

Accessory Trocar Insertion

Prevention and Recognition. Intra-abdominal injury is less likely to occur during insertion of the accessory trocars because they are inserted under direct observation. The structures most frequently injured are the inferior epigastric vessels that run lateral to the rectus muscles.[13] Nezhat and associates found that the most common complication of multipuncture operative laparoscopy was inferior epigastric vessel injury. Two methods are used to avoid injuring these vessels. First, the position of the superficial vessels often can be ascertained with transillumination of the abdominal wall, particularly in thin women. Second, the course of the inferior epigastric vessels can be seen through the parietal peritoneum laparoscopically. As the trocar is advanced through the abdominal wall, the direction of the trocar can be altered to avoid laceration.

Despite these safeguards, the inferior epigastric vessels can be injured intraoperatively. Long procedures associated with moving and dislocating the trocar sleeve, enlarging the trocar sleeve, inserting clamps and other instruments through accessory trocar incision sites, or enlargement of the incision to remove large tissue pieces may damage the anterior abdominal wall vessels. If a vessel is damaged, the surgeon may notice blood running down the cannula or abdominal wall hematoma may develop. The trocar sleeves may tamponade

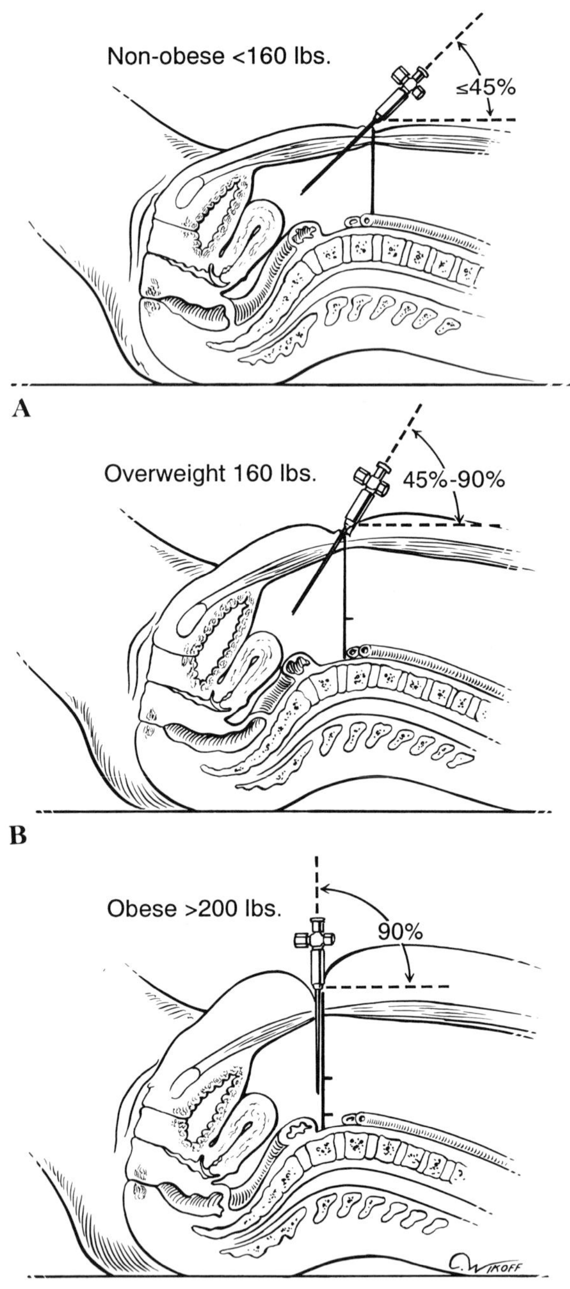

Figure 20-4 Angles of Veress needle and umbilical trocar insertion in an (A) non-obese, (B) overweight, and (C) obese patient.

bleeding from a small laceration that does not become apparent until the trocar sleeve is removed. Profuse bleeding may be observed from the incisional site or significant local swelling may be observed postoperatively.

The risk of complications increases if the trocar is not aimed toward the sacral hollow; it may go down the pelvic sidewall or puncture the posterior peritoneum. Injuries to iliac vessels are associated with profuse hemorrhage or a rapidly enlarging retroperitoneal hematoma, both requiring immediate laparotomy. Retroperitoneal bleeding may spread and accumulate before it is recognized. This injury occurs mostly in thin patients or those who have had abdominal surgery or lax abdominal walls.

When inserting the accessory trocars, sudden, uncontrolled entry or the use of excessive force may result in lacerations of the bladder, uterus, or bowel. Uterine lacerations are not life-threatening, and the bleeding usually is controlled easily. Bladder injury can occur if this organ is displaced because of previous laparotomy or if the accessory trocar is placed less than 4 cm above the pubic symphysis.

Management. Bleeding from an inferior epigastric artery can be controlled by sutures, electrocoagulation, or pressure (Figure 20-5). With the trocar in place, using 0 absorbable suture on a CT-1 needle, a figure-of-eight is placed on either side of the trocar. Alternatively, a straight needle can be passed transabdominally on the distal side of the trocar and pulled through the abdominal wall again using laparoscopic forceps. The suture is tied within the trocar incision and buried beneath the skin. The suture is removed within 24 hours postoperatively. If these two methods fail to control bleeding, the trocar incision can be extended and a grasping forceps used to apply pressure to the inferior epigastric artery to help find the bleeding point. Suture can be applied. A blunt instrument placed through a contralateral accessory trocar can be used to apply pressure to the bleeding point. Bipolar forceps may be applied at the source of the bleeding. A Foley catheter can be inserted through the 5-mm trocar sleeve of the involved side. The trocar sleeve is pulled up and the catheter bulb inflated. Upward traction is applied and maintained by placing a Kelly clamp on the catheter close to the skin and removing the upper part of the catheter. Finally, an expandable trocar can be inserted and used to apply pressure at the site from the skin and parietal surfaces.

Anesthesia

Most complications concerning the anesthesiologist result from the increased intra-abdominal pressures by the pneumoperitoneum, absorption of CO_2 gas or fluid, and Trendelenburg positioning. Vasovagal reaction and cardiac arrhythmias can develop from CO_2 absorption but can be avoided by administering atropine preoperatively. Difficul-

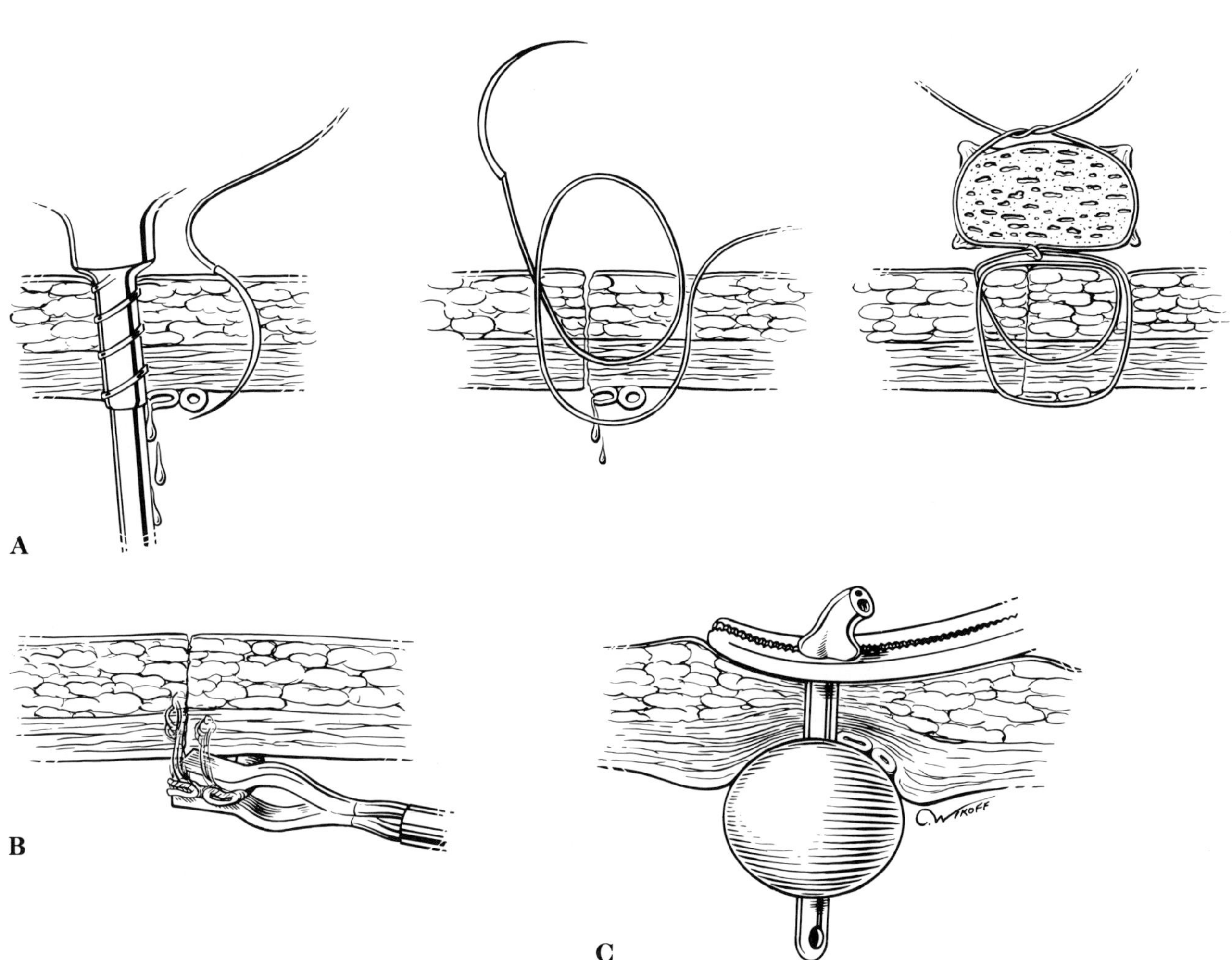

Figure 20-5 Methods to control bleeding resulting from inferior epigastric vessel injury. A, Figure-of-eight suture is placed on either side of the trocar and tied above the incision over a 4 × 4 sponge. The suture is removed 24 hours later. B, Bipolar forceps are introduced through the contralateral incision and the inferior epigastric vessels are coagulated above the peritoneum. C, A Foley catheter is inserted through the 5-mm trocar sleeve at the involved site. The sleeve is removed and the catheter bulb is inflated. Upward traction is applied and maintained by placing a Kelly clamp on the catheter close to the skin and removing the upper part of the catheter.

ties in ventilation result from steep Trendelenburg positioning, high intra-abdominal pressures, and obesity.

Fluid overload associated with hydrodissection, copious irrigation, or high molecular weight dextran used as a distention media for hysteroscopy can be avoided by accurately measuring input and output. Lavage with large volumes of room temperature irrigation fluid can be associated with hypothermia, so the fluid should be warmed or a heating blanket used.

Arrhythmias including junctional rhythm, bradycardia, bigeminy, and asystole have been associated with CO_2 insufflation of the abdomen. Bradycardia appears to result from pressure on the peritoneum with increased vagal response.

Electrosurgical Equipment

Equipment failure and improper use of electrosurgery during a procedure contribute to most injuries. Equipment malfunction is rarely the sole reason for injury. Rather, it is unfamiliarity with the equipment and the use of incompatible components. Often the first response to electrosurgical equipment failure is to increase the current, which further increases the risk of patient injury. If the equipment malfunctions, it is important to systematically check each component to localize the problem.

Even properly functioning equipment can result in injury. Tissue coagulation before its division or attempts to control a bleeding vessel can damage structures near the bipolar forceps if the surgeon fails to identify them (bowel, bladder, ureter, and large vessels). Although some injuries are evident intraoperatively, others become clinically apparent postoperatively. When unipolar current is used, the grounding pad must be applied, and mixed trocars (half plastic and half metal) that may contribute to burns should not be used.

Bleeding

Bleeding and hemorrhage are the cause of most emergency laparotomies. Nezhat and colleagues[1] reported an injury to the hypogastric artery managed laparoscopically with bipolar electrodesiccation. These authors performed three laparotomies to control bleeding following treatment of dense adhesions in their first 2000 operations, but only one in the last 5000. Bleeding occurs during sharp dissection of adhesions, transection of vessels during laser excision or dissection (the laser effectively coagulates very small vessels), uterosacral ablation, or with rough handling of tissues. Lacerations of the oviduct, mesosalpinx, and infundibulopelvic ligament can bleed profusely. Equipment, including unipolar or bipolar electrocoagulator, vasopressin, clips, sutures, and loop ligatures, should be on hand to help control bleeding. The choice of methods depends on the surgeon's preference. Most bleeding can be controlled with bipolar forceps. Infertility surgeons should use fine bipolar forceps to minimize thermal damage and adhesion formation. Pressure enables evacuation of blood and minimizes blood loss until the necessary equipment is placed in the abdomen.

The increased intra-abdominal pressure from CO_2 insufflation, the decreased venous pressure caused by Trendelenburg positioning, and retroperitoneal hematoma can tamponade bleeding from small or large vessels. When pressure gradients return to normal, bleeding into the retroperitoneal space may begin, eventually leading to hematoma and hypovolemic shock. All exposed vessels should be evaluated at the end of the procedure with the patient supine and intra-abdominal pressure reduced.[14] Pelvic sidewall blood clots should be evacuated before confirming complete hemostasis.

Complications Involving Specific Organs

Uterus

Complications involving the uterus include cervical lacerations or uterine perforation from sounding the uterus or use of the uterine dilator or uterine manipulator. Cervical lacerations are managed with pressure from a sponge stick or suture. Bleeding from uterine perforations is controlled with bipolar electrocoagulation. Occasionally, the uterus is repaired using laparoscopic suturing. A CO_2 laser beam can lacerate the uterine serosa and the uterus should not be used as a backstop.

Bladder Injuries

Prevention. Bladder injury is rare and usually occurs in patients who have had laparotomies[3] or whose bladder is not empty.[15] Under these conditions, sharp instruments such as trocars and uterine anteverters can perforate or lacerate the bladder, electricity and lasers can cause thermal injury, and blunt instruments can lacerate the bladder. Certain laparoscopic procedures increase the risk of bladder injury. The Veress needle can perforate a distended bladder. A misplaced Rubin's cannula can perforate the vagina and bladder with upward pressure.[16] Accessory trocar insertion can injure a full bladder, or one with distorted anatomy by previous pelvic surgery, endometriosis, or adhesions, or if insertion is less than 4 cm above the pubic symphysis. Coagulation or laser ablation of endometriosis implants or adhesiolysis in the anterior cul-de-sac can predispose the patient to bladder injury unless hydrodissection or a backstop is used with the CO_2 laser. During a laparoscopic hysterectomy (LH) or a laparoscopically assisted abdominal hysterectomy (LAVH), the bladder may be lacerated or torn if blunt dissection is used to free the bladder from the pubocervical fascia, particularly in women with prior cesarean, severe endometriosis, or lower segment myomas. Also, bladder injury can occur while entering and dissecting the space of Retzius before laparoscopic bladder neck suspension.

To prevent injuries, a Foley catheter is placed to drain the bladder. The position of the bladder should be assessed during the initial examination with the laparoscope. If the boundaries of the bladder are not clear, particularly when pelvic anatomy is distorted, the bladder should be filled with 350 mL normal saline to delineate its position. Care should be used when performing LH or LAVH and the assistant should push the uterus up during bladder dissection.

Recognition. Intraoperative recognition of a bladder injury is important to prevent long-term sequelae. Signs of intraoperative bladder injury include (1) air in the urinary catheter and bag during insufflation; (2) the bladder appears to be pushed by the accessory trocar as it is advanced through the abdominal wall; (3) blood in the urine; (4) urine drainage from the accessory trocar incision; (5) postoperative urinary retention, particularly if the amount of urine obtained during catheterization is less than anticipated; (6) postoperative signs of peritonitis; and (7) leakage of indigo carmine from the injured site. Because trocar injury often involves entry and exit punctures, locating both is important.

Some bladder complications become apparent postoperatively, particularly those caused by electrocoagulation. Signs and symptoms include decreased urine output, hematuria, suprapubic bruising, mass in the abdominal wall or pelvis, abdominal swelling, azotemia, or peritonitis. If a bladder injury is suspected, a retrograde cystogram may demonstrate a bladder leak.

Management. Small holes generally heal without sequelae. However, trocar injuries to the bladder dome require closure followed by urinary drainage for 5 to 7 days. Drainage promotes healing, encourages spontaneous closure, and minimizes further complications.

Lacerations may require a laparotomy, although some laparoscopists can repair the laceration laparoscopically. After identifying the injury and removing any endometriosis, adhesions or necrotic tissue, the laceration is repaired in one layer, using 0 polyglactin (Vicryl, Ethicon) or chromic suture. The suture is placed through the serosa, muscularis, and mucosa. Small injuries (less than 0.5 cm) may be repaired by placing one Endoloop around the injury. Cystoscopy is performed to be sure there is no damage to the ureteral orifices and the repair is watertight. In a series of eight intraoperative bladder injuries, five were repaired laparoscopically using one layer suturing (see Table 20-2).

Nezhat and associates[1] reported successful laparoscopic partial resection and repair of the bladder wall for severe vesical endometriosis without complication.[17] Recently, while removing an excised ovary through a 10-mm trocar, blood and CO_2 gas were noted in the urine bag. The trocar was removed and cystoscopy was performed immediately. A perforation was found on the anterior and posterior wall of the bladder dome. The ureteral orifices were not injured and there was no bleeding. A Foley catheter was inserted and remained for 7 days. Prophylactic antibiotics were given and after 7 days, a cystogram showed complete healing.

Ureter Injury

The development of the ureter is embryologically associated with the development of the female genital tract. This close association persists postnatally, predisposing women to ureteral injury.

Prevention. Knowledge of the ureter's path through the pelvis and the vulnerable points are key to preventing injuries (Figure 20-6). The intrapelvic segment of the ureter is near the broad ligament, ovaries, and uterosacral ligaments, and injuries occur often in these areas (Table 20-5).[18] The surgeon should note the ureter's course through the peritoneum. Endometriosis and severe pelvic adhesions can thicken the peritoneum, obscuring the location of the ureter, especially near the uterosacral ligaments.

If the ureter cannot be identified clearly through the peritoneum, it must be located by retroperitoneal dissection. Using hydrodissection, a horizontal incision is made in the peritoneum midway between the ovary and uterosacral ligament. The lower edge of the peritoneum is grasped and pulled medially. Blunt dissection with the suction-irrigator probe helps locate the ureter lateral to the peritoneum. If the peritoneum is involved with endometriosis and there is retroperitoneal fibrosis, the ureter can be attached to the peritoneum. The horizontal incision in the peritoneum is extended as necessary.

Until recently, most reported cases of ureteral injury during laparoscopic procedures involved electrocoagulation because it is the most reliable technique to arrest bleeding. As the use of stapling devices increases, additional injury to the ureters is being reported.[19–21]

Ureteral injury can occur during sharp dissection of an ovary adherent to the pelvic sidewall, in uterosacral transection, with ligation/transection/coagulation of the uterine arteries, when removing endometriotic implants or fibrosis from the ureter,[22–24] and while trying to control bleeding vessels. Nezhat and coworkers reported six ureteral injuries,[8] involving endometriosis and fibrosis (five) or adhesions (one). Four of the six injuries were intentional and were performed to treat partial or complete obstruction. Unrecognized anomalies in ureteral location may predispose the patient to injury.[25] To avoid such injuries, the tissue being destroyed or removed and the location of the ureter must be identified before irreversible action is taken. Meticulous and continuous attention to the location of the ureter will reduce complications.

Methods to protect the ureter include using hy-

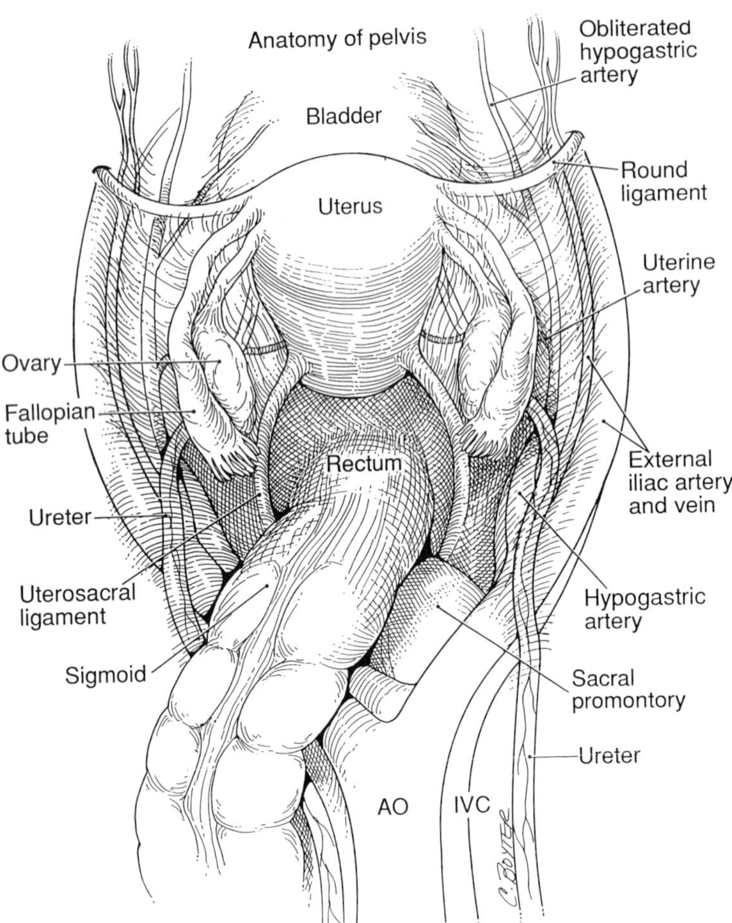

Figure 20-6 Knowledge of the ureter's path through the pelvis and its vulnerable points are key to preventing injuries.

drodissection and resecting affected peritoneum (Figure 20-7).[26] A small opening is made in the peritoneum and 50 to 100 mL lactated Ringer's is injected along the course of the ureter. This displaces the ureter laterally, providing a plane for safe ablation of endometriotic implants, lysis of adhesions, or resection of the involved peritoneum. The fluid absorbs the laser energy, decreasing the risk of thermal damage to underlying tissue.[27] This procedure is applicable only when the peritoneum is not densely adherent to the underlying ureter. During uterosacral transection, a backstop can be placed between the lateral aspect of the uterosacral ligament and ureter. Before using the bipolar forceps during adnexectomy, the infundibulopelvic ligament is put under traction to identify the ureter and avoid thermal damage.

TABLE 20-5 Laparoscopic Procedures Associated with Increased Risk of Ureteral Injury

Infundibulopelvic ligament/ovarian fossa
- Oophorectomy
- Lysis of pelvic sidewall adhesions
- Presacral neurectomy
- Endometriosis ablation
- Lysis of severe bowel adhesions

Ureteric canal
- Uterosacral nerve transection
- Uterosacral plication
- Hysterectomy

Cardinal ligament
- Hysterectomy
- Vaginal cuff closure

The routine use of preoperative intravenous pyelography is not recommended and no prospective study substantiates that this prevents ureteral injury. However, for selected patients, it may help diagnose ureteral obstruction and allow appropriate surgical planning. The routine use of ureteral catheters is not warranted, but we find it useful in cases of severe endometriosis and adhesions.

Recognition. It is reported that a favorite quote of Dr. Thomas Green of Boston was, "The venial sin is injury to the ureter; the mortal sin is failure of recognition."[28] Early recognition is critical to successful management. Intraoperative ureter

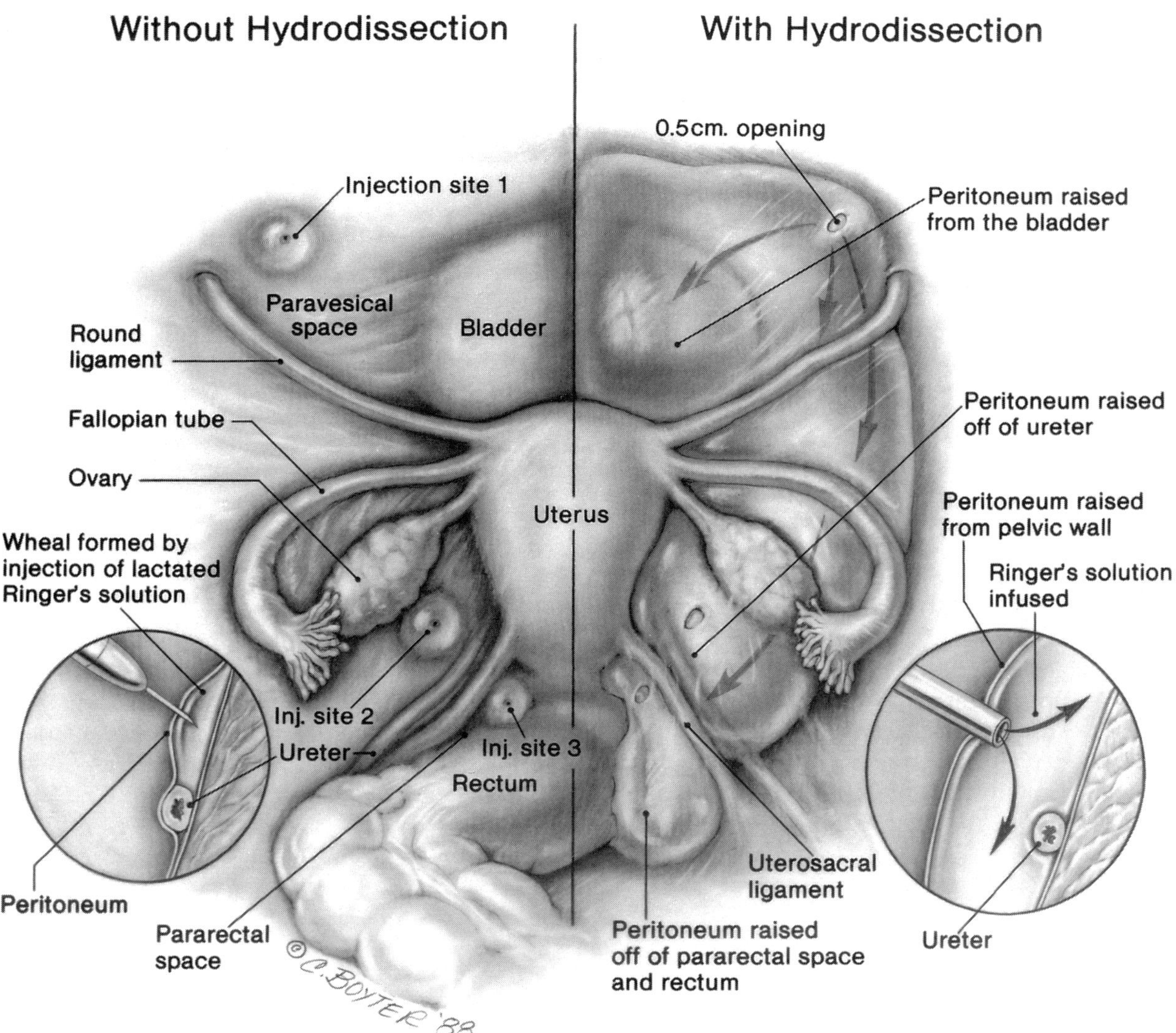

Figure 20-7 Methods to protect the ureter include using hydrodissection and resecting the affected peritoneum when treating endometriosis.

damage is suspected when urine leakage or blood-tinged urine is noted and indigo carmine dye is spilled intraperitoneally following intravenous administration. When surgical procedures involve the ureter, postoperative ureteral integrity can be ascertained by cystoscopy, ureteral catheterization, or intravenous retrograde pyelogram. Stenting of the ureter or repair by laparotomy generally is indicated, but laparoscopic repair of partial and full-thickness injuries is an option for some laparoscopists.[23,25]

Unfortunately, a diagnosis of ureteral injury usually is made postoperatively by intravenous pyelography.[18] Fever, flank pain, peritonitis, and abdominal distention within 48 to 72 hours postoperatively should alert the clinician to possible ureteral injury. Leukocytosis and hematuria may be present. Because the patient's symptoms may be indistinguishable from those of ileus or bowel injury, an intravenous pyelogram (IVP) is indispensable for differential diagnosis.

Management. Whether the discovery of ureteral complications is immediate or delayed, a urologist should be consulted. If the IVP indicates ureteral injury, initial therapy should involve attempts at either retrograde or antegrade stenting. Therapeutic options by laparotomy include ureteroureterostomy and ureteroneocystostomy. Both require stenting and drainage with a ureteral catheter. There have been several recent reports of conservative management of ureteral injuries as well as laparoscopic management. Winslow and associates[29] reported the conservative management of a patient who sustained an electrical burn injury to the left ureter secondary to laparoscopy performed for an infertility evaluation. Postoperative retrograde ureteral stenting was performed for 18 days. Following removal of the catheter, an IVP demonstrated grade III left hydronephrosis secondary to ureteral stricture, which had developed at the pelvic brim. The patient eventually underwent cystoscopy and left retrograde catheterization with placement of a J-stent. Her renal function improved markedly.

Gomel and James[25] reported ureteral injury that occurred during needle electrosurgical ablation of the left uterosacral ligament. While examining the pelvic structures at the end of the procedure, a transverse laceration was found over the anterior aspect of the ureter extending over one half of its circumference. Notably, the ureter was medial to the uterosacral ligament, a significant variation from its normal lateral position. The edges of the laceration appeared healthy with no blanching or irregularity. Interestingly, no leakage of blue-stained urine was observed after intravenous injection of methylene blue. A whistle-tip ureteral catheter was introduced through a cystoscope. The edges of the laceration were approximated with a single 4-0 plain catgut suture. Pelvic drainage was not used and the patient was given prophylactic antibiotics. Two weeks following the procedure, the stent was removed, and an IVP performed 10 weeks postoperatively did not indicate ureteral dilation or stenosis.

Nezhat and coworkers[30] managed a case of long-term ureteral obstruction caused by endometriosis and incidental partial resection of the ureter laparoscopically. The ureter's course was distorted by a 2-cm fibrotic nodule on the ureter, approximately 4 cm above the bladder, corresponding to the level of obstruction (Figure 20-8A). Hydrodissection aided in entering the retroperitoneal space at the pelvic brim. The ureter was dissected with the CO_2 laser (Figure 20-8B). Under cystoscopic guidance, a 7F ureteral catheter was passed through the ureterovesical junction (Figure 20-8C). The catheter was advanced through the proximal portion of the ureter to the left renal pelvis (Figure 20-8D). The edges of the ureter were reapproximated using four interrupted 4-0 polydioxanone sutures (Figure 20-8E). The postoperative course was uncomplicated and a postoperative IVP confirmed ureteral patency.

In one case, during the treatment of severe pelvic wall endometriosis, a 1.5-cm segment of the ureter was unintentionally, completely resected midway between the pelvic brim and ureterosacral ligament.[23] After identifying the location of the injury by injecting indigo carmine intravenously, the 2 to 3 cm of the proximal and distal ureteral ends were freed from the periureteral attachments. After the ends were approximated with a 4-0 polydioxanone suture (Ethicon), a stay ureteral stent was introduced cystoscopically and passed through the proximal end of the injury into the renal pelvis.[23] The stent was secured outside and the patient was placed on continuous drainage. The ureter was repaired by placing four 4-0 polydioxanone sutures at 12, 6, 9, and 3 o'clock. The lacerated edges were approximated. A Jackson-Pratt drain was inserted and an indwelling Foley catheter was introduced into the bladder. The duration of the entire procedure was 187 minutes, and the repair took 35 minutes. Cefoxitin (1 g) was given preoperatively and continued postoperatively (1 g q6h) until the patient was discharged from the hospital.

On the first postoperative day, there was no drainage from the Jackson-Pratt drain and it was removed. No postoperative complications were noted. The patient remained afebrile with normal renal function tests and sterile urine. Although the ureteral stent stayed in place, the Foley catheter was removed. The patient was discharged on the second postoperative day and prescribed prophylactic antibiotics (Septra DS). Six weeks postoperatively, the ureteral catheter was removed and no evidence of ureteral dilation or stenosis was found. An IVP revealed no leakage.

Of the four cases of partial resection or injury, one was during separation of the left ovary from the pelvic sidewall, which was involved with severe adhesions and endometriosis. The direction of the ureter was distorted, and despite retroperitoneal dissection, a 1-cm perforation was noted in the mid-pelvic area between the pelvic brim and uterosacral ligaments. After the ovary was removed, the ureter was freed and a ureteral stent was placed. The perforation was repaired with one 4-0 polydioxanone suture. No drainage was used. The patient was discharged the following day. The ureteral stent was removed 2 weeks later, after an IVP revealed that no leakage or stenosis was present.

The other three patients had severe right pelvic sidewall endometriosis with ureteral involvement, resulting in some degree of stenosis and hydroureter. The endometriosis and fibrosis were excised and removed, but required ureteral resection. In two cases, the ureter was repaired with two sutures. In one, the perforation was small and was managed by inserting the ureteral stent, which remained for approximately 2 weeks. For all six

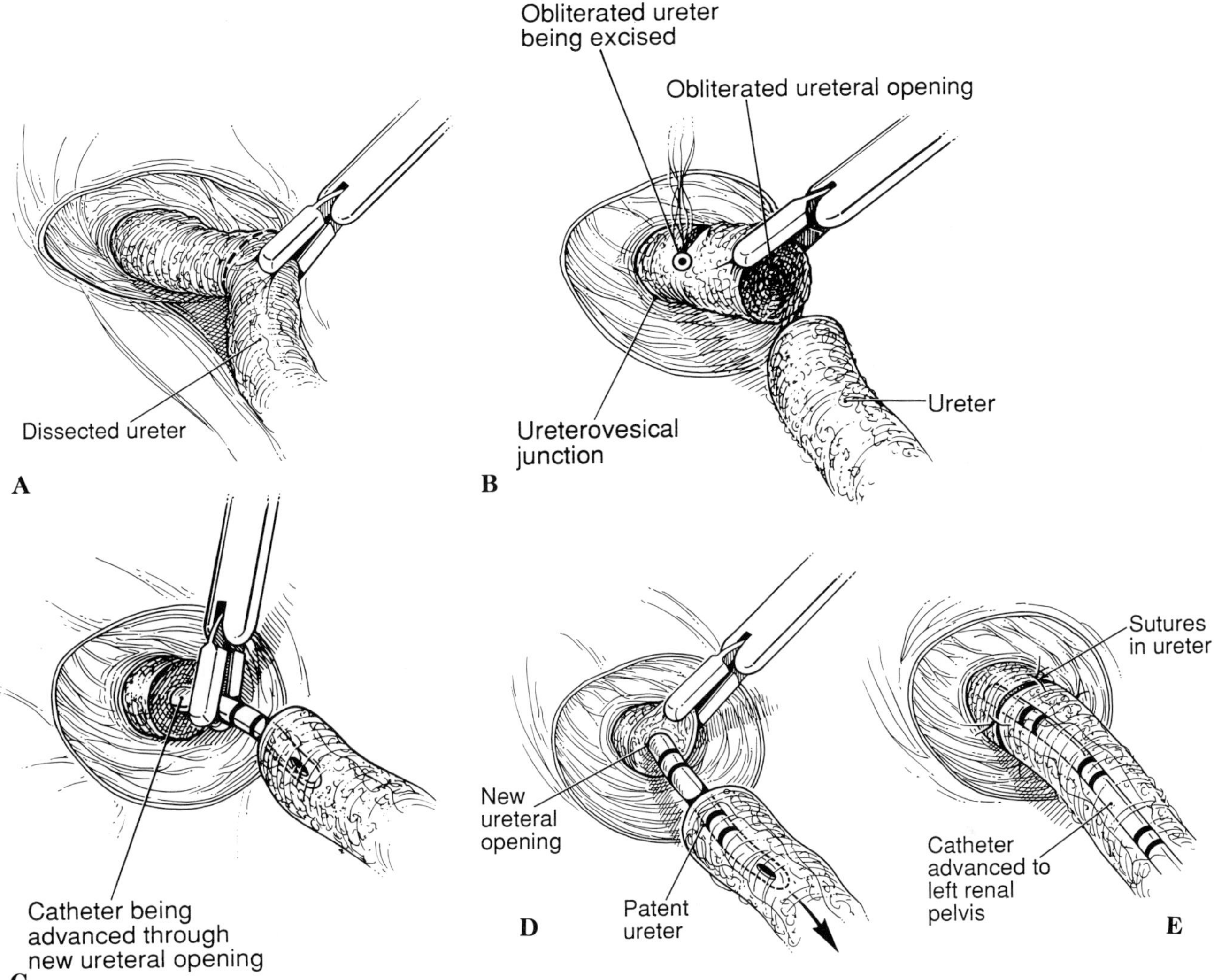

Figure 20-8 A, Ureterolysis is performed and the ureter involved with endometriosis and fibrosis is dissected and pulled medially. B, The obliterated portion of the ureter is excised with the CO_2 laser. C, Under cystoscopic guidance, a 7F ureteral catheter was passed through the ureterovesical junction. D, The catheter was advanced through the proximal portion of the ureter to the renal pelvis. E, The edges of the ureter were approximated at 12, 3, 6 and 9 o'clock using four interrupted 4-0 polydioxanone sutures.

cases, a 2- to 4-year follow-up has been conducted. To date, no long-term complications have been reported. A laparoscopist familiar with delicate laparoscopic suturing can repair ureteral injuries laparoscopically with good results.

Small Bowel

In general, small bowel injuries occur if the bowel is immobilized by adhesions.[8] The bowel can be injured during Veress needle or trocar insertion, bowel manipulation, or enterolysis. Electrosurgery and stray laser beams can result in unrecognized thermal injuries to the bowel. Injury to the gastrointestinal tract is a serious complication. Whether discovered intraoperatively or several days following surgery, small bowel injuries result in unplanned laparotomy, serious morbidity, and even death.[3]

Prevention. Direct mechanical injury to the gastrointestinal tract is less common than electrical injury. Intestinal lacerations can occur when using scissors, the laser, or electricity. Risk of injury is higher when adhesions are dense and tissue planes poorly defined. In addition, traction on the bowel with serrated graspers may result in abrasions and lacerations. A case of inadvertent small bowel biopsy, unfortunately diagnosed by the pathologist, has been reported.[31] Bowel inspection following sharp dissection or in the presence of bleeding or hematoma should alert the operator to bowel trauma. Manipulation of the bowel such as displacement of the bowel from the pelvis with a blunt metal probe is done with care, and blunt dissection of the bowel should be avoided. The bowel can be trapped in incisions, and as trocars are withdrawn, the patient is at risk of a small bowel obstruction.[32] For this reason, some advocate opening the valve of the umbilical trocar as it is withdrawn to prevent creation of a vacuum that may draw the bowel into the incision. Using a Z-track insertion eliminates this complication.[33]

Adhesions between the small bowel and anterior abdominal wall are associated with a risk of trocar injury, especially in those who have had a bowel resection or exploratory laparotomy for trauma. Women who undergo a second-look laparoscopy following treatment for ovarian carcinoma by laparotomy may have adhesions from previous abdominal surgery and generally have had an omentectomy and debulking with adhesion formation.[34]

Despite the use of open laparoscopy, bowel lacerations can occur on entering the peritoneum.[35] It is difficult to decide which patients should have an open laparoscopy. In a series of 22 patients who had small bowel injuries, all had previous laparotomies and small bowel adhesions.[1] Seven were trocar injuries, 13 occurred during adhesiolysis, and two during open laparoscopy (see Table 20-2).

When a patient is at risk for bowel adhesions, it is prudent to prepare her with a mechanical and antibiotic bowel preparation preoperatively to eliminate bowel contents, decompress the bowel, and prevent infection.

Recognition. Electrical injuries to the bowel are not always apparent intraoperatively or their appearance leads the surgeon to choose conservative management. Most intestinal burns less than 5 mm in diameter can be managed expectantly. If the area of blanching on the intestinal serosa exceeds 5 mm, the extent of thermal damage will probably exceed the apparent damage, and therapy should be instituted immediately. The actual area of injury can extend up to 5 cm from the apparent injury.[36]

If the small bowel has been lacerated by a trocar, the surgeon initially may view a mucosal surface or notice a foul smell when the laparoscope is inserted. Small bowel contents may be observed leaking from a laceration or a hematoma may be present on the small bowel serosa.

If the small bowel injury is not recognized intraoperatively, the patient generally presents on the third or fourth postoperative day with lower abdominal pain, mild fever, slight nausea, and anorexia. By the fifth or sixth postoperative day, symptoms include fever, severe abdominal pain, nausea, vomiting, constipation, increased white blood cell count, and peritonitis.[36] Radiographs reveal multiple air-fluid levels or air under the diaphragm.

Management. Complications from small bowel injury are related to the extent of damage and the time lapsed before the injury is discovered. Sharp trocar injuries to the bowel can be limited to the serosa or deep, involving the entire wall. Small punctures or superficial lacerations seal readily and require no further treatment, assuming that careful inspection of the affected bowel reveals no leakage of bowel contents or bleeding. Small (less than 5 mm) superficial lacerations need to be inspected to ensure that only the serosa is involved. In these cases, the patient may be treated conservatively and discharged the day of surgery with instructions to report any untoward reaction.

Patients with obvious peritoneal soiling require intervention and perhaps laparotomy. The bowel should be inspected on both sides to detect through-and-through injuries, especially if produced by a trocar. If only one entry is found and repaired, peritonitis may develop postoperatively. If the laparoscope has been inserted through the bowel laceration and laparotomy is performed, the defect is identified and closed by a purse-string suture as the laparoscope is withdrawn to minimize peritoneal contamination.[37,38]

Small bowel should be repaired in one or two layers by placing an initial row of interrupted sutures of 3-0 chromic catgut to approximate the mucosa and muscularis. A reinforcing layer of 3-0 silk Lembert sutures is used to approximate the muscularis and serosal edges.[39] All lacerations should be closed transversely to minimize the occurrence of stenosis of the bowel lumen. This closure is appropriate only if the laceration is less than one half the diameter of the bowel. If the laceration exceeds one half the diameter of the lumen, segmental resection and anastomosis should be performed. If the mesenteric blood supply is interrupted by the puncture, a resection must be performed regardless of the size or the length of the laceration to maintain blood supply to that particular segment of bowel.[37] Intraoperative consultation with a general surgeon is appropriate whenever significant bowel trauma occurs. Small bowel injuries caused by trocars or the CO_2 laser can be repaired in one layer using 3-0 silk or 4-0 polydioxanone without complication or laparotomy.[40] Injuries less than 2 cm (small or large bowel) may be repaired transversely or longitudinally (Figure 20-9); however, injuries over 2 cm should be repaired transversely. Following is a simple technique to repair bowel injuries caused by sharp instruments or the CO_2 laser if the perforation is less than 1 cm. After the edge of the perforation is cleaned of debris, a grasping forceps is used to bring the perforation inside a 4-0 polydioxanone or 0 polyglactin Endoloop suture and tie the loop around the perforation (Figures 20-10A and 20-10B). To evaluate the repair, the abdomen and posterior cul-de-sac are filled with lactated Ringer's (Figure 20-10C). A sigmoidoscope is used to insufflate the bowel, which is pushed under the fluid.[40] The presence of air bubbles indicates inadequate repair (Figure 20-10C, *inset*). We have used this technique to repair 12 cases of small and large bowel injuries without complication.

Following repair of a bowel laceration, the entire abdomen is irrigated. A nasogastric tube may be placed and removed when drainage has decreased, indicating that bowel function has resumed. The patient is not given anything by mouth until she passes flatus.

When possible bowel laceration becomes apparent after the patient has been discharged, conservative management is successful in patients who have not developed peritonitis.[36] In-hospital management consists of hydration, nothing by mouth, and close observation with white blood cell count and physical examination every 6 hours. Wheeless[36] reported that over one half the patients treated conservatively required no surgical intervention. Those whose condition deteriorated during observation underwent laparotomy and had no complications attributable to delayed surgery.

Immediate surgical intervention and possible laparotomy may be indicated in patients who present with fever, severe abdominal pain, nausea, vomiting, obstipation, or peritonitis, or in those whose clinical condition worsens. Surgical considerations for managing bowel injuries discovered postoperatively differ somewhat from those discovered and managed intraoperatively. The damaged bowel must be repaired or resected. In addition, resection of all necrotic tissue in the pelvis is mandatory even if this requires a hysterectomy and bilateral salpingo-oophorectomy. If burned or necrotic tissue, which has been bathed in intestinal contents, blood, or serum is not excised, a pelvic abscess will develop.[36]

Wheeless[36] presented a seven-point plan to manage patients with peritonitis secondary to bowel perforation.

1. Preoperative stabilization with fluids, electrolytes, and nasogastric suction
2. Exploratory laparotomy with repair or resection of the injured bowel
3. Resection of all necrotic tissue

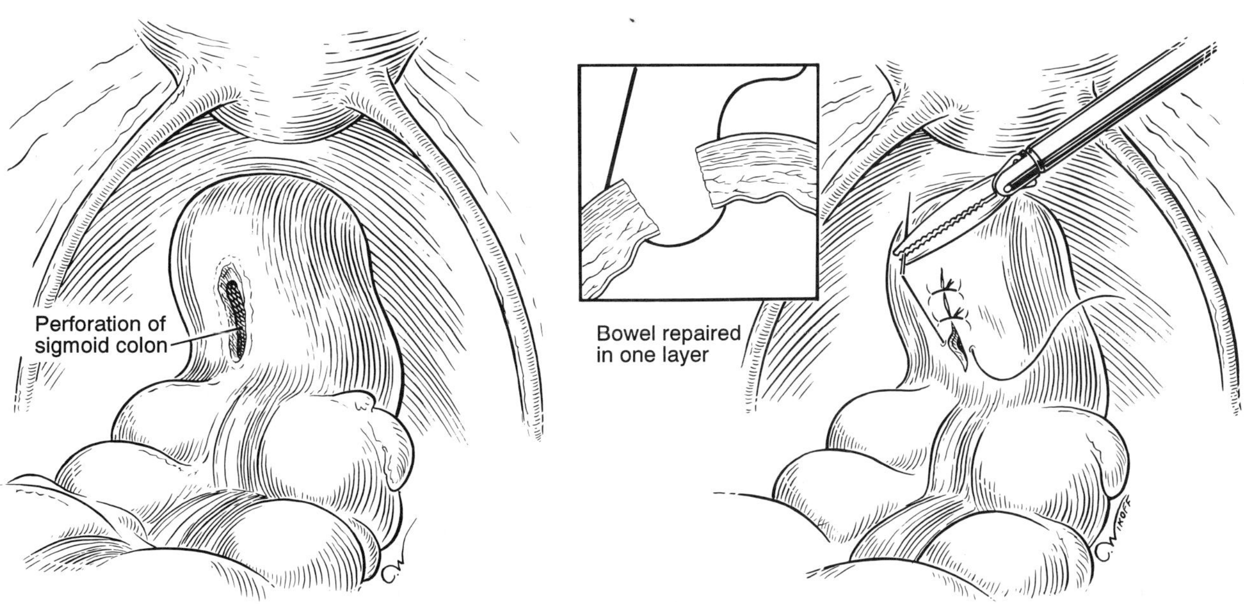

Figure 20-9 A, An injury to the rectosigmoid colon (less than 2 cm) during treatment of bowel endometriosis. B, The bowel is repaired in one layer longitudinally using 0 polyglactin suture (Vicryl, Ethicon).

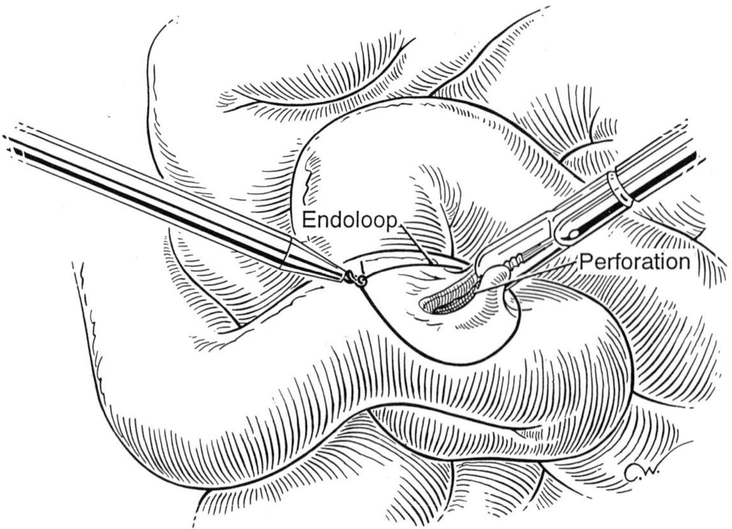

A

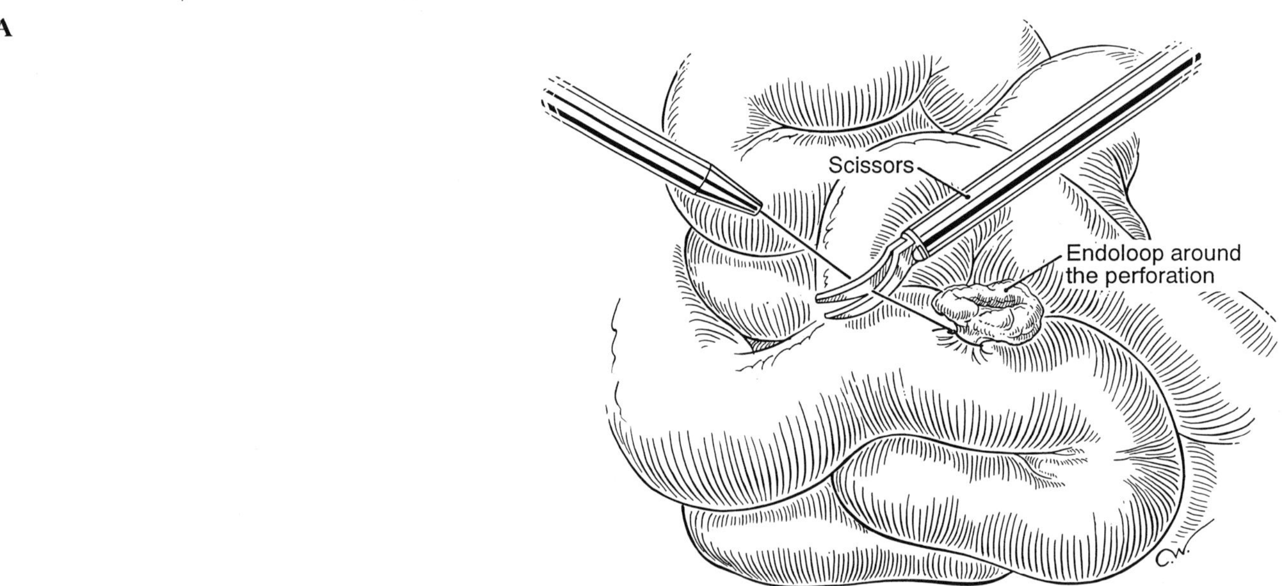

B

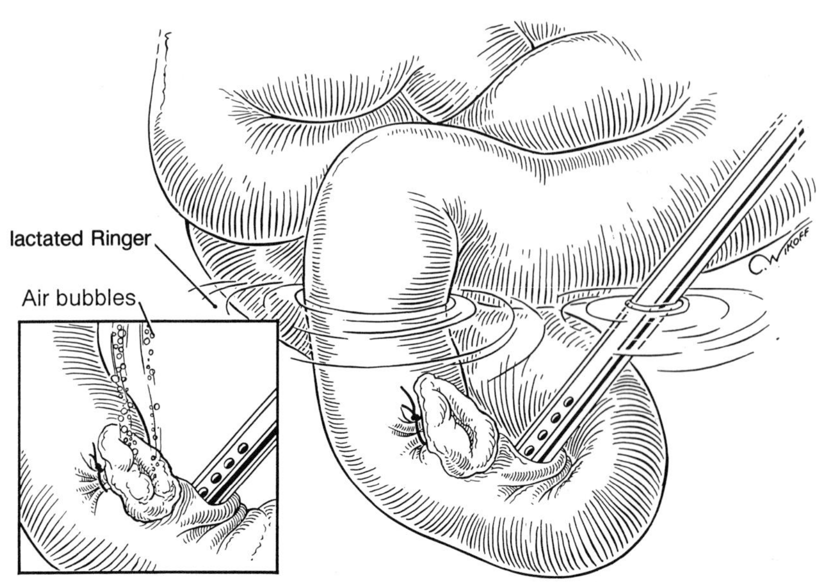

C

Figure 20-10 Repair of a small bowel perforation (less than 1 cm) with an Endoloop. A, Forceps are used to bring the perforation inside the loop of 4-0 polydioxanone or 0 polyglactin. B, The Endoloop is tied around the perforation, leaving an adequate stump. C, The repair is examined under fluid. The presence of air bubbles indicates inadequate repair.

4. Copious and repeated saline lavage of the abdomen
5. Pelvic drainage through the vagina using a closed drainage system
6. Aggressive antibiotic therapy
7. Embolus prophylaxis with minidose heparin (5000 U t.i.d.)

In a recent AAGL membership poll, the two deaths reported from 36,928 procedures were attributed to bowel injuries. In one instance the patient had extensive adhesions from the abdominal wall to the bowel. Although the bowel injury was recognized and repaired, the patient developed a persistent postoperative ileus and died of peritonitis. The second death was attributable to sepsis after an unrecognized small bowel perforation.[3]

Large Bowel

Colon entry is a major complication, particularly if the bowel is unprepared or if the injury is not recognized. Even small perforations, such as those from the Veress needle, require attention because the high bacterial concentration of minor leaks can cause infection and abscess formation.

Prevention. Factors that contribute to an increased risk of large bowel injuries include: (1) failure to establish an adequate pneumoperitoneum; (2) the use of dull trocars that require excessive force; (3) uncontrolled, sudden entry of sharp instruments; and (4) gastric distention. Poorly controlled or sudden trocar entry can result in rectosigmoid laceration. Gastric distention can displace the transverse colon toward the pelvis, where it can be punctured by the Veress needle or lacerated with the trocar. This complication can be eliminated by using a nasogastric tube intraoperatively.

The rectosigmoid colon can be injured if the depth of penetration by endometriosis is underestimated or the cul-de-sac is obliterated. When the rectum is adherent to the posterior aspect of the cervix or uterosacral ligaments, blunt dissection may lacerate the rectum. Sharp dissection with scissors or the CO_2 laser is recommended. The combination of high-power superpulse or ultrapulse CO_2 laser and hydrodissection is relatively safe for working around the bowel.

When the cul-de-sac is dissected, identification of the vagina and rectum is facilitated by placing a probe or an assistant's finger in both the vagina and rectum. Dissection should begin lateral to the uterosacral ligaments, where anatomy is less distorted, and proceed toward the obliterated cul-de-sac.[41,42] Similarly, when posterior culdotomy is performed for tissue removal or during laparoscopic hysterectomy, correct identification of vagina and rectum is important.[19,43]

When a difficult pelvic operation is contemplated, such as cul-de-sac nodularity in a patient with endometriosis or a history suggesting significant pelvic adhesions, preoperative bowel preparation is indicated.

Recognition. Perforation of the large bowel with the Veress needle can sometimes be recognized by the saline aspiration test; recovery of brownish fluid is pathognomonic. Fecal odor may be detected. If large bowel entry is suspected based on these two tests, the needle should be promptly withdrawn and another sterile Veress needle reinserted. Once the laparoscope is inserted, the entry site should be sought and examined. Because of the high bacterial concentration, minor leaks of fecal material into the peritoneal cavity can be the source of serious infection. Underwater examination is recommended following the treatment of severe endometriosis and adhesions of the rectum and rectosigmoid colon (see Figure 20-10C).

Large bowel injuries can be serious because they may not be recognized at surgery. Under these circumstances, the patient generally presents on the third or fourth postoperative day with lower abdominal pain, mild fever, slight nausea, and anorexia. By the fifth or sixth postoperative day, these symptoms progress to include fever, severe abdominal pain, nausea, vomiting, obstipation, increased leukocyte count, and peritonitis.[36] An upright x-ray may show changes consistent with an ileus.[44] The patient appears ill with no clear explanation.

Management. For small colonic wounds associated with minimal contamination, laparotomy with primary suture closure has been the accepted therapy. In addition, copious lavage of the peritoneal cavity, broad-spectrum antibiotics, and drainage minimize the risk of infection. Under the proper circumstances, a small wound to the colon may be closed through the laparoscope. This procedure was performed in 25 of 26 large bowel injuries without complication. Copious irrigation and antibiotic coverage are essential.

Electrical injury to the right colon is managed by resecting the injured segment and primary anastomosis. Diverting ileostomy facilitates healing and reduces morbidity and mortality. Injury to the descending colon, sigmoid, or rectum in unprepared bowel is not amenable to primary closure or resection with primary anastomosis. Diverting colostomy with resection of the injured portion is recommended.[45] Colonic lacerations in prepared bowel can be repaired laparoscopically after excising endometriosis nodules and identifying the extent of the laceration. A single-layered repair using 4-0 silk, 4-0 polydioxanone, or 0 polyglactin sutures is performed.

In a series of 100 consecutive rectosigmoid colon planned and unplanned enterotomies,[1] repair was completed with single layer suture and an Endoloop. Complications included one fistula and one pelvic infection with abscess. The fistula was managed by drainage under CT scan guidance and antibiotic therapy. The pelvic abscess was managed by drainage under CT scan guidance and laparoscopy after failed treatment with antibiotic therapy. Neither patient required laparotomy. Both patients underwent anterior bowel disk excision for full thickness endometriosis.

The knowledge that the bowel can be repaired successfully by laparoscopic techniques in the properly prepared patient should increase the confidence of the surgeon operating in the deep pelvis.

Postoperative Complications

Bleeding

Hemostasis appearing adequate before closure because of Trendelenburg position, high intra-abdominal pressures, and relative hypotension may change once the patient resumes an upright position. If the patient does not respond to intravenous hydration, a repeat hematocrit may suggest hemorrhage and physical examination may reveal abdominal distention.

Nezhat and colleagues reported 17 complications involving postoperative bleeding. Only three patients required laparotomy. Location of the bleeding included nine from the anterior abdominal wall (seven from the suprapubic incisions and two from the umbilical incision), three from the vaginal cuff postlaparoscopic and laparoscopic assisted vaginal hysterectomy, and five cases of intra-abdominal bleeding (see Table 20-2). Vaginal cuff bleeding was managed by vaginal repair and packing without re-exploration or transfusion.

Of five cases of intra-abdominal bleeding,[1] one was caused by persistent ectopic pregnancy, three resulted from a blood disorder, and no source of bleeding was found for the fifth. One patient with persistent ectopic pregnancy presented at another center with signs of intra-abdominal bleeding and underwent laparotomy. She had a leaking, persistent ectopic pregnancy, which was removed. Another patient who had storage pool disease presented with intra-abdominal bleeding 24 hours postoperatively. At laparoscopy, we were unable to locate the source of bleeding, so laparotomy was performed. However, laparotomy also failed to reveal the site. It was generalized oozing from the pelvic cavity. Postoperatively, she was treated with blood products and coagulation factors.

Small Bowel

In our series, we had six postoperative admissions due to small bowel complications (see Table 20-2). Only one required laparotomy. This patient developed peritonitis one day after laparoscopic treatment of endometriosis and adhesions. Exploratory laparotomy showed severe bowel strangulation due to a congenital malrotation of the mesentery, but no bowel perforation. She required extensive bowel resection and postoperative dietary adjustment.

Three patients with small bowel ileus were managed by conservative therapy and one underwent laparoscopy to rule out pelvic infection. One patient was admitted for hydration and antibiotic therapy for severe gastroenteritis.

Large Bowel

Postoperative large bowel complications occurred after unrecognized intraoperative bowel injuries, delayed necrosis caused by excessive thermal damage, and ischemia after enterotomy and bowel resection. Postoperative abdominal pain, fever, constipation, and peritoneal signs should alert the physician. Patients who had excessive posterior cul-de-sac dissection, treatment of endometriosis, and lysis of severe large bowel adhesions should be given specific instructions regarding the avoidance of constipation and not using an enema, which can contribute to bowel perforation.

In our series, we encountered five postoperative complications involving the large bowel (see Table 20-2). All patients had a history of rectal and rectosigmoid colon endometriosis and underwent different techniques of bowel resection. Two women developed leaks and pelvic infections. One required laparoscopic temporary colostomy with subsequent takedown and repair by laparotomy. One was managed by prolonged drainage under CT scan guidance and antibiotic therapy. One woman had a bowel stricture after complete segmental resection, requiring resection and reanastomosis by laparotomy. One patient developed a pelvic abscess and subsequently underwent right salpingo-oophorectomy. The abscess was drained laparoscopically and under CT scan guidance. One patient with a history of endometriosis and constipation and underwent anterior wedge resection of rectal endometriosis had an immediate postoperative rectal prolapse, which was reduced without surgical management. Her bowel symptoms persisted and she subsequently had a colectomy at another center.

Bladder and Ureter

Postoperative genitourinary complications can present with peritoneal signs such as small bowel ileus, peritonitis, abdominal and flank pain, or fistula formation. Thorough postoperative evaluation including IVP and cystogram, pelvic ultrasound or CT scan should be implemented if injury is suspected.

In our series we had three significant genitourinary complications, including one ureteral injury. One patient with a history of recent previous cervical conization underwent total laparoscopic hysterectomy and bilateral salpingo-oophorectomy. Three days postoperatively, she presented with right hydroureter and hydronephrosis with a ureterovaginal fistula. After placement of ureteral stents failed, she underwent laparoscopic evaluation. At that time, it was found that the distal portion of the right ureter had been obstructed by hemostatic suture. The suture apparently became loose and a fistula formed. Laparoscopic adhesiolysis and uterolysis were performed and the injury site was identified close to the bladder. After a ureteral stent was inserted cystoscopically, ureteroureterostomy was performed using 4-0 PDS. An abdominal drain was inserted and the patient was treated with antibiotic therapy. There were no postoperative complications. Follow-up studies showed mild stricture of the distal portion of the ureter, which responded to the conservative ureteral dilatation.

Two patients developed vesicovaginal fistulas. One patient underwent extensive pelvic adhesiolysis and removal of ovarian remnant from the rectum, right ureter, and bladder. Partial cystectomy was performed to remove the entire lesion. The bladder was repaired and drained with an indwelling Foley catheter. Unfortunately, the patient discontinued the Foley catheter less than a week postoperatively and she developed a vesicovaginal fistula one week later. The patient did not respond to prolonged bladder drainage and underwent laparoscopic vesicovaginal fistula repair successfully. She has been doing well since. The other woman developed a vesicovaginal fistula 2 weeks after total laparoscopic hysterectomy. She was managed with 2 weeks of bladder drainage and antibiotic therapy without sequelae.

Nerve Injuries

Common postoperative neurologic syndromes include sciatic nerve injury, brachial palsy (shoulder-hand syndrome), and perineal nerve palsy. Allowing the buttocks to protrude too far off the end of the operating table may cause back injury.

Shoulder Pain

The CO_2 commonly used for insufflation is a peritoneal irritant. Intraoperatively, this irritation can manifest itself as a vasovagal reaction. Postoperatively, residual gas accumulates under the diaphragm when an upright position is maintained, thus irritating the diaphragm. The pain is referred to the shoulder by the phrenic nerve.

Complete removal of intra-abdominal CO_2 is difficult but may be improved by leaving the patient in a Trendelenburg position. Pressure exerted on the abdomen toward the symphysis allows the gas trapped in the lower abdomen to be expressed through the umbilical or suprapubic trocars. If pain develops, the patient can assume a supine position and use a pillow to elevate the lower abdomen, allowing gas to accumulate in the pelvis.

Infection

Postoperative infection is unusual following laparoscopic procedures, although the risk appears to be higher following prolonged, intricate cases. Most infections are limited to skin or stitch abscesses and require incision and drainage. Occasionally, a pelvic infection occurs following tubal surgery, but it is not clear whether this is caused by a preexisting condition or contamination, or if it is secondary to tissue destruction and necrosis. Urinary tract infections can be caused by instrumentation or asymptomatic bacteria.

Nezhat and colleagues report six pelvic infections.[1] Only two required laparotomy for management. All infections except one occurred in patients who had bowel surgery for the treatment of severe endometriosis, bowel adhesions, appendectomy, and bowel resection. The patient had a history of pelvic infections that, in spite of prophylactic antibiotic therapy, she still developed a postoperative pelvic infection.

Incisional Hernia

Herniation of the omentum or small bowel at the umbilical incision site has been reported with 7-mm or larger trocars. Patients at increased risk are those who are very thin (especially those who are elderly), have chronic coughs, or have a history of hernias. Possible preventive measures, although not proven, include Z-track insertion, avoiding trocar insertion directly through the umbilicus, and careful withdrawal of the umbilical trocar.

A subclinical hernia with adhesions between the peritoneal incision site and bowel may place a patient at significant risk of bowel perforation should she require another laparoscopy. Some surgeons advocate removing the umbilical trocar under laparoscopic observation to avoid entrapment of the bowel or to remove the trocar with the valve open to avoid negative pressure, which could draw omentum or small bowel into the defect. Nezhat and colleagues report two incisional hernias in their series.[1] One involved the omentum and the other involved the small bowel. Neither required bowel resection.

Vaginal cuff dehiscence is a rare posthysterectomy complication that has been reported following both abdominal and vaginal hysterectomies, and may occur spontaneously or postcoitally. We recently noted vaginal cuff dehiscence following total laparoscopic hysterectomy in two women at 2 and 4 months postoperatively. Both women presented with vaginal bleeding and abdominal pain. One occurred following vaginal intercourse, and the other was apparently spontaneous. In one woman, a portion of the small bowel protruded into the vagina; the other woman had only opening of the vaginal cuff. In each case, repair was accomplished vaginally using 0 polydioxanone. Both women continue to do well.

Death

The AAGL 1979 membership survey, which involved primarily diagnostic laparoscopic procedures for tubal ligation, reported 2 deaths among 88,986 procedures, a death rate of 2/100,000.[2] Peterson and colleagues[46] identified 29 deaths (3.6/100,000) associated with tubal sterilization: 11 resulted from anesthesia, 7 were caused by sepsis following unrecognized bowel injury, 4 were caused by hemorrhage following major vessel laceration, 3 resulted from myocardial infarction, and 4 were related to other causes. Some deaths might have been prevented by using endotracheal intubation for general anesthesia, safer use of unipolar coagulation or use of alternative techniques, and careful insertion of the Veress needle and trocar.

As laparoscopic surgery has increased in complexity, the associated mortality rate increased to 5.4/100,000 procedures.[3] The 1988 AAGL membership survey, which concentrated on operative laparoscopic experience, reported 2 deaths in 36,928 procedures. In one instance the patient had extensive adhesions from the abdominal wall to the bowel. Although a bowel injury was recognized and repaired, the patient developed a persistent postoperative ileus and died of peritonitis. The second death was attributed to sepsis after an unrecognized small bowel perforation.

References

1. Nezhat F, Nezhat C, Nezhat CH. Complications of gynecologic operative laparoscopy in 6949 patients. Presented at the Society of Laparoendoscopic Surgeons Meeting, Seattle, WA, June 10-11, 1994.
2. Phillips JM, Hulka JF, Hulka B, et al. 1979 AAGL membership survey. *J Reprod Med.* 1981;26:529.
3. Peterson HB, Hulka JF, Phillips JM. American Association of Gynecologic Laparoscopists' 1988 membership survey on operative laparoscopy. *J Reprod Med.* 1990;35:587.
4. Lehmann-Willenbrock E, Riedel HH, Mecke H, et al. Pelviscopy/laparoscopy and its complications in Germany 1949–1988. *J Reprod Med.* 1992;37:671.
5. Levinson CJ, Hulka JF, Richardson DC. Laparoscopy. In: Schaefer G, Graber EA, eds. *Complications in Obstetric and Gynecologic Surgery.* Philadelphia: Harper & Row; 1981:281.
6. Querleu D, Chapron C, Chevallier L, et al. Complications of gynecologic laparoscopic surgery—a French multicenter collaborative study. *N Engl J Med.* 1993; Letter. 328:1355.
7. Soderstrom RM, Butler JC. A critical evaluation of complications in laparoscopy. *J Reprod Med.* 1973;10:245.
8. Nezhat C, Nezhat F, Nezhat CH. Operative laparoscopy (minimally invasive surgery): state of the art. *J Gynecol Surg.* 1992;8: 111–141.
9. Gomel V, Taylor PJ, Yuzpe AA, et al. Laparoscopy and hysteroscopy in gynecologic practice. Chicago: Yearbook Medical Publishers; 1986:56.
10. Metzger DA. Trocar injuries to the small intestine. In: Corfman RS, Diamond WP, DeCherney AH, eds. *Intra-abdominal Endoscopic Complications: Prevention, Recognition and Management.* Cambridge, MA: Blackwell Scientific Publications; 1993:50.
11. Nezhat FR, Silfen SL, Evans D, et al. Compar-

ison of direct insertion of disposable and standard reusable laparoscopic trocars and previous pneumoperitoneum with Veress needle. *Obstet Gynecol.* 1991;78:148.

12. Corson SL, Batzer FR, Gocial B, et al. Measurement of the force necessary to laparoscopic trocar entry. *J Reprod Med.* 1989; 34:282.
13. Pring DW. Inferior epigastric hemorrhage, an avoidable complication of laparoscopic clip sterilization. *Br J Obstet Gynaecol.* 1983; 90:480.
14. Nezhat C, Nezhat F, Winer W. Salpingectomy via laparoscopy: a new surgical approach. *J Laparosc Surg.* 1991;1:91–95.
15. Georgy FM, Fetterman HH, Chefetz MD. Complication of laparoscopy: two cases of perforated urinary bladder. *Am J Obstet Gynecol.* 1974;120:1121.
16. Sherer DM. Inadvertent transvaginal cystotomy during laparoscopy. *Int J Gynecol Obstet.* 1990;32:77.
17. Nezhat F, Nezhat C. Laparoscopic segmental bladder resection for endometriosis: a report of two cases. *Obstet Gynecol.* 1993;81: 882–884.
18. Granger DA, Soderstrom RM, Schiff SF, et al. Ureteral injuries at laparoscopy: insights into diagnosis, management and prevention. *Obstet Gynecol.* 1990;75:839.
19. Nezhat C, Nezhat F, Gordon S, et al. Laparoscopic versus abdominal hysterectomy. *J Reprod Med.* 1992;37:247–250.
20. Woodland MB. Ureter injury during laparoscopy-assisted vaginal hysterectomy with the endoscopic linear stapler. *Am J Obstet Gynecol.* 1992;176:756–757.
21. Nezhat C, Nezhat F, Bess O, et al. Injuries associated with the use of a linear stapler during operative laparoscopy: review of diagnosis, management and prevention. *J Gynecol Surg.* 1993;9:145.
22. Cheng YS. Ureteral injury resulting from laparoscopic fulguration of endometriotic implant. *Am J Obstet Gynecol.* 1976; 126:1045.
23. Nezhat C, Nezhat F. Laparoscopic repair of resected ureter during operative laparoscopy to treat endometriosis. A case report. *Obstet Gynecol.* 1992;80:543–544.
24. Chaffkin L, Luciano LA. Ureteral injuries. In: Corfman RS, Diamond WP, DeCherney AH, eds. *Complications of Laparoscopy and Hysteroscopy.* Cambridge, MA: Blackwell Scientific Publications; 1993:134.
25. Gomel V, James C. Intraoperative management of ureteral injury during operative laparoscopy. *Fertil Steril.* 1991;55:416.
26. Nezhat C, Nezhat F. Safe laser excision or vaporization of peritoneal endometriosis. *Fertil Steril.* 1989;52:149–151.
27. Cook AS, Rock JA. The role of laparoscopy in the treatment of endometriosis. *Fertil Steril.* 1991;55:663.
28. Nichols DH. *Clinical Problems, Injuries and Complications of Gynecologic Surgery.* 2d ed. Baltimore: Williams & Wilkins; 1988:181.
29. Winslow PH, Kreger R, Effesson B, et al. Conservative management of electrical burn injury of ureter secondary to laparoscopy. *Urology.* 1986;27:60.
30. Nezhat C, Nezhat F, Green B. Laparoscopic treatment of obstructed ureter due to endometriosis by resection and ureteroureterostomy. A case report. *J Urol.* 1992;148:865–868.
31. Gentile GP, Siegler AM. Inadvertent intentional biopsy during laparoscopy and hysteroscopy: a report of two cases. *Fertil Steril.* 1981;36:402.
32. Sauer M, Jarrett JC. Small bowel obstruction following diagnostic laparoscopy. *Fertil Steril.* 1984;42:653.
33. Corson SL, Bolognese RJ. Laparoscopy overview and results of a large series. *J Reprod Med.* 1972;9:148.
34. Loffer FD, Pent D. Indications, contraindications and complications of laparoscopy. *Obstet Gynecol Surv.* 1975;30:407.
35. Penfield AJ. However to prevent complications of open laparoscopy. *J Reprod Med.* 1985;30:660.
36. Wheeless CR. Gastrointestinal injuries associated with laparoscopy. In: Phillips JM, ed. *Endoscopy in Gynecology.* Santa Fe Springs, CA: American Association of Gynecologic Laparoscopists. 1978:317.
37. DeCherney AH. Laparoscopy with unexpected viscus penetration. In: Nichols DH, ed. *Clinical Problems, Injuries and Complications of Gynecologic Surgery.* Baltimore: Williams & Wilkins; 1988.
38. Corson SO, Batzer FR, Gocial B, et al. Measurement of the force necessary for laparoscopic trocar entry. *J Reprod Med.* 1989; 34:282.
39. Borton M. In: *Laparoscopic Complication: Prevention and Management.* Philadelphia, BC Decker; 1986.
40. Nezhat C, Nezhat F, Ambroze W, et al. Lapa-

roscopic repair of small bowel, colon, and rectal endometriosis: a report of twenty-six cases. *Surg Endosc.* 1993;7:88–89.

41. Nezhat C, Nezhat F, Pennington E. Laparoscopic treatment of lower colorectal and infiltrative rectovaginal septum endometriosis by the technique of videolaseroscopy. *Br J Obstet Gynaecol.* 1992;99:664–667.
42. Redwine D. Laparoscopic en bloc resection for treatment of the obliterated cul-de-sac in endometriosis. *J Reprod Med.* 1992;37:696.
43. Nezhat F, Brill AI, Nezhat CH, et al. Adhesion formation after endoscopic posterior colpotomy. *J Reprod Med.* 1993;38:534–536.
44. Thompson BH, Wheeless CR Jr. Gastrointestinal complications of laparoscopic sterilization. *Obstet Gynecol.* 1973;41:669.
45. Kirkpatrick JR, Rajpal SG. The injured colon: therapeutic considerations. *Am J Surg.* 1975;129:187.
46. Peterson HB, DeStefano F, Rubin GL, et al. Deaths attributable to tubal sterilization in the United States, 1977 to 1981. *Am J Obstet Gynecol.* 1983;146:135.

21

Questions and Answers

General Laparoscopy

1. What are the exact landmarks for the accessory puncture sites?

In operative laparoscopy, two lateral accessory trocars should be inserted approximately 4 to 5 cm above the symphysis pubis on a line midway between the abdominal midline and the iliac crest. Transilluminating the abdominal wall and direct observation through the laparoscope help to avoid the inferior epigastric arteries as the trocar enters the abdominal cavity.

2. How is the bowel displaced so that the pelvis may be observed?

Steep Trendelenburg positioning is the primary means of displacing the bowel and exposing peritoneal surfaces. In women with a deep pelvis, the bowel is displaced into the upper abdomen under direct vision, using a blunt probe or closed blunt grasping instrument to avoid lacerating the bowel or mesentery. It may be necessary to tilt the patient to the left, particularly for a presacral neurectomy and para-aortic node dissection in which the descending colon and rectosigmoid can make observation difficult. An additional trocar with a blunt tipped instrument may be used. Instruments can be inserted through a 5-mm trocar sleeve and fanned out in the abdomen to retract the bowel.

3. Are procedures such as treatment of endometriosis and adhesiolysis appropriate for freestanding surgery centers?

Any operating room in which operative laparoscopy is performed must be equipped fully for an emergency laparotomy.

4. What is the expected recovery time following laparoscopic oophorectomy, salpingectomy, and tubal operations for ectopic pregnancy?

Recovery after laparoscopic oophorectomy, ablation of endometriosis, salpingectomy, or laparoscopic treatment of ectopic pregnancy is generally less than one week. Full recovery depends on the procedure performed, its duration, postoperative pain, the patient's general health, and the nature of her work.

5. How do you modify the laparoscopic procedure for patients with previous pelvic operations?

For patients who have undergone an uncomplicated pelvic operation, there is no need to alter procedures from the surgeon's usual practice. However, in patients who have undergone bowel surgery or multiple laparotomies for gynecologic disease, or in patients who have had a ruptured appendix, an open laparoscopy, modification of primary trocar, or mapping technique should be considered (see Chapter 8). The incision and trocar insertion at open laparoscopy may take longer than standard laparoscopy.

6. Where do you inject the bowel for hydrodissection?

The bowel is covered with a peritoneal layer as are other pelvic-abdominal organs. When injecting the bowel to raise an implant of endometriosis, it is important to place the needle just underneath the bowel serosa. If the proper plane is entered, the fluid will quickly disperse under the serosa. If the needle is injected too far, a bleb will form and injection pressures will be high.

7. What happens to pneumoperitoneum when the suction-irrigator is used? Is the CO_2 gas released?

When suctioning fluid from the cul-de-sac, it is important to keep all the holes of the suction-irrigator beneath the level of the fluid to avoid removing pneumoperitoneum. If the suction-irrigator is positioned improperly, the CO_2 gas will be removed preferentially. However, with high-flow insufflators, pneumoperitoneum rarely is lost and quickly restored.

8. Do you keep a cannula and a tenaculum on the cervix at all times during the procedure?

It is important throughout the procedure to be able to manipulate the uterus for optimal observation. Different types of uterine manipulators are available. Depending on the laparoscopic procedure, digital examination, probes, and sponge stick applicators are used in the cul-de-sac for identification of structures during laparoscopy.

9. In elective cases, do you order a preoperative enema for better exposure of the cul-de-sac?

Patients with known or suspected endometriosis affecting the cul-de-sac or suspected intestinal adhesions, or those with previous bowel surgery or extensive gynecologic operative procedures should have a preoperative bowel preparation.

10. What irrigation pressure do you use?

Using the Nezhat-Dorsey hydrodissection pump, 200 to 300 mm Hg is used for routine irrigation. When hydrodissection is desired, up to 600 mm Hg is used.

11. How do you expose the back wall of the uterus in the area of the uterosacral ligament, particularly when the uterus is large or retroflexed?

One assistant holds the uterine manipulator so that the uterus is maximally anteverted. The other assistant takes a manipulating probe, places it behind the uterus, and further anteverts the uterus. This method usually provides the necessary exposure.

12. How do you defocus the HeNe beam during videolaseroscopy?

The HeNe beam and the laser beam can be defocused by using the switch on the coupler. If a direct coupler is used, defocusing is possible by loosening the coupler attached to the laparoscope.

13. To what extent is operative laparoscopy an outpatient procedure?

Most laparoscopic procedures (95%) can be done on a "same-day" basis. The decision to admit a patient overnight depends on the duration of the operation, degree of postoperative pain, nausea and vomiting, and the surgeon's concern about complications such as bleeding or bowel perforation. Laparoscopic hysterectomy, retropubic urethral suspension, radical hysterectomy, bowel resection, and lysis of extensive bowel adhesions may require additional hospitalization.

14. How do you minimize the chance of vascular injury when making the suprapubic accessory trocar incisions?

Three methods reduce the chance of vascular injury during the placement of the accessory trocars. First, the operator transilluminates the abdominal wall with the laparoscope to check for superficial vessels. The inferior epigastric artery and vein often are seen beneath the peritoneum running parallel to the lateral border of the rectus muscle. The operator can alter the trocar's trajectory to avoid lacerating these vessels. This method is useful in thin individuals. Second, once the trocar has been inserted into the stab incision, the operator examines the abdominal wall through the laparoscope where the trocar indents the abdominal wall. Third, the inferior hypogastric vessels are always lateral to the umbilical ligaments. Placing the accessory trocars medial or 2 to 3 cm lateral to the umbilical ligaments will avoid injuring these vessels.

15. Is there any reason to use hydroflotation at the end of laparoscopic procedures?

Hydroflotation involves filling the pelvis with fluid for three purposes: to locate bleeding points, to ascertain the health of the fimbria, and to look for adhesions that were missed previously. This procedure is done with the patient in the supine position.

16. Should we be worried about the laser plume and char as possible carcinogens?

As of January 1993, no data have been published to link the laser plume or char to carcinogenesis. However, intact DNA has been found in these laser by-products and until additional information is available, all laser plume should be evacuated in filtered containers, and the release of laser smoke into the operating room should be minimized.

17. Does elevating the abdomen with towel clips facilitate insertion of the Veress needle?

Elevating the abdominal wall with towel clips increases the distance between the abdominal wall and the structures immediately below, such as the spine, sacral promontory, and aorta. In normal-sized individuals, this may be necessary. In obese individuals (body mass index of 30 or greater), it provides a margin of safety that significantly decreases complications.

18. What creates the pressure for hydrodissection?

The Nezhat-Dorsey pump or a similar apparatus is ideal for continuous controlled water pressure. A blood pressure cuff does not generate sufficient pressure for hydrodissection.

19. It is reported that most laparoscopic injuries occur with the Veress needle. Is this because it is the first probe in the abdomen?

The Veress needle is inserted when there is no pneumoperitoneum and it can puncture or lacerate an internal structure. Most major blood vessel injuries during laparoscopy are caused by the Veress needle.

20. What adjuvants do you use to decrease adhesion formation?

Unfortunately, there is no ideal method at present for the prevention of adhesion formation or reformation. Some studies have shown Interceed to be effective for adhesion reduction in laparotomy, but no data are available for laparoscopy at present. On occasion, we have used Gore-Tex Surgical membrane (G.L. Gore, Albuquerque, NM) for extensive adhesions. Keeping the operative field moist seems to be effective.

21. With hydrodissection, do you require an intake-output sheet?

The fluid injected for hydrodissection usually does not amount to more than 500 mL and will be eliminated postoperatively. For a patient in whom monitoring fluid status is indicated (such as a cardiac patient or an elderly patient), intake-output charting is essential.

22. What irrigating fluid do you use during operative laparoscopy?

Warmed lactated Ringer's solution.

23. How much fluid do you use in a typical one-hour case?

If a procedure involves extensive use of the CO_2 laser, it is not uncommon to use 5 to 10 L of fluid.

24. Which instruments do you manipulate and which are held by the assistant?

The coordination between the surgeon and assistant is crucial to the smooth performance of surgery. If the surgery is performed with trained assistants, the surgeon holds the videolaparoscope, laser, and the suction-irrigator. The grasping instruments are held by the assistant. In training programs for residents and fellows, these individuals are more involved as assistants. With a new resident, the operator holds a suction-irrigator, the laser, and the videolaparoscope, while the resident grasps certain structures to improve vision. This enhances the residents' hand-eye coordination and allows them to eventually use the grasper, laser, and videolaparoscope simultaneously. At the most advanced teaching level, the resident or fellow holds the laser, videolaparoscope, and the suction-irrigator, and the teacher-assistant helps with the grasping instrument.

25. Are prophylactic antibiotics advisable for all laparoscopic procedures?

Perioperative antibiotics (Ancef, ampicillin, or doxycycline) are advised. The uterine manipulator placed within the cervical canal may contaminate the uterine cavity, placing the patient at risk for an upper genital tract infection. Individuals with prior tubal damage from pelvic inflammatory disease are at risk for postoperative infection. If evidence of previous tubal infection is found at laparoscopy, doxycycline is prescribed for one week following surgery.

26. What do you tell patients who believe an annual CA-125 determination should be done with Pap smears and mammography?

In a postmenopausal patient whose family has a history of ovarian cancer, CA-125 levels may help detect it in the early stages. However, many benign gynecologic disorders are associated with elevated CA-125 levels, including fibroids, endometriosis, and salpingitis, that could lead to unnecessary concern and intervention. Therefore, a CA-125 assay is not recommended as part of an annual examination. In selected patients with an adnexal mass, CA-125 and other tumor markers can serve as a baseline in future treatments.

27. Is the disposable or reusable suction-irrigator device better?

Both perform well, although the reusables are prone to leakage and spring failure. Reusables cost less than disposables.

28. Do you avoid superpulse to minimize bleeding?

The superpulse mode allows the laser to function as a sharp knife or scissors and is ineffective at coagulating. If sharp dissection is desired, the superpulse mode should be used with the highest power setting with which the operator feels comfortable.

29. When using the CO_2 laser, are glasses necessary?

If the procedure is performed as an open case, safety glasses must be used. If the laser is used endoscopically, glasses are not necessary. However, there are reasons to wear protective goggles, including protection from contamination by bodily fluids.

30. What is the surgeon's ideal position when performing operative laparoscopy?

The operator should use the dominant hand to hold the laparoscope so that it does not twist. The other hand manipulates the suction-irrigator or other accessory instruments. Alternatively, the assistant holds the laparoscope while the surgeon manipulates both instruments in the accessory trocars.

31. Which patients are at highest risk during operative laparoscopy?

The procedure is potentially hazardous in patients who have had extensive abdominal and pelvic bowel adhesions, history of multiple pelvic and abdominal procedures, and in obese patients.

32. Should a patient always be intubated prior to laparoscopic surgery?

Because of high intra-abdominal pressures and the need for controlled ventilation, the patient must be intubated. This protects against intraoperative gastric aspiration. In addition, the patient generally is given muscle relaxants, which require intubation.

33. What causes shoulder pain following laparoscopy?

The CO_2 collects under the diaphragm causing pain referred to the shoulder. Most gas is eliminated by applying abdominal pressure as the trocars are removed.

34. What was the first use of laparoscopy in gynecology?

It was used to diagnose tubal pregnancy. (Hope RB. Differential diagnosis of ectopic gestation by peritoneumoscopy. *Surg Gynecol Obstet.* 1937;64:229.)

35. What is the preferred viewing angle of the laparoscope for operative procedures?

0 degree laparoscope

36. Who first described a gaseous medium to distend the uterine cavity?

Rubin IC. Uterine endoscopy with uterine insufflation. *Am J Obstet Gynecol.* 1925; 10:313.

37. What and when was the first published use of hysteroscopy?

Postmenopausal bleeding; Panteleoni DC. Endoscopic examination of the cavity of the womb. *Med Press Circ.* 1869;8:26.

Appendectomy

38. Do you recommend performing an appendectomy without the laser?

Laparoscopic appendectomy does not require the laser. Endoloop sutures (Ethicon) or the Endo GIA stapler are alternatives. Either Betadine or bipolar electrocoagulation can sterilize the appendiceal stump.

39. Please discuss the complications of appendectomy associated with laparoscopic ovarian cystectomy.

When performing an appendectomy with other pelvic procedures, fecal contamination of the appendiceal stump can result in a pelvic or an ovarian infection, if the ovaries are open for cystectomy or other procedures. However, incidental appendectomies have been performed during pelvic procedures by laparotomy for decades, without complications. Assuming that optimal technique and copious irrigation of the pelvis are performed, there is little reason for concern.

Colpotomy

40. If a colpotomy is necessary to remove a large fibroid or ovary, what postoperative instructions are given to the patient as far as lifting, intercourse, etc.? Are prophylactic antibiotics administered? What kind and for how long?

If a colpotomy is made to remove tissue, the patient is instructed to avoid intercourse for 4 to 6 weeks to allow the incision to heal. Heavy lifting is discouraged for the same period. Perioperative prophylactic antibiotics (ampicillin, Ancef, or doxycycline) are suggested to prevent infection related to the colpotomy.

41. To perform a colpotomy, do you approach abdominally or vaginally?

The colpotomy can be performed by several methods. A sponge stick is inserted in the vagina and pressure is applied to the posterior fornix so the stretched cul-de-sac can be seen easily through the laparoscope. Using the CO_2 laser, monopolar scissors or needle electrode, the vagina is incised abdominally. Once the incision is made, the sponge stick is left in place to prevent the escape of CO_2.

Cystectomy

42. Is it necessary to perform a peritoneal washing before puncturing an ovarian cyst?

Because any cyst may be malignant, a peritoneal washing is essential. The gross characteristics should not be suspicious for malignancy. If the fluid volume is low, normal heparin is added to the pelvis and aspirated. The peritoneal fluid or washings are sent for cytologic examination. Only after the washings have been obtained can the cyst be punctured.

43. Is bipolar electrocoagulation necessary for ovarian cystectomy?

Generally, when the cyst capsule is removed from the ovary, the contraction of the ovarian capsule provides significant hemostasis. Bleeding can occur at the base, particularly if the cyst was close to the hilum. Under these circumstances, a needle electrode or a fine bipolar forceps can be used to minimize thermal damage.

44. What is the largest ovarian cyst that can be removed without suturing the defect?

Once cyst contents are aspirated, the ovarian cortex shrinks rapidly. There are few reasons to suture the ovary. In fact, placement of ovarian sutures contributes significantly to adhesion formation. Although it may be necessary to place one or two fine (5-0) monofilament sutures to reapproximate the edges of the ovary, the use of suture should be minimized.

45. What size adnexal mass is too large for laparoscopic surgery?

We have performed ovarian cystectomies on ovaries as large as 25 cm. The limit depends on the ability to see the entire ovarian cyst to rule out excrescences and the possibility of ovarian cancer.

46. How is a cystic teratoma managed laparoscopically?

A cystic teratoma contains sebaceous material that is irritating to peritoneal surfaces and can cause chemical peritonitis and possible adhesions. A colpotomy can be made through which the cyst is incised and drained and its capsule removed. These same procedures can be performed through a minilaparotomy incision. The cyst wall is punctured and the contents rapidly aspirated. The wall is removed, placed in an Endobag, and removed through the cul-de-sac or an accessory trocar incision. Following removal, it is critical to irrigate the pelvis copiously with 5 to 10 L of warm lactated Ringer's. The sebaceous material is less dense than water and will float, facilitating removal. Occasionally, when the cyst is mainly solid, it can be removed intact without rupturing.

47. How do you perform laser drilling of the ovary?

The procedure involves puncturing several cysts with the CO_2 laser, fiber laser, or electrode to ablate the cyst wall and a thin layer of surrounding stroma. Using an energy source with a high-power density and limiting the number of holes to 15 to 20 minimizes the thermal damage to the ovarian cortex, preventing adhesion formation and excessive destruction of the ovarian follicles. There are few indications for laser drilling of the ovary. The idea behind the procedure is to puncture as many small cysts as possible to decrease the amount of androgen produced by the ovarian stroma. This procedure may cause postoperative adhesions and may compromise the woman's fertility. In women who show resistance to medical induction of ovulation, drilling can improve response to these medications, or even result in spontaneous ovulation.

Tube

48. Do you advocate postpartum laparoscopic tubal sterilization?

Immediate postpartum sterilization is performed when the uterus is approximately 20 weeks in size and fills the entire pelvis, rendering insertion of the Veress needle and laparoscopic trocar difficult. Making the subumbilical minilaparotomy incision is fast and easy; often it can be performed under regional anesthesia. There is no advantage to performing postpartum tubal sterilization laparoscopically.

49. How is salpingectomy performed?

The tube is removed by coagulating and cutting its attachments to the mesosalpinx and its attachment to the uterus.

50. Have you performed tubal reversal by laparoscopy?

The ability to perform laparoscopic tubal reversal is limited by the fine suture and needles required for anastomosis. However, it is possible to prepare the tubes through the laparoscope and either bring the ends through a minilaparotomy incision or bring the entire uterus out to perform the anastomosis under the operating microscope, using 8-0 polydioxanone suture.

51. Do you use the CO_2 laser to repair hydrosalpinges?

A number of methods and instruments can be used to perform neosalpingostomy. The CO_2 laser can cut and coagulate simultaneously. It can be used also to flare the tubes when set at 10 W with a defocused beam. The hydrosalpinges also can be cut with operating scissors, and bleeding points specifically coagulated using the fine bipolar electrocoagulator.

Radical Hysterectomy

52. How long is a patient hospitalized after radical hysterectomy?

Early in our experience, we kept women for 48 hours. Recently, some women have been discharged the following day because there is little manipulation of the bowel and function returns promptly; patients ambulate within 12 hours.

Ectopic Pregnancy

53. The demonstration videos seem to show that removing an ectopic pregnancy appears less bloody than during a laparotomy. Why?

A dilute Pitressin solution (1 ampule of 20 U in 100 mL lactated Ringer's) is injected into the mesosalpinx. This eliminates most bleeding. In addition, the pneumoperitoneum increases the intra-abdominal pressure and tamponades small blood vessels.

54. When treating ectopic pregnancies laparoscopically, can electrocoagulation be used to open the tube?

Electrosurgery is an excellent modality for coagulating vessels along the most distended portion of the antimesenteric part of the tube. Once the area is coagulated, laparoscopic scissors or a needle electrode can be used to open the tube. A monopolar scissors can be used to coagulate and open the tube in one motion.

55. How well does needle tip electrocoagulation work in treating ectopic pregnancy and ovarian cystectomies?

The needle tip electrode is excellent for performing laparoscopic procedures. In some instances it can replace the laser. The needle tip should be used in the cutting mode, and should barely touch the tissue surface. With electrosurgery, thermal damage may spread if large tips are used on large surface areas in contact with tissue. It is important to remain aware of the location of underlying or adjacent structures.

56. Are there any sizes or locations of ectopic pregnancies that you would not treat through the laparoscope?

Whether to do a certain ectopic laparoscopically depends primarily on the surgeon's skill and experience and the patient's stability. Salpingectomies and other conservative procedures have been described to treat varying sizes and locations of ectopic pregnancy.

57. Explain the procedure for treating a ruptured ectopic.

Ruptured ectopics do not necessarily warrant a laparotomy. If the patient is hemodynamically stable and initial laparoscopic examination indicates a moderate blood loss, it may be possible to control bleeding laparoscopically and perform any indicated procedures. However, in an unstable patient who has a large hemoperitoneum, laparotomy is the better choice. Managing ruptured ectopic pregnancies involves examining the pelvis, localizing the ectopic, aspirating blood and clots, localizing and controlling the bleeding points, and performing either salpingectomy or salpingostomy. In rare situations, an oophorectomy is performed concurrently. Controlling bleeding is the most critical part of the procedure, and several methods can be attempted sequentially to achieve hemostasis: (1) identification of the maximal bleeding point followed by bipolar electrodesiccation, (2) injection of the mesosalpinx with dilute vasopressin, (3) electrodesiccation of vessels in the mesosalpinx, (4) partial or complete salpingectomy, depending on the portion of tube involved and the patient's desire for fertility.

58. In a small ectopic pregnancy, why not use bipolar forceps to coagulate the tube and the pregnancy similar to a tubal ligation by fulguration (assuming that the patient does not desire future fertility)?

Electrocoagulation of the ectopic pregnancy and involved tube can treat a small ectopic pregnancy. However, not all tubal bulges are ectopic pregnancies, and the presence of a blood clot may complicate the precise location of the trophoblast. Therefore, performing either a segmental resection or salpingostomy is recommended to verify the location of the ectopic pregnancy and maximize the chances for complete treatment.

59. What is the usual or average charge for laparoscopic treatment of ectopic pregnancy compared to the same treatment by laparotomy?

The charge for the treatment of ectopic pregnancy should be the same for laparotomy or laparoscopy. Because laparoscopic procedures require additional skill and training, some think the charge should be higher. However, the procedure is the same, regardless of the method of access.

60. Do you perform adhesiolysis during laparoscopic surgery for ectopic pregnancy?

Depending on the patient's stability and the available equipment, adhesions should be managed at that time, particularly in a woman who desires future fertility. In a woman who desires sterilization, adhesiolysis would be performed only if she also had pelvic pain or there was concern about possible bowel obstruction.

61. Where do tubal pregnancies implant?

They implant either intraluminally or in the tubal wall.

62. Are serial β-human chorionic gonadotropin (β-hCG) titers indicated following laparoscopic surgery for ectopic pregnancy in all patients?

Without exception, the patient returns for a serum β-hCG one week postoperatively to ascertain resolution of the ectopic gestation. The β-hCG level should be either undetectable or very low. If it is above 20 mIU/mL, a repeat blood test is ordered one to 2 weeks later when the β-hCG should be undetectable.

Endometriosis

63. Young women with mild endometriosis and pain do not seem to get relief from laparoscopic ablation of implants. Do any data support routine postoperative treatment with oral contraceptives? Are there data on long-term fertility prognosis for these patients?

In young women, mild endometriosis may be understaged because clear vesicular or red-appearing endometriosis is missed. Because only visible endometriosis is identifiable and treated, ablation sometimes is unsuccessful in these young women. Many suffer from primary dysmenorrhea that may not respond to oral contraceptives or nonsteroidal anti-inflammatory agents. Hormonal suppressive therapy will diminish dysmenorrhea, but pain will return promptly after medication is terminated. In young women with unresponsive dysmenorrhea, a uterosacral transection or presacral neurectomy should be considered at initial laparoscopy. No reports in the literature suggest that oral contraceptives prevent or alter the progression of endometriosis. If oral contraceptives are used, the optimal time to begin treatment is immediately after surgical ablation of implants or during the last week of hormonal suppressive therapy. The preferred pill is one which the patient will tolerate with minimal subjective symptoms and breakthrough bleeding. There is no demonstrated advantage of high-dose progestin pills over low-dose pills.

64. Is there any place for uterine suspension in the laparoscopic treatment of endometriosis?

In women with severe cul-de-sac disease requiring extensive dissection of that area, uterine suspension may prevent adhesion reformation.

This procedure may benefit women who complain of severe dyspareunia. On pelvic examination, the uterus is retroverted and pressure on the uterine-cervical junction reproduces the dyspareunia. If no other cul-de-sac disease is found at laparoscopic examination, uterine suspension may be warranted. It is not recommended as a routine procedure for uterine retrodisplacement because attaching the round ligaments to the fascia may cause the patient significant postoperative pain for 2 to 3 weeks.

65. Why excise endometriosis implants instead of ablating them with the laser?

Superficial endometriosis is treated optimally by ablation. If large areas of peritoneum are involved with endometriosis or if a woman has recurrent endometriosis in an area previously ablated, it may be better to excise that entire area of peritoneum. In particular, areas with scarring or fibrosis should be excised because there may be endometriosis beneath them. One concern in laser ablation or excising large areas of peritoneum is the chance of adhesion formation. Animal studies indicate that these areas are reperitonealized in 24 to 48 hours and that adhesion formation is low. However, the surgeon should be cautious particularly when excising areas of peritoneum which are opposed, that is, the anterior cul-de-sac.

66. What types of preoperative work-up do you recommend for patients with severe endometriosis, particularly when the rectum may be involved?

In women with bowel symptoms such as dyschezia, tenesmus, or cyclic rectal bleeding without hemorrhoids or rectal fissures, a sigmoidoscopic examination is indicated around the time of menstruation, when implants are more visible. However, many women do not demonstrate rectal lesions, but at laparoscopy or laparotomy significant bowel involvement is seen. A negative sigmoidoscopy does not rule out bowel involvement. In patients who have significant rectovaginal nodularity on physical examination, a preoperative bowel preparation is used (Go-LYTELY or magnesium citrate) and antibiotics and Fleet enemas are administered the day of surgery. Consultation with a general surgeon experienced in laparoscopic bowel resections also is indicated. A preoperative ultrasound can assess the ovaries for endometriomas. Preoperative hormonal suppressive therapy can be useful in decreasing the inflammation, bleeding, and possible postoperative adhesion formation.

67. How do you know where to place the hydrodissection needle when removing an endometrioma?

Generally, after the ovarian capsule is punctured and the cyst contents removed, the border between the ovarian stroma and the cyst capsule is clear. If differentiation is not possible, the cyst is opened with laparoscopic scissors or CO_2 laser. The hydrodissection needle is inserted between these two structures and a plane is developed using hydrodissection.

68. How do you prevent recurring endometriosis?

The clinical course of endometriosis is difficult to predict and few studies exist to guide the prevention of recurrence. Postoperative hormonal suppressive therapy is indicated for pelvic pain or residual endometriosis although it may not enhance fertility. Theoretically, oral contraceptives can reduce the recurrence of endometriosis because of the light menses associated with their use. Some physicians treat endometriosis as it recurs symptomatically; others treat it prophylactically.

69. Do you monitor postoperative CA-125 levels as follow-up for the recurrence of endometriosis?

CA-125 is not useful in diagnosing endometriosis and there is no reason to routinely obtain CA-125 levels in patients being followed for endometriosis.

70. After aggressive excision of endometriosis, how long is it before implants recur?

Little is known about the natural history of endometriosis, although 10% to 25% of all biopsies obtained from normal-appearing peritoneum show histologic evidence of endometriosis. However, only visible implants are treated surgically. The implants not grossly visible at initial laparoscopy can become visible later and be counted as a recurrence. The length of this interval is unknown. Another measure of implant recurrence is the return of pain after laparoscopic treatment of endometriosis. Again, this interval varies, depending on factors such as adhesion formation and whether a presacral neurectomy or uterosacral transection was performed.

71. How do you manage a peritoneal defect or window that may be associated with endometriosis? What do you advise for a peritoneal defect without other evidence of endometriosis?

When a peritoneal defect is found in a patient with suspected endometriosis, endometriosis will likely be found at the base of the defect. The tissue in the defect should be grasped in the center of the peritoneum and excised, either with scissors or the laser. If the defect is close to large blood vessels or the ureter, hydrodissection is indicated. In women with pain, a peritoneal defect should be excised if it corresponds to the location of the pain and if no other cause can be found.

72. Do you prescribe postoperative gonadotropin-releasing hormone (GnRH) agonist if all visible endometriosis has been excised?

If a patient has laser ablation of endometriosis because of pelvic pain or infertility and all visible evidence of the disease is treated, postoperative hormonal treatment is not indicated. If the patient's pain is not relieved, the GnRH agonist or other hormonal suppressive therapy is considered.

73. After vaporizing endometriosis, is much carbon left behind? Will it be visible at second-look surgery? How do you reduce or eliminate it?

The presence of carbon increases with low-power settings of the laser. This carbon must be removed with the suction-irrigator and gentle abrasion for several reasons. (1) The carbon will remain on the peritoneum and in a second-look surgery may be mistaken for endometriosis. (2) Carbon left on the tissue will make it difficult to continue with laser vaporization because the carbon particles will pick up some of the laser energy and super heat. This changes the laser's operating characteristics. (3) Char makes it difficult to determine if all endometriosis has been ablated.

Hysterectomy

74. How do laparoscopic hysterectomy (LH) and laparoscopically assisted vaginal hysterectomy (LAVH) compare to vaginal hysterectomy and total abdominal hysterectomy (TAH) regarding postoperative pain?

It has been demonstrated that LH and LAVH are associated with a shorter hospital stay and patients require less pain medication compared to TAH. However, women who undergo LAVH require more pain medication during the immediate postoperative period than those who have a vaginal hysterectomy (Stovall or Summitt).

75. How long does the patient stay in the hospital after LAVH?

Approximately 30% of patients can leave the hospital on the first postoperative day; others are discharged in 2 or 3 days. The criteria for discharge include the patient's ability to tolerate a regular diet and to ambulate, and the absence of sequelae.

76. Please comment on the multifire stapler and its use in laparoscopic hysterectomy.

The multifire GIA stapler can clamp and cut tissue efficiently. The device places six rows of small titanium staples and cuts the tissue, leaving three rows of staples on either side of the transected pedicle. This rapid-firing device leaves essentially bloodless pedicles. However, the instrument is disposable and costs approximately $500.00. Each round of staples costs $100. The benefit of decreased hospitalization time with LAVH is exceeded by the cost of using disposable instruments. The ureter must be identified before firing the device.

77. Describe the ligation of the infundibulopelvic ligament.

There are many approaches to the infundibulopelvic ligament, depending on the anatomy and whether the operator wants to proceed from the uterine ovarian ligament to the infundibulopelvic ligament with dissection, or tie off the ligament first. The safest way to ligate the ligament is to identify the ureter before isolating the vessels of the ligament. The vessels are desiccated with a bipolar electrocoagulator and divided. A suture can be applied to the ligament through openings made in the peritoneum over the infundibulopelvic ligament and 2 ligatures are applied.

Laser

78. Please discuss the laser settings: wattage, spot size, focus, superpulse, and ultrapulse.

The number of watts determines the amount of power used. The spot size determines power density, that is, over what surface area this energy is dispersed. Given the same wattage, a larger spot size produces a lower power density. The focus of the laser beam determines the efficiency of the energy transmitted to the tissue. A small spot size and a high power setting allow efficient energy transmission, and therefore a clean cutting mode. However, if the spot size is large or the power density low, the energy is distributed inefficiently. In this case, a significant warming effect occurs that is more effective for coagulation or tissue desiccation and contraction (such as flaring the tubal serosa for a neosalpingostomy). If a cutting mode is desired, low power densities result in increased thermal damage, tissue necrosis, and adhesion formation. The superpulse and ultrapulse modes (Coherent, Palo Alto, CA 5000 series) deliver energy as a pulse, with the amount of mean energy delivered remaining constant. However, because power is delivered intermittently, higher peak power densities, and therefore higher performance levels can be achieved.

79. Please discuss the superpulse and ultrapulse modes. What are the indications and advantages?

Superpulse uses the power from the laser in a pulse rather than continuous mode. Although the average power emitted over any given time interval is the same with a pulsed or continuous mode, the effective power from the pulsed mode is greater because of the increased power density delivered with each pulse of laser energy. Superpulse and ultrapulse cut through tissue quickly and with little thermal damage but minimal coagulation. Superpulse and ultrapulse are indicated for cutting avascular tissue, such as adnexal adhesions, or to open ovarian cysts or hydrosalpinges when minimal thermal injury is desired.

80. Can you use the Nd:YAG laser without sequelae when fulgurating lesions on the bladder?

Any laser can injure tissue adjacent to and beneath the area being treated. The risk of injury depends on several factors, including power density and wavelength of the laser. The Nd:YAG laser penetrates deeper than the visible effect and is more likely to damage underlying tissue such as the bladder. The Nd:YAG laser ablates several millimeters of tissue, so it is appropriate for endometrial ablation if penetration depth is an advantage.

81. How do you decide which laser to use during surgery?

The CO_2 laser penetrates the least of all lasers, making it ideal for delicate structures such as the ureter, bladder, and peritoneum, that is, "you see what you get." It can produce very high power densities with ultrapulse delivery. The CO_2 laser can be delivered directly through the laparoscope and requires one less accessory trocar. Fiber lasers are slower than the CO_2 laser because of the differential absorption by pigmented tissues. This may contribute to the increased thermal damage and risk of adhesion formation found with these lasers.

82. Is hydrodissection effective with KTP or Nd:YAG to protect sensitive structures?

Hydrodissection is effective only with the CO_2 laser. KTP and Nd:YAG laser energy is not absorbed by water so hydrodissection will not protect underlying structures.

83. Please discuss your position on the use of a beam splitter-type camera?

This camera splits the image to deliver 40% of light directly through the laparoscope and 60% to the TV monitor. This significantly reduces the quality of both images. However, if the surgeon has difficulty operating from the monitor, the beam splitter is a good alternative, allowing direct observation for the surgeon and monitor view for the assistant. Operating directly through the laparoscope is tiresome, offers limited magnification, and is associated with impaired observation. The clearer, magnified image on the video monitor allows the gynecologist to operate in an upright, comfortable position.

84. What characteristics of laparoscopic surgery help prevent adhesions?

Tissue is irrigated constantly, does not contact talc, and is handled minimally. Very few sutures are placed. All of these reduce adhesion formation. Other factors that help minimize adhesion formation are hemostasis and appropriate settings for electrocoagulators and high power settings for lasers. The smallest bipolar electrocoagulator should be used, and only the isolated vessels should be grasped to reduce thermal damage to surrounding tissue.

85. Do you use the KTP laser for myomectomies?

A laser is not essential for performing myomectomies. The basic instruments required include one to simultaneously incise and coagulate the myometrium over the fibroid, an instrument for blunt dissection, and a bipolar electrocoagulator to control bleeding. The surgeon can use CO_2 or KTP laser to make the initial incision through the uterine serosa to facilitate dissection of fibers attached to the myoma.

86. What power setting do you use for the CO_2 laser during operative laparoscopy?

When using the ultrapulse CO_2 laser, gynecologists should use the highest power setting with which they are comfortable. High settings decrease thermal damage to surrounding tissue and laser plume and make the procedure more efficient.

87. Do you think that the laser will supplant the use of electrosurgery in laparoscopic surgery?

Many instruments are used to perform laparoscopic surgery. The CO_2 laser and electrosurgery are complementary and extend the endoscopist's ability. Some procedures are better suited to the CO_2 laser and others to electrocoagulation. The CO_2 laser's major advantages are its reproducible and predictable thermal properties and its ability to be used through the operating channel of the laparoscope. This reduces the number of accessory ports.

88. At a power of 25 W and an effective laser beam diameter of 2 mm, what is the average power density?

To calculate the power density (W/cm^2) the following formula is used:

$$PD = \frac{P \times 400}{\pi \times d^2} = \frac{25 \times 400}{\pi \times 4} = 7.96 \text{ W/cm}^2$$

89. What is the minimal depth of thermal necrosis produced by a CO_2 laser beam?

100 μm.

90. Does ordinary glass stop any kind of laser beam?

Yes, the CO_2 laser beam.

Myomectomy

91. What happens to the small fragments of myoma that are not collected?

Fragments of tissue left behind can undergo necrosis, causing peritonitis and possible adhesion formation. All tissue and fragments must be removed from the abdomen at the time of surgery.

92. At times you can see 2- to 3-mm whitish patches on the surface of the uterus when doing a laparoscopy. What are they?

These patches result from inflammatory processes such as pelvic inflammatory disease, endometriosis, or tuberculosis. If the nature of the patches is in question, a biopsy should be taken.

93. Do you consider laparoscopic myomectomy to be contraindicated by a certain size or location of a fibroid?

Whether a fibroid can or should be removed laparoscopically depends on its location and size. Small and moderate-size pedunculated fibroids (less than 5 cm) are easiest to remove, regardless of location. Large intramural fibroids (greater than 5 cm) located in the broad ligament are difficult to remove. One concern when performing endoscopic myomectomies is sufficient closure of the defect so that fistula formation is prevented and myometrial integrity is ensured for future childbearing. Performing a minilaparotomy incision to close the uterine incision is recommended, particularly for large intramural fibroids.

94. What do you think of a trial of labor in a patient with previous multiple myomectomy?

If all fibroids were serosal or pedunculated, then a trial of labor is indicated. However, with intramural fibroids, uterine integrity has been compromised and an elective cesarean delivery would be indicated, whether the myomectomy was performed by laparotomy or laparoscopy.

95. Do you suture the myometrium after myomectomy?

Patients in whom the myometrial defect is not repaired have significant uterine defects on second-look laparoscopy, including endometrial-serosal fistulas. When the defect is sutured, a better cosmetic appearance is noted and presumably better myometrial strength and integrity. However, if suture is used, adhesion formation increases significantly. Approximating the myometrium with suture to ensure uterine integrity or allowing the defect to heal spontaneously to avoid adhesion formation is controversial, particularly for women of childbearing age. Although the myometrium can be closed endoscopically with sutures, the quality of the closure may impede optimal healing. We suggest making a small minilaparotomy incision to close large myometrial defects directly.

Presacral Neurectomy and Uterosacral Transection

96. Do you recommend cutting the uterosacral ligaments in cases of pelvic pain?

Uterosacral ligament transection is only effective with central pain caused by uterine cramping or severe dysmenorrhea. Adnexal and other pelvic pain is not transmitted through the hypogastric plexus, and other causes should be considered. The uterosacral ligaments are ablated if they are involved with endometriosis.

97. How difficult is it to reach the presacral area?

With maximal Trendelenburg position and with the bowel pushed from the cul-de-sac, the presacral area is accessible in most patients. For some, a third accessory trocar is inserted in the midline to hold the descending colon out of the operative field.

Uterine Suspension

98. For uterine suspension, where are incisions placed and through which puncture sites?

If the accessory trocar incisions are placed 4 to 5 cm above the symphysis, midway between the midline of the abdomen and the iliac crest, the round ligament is grasped and brought through the incisions. The pneumoperitoneum is decreased to minimize the traction applied to the round ligaments to avoid tearing and bleeding. Occasionally graspers are inadequate for this maneuver; a Kocher or Kelly clamp can be inserted through the incision to grasp the round ligament. The remainder of the pneumoperitoneum is allowed to escape and the round ligament is sutured to the fascia.

Medication

99. When do you use GnRH agonists?

GnRH agonists can shrink fibroids, making them more amenable to laparoscopic removal, decrease the intraoperative bleeding, and also stop menstruation and abnormal bleeding. They can be used as a pretreatment for treatment of severe endometriosis. The use of GnRH agonists before laparoscopic ablation of endometriosis is controversial. Preoperative use of GnRH agonists does make the implants less visible, and therefore more difficult to treat. One to 2 months of preoperative GnRH agonists may decrease the chance of confusing a hemorrhagic corpus luteum cyst with an endometrioma. There is no reason to remove hemorrhagic corpus luteum cysts. Another indication for preoperative use of GnRH agonists is that they may act synergistically with ablation to provide patients with longer term pain relief.

100. Do you use furosemide in the operating room?

If fluid overload is suspected during a hysteroscopic procedure, the patient's electrolytes are evaluated. Furosemide is administered if indicated by a difference in input and output greater than 500 mL and the suspicion of fluid overload, but its routine use is unnecessary.

Injury

101. If the bladder dome is injured with a 5-mm trocar without active bleeding, is it necessary to repair the bladder or is drainage adequate, and for how many days?

If the bladder is injured with a single puncture of a 5-mm trocar, neither are necessary. However, more conservative management would require placing a single absorbable suture and draining the bladder for 3 to 7 days.

At CSPS a bladder dome injury with a 10-mm trocar was managed without suturing. After cystoscopy was performed to ensure that the ureteral orifices were not injured and there was no bleeding, the bladder was drained and prophylactic antibiotics were prescribed for 7 days. A cystogram was performed, which revealed complete healing of the bladder with no sequelae.

102. How do you manage intestinal perforation and fecal contamination during laparoscopy?

Under these circumstances the gynecologist should immediately consult a general surgeon. In patients without a prior bowel prep and depending on the type of injury, laparotomy with closure of the defect and placement of a temporary diverting colostomy has been recommended. In patients with a prior bowel prep, the injury can be managed by closure of the intestine, copious irrigation, and antibiotic coverage. We have performed the repair endoscopically, avoiding a colostomy, and patients recovered without sequelae.

103. How do you verify that the bladder and ureter have not been injured during operative laparoscopy for endometriosis?

Throughout any pelvic operation, the location of the ureter must be identified. If there is any concern about ureteral injury, indigo carmine is given intravenously and the injured site is examined for evidence of extravasation. A cystoscope can be inserted to look for evidence of blue dye exiting the ureteral orifices. An intraoperative intravenous pyelogram (IVP) can be performed to look for leakage. These procedures help identify ureteral damage. However, ureteral damage may not be suspected and the above tests may not show any damage. The patient may present several days or weeks postoperatively, often with complaints of malaise, ileus, flank pain, pelvic pain, etc. The physician should obtain an IVP in patients with these symptoms. When using the CO_2 laser on or near the bladder, it is important to use hydrodissection. If laceration is suspected, the bladder can be filled with sterile milk, which will leak from a defect.

INTRODUCTION TO THE COLOR APPENDIX

This color atlas is divided into several parts. The first eight parts consist of illustrations that were selected because they were considered to be classic photos and in some cases, serve to amplify the descriptions of procedures found in the text. The last section of illustrations are color versions of figures that have appeared in the text in black and white.

The atlas shows several varieties of ovarian cysts encountered during diagnostic laparoscopy that were subsequently treated endoscopically. Types of endometriomas described in the text are also included, and the result of ovarian "drilling" of polycystic ovaries is characteristic of the procedure. The technique of a laparoscopic myomectomy is shown in five illustrations.

COLOR ATLAS

OVARIAN CYST

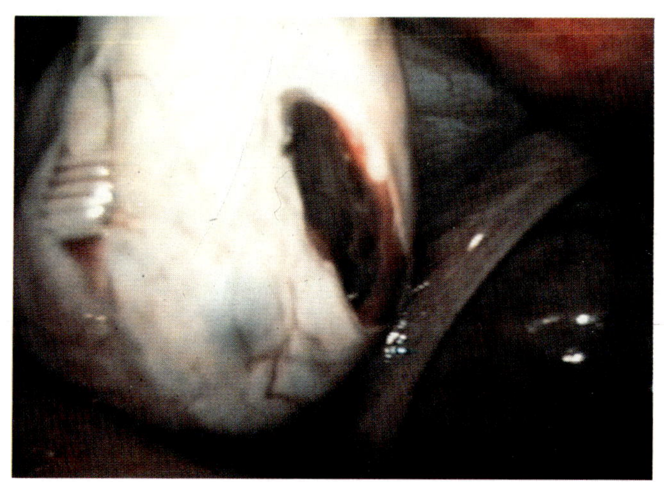

1. **Cystic hemorrhagic corpus luteum.**

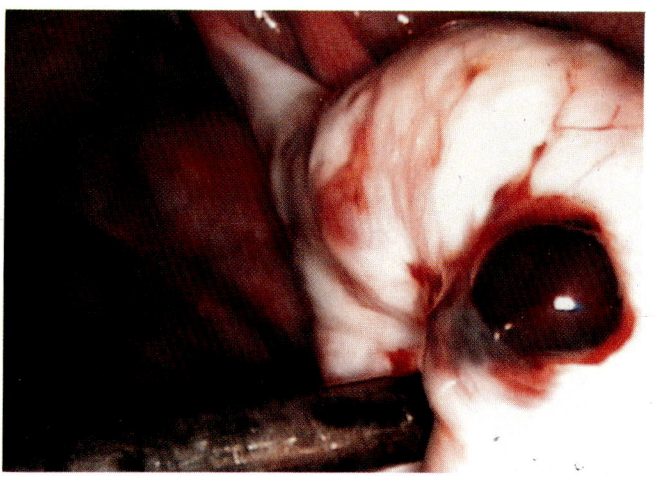

2. **Type I endometrioma.**

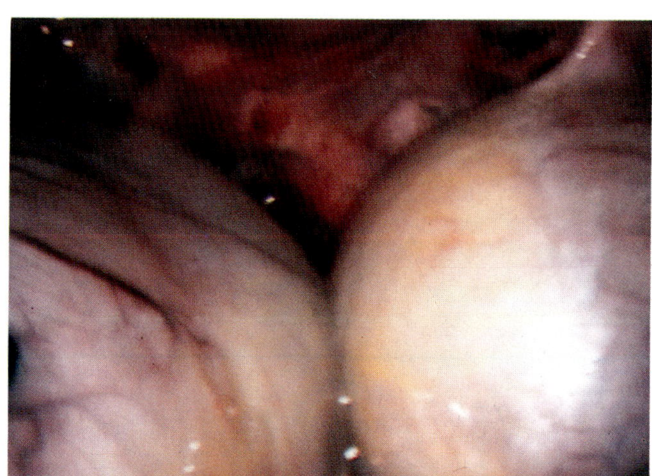

3. **Bilateral endometriomas, Type IIA.**

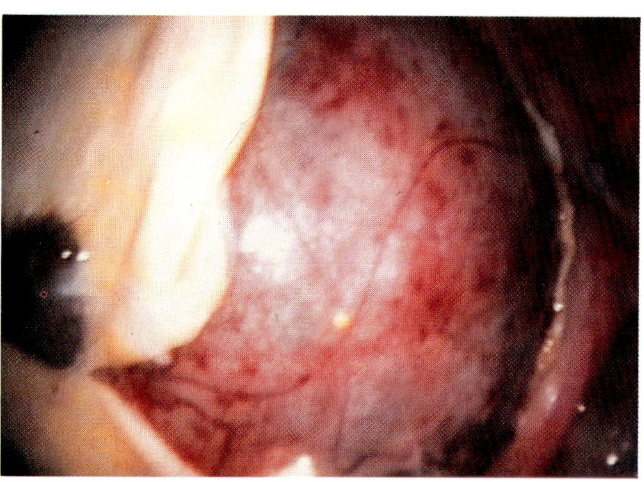

4. **Endometriosis limited to the ovarian cortex, Type IIA.**

OVARIAN CYST

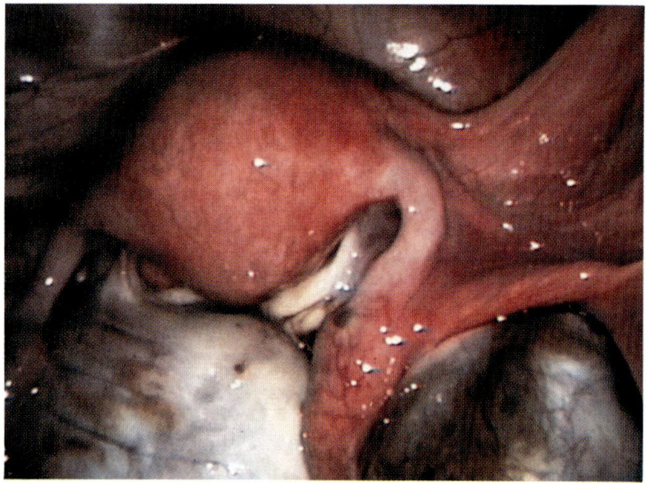

5. Bilateral endometriomas are noted, Type IIC.

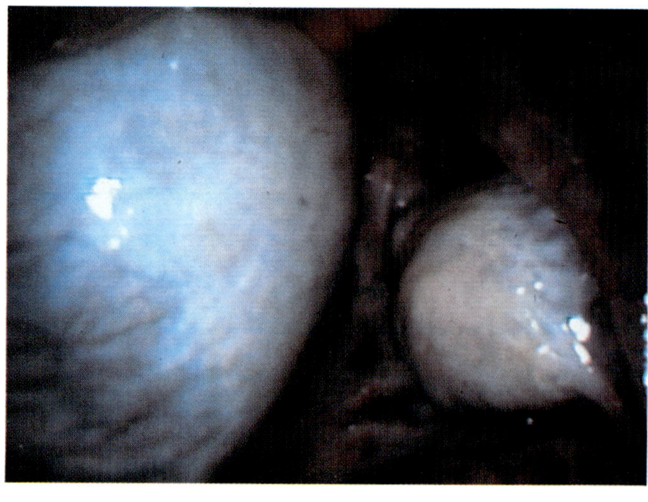

6. Cystic teratomas were found in both of these ovaries.

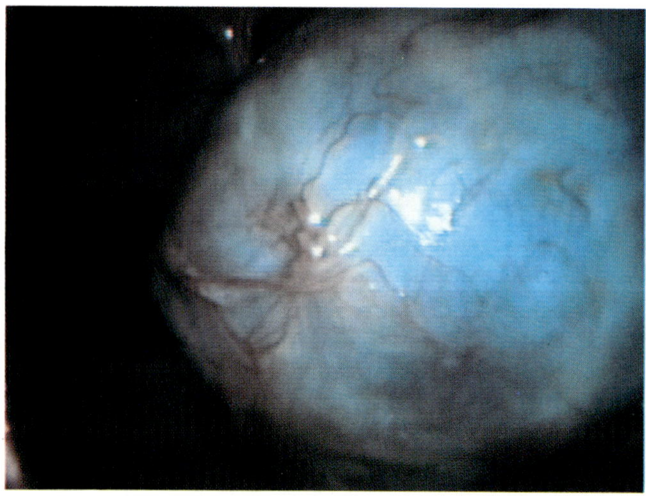

7. Benign serous cystadenoma was found on histologic examination.

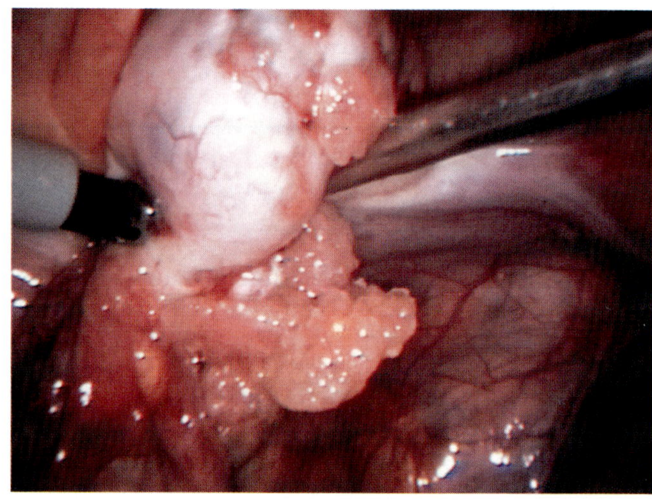

8. Ovarian cancer is noted with excrescences.

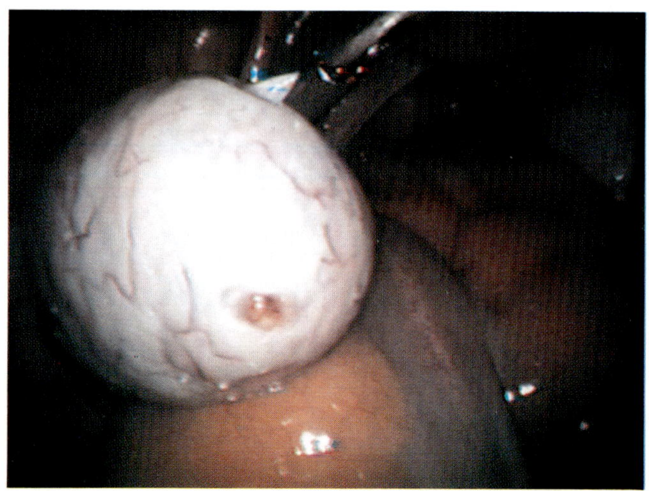

9. Polycystic ovary is seen with characteristic superficial blood vessels.

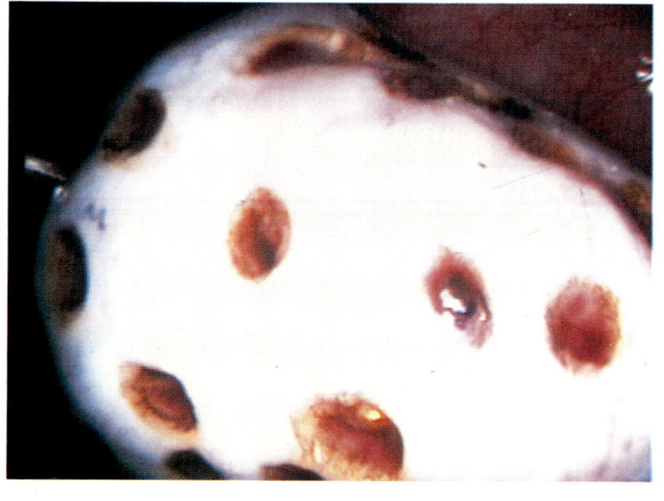

10. The ovary is seen after "drilling" with the CO_2 laser.

MYOMECTOMY

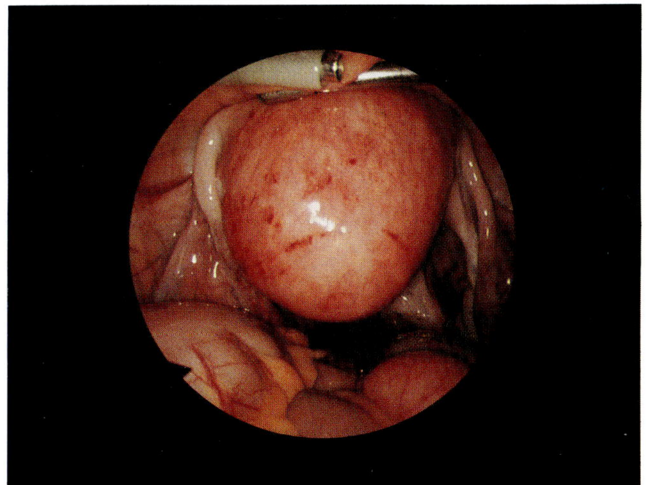

11. Posterior intramural myoma.

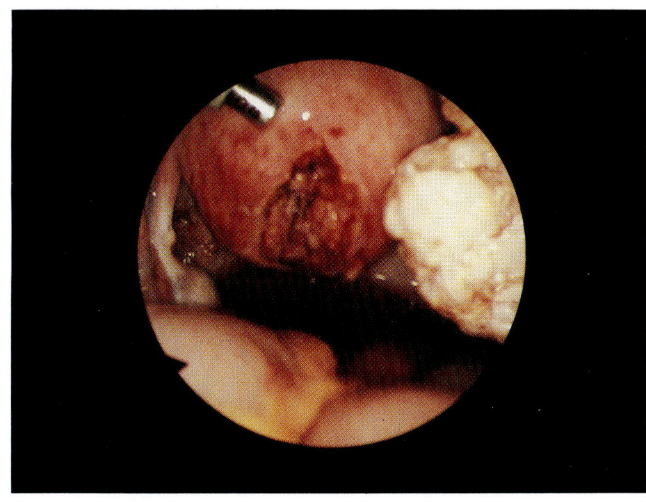

12. An incision was made over the myoma through the serosa and myometrium.

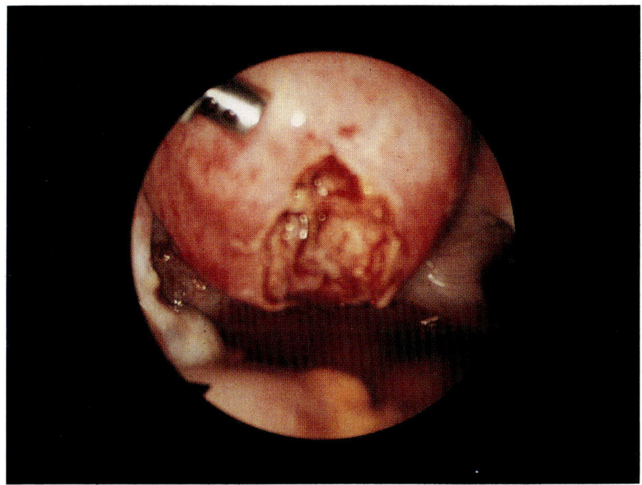

13. A portion of the myoma is seen at the base of the incision.

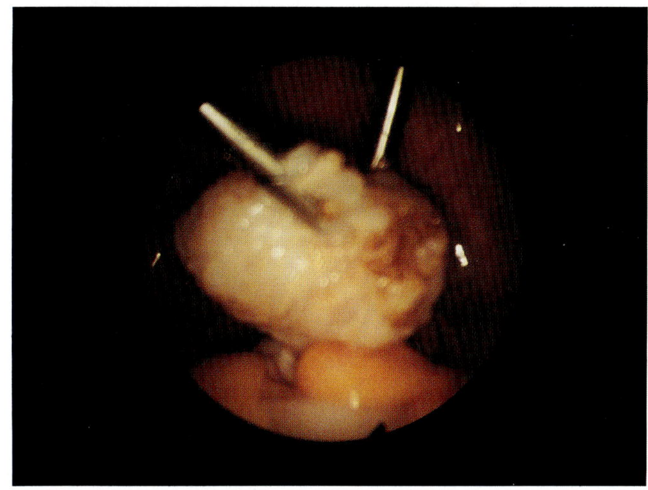

14. A laparoscopic myomectomy was done.

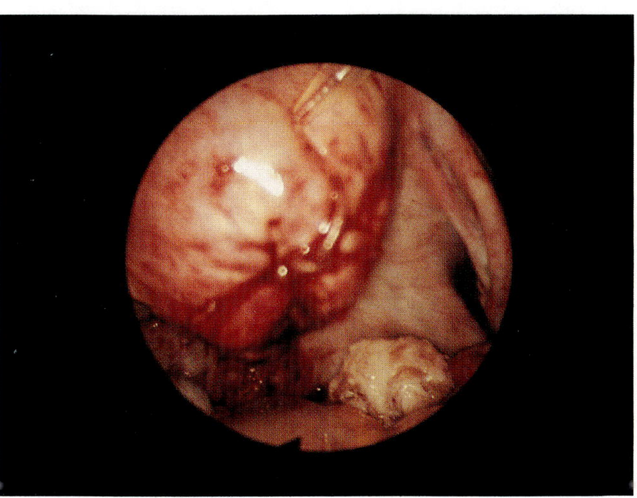

15. The uterine defect was closed in a single layer with O-Vicryl.

LUNA

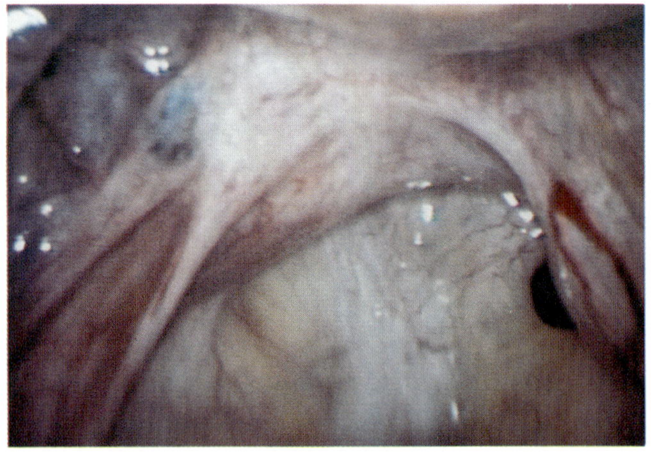

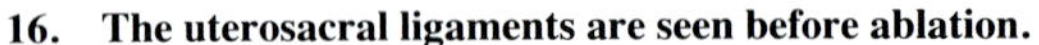

16. The uterosacral ligaments are seen before ablation.

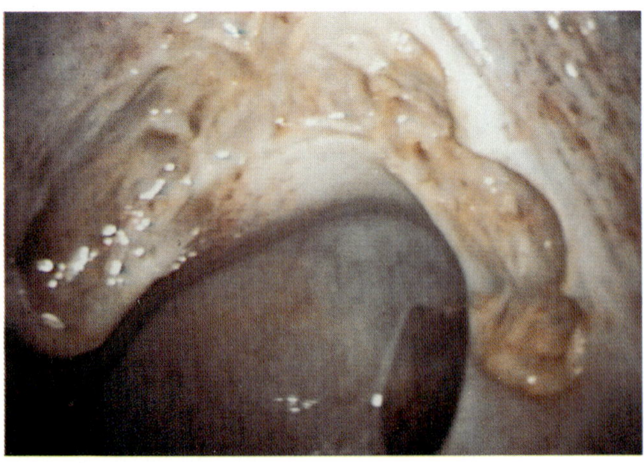

17. After ablation of the uterosacral ligaments.

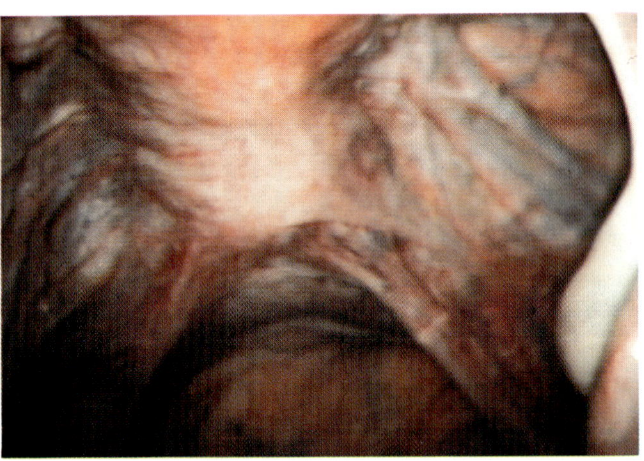

18. Two years later the area of ablation has healed without adhesions.

PELVIC SIDE WALL ANATOMY

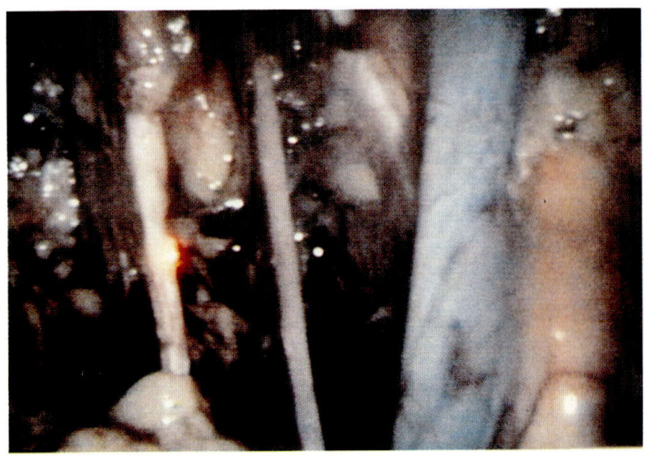

19. External iliac artery and vein are seen on the right; the obturator nerve is in the middle; the obliterated hypogastric artery is on the left.

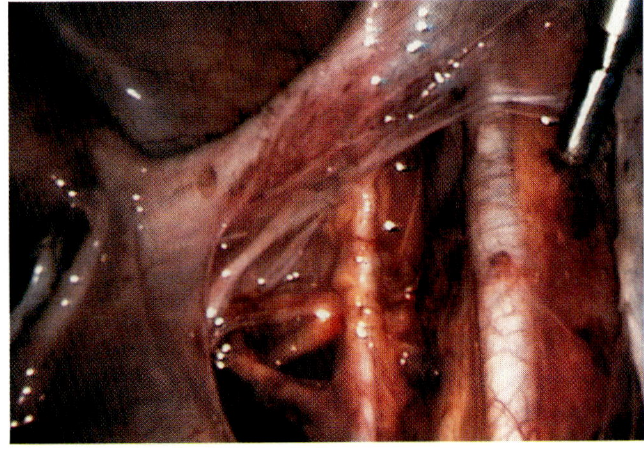

20. The uterine artery has been dissected from the hypogastric artery. The external iliac artery is on the right; the right round ligament appears in the foreground; the infundibulopelvic ligament is medial.

ECTOPIC PREGNANCY

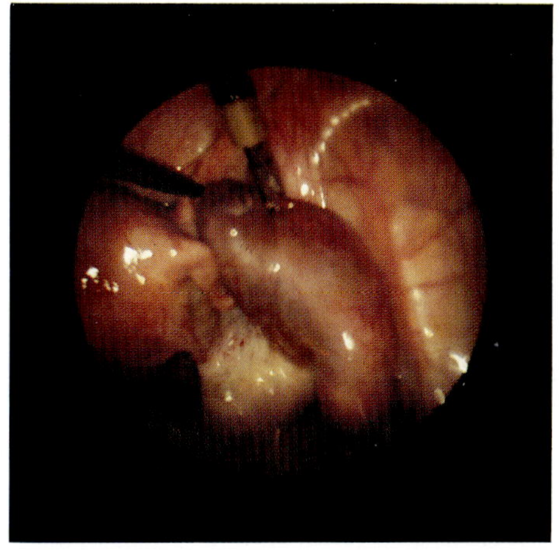

21. Unruptured ampullary pregnancy.

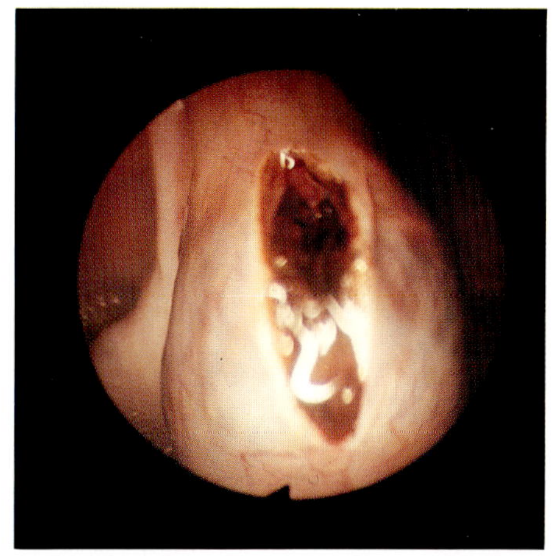

22. A linear tubal incision reveals the products of conception.

FULL THICKNESS ENDOMETRIOSIS OF THE BOWEL AND REPAIR

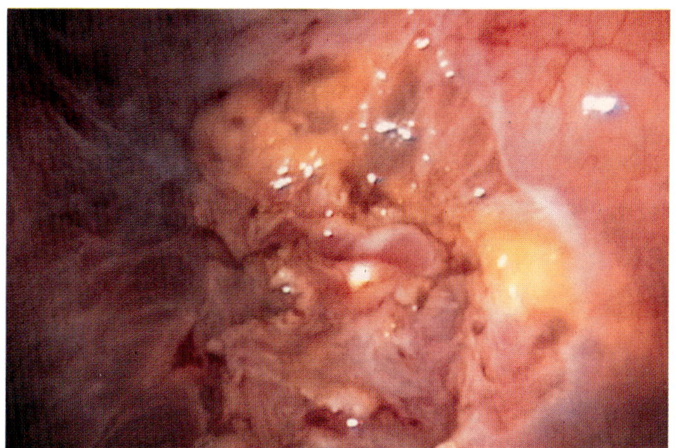

23. Rectal endometriosis has been excised and the rectal mucosa is seen.

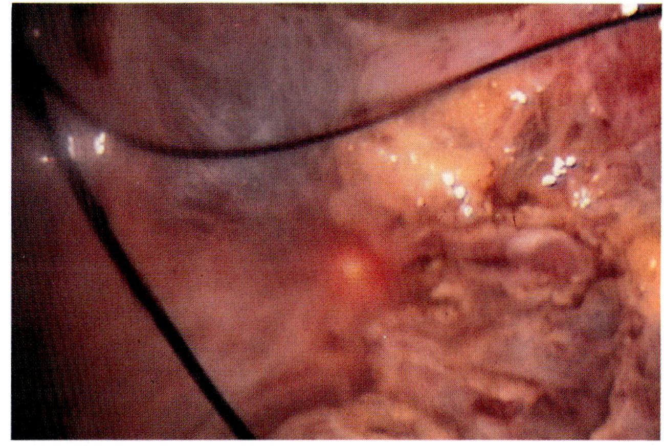

24. An Endoloop-PDS suture has been inserted into the area.

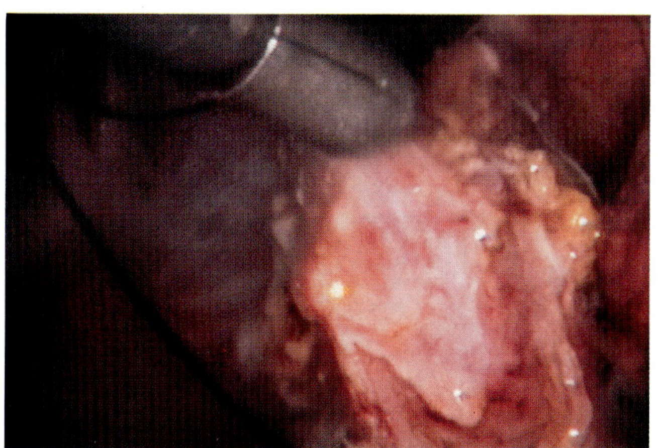

25. The rectal opening is brought inside of the loop.

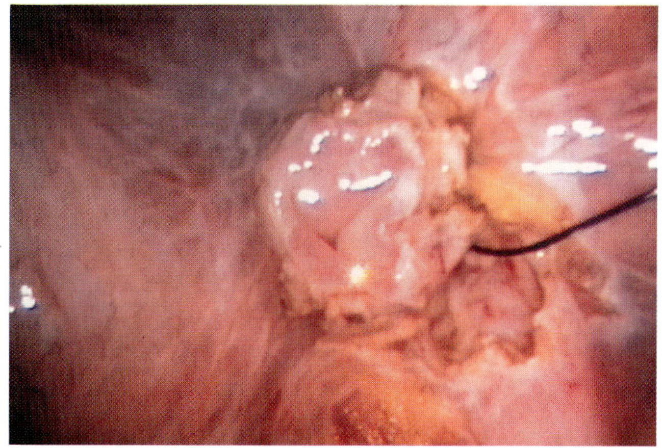

26. The perforation was repaired and examined under fluid after injecting air into the rectum to check for leakage.

FULL THICKNESS ENDOMETRIOSIS OF THE BOWEL AND REPAIR

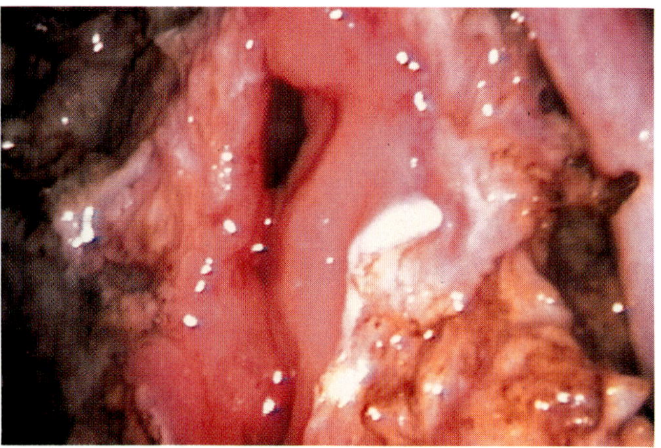

27. Another technique for laparoscopic rectal repair. The extensive full thickness rectal endometriosis has been removed.

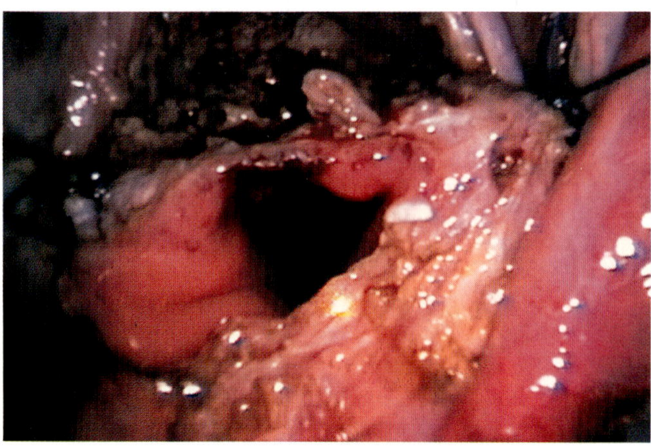

28. Two sutures were applied at the angles and the incision was transformed into a horizontal opening.

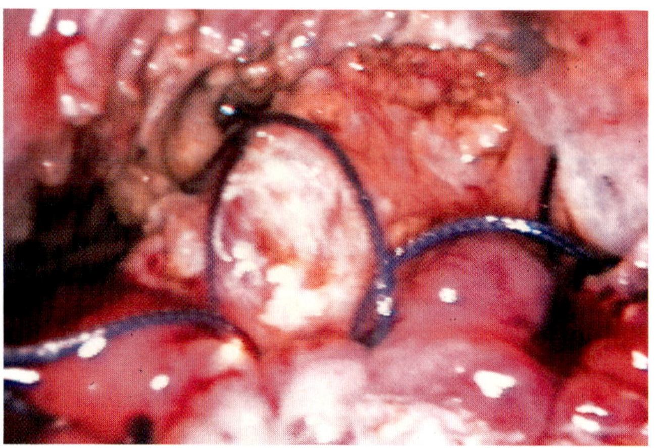

29. The incision was repaired with interrupted O-Vicryl sutures.

ENDOMETRIOSIS

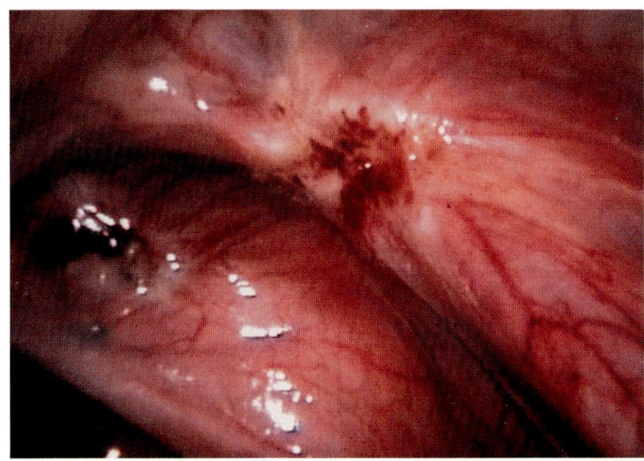

30. Endometrial implants are seen over the ureter.

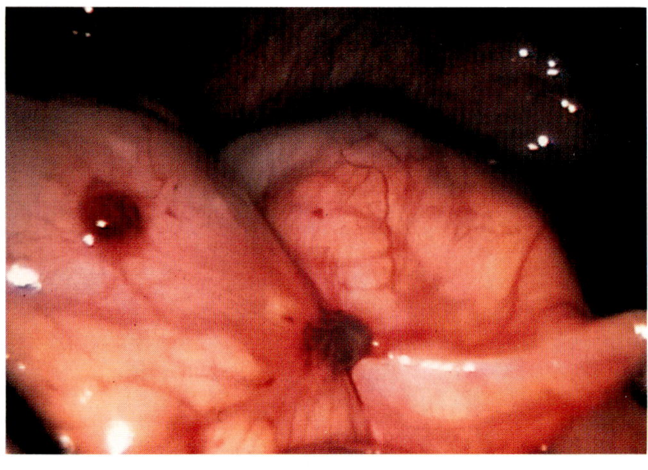

31. Rectosigmoid involved with endometriosis.

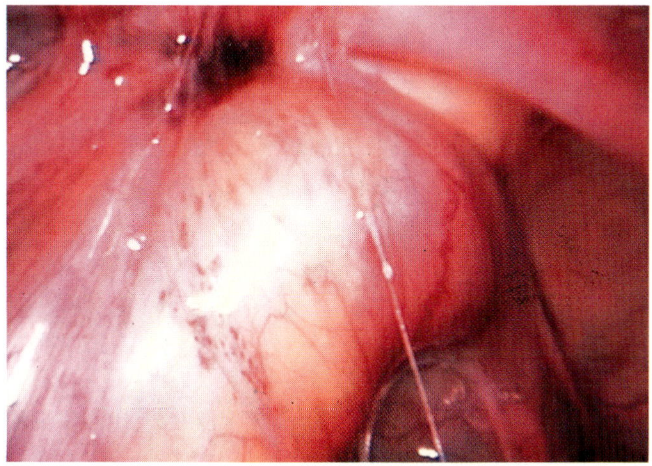

32. Rectal endometriosis is attached to the uterosacral ligament.

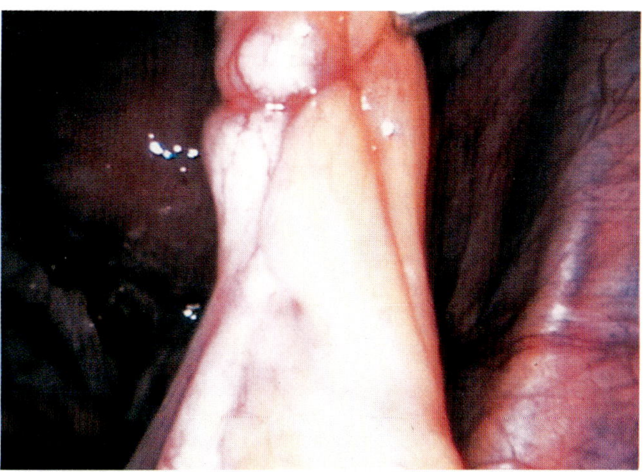

33. Appendix was involved with endometriosis.

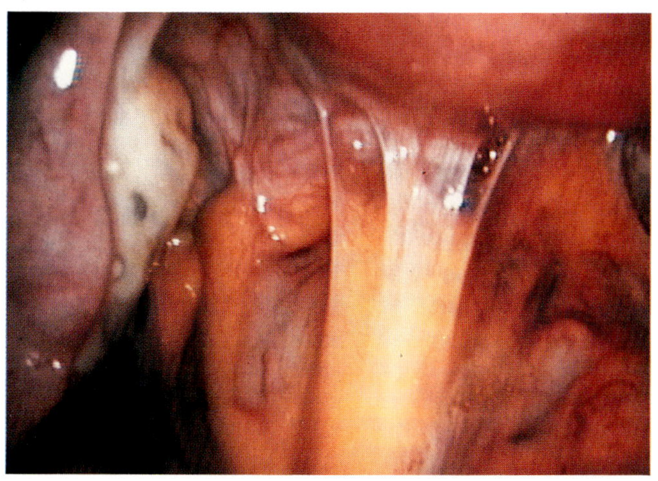

34. Cul-de-sac has been obliterated with endometrial implants and adhesions.

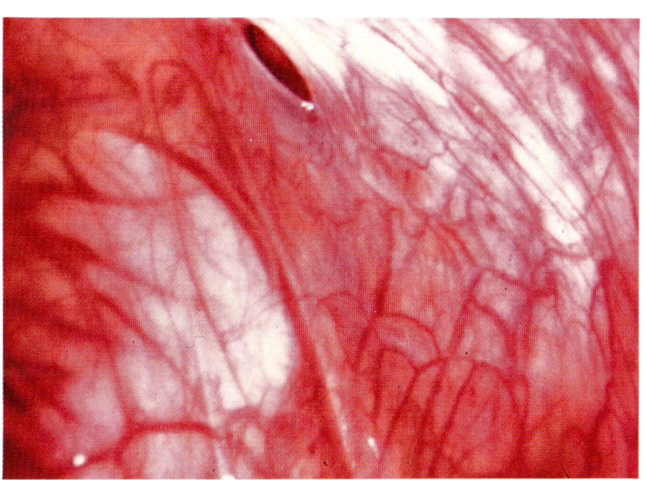

35. Opening of deep peritoneal defect which contained endometriosis.

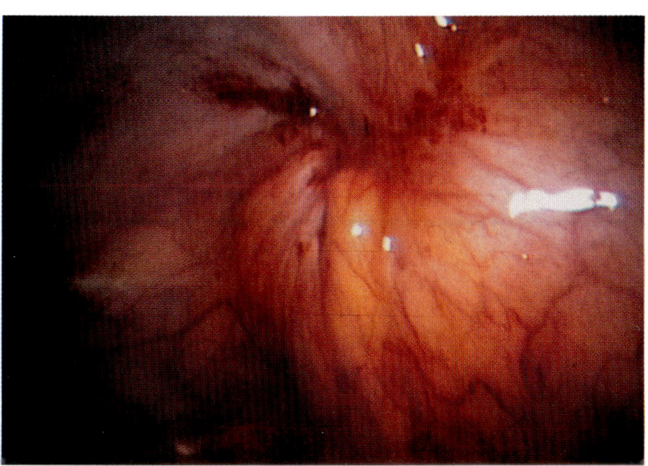

36. Severe infiltrative rectovaginal endometriosis.

ENDOMETRIOSIS

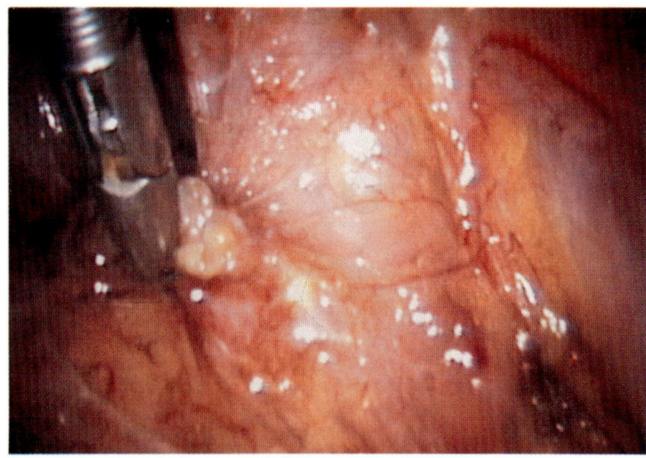

37. Wide and deep dissection is required to completely remove the lesion.

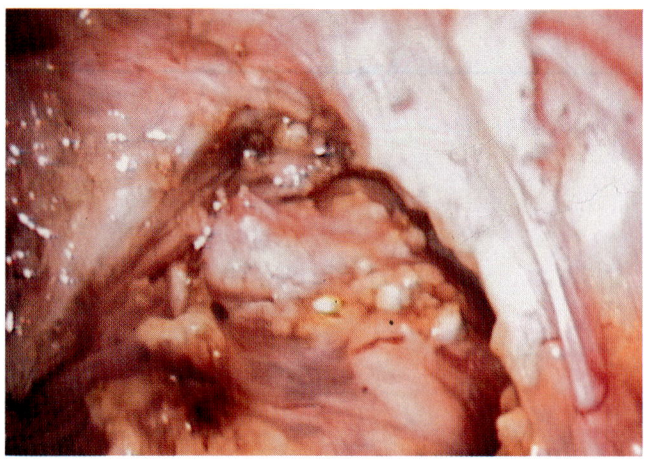

38. Posterior cul-de-sac is seen after removal of the lesion.

BLADDER ENDOMETRIOSIS

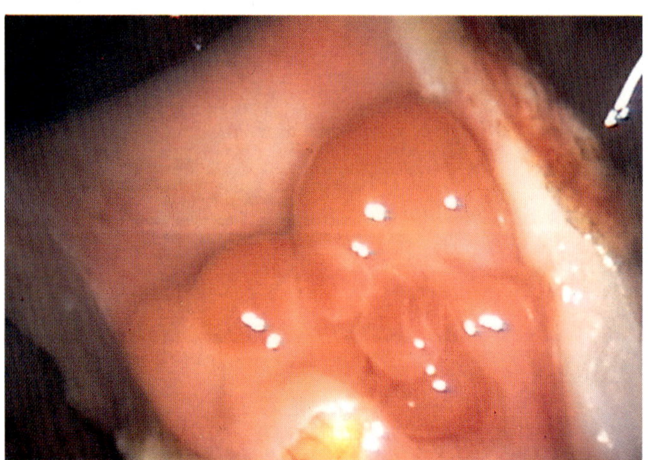

39. Endometriosis is seen in the bladder after a laparoscopic cystotomy.

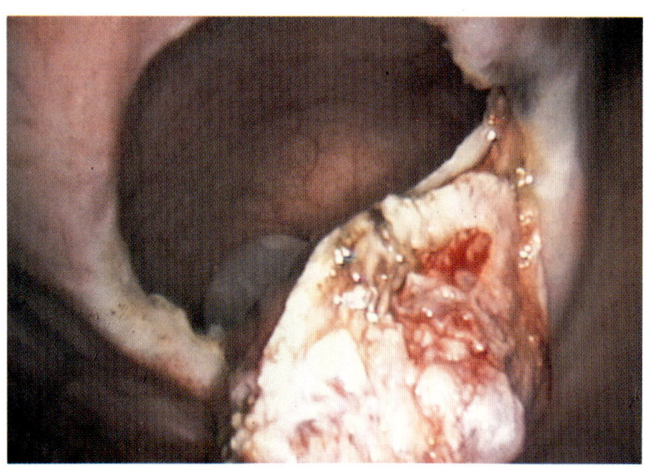

40. Endometriosis was removed after a partial cystectomy.

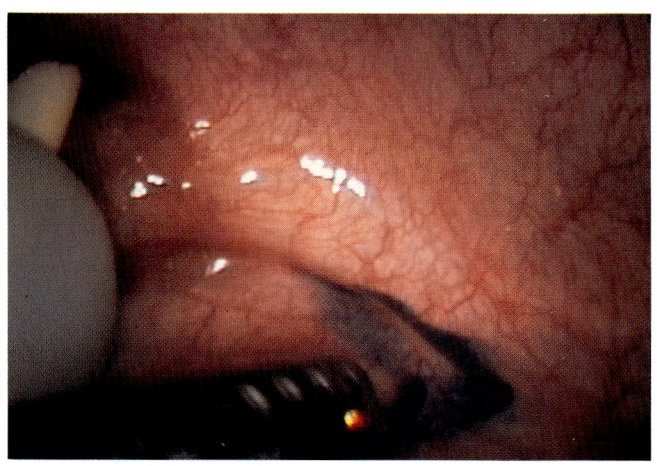

41. Indigo carmine was injected intravenously and is seen in the bladder showing intact ureteral orifices.

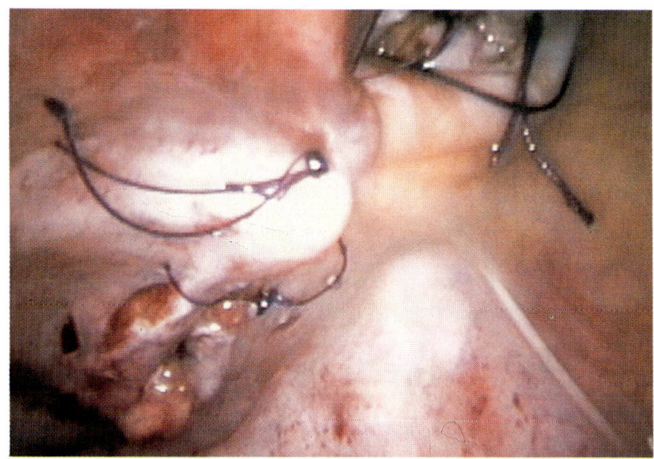

42. Bladder was repaired with a single layer of O-Vicryl sutures.

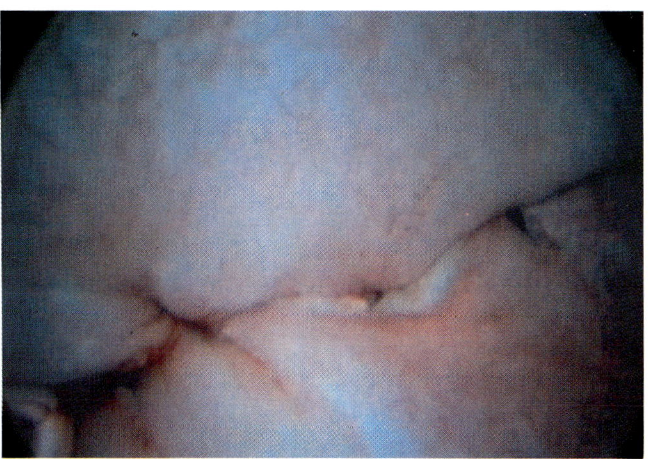

43. Cystoscopy was done right after repair.

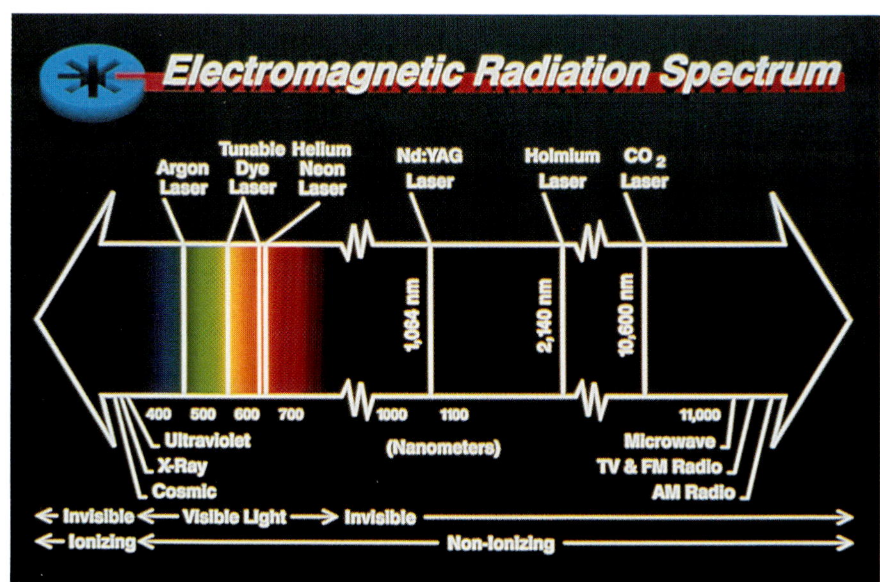

44. Laser light is unique and uniform unlike regular light, which is divided into the colors of the spectrum.

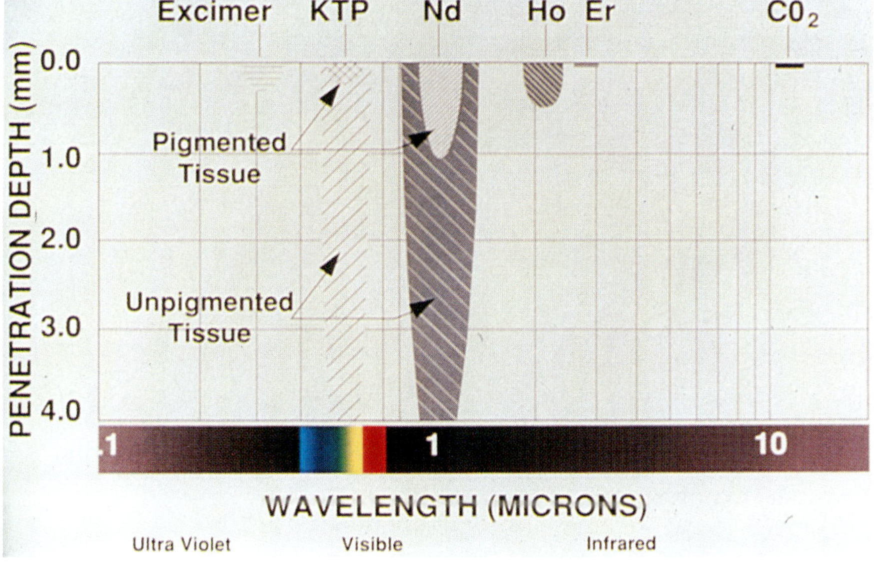

45. Argon, KTP, and Nd-YAG lasers are absorbed by pigmented tissues containing hemoglobin but pass through water and clear tissues.

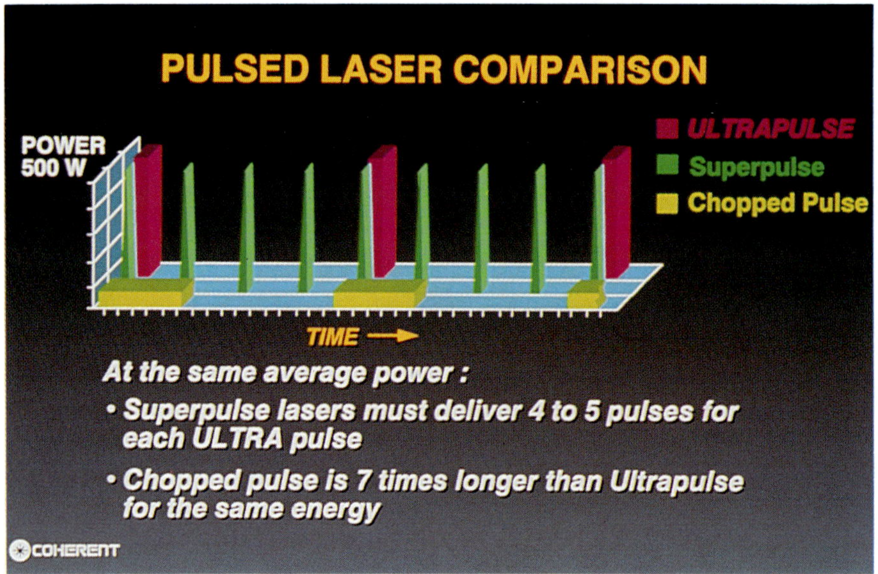

46. Comparison of ultrapulse, superpulse, and chopped pulse modes.

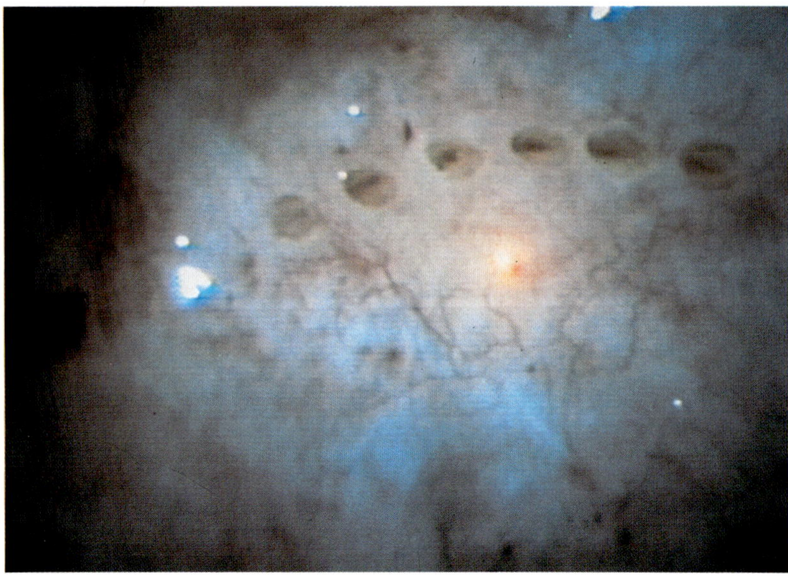

47. The new ultrapulse laser eliminates the "thermal blooming" effect and side effects such as the formation of charred tissue.

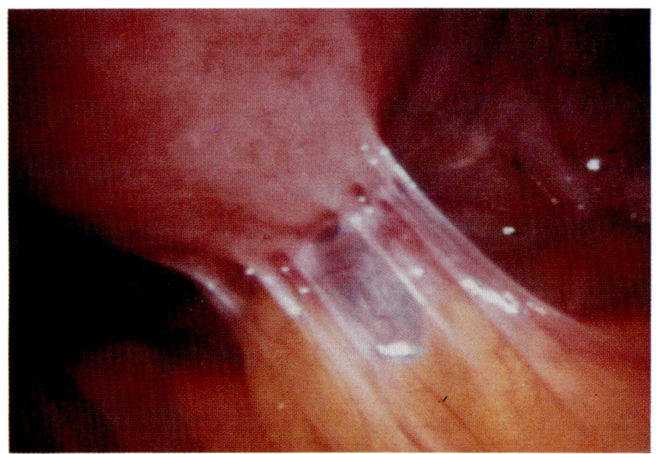

48. Avascular adhesions between the uterus and omentum are put under stretch before dissection with scissors.

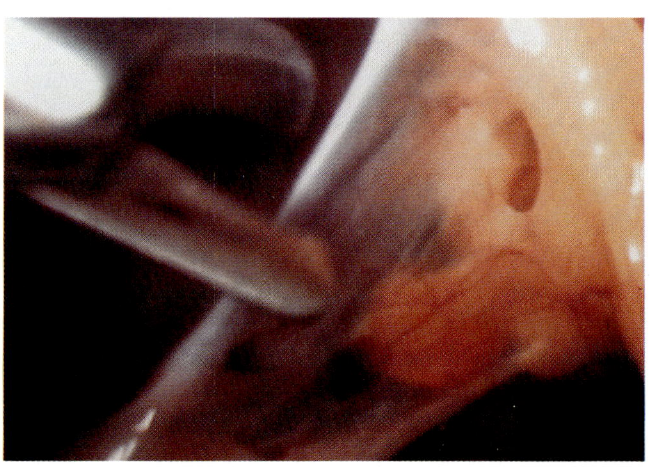

49. Avascular adhesions are dissected with scissors.

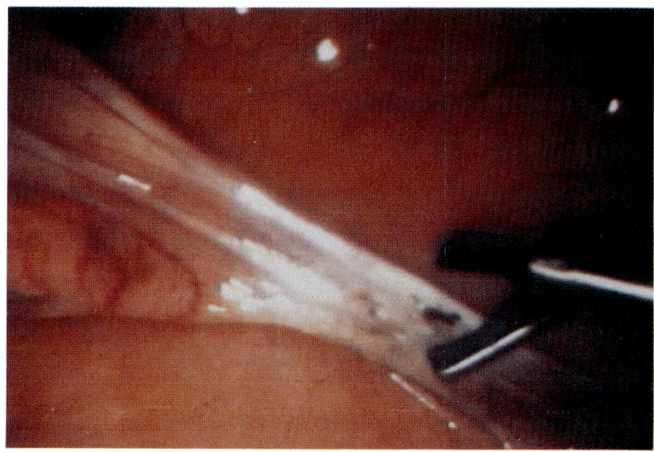

50. Thick, vascular adhesions are coagulated before dissection.

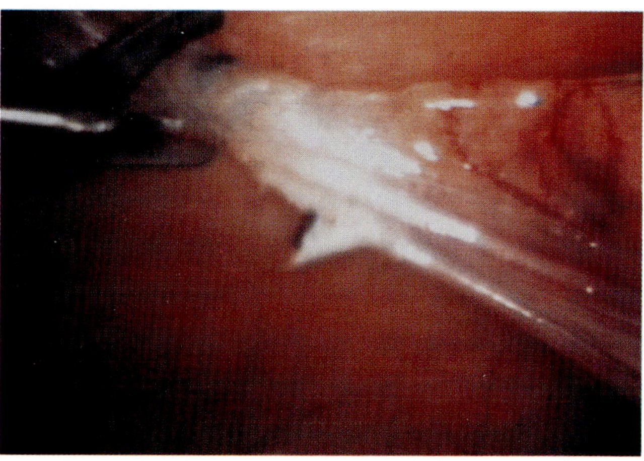

51. A coagulated vascular adhesion is lysed with scissors.

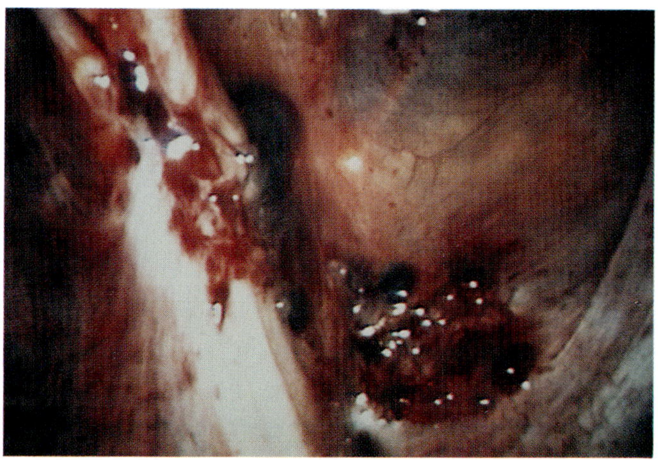

52. Powder burn lesions represent foci of inactive disease containing "burned out" stroma and glands embedded in hemosiderin deposits.

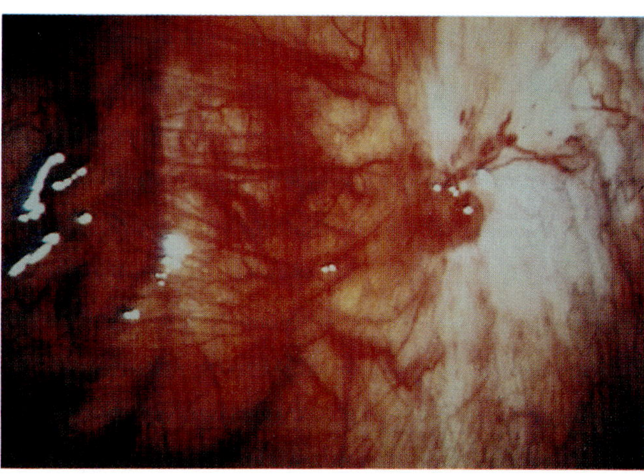

53. Atypical and nonpigmented lesions, seen as clear vesicles, pink vascular patterns, white scarred lesions, red lesions, yellow-brown patches, and peritoneal windows, represent active endometriosis.

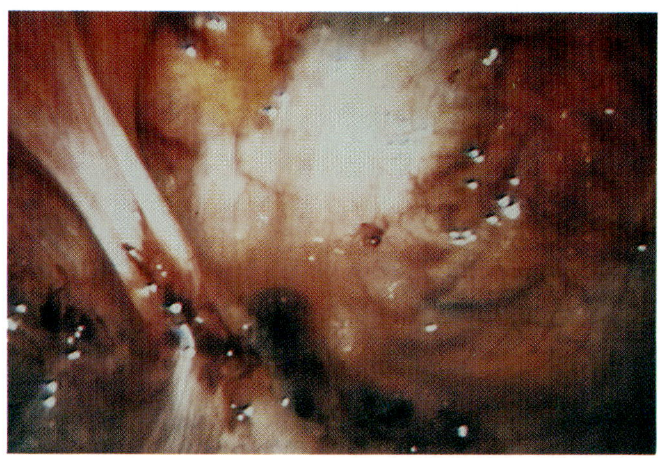

54. These lesions progress to an intermediate depth, become inactive, or infiltrate deeper (usually more than 5 mm).

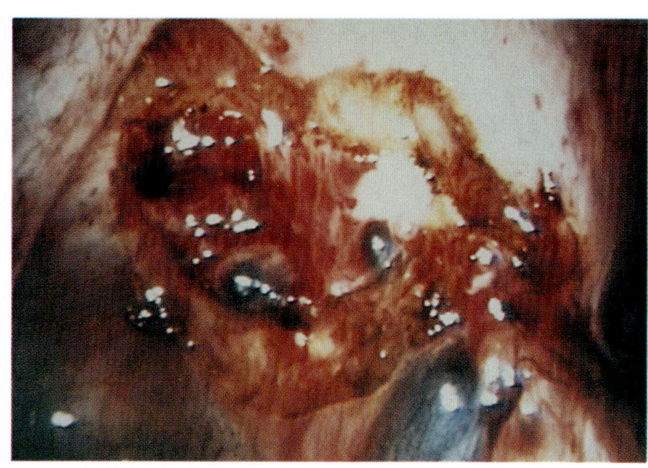

55. Superficial peritoneal endometriosis is vaporized with laser, coagulated with monopolar or bipolar current, or excised.

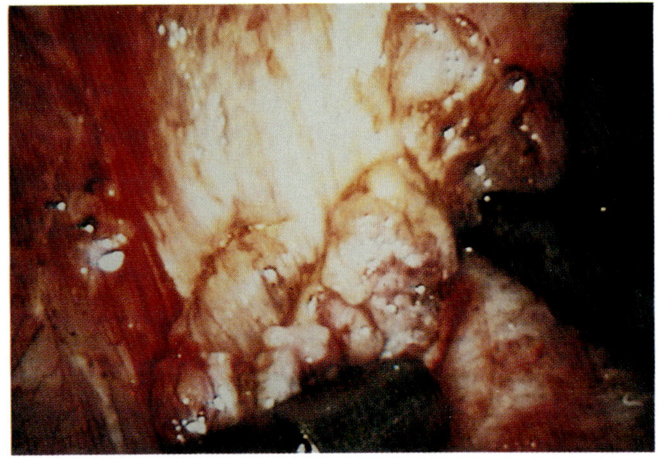

56. After an incision is made around the lesion, it is elevated with a grasping forceps and either cut or vaporized with CO_2 laser.

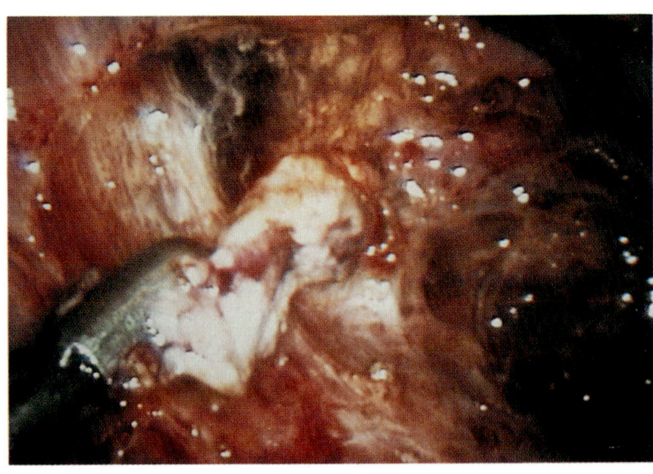

57. A wide dissection is necessary to be able to remove the entire lesion.

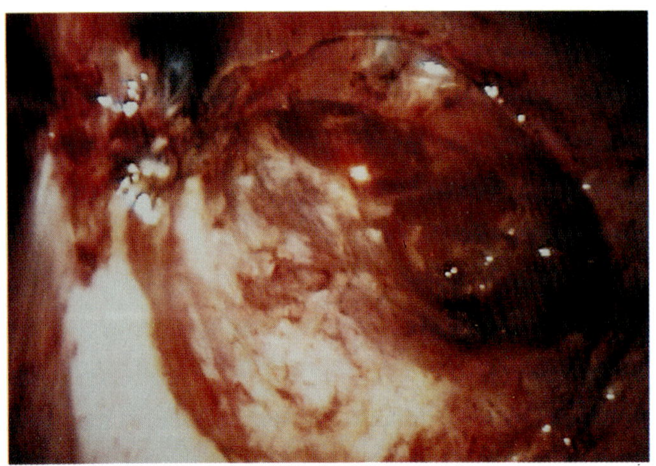

58. Posterior cul-de-sac and right uterosacral ligament after the fibrotic lesion is removed.

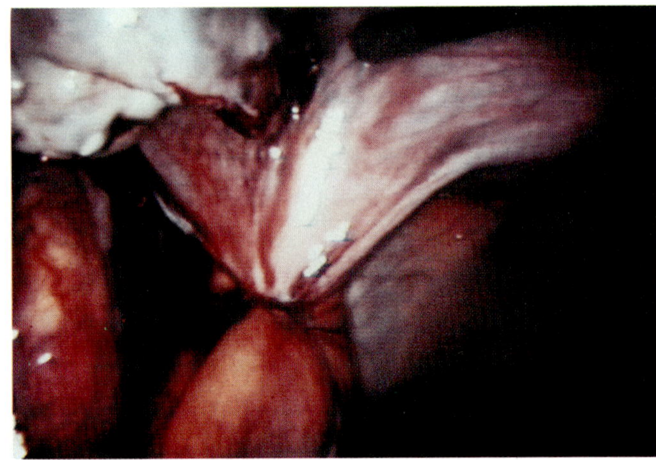

59. At laparoscopy, we found a 3- to 4-cm fibrotic nodule over the left ureter approximately 4 cm above the bladder, distorting the course of the ureter.

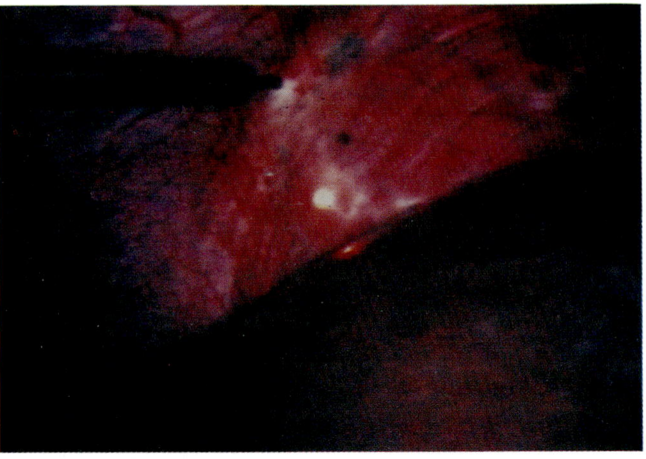

60. Endometriotic lesions on the diaphragm above the liver.

INDEX

Page numbers followed by t refer to tables; page numbers in italics refer to figures.

Abdominal aorta, palpation of, 81, *83*
Abdominal wall, 1
  assessing, for intestinal adhesions, 90
  attachment of bowel to, 90, *91*
  vascular injury, 287
Abscess, tubo-ovarian, 185, 186–188. (*See also* Tubo-ovarian abscess.)
Adenomyosis, 213, *214*
Adhesiolysis, 59, 68t, 99–104
  bowel preparation for, 80, 99
  in fimbrioplasty, 190, 192, *193*
  freestanding surgery centers and, 311
  intestinal injury during, 99, *102*
    repair of, *103*
  technique for, 99, *100, 101, 102–103*
  therapeutic efficacy of, 122
  during treatment for ectopic pregnancy, 317
  underwater, 142
Adhesion(s)
  adnexectomy with, 176–177, *177*
  after wedge resection, by laparotomy, 179, 179t
  avascular, 99, *101*
  bowel, *92*, 126
  coagulation of, CO_2 laser, 99
  filmy, 99
  formation of. (*see* Adhesion formation.)
  infertility and, 97
  intestinal, 90, 126
    assessing abdominal wall for, 90
    severing of, 99, 126
  vascular, coagulated, 99, *101*
Adhesion formation, 97
  after laparotomy, 89t
  chemotherapy and, 89
  factors promoting, 89, 97, 98t
  peritonitis and, 89
  Pfannenstiel incision and, 89, 89t
  postoperative, 89t, 97
    detection of, 90
    incidence of, 89t
    laser surgery vs. electrosurgery for, 67t
    prevention of, 207–208, 320
  prevention of, 97–99, 99t
    antihistamines in the, 98, 99t
    corticosteroids in the, 98, 99t
    dextran in the, 98, 99t
    surgical membranes in the, 98–99, 99t
    in tubal surgery, 188, 189t
  radiation therapy and, 89
  suturing and, 158, 159t
  in tubal surgery, 198, 200
    prevention of, 188, 189t
Adnexal torsion, 181
Ampicillin, 71
Anastomosis, tubal, 198
Anastomosis, tubal surgery for, 198, 200
ANECTINE, 74
Anesthesia, 71–75. (*See also* Laparoscopy, anesthesia during.)
  epidural, 73
  maintenance of, 74
Antibiotics, 313
  preoperative, 71
Antihistamines, adhesion formation and, 98, 99t
Antiinflammatory drugs, nonsteroidal, 74
Appendectomy, 239–243
  laparoscopic, 239–243
    indications for, 243
    outcome of, 243t
    prophylactic, 239–240
    rationale for, 239
    stapling devices for, 241, *242*
    technique for, 240–243, *240, 241, 242*
Appendicitis, 239, 243
  histologic findings in, 239
Appendix, in endometriosis, 125, 134
Argon lasers, 47
  delivery systems of, 54
  models of, 54
  physical characteristics and properties of, 49t, 54
Aspiration/injection needle, 28–29, *29*
Atracurium, 74

Beta-blockers, 71
Bladder injury. (*See* Urinary bladder injury.)
Bladder reflection, 59
Bleeding, 296, 306
  control of, 156, *157*
  para-aortic lymphadenectomy and, 278
  postmenopausal, 314
  presacral neurectomy and excessive, 250
  superpulse mode and, 314
Bowel adhesions, 126
Bowel displacement, for pelvis observation, 311
Bowel distention, secondary to obstruction, 89
Bowel endometriosis. (*see* Gastrointestinal endometriosis.)
Bowel injury, 305–306, 322. (*See also* Intestinal injury.)
  prevention of, 301–302
Bowel preparation, 79–80, 80t
  for adhesiolysis, 99
  one-day, 80t
  three-day, 80t
Bowel resection, 61
  in gastrointestinal endometriosis, 134–137, *135*, *136*, *137*, *138*, *139*, *140*, *141*
Breast cancer, oophorectomy in, 167
Burch procedure, 255, 260, 262

CA-125 antigen, 313
  ovarian cysts and, 150t, 152
  postoperative monitoring of, 318
Camera equipment, 18–24
  beam splitter-type, 320
  charged coupled device in, 19
  chip-on-stick, 22
  in endoscopic surgery, 18–24. (*See also* Videolaseroscopy.)
    history of, 19, *19*
  light sources for, 22
  operation of, 19–21
Capacitative coupling, 58, *59*
  thermal injury from, 58
Carcinogenesis, laser by-product and, 312–313
Cardiac arrhythmias, laparoscopy and, 75
Cavitational Ultrasonic Surgical Aspirator, 61. (*See* also Ultrasonic surgery.)
Cervical cancer, 274
  pelvic lymphadenectomy in, 273
  staging of, operative laparoscopy in, 274, 284t
Char, 312–313, 319
Chemotherapy, 275
  adhesion formation and, 89
  port placement for, 276
Cholecystectomy, ultrasonic surgery for, 61
Chromopertubation, 94, *192*
  in fimbrioplasty, 191
  neosalpingostomy and, 192, *193*
Civil liability. (*see* Malpractice.)
Clip applicators, 30, *32*
Coaptive coagulation, 60
Cohen cannula, 30
CO_2 laser, 15, *16*
  adhesiolysis with, 68t
  adhesion coagulation with, 99
  delivery system of, 52–54
  embolus associated with, 75
  most efective use of, 55, 68
  Nd-YAG laser vs., 66–67
  ovariolysis using, *101*
  physical characteristics and properties of, 49t, 52, 53, 54
  power density of, 51
  problems associated with delivery of, 51–52
  safety glasses and, 314
  salpingostomy with, 111, *112–113*, *114*, *115–116*, *117*
  setting for, 321
  speed of transection with, 68t
  superpulse mode of, 51, 209
    bleeding and, 314
  "thermal blooming effect" and, 52, *52*
  thermal injury with, 51
    depth of, 68t, 321
  ultrapulse mode of, 51
    in laparoscopic myomectomy, 209, *209*
    in tubal surgery, *193*, *194*
"Cold light" concept, 1
Colonoscopy, 4, 133
Colpotomy, 315
  patient instructions following, 314–315
  risks associated with, 178
  vaginal closure of, 179
Complications
    bleeding as, *296*
    electrosurgical, 295–296
    gastrointestinal, 288t
    gynecologic, 289t
    incidence of, 287, 288t
    intraoperative, 289–306
    management by laparotomy, 287
    large bowel injury, 301–306
    postoperative, 306–308
    prevention of, 287–288
    procedural failure leading to, 289–296
    small bowel injury, 301–305
    ureteral injury during, 297–301
    urinary bladder, 296–297
    urogenital, 288t
    uterine, 296
    vascular, 288t
    Veress needle, 289–291
Computed tomography, of ovarian cysts, 152
Constipation, 140
Containment bag, 121–122
Corticosteroids, adhesion formation and, 98, 99t
Coupler, Coherent-Nezhat, 53
Coupling lenses, 53, *53*
Cul-de-sac, intestinal
  enema for exposure of, 312
  restoration, in gastrointestinal endometriosis, 137–140, *139*, *140*, *141*

Culdoscope, 1
Culdotomy, 164, *164*
  anterior, *231*
  antibiotic preparation for, 163
  in hysterectomy, 224, 225
  posterior, *232*
CUSA. (*See* Cavitational Ultrasonic Surgical Aspirator.)
Cyst(s), 159t
  chocolate, 159
  ovarian. [*See* Ovarian cyst(s).]
Cystectomy, 60
  ovarian, 153, 155–160. (*See also* Ovarian cystectomy.)
  ultrasonic surgery for, 61
Cystic teratoma, 315

Demerol, 71, 74
DEPO-PROVERA, 123
Dextran, adhesion formation and, 98, 99t
Diabetes mellitus, tubo-ovarian abscesses and, 188
Diaphragmatic endometriosis, 140–142, *141*
  hormone therapy for, 142
  postoperative follow-up in, 141–142
Diarrhea, 140
Dihydroporphyrin ether, 143
Dilation, instruments for, 41
Direct coupling of electricity, thermal injury from, 59
Dyschezia, 140
Dysgenetic gonads, removal of, 175–176, *176*
Dysmenorrhea, 317
  endometriosis and, 317
  presacral neurectomy for, 315

Ecchymosis, skin, 140
Ectopic pregnancy, 107–118
  ampullary, *108*
  cornual, *108*, 114, 117
  diagnosis of, 1, 107–109, 314
    human chorionic gonadotropin in, beta, 107–108
    progesterone in, 108–109
    transvaginal sonography in, 107
  endoscopic surgery for, 111
  ethnicity and, 107
  fimbrial, *109*
  implantation in, 317
  incidence of, 107
  infertility and, 185
  interstitial, *108*, 114, 117
    differential diagnosis of, 114
    laparotomy for, 117
    management of, 114
  intrauterine gestational sac in, 110
  isthmic, *108*
  laparoscopy vs. laparotomy for, 110t, 316
  maternal deaths attributed to, 107
  methotrexate in, 117–118
  nonsurgical management of, 117–118
  physical findings in, 109–110, 110t
  prostaglandin sulprostone vs. methotrexate for, 118
  risk factors for, 107, 109t
  ruptured
    salpingectomy for, 196
    treatment of, 316–317
  salpingectomy for, 196
  sexually transmitted disease and, 107
  sites of, 107, *108*, *109*
  symptoms of, 109, 110t
  treatment for, 110–114
    adhesiolysis during, 317
    charge for, 317
    human chorionic gonadotropin after, monitoring of, 317
    laparoscopic approach, 111–114, 316, 317
    nonsurgical, 117–118
  tubal operations and, 107, 196
  tubal operations for. (*See also* Tubal surgery.)
    recovery time after, 107
  varying sizes and locations of, treatment for, 316
Edema, pulmonary, 75
Electrical currents, *59*
  alternating, 57, *58*
  coagulating, 58
  cutting, 57, *59*
    characteristics of, 59
    clinical applications of, 59, *60*
  direct, 57, *58*
Electrical energy, 57, 58t
  capacitative coupling of, 58, *59*
  currents of. (*See* Electrical currents.)
  measurement of, 57
  wave forms of, types of, 57–58, *58*
Electrocoagulation. (*See also* Electrosurgery.)
  in ectopic pregnancy, 316, 317
  needle tip, 316
Electrogenerators, 57
  with bipolar forceps, 30, *31*
Electrosurgery, 57–63
  activation of electrode in, 59, *60*
  alternating current in, 57, *58*
  bipolar systems in, 58–59
    stapling devices as alternative to, 197
  clinical applications of, 59
  desiccation in, 59–60
    clinical application of, 60
    extent of lateral damage with, *60*
    hemostasis during, 60
  direct coupling of current in, 62–63
  electrical energy source in, 57
  electrogenerators recommended for, 57
  in forceps, bipolar vs. monopolar, 60
  fulguration in, *61*
    after cystectomy, 60
    after myomectomy, 60
  insulation failure in, 62
  laser surgery vs., 65–68, 321
    for fibrosis at site of injury, 67t
    for infertility, tuboperitoneal causes of, 68
    in ovariectomy, 65–66, *66*

Electrosurgery (*Continued*)
postoperative adhesions in, 67t
thermal injury in, depth of, 65, 67t
tissue effects in, 65–66, 66t
for tubal disease, 192t
reduction of adhesions with, 68t
safe use of, 62–63
speed of transection with, 68t
thermal injury from, 58–59, 63, 68t
in tubal sterilization, 57
unipolar systems in, 58–59
vaporization in, 59
voltage in, measurement of, 57
Embolus, CO_2 laser associated with, 75
Endoknot cannula, *35*
Endoloop suture, 32, *33*
as alternative to laser, 314
in oophorectomy, 174–175, *175*
in salpingectomy, 197–198, *198*, *199*
in salpingo-oophorectomy, 175, *176*
Endometrial cancer, 275–285
laparoscopic management of, 275–285
chemotherapy and, 276
disadvantage of, 285
para-aortic lymphadenectomy in, 276, *277*, 278, *278*
pelvic lymphadenectomy in, 278–279, *280*
radiation therapy and, 276
radical hysterectomy in, 273, 274, 279, *280–281*, 282, 284–285
radiation therapy and, 270
staging of, 275
Endometriomas, 159t. (*See also* Endometriosis.)
classification of, 158–160, *159*, 160t
medical management of, 160
surgical management of, 160–164, *162*, *163*
placement of hydrodissection needle in, 318
Endometriosis, 121–143
appendix involvement with, 125, 134
bladder, *132*, 132–133, *133*, *134*
bowel involvement with, 318
clinical appearance of, 124t, 124–125
cul-de-sac obliteration in, 131
deep retroperitoneal, 125
diagnosis of, 125
diaphragmatic, 140–142, *141*
dysmenorrhea and, 317
excision vs. ablation for, 318
exercise and, 142
freestanding surgery centers and, 311
gastrointestinal, 133–140
appendiceal involvement in, 134
bowel resection in, 134–137, *135*, *136*, *137*, *138*, *139*, *140*, *141*
colonoscopy in, 133
cul-de-sac restoration in, 137–140, *139*, *140*, *141*
history of, 133
proctoscopy in, 133
symptoms of, 133
history of, 121
surgical, 121–122
hysterectomy for, 123, 226–236
cardinal ligament in, 227, 230, *231*
culdotomy in, with cuff closure, 230, *231*, *232*
dissection of rectosigmoid colon-uterine attachment in, 226, *226*, *227*, *228*
final laparoscopic evaluation in, 233
Moschcowitz procedure during, 232–233
procedure for, 227, *228–229*, *230*
recurrence rate after, 123
laparoscopy for, 121–143
dihydroporphyrin ether and, 143
histologic findings in, 124, *124*, 124t, *125*
laparotomy vs., 122t, 122–123
photodynamics in, 143
restoration of tubo-ovarian anatomy after, 142
technique of, 126–142
oral contraceptives and, 317
ovarian, 59, 126–129. (*See also* Ovarian endometriosis.)
ultrasonic surgery for, 61
pain management of, 142
peritoneal, 126
treatment of, hydrodissection pump in, 126, *127*
peritoneal defect and, management of, 318–319
recovery time after ablation of, 311
rectosigmoid colon-uterine attachment in, 226, *226*
recurrence of, 318
estrogen replacement therapy and, 123, 142
minimizing, 142–143
risk factors for, 142
salpingo-oophorectomy for, 123
surgery for, 123–125
conservative, 123–125
gonadotropin-releasing hormone after, 319
hormone replacement therapy after, 123
radical, 123
recurrence rate after, 124
ureteral, 129–131, *130*, *131*
uterine suspension for, 317–318
Endoscope, 21–22
Endoscopic surgery, 4
camera equipment in, 18–24
for ectopic pregnancy, 111
lasers in, 47–54
Enema, preoperative, 312
Enflurane, 74
Enterorrhaphy, 99
Epigastric vessels, 87, *88*
bleeding from, control of, 294, *295*
Equipment, for laparoscopy, 15–45. (*See also* Laparoscopy, equipment for.)
Esophagogastroduodenoscopy, 4
ESTRACE, 123
Estrogen, 123
Exercise, endometriosis and, 142
Extracorporeal knot tying, *34*, 34–35, *35*
uterine repair using, 210, *211*
Extracorporeal pretied suture knot, 35–36, *36*, *37*

Fallope rings, in uterine suspension, 215, *215*
Fentanyl, *74*
  ibuprofen vs., for postoperative pain, 74, *74*
Fiberoptics, monitoring of laser surgery with, 54
Fibroids. (*See* Uterine leiomyomas.)
Fimbriolysis, 99, 101
Fimbrioplasty, 190, 191, *193*
  adhesiolysis in, 190, *193*
  chromopertubation in, 191, 192, *193*
  pregnancy rate after, 185
  steps in performing, *193*
Fistula. (*See also* Vesicovaginal fistula.)
  uteroperitoneal, 216
Fluid management, in laparoscopy, 75
FORANE, 74
Forceps, 26–27, *27*
  biopsy, 28, *29*
  bipolar, *31*, *304*
    control of bleeding with, 156, *157*
    electrogenerator and, 30, *31*
    monopolar vs., in electrosurgery, 60
  fine, *28*
  spoon, *31*
Fulguration, 60, *61*, 62'
Furosemide, intraoperative, 75, 322

Gentamicin, 71
Glycopyrrolate, 74
Gonadotropin-releasing hormone, 319
  analogs, postoperative, 160
  indications for, 322
  preoperative, 263, 264
Graspers, 30, *31*
  specialized, 37
Gynecologic malignancy, 273–285
  cervical cancer. (*See also* Cervical cancer.)
  endometrial cancer, 275–285. (*See also* Endometrial cancer.)
  historical perspectives on management of, 273
  informed consent for management of, 273–274
  ovarian cancer, 274–275. (*See also* Ovarian cancer.)
  para-aortic lymphadenectomy in, 276, *277*, 278, *278*
  pelvic lymphadenectomy, 274, 278–279, *280*
  radical hysterectomy in, 273, 274, 279, *280–281*, 282, 284–285
  second-look laparoscopy in, 275
Gynecologic surgery, lasers in, 47, 49, 49t, 54–55

Hemostasis, 60, 61
Hernia, 87, 307–308
  repair of, ultrasonic surgery for, 61
Hopkins rod lens system, laparoscope with, 16
Hormone therapy, 123
  for diaphragmatic endometriosis, 142
  for ovarian cysts, 152
Human chorionic gonadotropin, beta, in ectopic pregnancy, 107–108
HUMI manipulator, 30
Hydrodissection
  injection of bowel and, 311
  intake-output charting with, 313
  in ovarian cyst removal, 157, *157*
  in peritoneal endometriosis, treatment of, 126, *127*
  in tubo-ovarian abscess, 187, *187*
  in ureteral endometriosis, 129, *318*
Hydrodissection pump, 24–26, *25*, *26*
  generation of pressure and, 313
  Nezhat-Dorsey, *24*, 312
  position in operating room of, 43
Hydroflotation, 312
Hydrosalpinges, 316. (*See also* Neosalpingostomy.)
  etiology of, 189
  identification of, *193*
  recurrent, 196
Hypotension, 95
Hysterectomy, 4, 216–226
  abdominal, 206–207, 207t
    laparoscopic hysterectomy vs., 234
  abdominal myomectomy vs., 206–207, 207t
  adnexectomy during, 219, 221, *221*
  basic steps of, 218t
  bladder flap during, development of, *221*, 221–222, *222*, *223*, *224*
  cardinal ligament in, 222–224, *225*, 227, 230, 231
  complications after, 236t
  culdotomy during, 224, *225*
    with cuff closure, 230, *231*, *232*
  for endometriosis, 123, 226–236. (*See also* Endometriosis, hysterectomy for.)
  additional procedures performed during, 235t
  hormone replacement therapy after, 123
  indications for, 217, 217t
  laparoscopic
    abdominal hysterectomy vs., 234
    multifire stapler in, 319
    subtotal, 218, 233–234, 235t
    total, 218, 231–232, *232*, 233, 235t, 319
    urinary bladder injury during, 296
    vaginally assisted, 218, 235t, 319
      hospital stay for, 319
  laparoscopically assisted, 218, 319
    urinary bladder injury during, 296
  laparoscopic myomectomy vs., 206–207, 207t
  for large myomas, 234
  operative technique for, 218–219
  pelvic lymphadenectomy and, 222, 228
  positioning of patient for, 218
  preoperative evaluation for, 218
  prevalence of, 216
  radical. (*see* Radical hysterectomy.)
  ureteral evaluation and dissection in, 219, *219*, *220*
  uterine vessels in, 222, *224*
    electrodesiccation, *224*
  vaginal, 217, 217t
    laparoscopically assisted, 217, 217t, 218, 235t
  vaginal portion of, 224
  vaginal vault prolapse after, 262

Hysterosalpingography, 79
  salpingoscopy vs., 194, 195, 195t
Hysteroscopy, diagnostic, 80
  for postmenopausal bleeding, 314

Ibuprofen, fentanyl vs., for postoperative pain, 74, *74*
"Iceberg" lesion, 125
INDERAL, 71
Infection, postoperative, 307
Infertility, 179–180
  adhesions associated with, 97
  chromopertubation in, 94
  ectopic pregnancy and, 185
  pelvic inflammatory disease and, 185
  peritonitis and, 185
  treatment of, 179–180
  tubal peritonitis, caused by, 68, 185
  uterine leiomyomas and, 261
Informed consent, 7–14
  adequacy of, 8
  concept of, 7
  essentials of, 7–8
  exceptions to, 8–8
  forms for, *10–13*
  gynecologic malignancy, for, 369
Infundibulopelvic ligament, *178*
  ligation of, 182, 319
  in oophorectomy, 169–170
    by retroperitoneal dissection, *177*
  pretied sutures for, placement of, 182
Instruments. (*See also* specific instruments.)
  disposable, 15
  essential, 15–30
  operating room, 41–45
  reusable, 15
  specialized, 30–41
Insufflator, 18, *18*
Intestinal adhesions, 90
  assessing abdominal wall for, 90
  severing of, 99, 126
Intestinal endometriosis. (*See* Gastrointestinal endometriosis.)
Intestinal injury. (*See also* Bowel injury.)
  during adhesiolysis, 99, *102*
    repair of, *103*
Intracorporeal knot tying, 36, *38–39*
Intubation, 314
In vitro fertilization, 185
Irrigating fluid, 313
Isoflurane, 74

Ketorolac, 74, 75
Kidney biopsy, ultrasonic surgery for, 61
KTP lasers, 47
  delivery systems of, 54
  hydrodissection and, 320
  for myomectomy, 320
  physical properties and characteristics of, 49t, 54

Laparoscope, 15, *16*
  with Hopkins rod lens system, 16
Laparoscopic surgery. (*see* Laparoscopy.)
Laparoscopy
  adhesiolysis with, 99–104. (*See also* Adhesiolysis.)
  anesthesia during, 71–75
    complications from, 294–295
    considerations specific for, 71, 73
    induction and maintenance of, 73–74
    narcotics and, 74, 75
    nausea from, management of, 75
    recovery after, 75
    regional vs. general, 73
  as an outpatient procedure, 312
  for appendectomy, 303–307
  bleeding during, 296
  bowel preparation for, 79–80
  cardiac arrhythmias and, 75
  CO_2 embolus and, 75
  complications of (*see* Complications)
  consent for, informed, 7–14. (*See also* Informed consent.)
  contraindications to, 288–289, 289t
    bowel distention as, 89
  credentialing guidelines for, 3
  diagnostic, 125–126, 185–186
  electrosurgery during. (*see* Electrosurgery.)
  for endometriosis, 121–143. (*See also* Endometriosis, laparoscopy for.)
    histologic findings in, 124, *124*, 124t, *125*
    pregnancy rates after, 122t
  equipment for, 15–45. (*See also* specific instruments.)
    disposable, 15
    essential, 15–30
    operating room, 41–45
    reusable, 15
    specialized, 30–41
  fluid management in, 75
  in freestanding surgery centers, 311
  for gynecologic malignancy, 273–285
    cervical cancer, 273
    endometrial cancer, 275–285
    ovarian cancer, 274–275
  in gynecology, first use of, 314
  history of, 1–2
  hydroflotation and, 312
  hysterectomy by. (*see* Hysterectomy.)
  hysteroscopy before, 80
  intestinal activity during, spontaneous, 74
  intubation prior to, 314
  irrigating fluid for, 313
  laparotomy vs., 110t, 122t, 122–123, 192t, 289
  malpractice and. (*see* Malpractice.)
  minilaparotomy and, 262
  mortality rates for, 288t, 308
  muscle relaxation during, 74
  myomectomy by. (*see* Myomectomy, laparoscopic.)
  nitrous oxide in, 74
  open, 86–87

closed vs., 87
complications of, 87
operating room set-up for, 41–44, *43*, *44*
ovarian drilling by, *180*, 180–181
ovarian remnant syndrome and, 182
ovarian wedge resection by, 179–181
pain management after, 74
ibuprofen vs. fentanyl for, 74, *74*
narcotics for, 74
prophylatic NSAIDs for, 74
patient education for, 7–14
patient expectations for, 7
patient preparation for, 80
patients at risk during, 314
for patients with previous pelvic surgery, 89–92, 311
for pelvic inflammatory disease, 185–186
pneumoperitoneum in, establishment of, 85
position of patient for, 80
postoperative care, 94
postoperative problems, 94–95
preinduction medications for, 71
preoperative antibiotics in, for mitral valve prolapse, 71
preoperative evaluation in, 71, 79–80
for ovarian cysts, 151–152
preparation for, 71
presacral neurectomy by, 247–248, 249–250
pulmonary edema and, 75
for salpingitis, diagnosis of, 186
salpingoscopy by, 195–196, *196*
second-look, 219
after presacral neurectomy, 222
for endometriosis, 142
for tubo-ovarian abscess, 187
specimen retrieval during, 37, *40*, 40–41, *41*
technique
for endometriosis, 126–142
bladder, *132*, 132–133, *133*, *134*
diaphragmatic, 140–142
gastrointestinal, 133–140
genitourinary, 129–133
ovarian, 126–129
peritoneal, 126, *127*, *128*
ureteral, 129–131, *130*, *131*
termination procedures in, 44–45
Trendelenburg position in, 71, *72*, 73
tubo-ovarian abscesses, *131*, 186–188, *187*
tubal anastomosis by, 198, 200
ultrasonic surgery in. (*see* Ultrasonic surgery.)
uterine manipulation during, 312
vaginal vault suspension by, 263–268
vesicovaginal fistula repair by, 268, *268*, *269*, 270
Laparotomy
adhesions after, 89t
for ectopic pregnancy, interstitial, 117
for endometriosis
pregnancy rates after, 122t
instruments for, 37
laparoscopy vs, 110t, 110–111, 122t, 122–123
laparoscopy vs., 192t, 289
for management of laparoscopic complications, 287
myomectomy by. (*see* Myomectomy, by laparotomy.)
ovarian wedge resection by, 179
adhesions after, 179, 179t
for tubo-ovarian abscesses, 188
for urinary bladder repair, 297
videolaseroscopy vs., 4
Large bowel injury, 305–306
management of, 305–306
postoperative, 306–307
prevention of, 305
recognition of, 305
Laser(s). (*See also* Laser surgery.)
beam of. [*see* Laser(s), light energy of.]
by-products of, carcinogenesis and, 312–313
characteristics of, 49t
components of, 50–52
coupling lenses of, 53, *53*
CO_2 vs. Nd-YAG, 66–67
delivery systems of, 52–54
fiber, 54
Endoloop suture as alternative to, 314
in endoscopic surgery, 47–54
in gynecologic surgery, 47, 49, 49t, 54–55
history of, 47
light energy of, 321
characteristics of, 47, *48*
glass and, 321
mode of delivery of, 50–52
comparisons of, 50, *50*, *51*
source of, 47, *48*
thermal injury and, 51
physical properties of, 47–50, 49t
position in operating room of, 44
power density delivered by, 47–49
resonator cavity of, 50, *50*
selection of, 320
settings on, 319–320
substances used in, electromagnetic spectrum of, *48*
tissue effects of, 49, 49t
Laser surgery. [*See also* Laser(s).]
electrosurgery vs., 65–68, 321
for fibrosis at site of injury, 67t
for infertility, tuboperitoneal causes of, 68
in ovariectomy, 65–66, *66*
for postoperative lesions, 67t
thermal injury in, depth of, 65, 67t
tissue effects in, 65–66, 66t
for tubal disease, 192t
monitoring of, with fiberoptics, 54
mortality and, 55
Latzko's technique, for vesicovaginal fistula repair, 268
Leiomyomas, uterine. (*see* Uterine leiomyomas.)
Light sources, 321
for videolaserscopy, 22, *22*
position in operating room of, 43
Liver biopsy, ultrasonic surgery for, 61

Lymphadenectomy
  para-aortic, 276, *277*, 278, *278*
  pelvic, 273
    in cervical cancer, 274
    in endometrial cancer, 278–279, *280*
Lymph node, pelvic, ultrasonic surgery for, 61

Magnetic resonance imaging, of ovarian cyst, 152
Malpractice, 9–10
Marshall-Marchetti-Krantz procedure, 255, *260*
  otoses and, 262
Medroxyprogesterone acetate, 123
Methotrexate, 117–118
  prostaglandin sulprostone vs., for ectopic pregnancy, 117–118
Midazolam, 71
"Mill-wheel murmur," 75
Mitral valve prolapse, preoperative antibiotics for, 71
Monitor, video, 23
  position in operating room of, 43
Morcellator, tissue, 37
Morphine, 74
Mortality, 55
  hysterectomy and, radical, 370
Moschcowitz procedure, 232–233, 262
  in retropubic urethral suspension, 257, 260
  in vaginal vault suspension, 263, *264*
Muscle relaxation, during laparoscopy, 74
Mutifire stapler, 319
Myoma screw, 36, 265, *266*
Myomectomy, 205–213
  abdominal, 206–207, 207t
  fragments of tissue after, 321
  fulguration after, 60
  KTP lasers for, 320
  labor after, 321
  laparoscopic, 205, 206t, 321
    abdominal myomectomy vs., 206–207, 207t
    excision of myomas in, 208–211, *209*, *210*, *211*
    hysterectomy vs., 206–207, 207t
    minilaparotomy and, 206
    monitoring of ureter during, 211
    removal of myomas in, 211–212, *212*, *213*
    uteroperitoneal fistulas after, 206
  laparoscopically assisted, 205, 206t
    criteria for, 206
    maintaining uterine wall integrity in, 208
    minimizing blood loss in, 207
    preventing postoperative adhesions in, 207–208
  by laparotomy, 205, 206t
  suturing myometrium following, 321
  types of, comparison of, 205–206
  ultrasonic surgery for, 61

Narcotics, 71, 74
  emetic effects of, 74
  respiratory effects of, 75
Nausea, postoperative, 94
  management of, 75
  pain management and, 75
Nd-YAG laser, 47
  CO_2 laser vs., 66–67
  cutting ability of, 67
  delivery systems of, 54
  hydrodissection and, 320
  physical properties and characteristics of, 49t, 54–55
  reduction of adhesions with, 68t
  speed of transection of, 68t
  thermal injury with, 67
    depth of, 68t
Needle, aspiration/injection, 28–29, *29*
Needle-holders, 37, *40*
Neodymium-yttrium aluminum garnet laser. (*see* Nd-YAG laser.)
Neosalpingostomy, 192–193, *194*, *195*, 316
  chromotubation and, 192, *193*
Neostigmine, 74
Nerve injuries, 307
Neurectomy, presacral, 245–251. (*See also* Presacral neurectomy.)
Nezhat-Dorsey hydrodissection pump, *24*
  in ovariolysis, *101*
Nitrous oxide, in laparoscopy, 74
Nonsteroidal antiiflammatory drugs, 74
NORCURON, 74

Obese patients, 88–89
  insertion of Veress needle in, 81, *83*
  para-aortic lymphadenectomy in, 279
Olshausen uterine suspension, modified, 216, *216*
Oophorectomy, 163–164
  in advanced breast cancer, 167
  in early ovarian cancer, 167
  by Endoligature, 174–175, *175*
  exposure and manipulation of ovary in, 167, 169
  indications for, 167, 169–170
  infundibulopelvic ligament in, management of, 169–170
  recovery time after, 311
  by retroperitoneal dissection, 177, *177*
  technique for, 170, *170*, *171*
  tissue removal in, 178–179
  ureteral injury and, 298t
Oral contraceptives, endometriosis and, 317
Ovarian biopsy, 1
Ovarian cancer, 274–275
  adnexal mass with, 149
  advanced, 149
  age and, 152–153
  chemotherapy for, 275
  incidence of, 149
  oophorectomy in early, 167
  ovarian cysts and, 149, 150t, 151, 151t
  second-look laparoscopy in, 275
  staging of, 149
    laparoscopy in, 273, 274–275, *279*
    para-aortic lymphadenectomy for, 278, *279*
  tubo-ovarian abscesses and, 188

Ovarian cyst(s), 149–164
  aspiration of, *29*, 152
    before cystectomy, 153
  CA-125 antigen and, 150t, 152
  computed tomography of, 152
  hormone therapy for, 152
  intraoperative evaluation of, 153
  laparoscopy for, 149–164
    preoperative evaluation in, 151–152
  magnetic resonance imaging of, 152
  malignancy and, 149, 150t, 151, 151t
  premenopausal, 152–153, 153t
  preoperative evaluation for, 152–153, 153t
  size of, cystectomy and, 315
  ultrasonography of, 150t, 151
Ovarian cystectomy, 153, 155–160
  appendectomy with, complications associated with, 314
  approximation of ovarian edges in, 157–158, *158*, *159*
  biopsy specimen from, 155
  control of bleeding in, 156, *157*
  cyst aspiration before, 153, 155, *155*
  cyst size and, 315
  electrocoagulation for, bipolar, 315
  hydrodissection in, 155, *156*, *157*
  partial oophorectomy in, for large cysts, 156, *157*
  peritoneal cell washing prior to, 315
  removal of capsule from stroma in, 155–156, *156*
  removal of cystic mass in, *163*, 163–164, *164*
  suction-irrigator in, 157, *158*, 162
  suturing in, 315
  vasopressin in, 155
Ovarian drilling, *180*, 180–181, 315
  adhesions following, 180, 180t
  ovarian wedge resection vs., 180, 180t
  procedure for, *180*, 180–181
Ovarian endometriosis, 59, 126–129
  histopathologic classification in, 159–160, *160*, 160t
  history of, 158
  resection of, 126–129, 160
  vaporization of, 59
Ovarian remnant syndrome, 175, 181–182
  diagnosis of, 182
  factors associated with, 182
  laparoscopy and, 182
  preoperative preparation for removal of, 182
  prevention of, 182
  ultrasonography in, 182
Ovarian surgery. (*See* Ovarian cystectomy; Salpingo-oophorectomy); (*See also* Oophorectomy)
  biopsy specimen from, 167, *169*
  bleeding in, control of, 167, *169*
  immobilization of ovary in, 167, *168*
  uterine manipulation in, 167, 169
Ovarian torsion, 181, *181*
  gangrene and, 181
Ovarian wedge resection, 179–181
  laparoscopic ovarian drilling vs., 180, 180t
  by laparoscopy, 179–181
  results of, 179, 179t
Ovariolysis, *101*
Ovary. (*See also* Ovarian *terms*.)
  laser drilling of, 315
  removal of, in oophorectomy, 178–179
  residual, 167, 177–178
  streak, removal of, 175–176, *176*

Pain management, 74. (*See also* Presacral neurectomy.)
  in endometriosis, 142
  ibuprofen vs. fentanyl for, 74, *74*
  narcotics for, 74
  nausea and, 75
  postoperative, 95
  prophylactic NSAIDs for, 74, 95
Para-aortic lymphadenectomy, 276, *277*, 278, *278*
  bleeding and, 278
  in obese patients, 278
  videolaparoscopy in, 276
Pararectal space, development of, *280*, *281*
Paravaginal fascia, 258–259, *258*, *259*
Paravesical space, development of, *280*, *281*
Patient education, for laparoscopy, 7–14. (*See also* Informed consent.)
Patient expectations, for laparoscopy, 7
Pelvic anatomy, *277*
Pelvic exploration, *93*, 93–94
Pelvic inflammatory disease, 185–188
  antibiotic treatment of, 186, 186t
  diagnosis of, laparoscopic, 185–186
  differential diagnosis of, 186, 186t
  ectopic pregnancy and, 185
  hospital admission for, 186, 186t
  infertility and, 185
  inpatient treatment of, 186, 186t
  outpatient treatment of, 186, 186t
  primary sequelae in, 185
  sexually transmitted disease and, 185
Pelvic lymphadenectomy, 273
  in cervical cancer, 274
  in endometrial cancer, 278–279, *280*
  history of, 273
  hysterectomy and, 278, 284
  radiation therapy and, 274
Pelvic pain, 97
Pelvic surgery. (*See also* specific procedures.)
  previous laparoscopy for patients with, 89–92, 311
  reconstructive, 255–270. (*See also* Reconstructive pelvic surgery.)
PENTOTHAL, 73
Peritoneal biopsy, technique for, 274
Peritonitis, 162
  adhesion formation and, 89
  infertility and, 185
  small bowel injury and, 303
Pfannenstiel incision, adhesion formation and, 89, 89t, 90t
Phacoemulsifier, 61

Pneumoperitoneum
establishment of, 85, 291–292
avoiding injury in, 291
in patients at risk for adhesions, 91, *92*
release of, 94
suction-irrigator pump and, 312
Veress needle insertion and, 313
Polycystic ovarian disease. [*see* Ovarian cyst(s).]
Pregnancy, 122, 122t
after fimbrioplasty, 185
after tubal anastomosis, 198
following tuboplasty, 189
presacral neurectomy and, 250
tubal. (*see* Ectopic pregnancy.)
Presacral neurectomy, 245–251, *252*
anatomical considerations in, 245–246
sacral promontory, 246, 247–248
bleeding and, excessive, 250
complications of, 250–251
constipation and, 250
history of, 245
indications for, 247
instrument placement for, *246*, 247
labor and, painless, 250
laparoscopic, 247–248, 249–250
mortality rate of, 251
pregnancy rates and, 250
results of, 245, 248–250, 249t
second-look laparoscopy after, 278
technique for, 247–248, *247*, *248*, *249*
ureteral injury and, 298t
uterosacral transection as an alternative to, 322
Proctoscopy, 133
Progesterone, in ectopic pregnancy, 108–109
Progestins, 123
Prostaglandin sulprostone, methotrexate vs., 118
Pulmonary edema, laparoscopy and, 75

Radiation therapy, 276
adhesion formation and, 89
pelvic lymphadenectomy and, 274
Radical hysterectomy, 273, 274
completion of, 282
complications of, 274
for endometriosis, 123
for gynecologic malignancy, 274
hospitalization following, 284, 316
mortality rate for, 274, 285
technique for, 279, *280–281*, 282, *283*, 284–285
urinary tract infection after, 284
vaginal, 284
Reconstructive pelvic surgery, 255–270
retropubic urethral suspension, 255–262. (*See also* Retropubic urethral suspension.)
vaginal vault suspension, 262–268. (*See also* Vaginal vault suspension.)
vesicovaginal fistula repair, 268–270. (*See also* Vesicovaginal fistula repair.)
Rectal endometrioisis. (*see* Gastrointestinal endometriosis.)
Rectal prolapse, 140
Rectovaginal space, development of, *280*
Residual ovary syndrome, 167, 177–178
Retropubic cystourethropexy. (*see* Retropubic urethral suspension.)
Retropubic urethral suspension, 255–262
antibiotics and, 260
complications of, 260, 260t
follow-up in, 259–260
hospital stay for, 261, 261t
Moschcowitz procedure in, 257, 260
operative time for, 260
paravaginal fascia in, 258–259
identification of, 258
suturing of, *258*, *259*
patient position in, *256*
in postmenopausal women, 255
postoperative care in, 259–260
preoperative evaluation for, 255
results of, 260–262, 261t
Retzius space in, *257*, 257–258
technique for, 255, *256*, *257*, 257–260, *258*, *259*, *260*
Retzius space, *257*, 257–258
Rudimentary uterine horn, noncommunicating, 213–214

Sacral colpopexy. (*see* Vaginal vault suspension.)
Sacral promontory, palpation of, 81, *83*
Safety glasses, 314
Salpingectomy, 196–198
for ectopic pregnancy, 196
elecrocoagulation in, 196–197, *197*
by endoloop suture, 197–198, *198*, *199*
for hydrosalpinges, 196
indications for, 196
recovery time after, 311
technique for, 316
Salpingitis, diagnosis of, 186
Salpingo-oophorectomy, 163–164
for endometriosis, 123
stapling device in, 171, 173–174, *174*
technique for, 170–171, *172*, *173*
Salpingo-ovariolysis, 101
Salpingoscopy, 193–196, *195*
hysterosalpingography vs., 194, 195, 195t
laparoscopic, 195–196, *196*
complications of, 196
indications for, 195–196
technique for, 196, *196*
Salpingostomy, with CO_2 laser, 111, *112–113*, *114*, *115–116*, *117*
Scissors, 27–28, *28*
with unipolar electrocoagulation capability, 27, *29*
Sexually transmitted disease, 185
ectopic pregnancy and, 107
Shoulder pain, 307
etiology of, 94–95, 314

management of, 95
prevalence of, decrease in, 94
Skin ecchymosis, 140
Small bowel injury, 301–305
management of, 302–303, *303*, *304*
peritonitis secondary to, 303
postoperative, 306
prevention of, 301–302
recognition of, 302
Sonography, transvaginal, in ectopic pregnancy, 107
Specimen retrieval, during laparoscopy, 37, *40*, 40–41, *41*
Stapler. (*See* Stapling device.)
Stapling device, 30, 32, *32*, *33*
as alternative to electrocoagulation, 197
mutifire, 114, 319
in salpingectomy, 197, *198*
in salpingo-oophorectomy, 171, 173–174, *174*
Succinylcholine, 74
Suction-irrigator pump, 24–26
pneumoperitoneum and, 312
probes for, *25*
fibroid removal using, 209, *210*
in neosalpingostomy, 192
in ovarian cystectomy, 157, *158*, 162
"Quick-Disconnect," 25, *25*
in tubal surgery, 186, *187*
trumpet valve for, 24, *25*
SUFENTA, 71, 74
Sufetanil, 71, 74
Superpulse mode, 51, 320
bleeding and, 314
Surgery centers, freestanding, 311
Surgical membranes, adhesion formation and, 98–99, 99t
Suture(s), 32–36
endoloop, 32, *33*
material for, 32
purse-string, *126*
traction, *138*
in tubal surgery, 189
Suturing
adhesion formation and, 158, 159t
extracorporeal knot tying, *34*, 34–35, *35*
extracorporeal pretied suture knot, 35–36, *36*, *37*
intracorporeal knot tying, 36, *38–39*
material for, 32
in ovarian cystectomy, 315

Teratomas, 156–157
benign cystic, 162–163, 315
surgical management of, 156–158, *157*, *158*
"Thermal blooming effect," 52, *52*
Thermal injury, depth of, 65, 67t, 68t, 321
Thiopental sodium, 73–74
Tissue morcellator, 37
TORADOL, 74, 75
TRACRIUM, 74
Transvaginal sonography, 79
in ectopic pregnancy, 107
Trendelenburg position, 71, *72*, 73
cardiac function and, 71, *72*, 73, *73*
30-degree, 94
placement of Veress needle and, 81, *82*
repositioning of abdominal contents in, *72*
Trocar, *81*, 85–89
accessory, 87–88
avoiding vascular injury during insertion of, 312
placement of, *88*, 293, 311
for uterine suspension, 322
single site for, 95
three sites for, 95
two sites for, 95
disposable, 16
with inflatable balloon, 16, *17*
insertion of, 84–85, *85*, 292, *293*
adhesions and, 292, *293*
"blind," 87
direct, 86
in obese patients, 88–89, 292, *294*
in patients with previous laparotomy, 89–91, *92*
mapping the abdomen in, 91, *92*
pneumoperitoneum and, 85
techniques for, 85–86
primary, 16, *17*, 18
with retention screw, 16, *17*
reusable, 16, *17*
disposable vs., 86t
secondary, 18
Tubal anastomosis, 198, 200
pregnancy after, 198
Tubal disease, 185. (*See also* Tubal surgery.)
classification of, 190t
electrosurgery vs. laser surgery for, 192t
laparotomy vs. laparoscopy for, 192t
laser surgery vs. electrosurgery for, 192t
macrosurgery vs. microsurgery for, 191t
predisposing factors for, 185
salpingectomy in, 196–198. (*See also* Salpingectomy.)
Tubal pregnancy. (*see* Ectopic pregnancy.)
Tubal sterilization, 57
postpartum, 315–316
reversal of, 200, 316
Tubal surgery, 185–200. (*See also* Tubo-ovarian abscess, laparoscopy for; Tuboplasty.)
anastomosis in, 198, 200
for distal occulsion, 189–190, 192–193
ectopic pregnancy and, 107
efficacy of, 189, 191t
fimbrioplasty, 190, 192. (*See also* Fimbrioplasty.)
handling fallopian tubes of, 188, *189*
macro vs. micro, 191t
magnification in, 188
neosalpingostomy, 192–193
principles of, 188, 188t
prophylactic antibiotics in, 189

Tubal surgery (*Continued*)
- salpingoscopy in, 193–196, *195*, *196*. (*See also* Salpingoscopy.)
- sutures in, 189

Tuberculosis, 1
Tubo-ovarian abscess, 186–188
- diabetes mellitus and, 188
- laparoscopy for, 186–188
  - hydrodissection in, 187, *187*
  - second-look, 187
  - suction-irrigator probe in, 186, *187*
- laparotomy for, 188
- ovarian cancer and, 188
- pelvic inflammatory disease and, 185
- treatment of, 186–188

Tuboplasty. (*See* Tubal surgery.)

Ultrapulse laser, 51, *51*, 320
- control panel for, *52*
- in laparoscopic myomectomy, 265, *265*
- "thermal blooming effect" and, 52
- in tubal surgery, *193*, *194*

Ultrasonic surgery, 61
Ultrasonography, *154*
- of ovarian cysts, 150t, 151
- in ovarian remnant syndrome, 182
- surgical. (*see* Ultrasonic surgery.)

Ureteral endometriosis, 129–131, *130*, *131*
- CO_2 laser dissection in, 129, *130*
- hydrodissection in, 129
- incidence of, 129
- obstruction in, 129–131
- postoperative follow-up in, 131, *131*
- ureteral stent in, insertion of, 130, *131*

Ureteral injury, 297–301
- electrocoagulation and, 297
- incidence of, after radical hysterectomy, 370
- laparoscopic procedures associated with, 298t
- management of, 299–301, *301*
- oophorectomy and, 298t
- prevention of, 297–298, *299*
- recognition of, 298–299
- verification of, 323

Ureteral obstruction, uterine leiomyomas and, 261, 262t
Urinary bladder endometriosis, *132*, 132–133, *133*, *134*
Urinary bladder injury, 296–297, 322
- management of, 297
- prevention of, 296
- recognition of, 296–297
- verification of, 323

Urinary retention, 140
URISPAS, 339
Uterine horn, noncommunicating, rudimentary, 269–270
Uterine injury, 296
Uterine insufflation, 314
Uterine leiomyomas. (*See* also Myomectomy.)
- indications for treatment of, 261, 262t
- infertility and, 261
- intramural, 208
- large, hysterectomy for, 290
- morcellation of, *269*
- pedunculated, 264, 269
- subserosal, 208
- symptoms associated with, 261
- ureteral obstruction and, 261, 262t

Uterine manipulation, 30, *30*
- during laparoscopy, 312
- large or retroflexed, 312
- in ovarian surgery, 167, 169

Uterine manipulators, 30, *30*
Uterine surgery, 205–236
- for adenomyosis, 213, *214*
- hysterectomy, 216–226. (*See also* Hysterectomy.)
- myomectomy. (*see* Myomectomy.)
- preoperative evaluation of, 205
- for rudimentary uterine horn, noncommunicating, 213–214
- uterine suspension, *215*, 215–216, *216*. (*See also* Uterine suspension.)

Uterine suspension, *215*, 215–216, *216*
- for endometriosis, 247–248
- fallope rings in, 215, *215*
- indications for, 215
- Olshausen, modified, 216, *216*
- placement of accessory trocar for, 322
- ventrosuspension of round ligament in, 215–216, *216*

Uteroperitoneal fistula, after laparoscopic myomectomy, 216
Uterosacral ablation. (*see* Uterosacral transection.)
Uterosacral transection, 251, *252*, 253
- as an alternative to presacral neurectomy, 251
- complications of, 253
- for dysmenorrhea, 317
- results of, 251
- technique for, 251, *252*

Vaginal cuff closure, ureteral injury and, 298t
Vaginal vault prolapse, 262–263
- surgery for. (*see* Vaginal vault suspension.)

Vaginal vault suspension, *263*, 263–268, *264*, *265*
- avoiding anatomic injury in, 263–264
- bleeding in, 267
- extracorporeal knot tying in, 264, *265*
- Moschcowitz procedure in, 263, *264*
- patient history and, 266t
- postoperative care in, 265, 267
- results of, 267, 267t

Vagotomy, ultrasonic surgery for, 61
Vancomycin, 71
Vaporization, of ovarian endometriosis, 59
Vecuronium, 74
Veress needle, 18, *18*
- insertion of, 81, *82*, *83*
  - "blind," 87
  - facilitation of, 313
  - in obese patient, 81, *83*

pneumoperitoneum and, 313
trocar insertion vs., 86, 86t
placement of, 80–85, 233–235, *234*, *235*
infraumbilical approach for, 81, *81*
in obese patients, 81, *83*, 84
transabdominal approach for, 83, *84*
transcervical approach for, 83, *84*
transvaginal approach for, 82–83, *84*
Trendelenburg position and, 81, *82*, 289, *290*
umbilicus in, 81, *81*
verification for correct, 81–82, *84*, 84t
VERSED, 71
Vesicovaginal fistula, 307
incidence of, after radical hysterectomy, 218
Vesicovaginal fistula repair, 268, *269*, *270*
Videolaseroscopy, 2, 15
camera box for, 23, *23*
camera for, 22–23
in endometriosis, 2
endoscopes in, 21–22
focusing HeNe beam during, 312
future of, 23–24
history of, 19
laparotomy vs., 4
light sources for, 22, *22*
monitor for, 23
operation of, 19–21
ovarian drilling by, 180
troubleshooting techniques for, 23
Video recording, 44
Vomiting, postoperative, 94

Xenon light source, *22*

ISBN 0-07-105422-7